Basic & Clinical
Biostatistics

third edition

Beth Dawson, PhD
Professor and Chief
Informatics, Biostatistics & Research
Department of Internal Medicine
Southern Illinois University
School of Medicine
Springfield, Illinois

Robert G. Trapp, MD
Medical Director
The Arthritis Center
Springfield, Illinois
Formerly
Assistant Professor and Chief of Rheumatology
Department of Internal Medicine
Southern Illinois University
School of Medicine
Springfield, Illinois

Lange Medical Books/McGraw-Hill
Medical Publishing Division

New York St. Louis San Francisco Auckland Bogotá Caracas Lisbon
London Madrid Mexico City Milan Montreal New Delhi San Juan
Singapore Sydney Tokyo Toronto

McGraw-Hill

A Division of The McGraw·Hill Companies

Basic & Clinical Biostatistics, Third Edition

Copyright © 2001 by The McGraw-Hill Companies, Inc. Copyright © 1994, 1991 by Appleton & Lange. All rights reserved. Printed in the United States of America. Except as permitted under the United States Copyright Act of 1976, no part of this publication may be reproduced or distributed in any form or by any means, or stored in a data base or retrieval system, without the prior written permission of the publisher.

2 3 4 5 6 7 8 9 0 QPD QPD 0 9 8 7 6 5 4 3 2 1

Set ISBN: 0-8385-0510-4

Book code: 0-07-137052-8

CD-ROM code: 0-07-137053-6

ISSN: 1045-5523

This book was set in Times Roman by Pine Tree Composition, Inc.
The editors were Janet Foltin, Harriet Lebowitz, and Nicky Panton.
The production supervisor was Catherine Saggese.
The cover designer was Mary Skudlarek.
The index was prepared by Coughlin Indexing Services, Inc.
Quebecor/Dubuque was printer and binder.

This book is printed on acid-free paper.

Table of Contents

Preface

Basic and Clinical Biostatistics introduces the medical student, researcher, or practitioner to the study of statistics applied to medicine and other disciplines in the health field. The authors, a statistician who is a professor in a department of medicine and a practicing physician who participates in numerous clinical trials, have incorporated their experiences in medicine and statistics to develop a comprehensive text. We cover the *basics* of biostatistics and quantitative methods in epidemiology and the *clinical* applications in evidence-based medicine and the decision-making methods. We particularly emphasize study design and interpretation of results of research.

OBJECTIVE

Our primary objective is to provide the resources to help the reader become an informed user and consumer of statistics, and we have endeavored to make our presentation lively and interesting. You can expect to achieve the following goals:

- Develop sound judgment about data applicable to clinical care.
- Read the clinical literature critically, understanding potential errors and fallacies contained therein, and apply confidently the results of medical studies to patient care.
- Interpret commonly used vital statistics and understand the ramifications of epidemiologic information for patient care and prevention of disease.
- Reach correct conclusions about diagnostic procedures and laboratory test results.
- Interpret manufacturers' information about drugs, instruments, and equipment.
- Evaluate study protocols and articles submitted for publication and actively participate in clinical research.
- Develop familiarity with well-known statistical software and interpret the computer output.

APPROACH & DISTINGUISHING FEATURES

We have attempted to keep the practitioner's interests, needs, and perspectives in mind. Thus, our approach embraces the following features:

- A genuine medical context is offered for the subject matter. After the introduction to different kinds of studies is presented in Chapter 2, subsequent chapters begin with several *presenting problems*—discussions of studies that have been published in the medical literature. These illustrate the methods discussed in the chapter and in some instances are continued through several chapters and in the exercises to develop a particular line of reasoning more fully.
- Actual data from the presenting problems are used to illustrate the statistical methods.
- A focus on concepts is accomplished by using computer programs to analyze data and by presenting statistical calculations only to illustrate the logic behind certain statistical methods.
- The importance of sample size (power analysis) is emphasized and computer programs to estimate sample size are illustrated.
- Information is organized from the perspective of the research question being asked.
- Terms are defined within the relevant text, whenever practical, because biostatistics may be a new language to you. In addition, a glossary of statistical and epidemiologic terms is provided at the end of the book.
- A table of all symbols used in the book is provided on the inside back cover.
- A simple classification scheme of study designs used in clinical research is discussed (Chapter 2). We employ this scheme throughout the book as we discuss the presenting problems.
- Flowcharts are used to relate research questions to appropriate statistical methods (inside front cover and Appendix C).

- A step-by-step explanation of how to read the medical literature critically (Chapter 13)—a necessity for the modern health professional—is provided.
- Evidence-based medicine and decision making are addressed in a clinical context (Chapters 11 and 12). Clinicians will be called upon increasingly to make decisions based on statistical information.
- The reference section is divided into three categories to facilitate the search for the sources of a presenting problem or for a text or an article on a specific topic.
- Numerous end-of-chapter exercises (Chapters 2 through 12) and their complete solutions (Appendix B) are provided.
- A post-test of multiple-choice questions (Chapter 13) similar to those used in course final examinations or licensure examinations is included.

We made several important enhancements to the third edition. We updated the majority of presenting problems and, through the generosity of the authors of these studies, have been able to use the actual data to illustrate the statistical methods and design issues. One of the most exciting additions is the inclusion of the NCSS software, a commonly used statistical package, and the associated PASS program for estimating sample sizes. This software contains all of the procedures used in this text, and the procedures can be used to analyze your own studies. The data sets from the presenting problems have been placed on the CD-ROM. Please refer to the instructions immediately following the Acknowledgments entitled "Using the CD-ROM" for information about how to find the documentation on the programs and data sets on the CD-ROM.

Rethinking the way investigators ask research questions prompted us to reorganize some of the chapters to correspond with this logic, as opposed to the traditional organization of texts based strictly on statistical methods. We included or significantly enhanced the discussion of several topics, including evidenced-based medicine (Chapters 3 and 11), the comparison of correlation coefficients (Chapter 8), studies with repeated measures over time (Chapter 7), and the logistic regression and Cox proportional hazard models (Chapter 10).

We have established a Web page (http://www.clinicalbiostatistics.com), where we will post updates and other items of interest. You may also wish to take a look at the NCSS Web site (http://www.ncss.com) for new developments.

Beth Dawson, PhD
Robert G. Trapp, MD
October 2000

Acknowledgments

As we worked on the first, second, and third editions of this book, we were very grateful for the enthusiastic support of the current and former staff of Lange Medical Publications. With the acquisition of the Lange series by McGraw-Hill, we have been doubly fortunate for their excellent editorial staff and increased marketing capabilities. In preparing the third edition, we have been privileged to have the encouragement and support of Janet Foltin, Editor, Lange Medical Publications. Harriet Lebowitz, Senior Development Editor, has been the person to whom we have gone with editing questions and requests, and working with her has been exceptionally pleasant. We owe a special debt of thanks to the primary copyeditor, Linda Davoli, for her commitment to improve the readability of the text; she made important substantive and stylistic suggestions. We also appreciate the fine artwork by the previous Manager of Art Services, Eve Siegel, the current Manager of Art Services, Charissa Baker, and the art illustrator, Laura Pardi Duprey.

In order to use actual published studies to illustrate statistical concepts and methods, we asked many authors and journal editors for their permission to use their data, cite their published article, and sometimes reproduce tables or graphs. We wish to express our sincere appreciation to all the authors and journal editors for their generosity in sharing with us the results of their scholarly endeavors. We hope readers will consult the full articles that we have used as the basis for presenting problems and illustrations to enhance their understanding of medicine as well as the application of statistics in medicine. In particular, we want to acknowledge and thank the following investigators who sent us their data or subsets thereof:

AV Alexandrov and colleagues
K Bajwa, E Szabo, and CM Kjellstrand
JT Benson, V Lucente, and E McClellan
A Birtch
JM Crook and colleagues
CT D'Angio, WM Maniscalco, and ME Pichichero
BA Dennison, HL Rockwell, and SL Baker
DA Gelber and colleagues
M Gelkopf, M Sigal, and R Kramer
MA Gonzalo and colleagues
DC Good and colleagues
DM Harper
R Hébert, C Brayne, and D Spiegelhalter
AS Henderson and colleagues
PC Hindmarsh and CGD Brook
LG Hodgson and SJ Cutler
M Irwin and colleagues
JM Nesselroad and colleagues
CA Soderstrom and colleagues

In addition, we sincerely appreciate the cooperation of the journals in which this scholarly work appeared and the *Biometrika* trustees for permission to reproduce statistical tables.

Today, all researchers use computers to analyze data, and graphics from computer programs are often published in journal articles. We believe clinicians should have experience reading and interpreting the results of computer analysis. We are especially indebted to Jerry Hintze, the author of NCSS and PASS software, for working with us and to be able to offer our readers this software package along with the text. Dr. Hintze also placed the data from the presenting problems on the CD-ROM. Several other producers of statistical software were kind enough to provide their software so that we could present output from them as well. Our sincere thanks go to SPSS, Sample Power, and SYSTAT, all from SPSS Inc.; JMP from SAS Institute, Inc.; Dr. Janet Elashoff of nQuery Advisor; Visual Statistics from McGraw-Hill, Inc.; ConStatS from Tufts College; and Data Analysis from TreeAge.

Earlier editions of this book profited greatly from the critical insight of colleagues who made suggestions and constructive comments. For this third edition, we especially want to thank Drs. Gerald Arnold, Robert Bussing, Patricia Hopkins-Price, Paul Kolm, and Sherry Robinson, and Randall Robbs for their reviews of chapters, and W. J. Hall for his comprehensive comments.

The revisions for the third edition were extensive, and above all we thank Dr. David Steward, Chair of the Department of Medicine at Southern Illinois University School of Medicine, for his support, encouragement, and patience. We also appreciate the important assistance of our staff, in particular Ms. Ximena Nagasato, Aneeta Shailesh, Diane Dow, and Marilyn Clarke.

Finally, we express our gratitude for the encouragement from our families, in particular Gregory and Curtis Dawson, Dr. Timothy Sawers, Ms. Dorothy Trapp, and Matthew, Caitlin, Leanne, and Claire Trapp.

Using the CD-ROM

This section contains information on how to use the CD-ROM that accompanies this text. We suggest that you refer to our Web site (http://www.clinicalbiostatics.com) for updates of this information.

The CD-ROM contains the data sets from the presenting problems, the NCSS statistical programs, and the PASS power analysis programs, as well as instructions on how to use them. The NCSS and PASS programs are installed together. After installation, clicking on the NCSS icon opens that program, and PASS is one of the options on the menu bar, along with Analysis, Graphics, and so forth.

If you are new to the NCSS programs, we have some suggestions for getting started. First, on the CD itself there are several useful files. The Readme.txt file has information on installing NCSS and PASS. In the NCSS folder on the CD-ROM, the Readme.wri file informs you that it is possible to print the documentation contained in the DOCS directory, which is in the NCSS folder.

We highly recommend that you print some of the files in the DOCS directory to help you get started with NCSS. First, click on the _read_me.txt in the DOCS directory to obtain instructions on printing the files and a list of the documentation for NCSS and PASS. The DOCS directory contains a copy of all NCSS and PASS documentation in PDF (Adobe Acrobat) format. (A copy of Adobe Acrobat Reader 4.0 is contained in this directory as well, and the _read_me.txt file contains instructions on how to install it if you need to do so.) The _read_me.txt file contains a list of the PDF files and the chapters they document. Note especially the files listed under the heading QUICK START & SELF HELP MANUAL; these files are available **only** in PDF format on the CD-ROM and are not installed with the program itself. We strongly suggest that you print the first six files, because they give you a step-by-step introduction to NCSS. Other chapters may be printed now or later, as you need them. Except for the QUICK START & SELF HELP MANUAL, all manuals are installed with the program and available in the Help menu in NCSS.

Once you have installed NCSS and started the program, the first step is either to enter data (described in Chapter 2 of the QUICK START & SELF HELP MANUAL) or to open an existing data file. The data files used in the text are contained in a single folder called Dawson, included in the Data folder (in the NCSS folder). To open a specific data file, click on File on the menu bar and then click on the Open command. Open the Data folder and then the Dawson folder, and, after that, locate the data file you wish to use. All data files are listed by the last name of the first author of the study, and the data in NCSS format has an .s0 extension. For example, the Dennison data file in NCSS format is called Dennison.s0.

The documentation for each data set is in the Dawson folder in a file named (author) readme.txt, where "author" is the last name of the first author of the study. The documentation lists the variables in the data file and the meaning of the values of the variables. For example, the documentation for the Gelber data is contained in Gelber readme.txt. To view the documentation, open the Notepad (by clicking on Start, Programs, then Accessories).

The data files are provided in other formats as well. The Microsoft Excel format has an .xls extension, the SPSS format has a .sav extension, and a space-delimited ascii text file has a .txt extension. These additional formats are also contained in the Dawson folder.

For some of the illustrations in the text, especially in the early chapters, we have designed templates that can be loaded in NCSS to run the example. Accordingly, a special template named Benson has been stored with the two-sample *t* test procedure to correspond with the Benson study data used in Chapter 6 to illustrate the two-sample *t* test. To activate the template, click on the Template tab in the two-sample *t* test procedure, highlight the template file named Benson and click on the Load Template button. Then, click on the blue arrow in the upper left corner of the procedure window to run the example illustrated in the text. When we have designed a template for a given data set, we note that information in the (author) readme.txt file, alerting you to look for it.

The CD-ROM also has a folder named Calculations. This folder contains a number of excel programs to calculate difficult-to-find statistics, such as comparing two correlation coefficients. Using these programs is not required; they are included only for your convenience.

The CD-ROM included with this text is designed to run under Microsoft Windows. If you are using a Macintosh computer, we suggest you obtain one of the software products that runs Windows software on Macintosh computers, such as Virtual PC from Connectix.

All of the above information is contained in a file called Dawson readme.txt in the Dawson folder. We hope you enjoy using the data files and the NCSS and PASS programs.

Introduction to Medical Research

The goal of this text is to provide you with the tools and skills you need to be a smart user and consumer of medical statistics. This goal has guided us in the selection of material and in the presentation of information. This chapter outlines the reasons physicians, medical students, and others in the health care field should know biostatistics. It also describes how the book is organized, what you can expect to find in each chapter, and how you can use it most profitably.

1.1 THE SCOPE OF BIOSTATISTICS & EPIDEMIOLOGY

The word "statistics" has several meanings: data or numbers, the process of analyzing the data, and the description of a field of study. It derives from the Latin word *status,* meaning "manner of standing" or "position." Statistics were first used by tax assessors to collect information for determining assets and assessing taxes—an unfortunate beginning and one the profession has not entirely lived down.

Everyone is familiar with the statistics used in baseball and other sports, such as a baseball player's batting average, a bowler's game point average, and a basketball player's free-throw percentage. In medicine, some of the statistics most often encountered are called means, standard deviations, proportions, and rates. Working with statistics involves using statistical methods that summarize data (to obtain, for example, means and standard deviations) and using statistical procedures to reach certain conclusions that can be applied to patient care or public health planning. The subject area of statistics is the set of all the statistical methods and procedures used by those who work with statistics. The application of statistics is broad indeed and includes business, marketing, economics, agriculture, education, psychology, sociology, anthropology, and biology, in addition to our special interest, medicine and other health care disciplines. Here we use the terms **biostatistics** and **biometrics** to refer to the application of statistics in the health-related fields.

Although the focus of this text is biostatistics, some topics related to epidemiology are included as well. These topics and others specific to epidemiology are discussed in more detail in the companion book, *Medical Epidemiology* (Greenberg, 1996). The term "epidemiology" refers to the study of health and illness in human populations, or, more precisely, to the patterns of health or disease and the factors that influence these patterns; it is based on the Greek words for "upon" (*epi*) and "people" (*demos*). Once knowledge of the epidemiology of a disease is available, it is used to understand the cause of the disease, determine public health policy, and plan treatment. The application of population-based information to decision making about individual patients is often referred to as **clinical epidemiology** and, more recently, **evidence-based medicine.** The tools and methods of biostatistics are an integral part of these disciplines.

1.2 BIOSTATISTICS IN MEDICINE

Clinicians must evaluate and use new information throughout their lives. The skills you learn in this text will assist in this process because they concern modern knowledge acquisition methods. In the following subsections, we list the most important reasons for learning biostatistics. (The most widely applicable reasons are mentioned first.)

1.2.1 Evaluating the Literature

Reading the literature begins early in the training of health professionals and continues throughout their careers. They must therefore understand biostatistics to decide whether they can believe the results presented in the literature. Journal editors try to screen out articles that are improperly designed or analyzed, but few of them have formal statistical training and they naturally focus on the content of the research rather than the method. Generally, investigators for large, expensive studies consult statisticians in project design and data analysis, especially for research funded by the National Institutes of Health and other national agencies and foundations. Even then it is important to be aware of possible shortcomings in the way a study is designed and carried out. In smaller research projects, investigators consult with statisticians less frequently, either because the investigator is not aware of the need for statistical assistance or because the biostatistical resources are not readily available or affordable. The advent of easy-to-use computer programs to perform statistical analysis has been important in promoting the use of more relevant methods that are often more computationally complex. This same accessibility, however, has enabled people without the training or expertise in statistical methodology to report complicated analyses when they are not always appropriate.

The problems with studies in the medical literature have been amply documented, and we give only a few illustrations here. Williamson, Goldschmidt, and Colton (1986) reviewed 28 articles (published in the medical literature) that had assessed the scientific adequacy of study designs, data collection, and statistical methods in more than 4200 published medical reports. The reports assessed drug trials and surgical, psychotherapeutic, and diagnostic procedures published in more than 30 journals, many of them well known and prestigious. For example, the *British Medical Journal,* the *Journal of the American Medical Association,* the *New England Journal of Medicine,* the *Canadian Medical Association Journal,* the *Lancet,* the *American Journal of Psychiatry, Annals of Internal Medicine, Archives of Neurology and Psychiatry,* the *Journal of Nervous and Mental Disease,* and *Psychiatric Quarterly* were all included in three or more assessment articles. Williamson and his colleagues determined that, on the average, only about 20% of 4235 research reports met the assessors' criteria for validity. Eight of the assessment articles had gone a step further and looked at the relationship between the frequency of positive findings and the adequacy of the methods used in research reports. In the research reports evaluated in these eight articles, approximately 80% of those that were inadequately designed and analyzed had reported positive findings; however, only 25% of those that were adequately designed and analyzed had positive findings. Thus, evidence indicates that positive findings are reported more often in poorly conducted studies than in well-conducted ones.

Other articles indicate that the problems cited by Williamson and colleagues (1986) have not improved substantially. For example, Avram and associates (1985) found that only 15% of more than 200 articles in two anesthesiology journals were without major errors in analysis or design. Continuing problems prompted DerSimonian and coworkers (1982) to take a slightly different approach. They reviewed articles in four leading medical journals: *British Medical Journal,* the *Lancet,* the *Journal of the American Medical Association,* and the *New England Journal of Medicine.* They defined ten elementary aspects that authors of medical journal articles should include in their report of clinical trials, some of which are eligibility criteria for entering the study, the patient randomization method, statistical tests used, mention of patients lost to follow-up, and use of open or blind study designs. The authors did not attempt to determine whether these actions were properly done in the study but merely whether they were reported for the reader's information. The percentage of articles that reported these elementary facts ranged from 12% to 93%, depending on the particular aspect.

These findings are distressing, because physicians depend heavily on the medical literature to stay up to date. Furthermore, there is evidence that the use of statistics has continued to increase. For instance, the percentage of original papers in the *New England Journal of Medicine* with statistical methods (more than merely descriptive statistics) increased from 73% in 1978–1979 to 89% in 1990 (Altman, 1991b). Medical journal editors have generally responded positively to these problems and have been willing to publish articles that discuss shortcomings in study design and analysis (eg, see Garfunkle, 1986). Several journals, such as the *New England Journal of Medicine,* the *Journal of the American Medical Association,* and the *British Medical Journal,* have carried series of articles on study design and statistical methods. Some of the articles have been published in a separate monograph (eg, Bailar and Mosteller, 1992; Greenhalgh, 1997b).

Journals have also published a number of articles that suggest how practitioners could better report their research findings. We agree with many of these recommendations, but we firmly believe that we, as readers, must assume the responsibility for determining whether the results of a published study are valid. Our development of this book has been guided by the study designs and statistical methods found primarily in the medical literature, and we have selected topics to provide the skills needed to determine whether a study is valid and should be believed. Chapter 13 focuses specifically on how to read the medical literature and provides checklists for flaws in studies and problems in analysis.

1.2.2 Applying Study Results to Patient Care

Applying the results of research to patient care is the major reason practicing clinicians read the medical literature. They want to know which diagnostic procedures are best, which methods of treatment are optimal, and how the treatment regimen should be designed and implemented. Of course, they also read journals to stay aware and up to date in medicine in general as well as in their specific area of interest. Chapters 11 and 12 discuss techniques for applying the concepts of earlier chapters to decisions about the care of individual patients.

1.2.2.a Interpreting Vital Statistics: Physicians must be able to interpret vital statistics in order to diagnose and treat patients effectively. Vital statistics are based on data collected from the ongoing recording of vital events, such as births and deaths. A basic understanding of how vital statistics are determined, what they mean, and how they are used facilitates their use. Chapter 3 provides information on these statistics.

1.2.2.b Understanding Epidemiologic Problems: Practitioners must understand epidemiologic problems because this information helps them make diagnoses and develop management plans for patients. Epidemiologic data reveal the prevalence of a disease, its variation by season of the year and by geographic location, and its relation to certain risk factors. In addition, epidemiologic information helps society make informed decisions about the deployment of health resources, for example, whether a community should begin a surveillance program, whether a screening program is warranted and can be designed to be efficient and effective, and whether community resources should be used for specific health problems such as immunization programs or prenatal care. Describing and using data in making decisions are highlighted in Chapters 3, 4, 11, and 12.

1.2.2.c Interpreting Information about Drugs and Equipment: Physicians continually evaluate information about drugs and medical instruments and equipment. This material may be provided by company representatives, sent through the mail, or published in journals. Because of the high cost of developing drugs and medical instruments, companies do all they can to recoup their investments. To sell their products, a company must convince physicians that its products are better than those of its competitors. To make its points, it uses graphs, charts, and the results of studies comparing its products with others on the market. Every chapter in this text is related to the skills needed to evaluate these materials, but Chapters 2, 3, and 13 are especially relevant.

1.2.2.d Using Diagnostic Procedures: Identifying the correct diagnostic procedure to use is a necessity in making decisions about patient care. In addition to knowing the prevalence of a given disease, physicians must be aware of the sensitivity of a diagnostic test in detecting the disease when it is present and the frequency with which the test correctly indicates no disease in a well person. These characteristics are called the sensitivity and specificity of a diagnostic test. Information in Chapters 4 and 11 relates particularly to skills for interpreting diagnostic tests.

1.2.2.e Being Informed: Keeping abreast of current trends and being critical about data are more general skills and ones that are difficult to measure. These skills are also not easy for physicians to acquire, because many responsibilities compete for their time. One of the byproducts of working through this text is a heightened awareness of the many threats to the validity of information, that is, the importance of being alert for statements that do not seem quite right.

1.2.2.f Evaluating Study Protocols and Articles: Physicians and others in the health field who are associated with universities, medical schools, or major clinics are often called on to evaluate material submitted for publication in medical journals and to decide whether it should be published. Physicians, of course, have the expertise to evaluate the medical content of a protocol or article, but they often feel uncomfortable about critiquing the design and statistical methods of a study. No study, however important, will provide valid information about the practice of medicine and future research unless it is properly designed and analyzed. Careful attention to the concepts covered in this text will provide physicians with many of the skills necessary for evaluating the design of studies.

1.2.2.g Participating in or Directing Research Projects: Clinicians participating in research will find knowledge about biostatistics and research methods indispensable. The comprehensive coverage of topics in this text should provide most clinicians with the information they need to be active participants in all aspects of research.

Directing research projects also calls for some expertise in biostatistics. This text may not be detailed enough in some areas for project directors. In our discussions of more advanced topics, however, we frequently provide references to other resources for those interested in pursuing a subject in greater depth.

1.3 THE DESIGN OF THIS BOOK

We consider this text to be both *basic* and *clinical* because we emphasize both the basic concepts of biostatistics and the use of these concepts in clinical decision making. We have designed a comprehensive text covering the traditional topics in biostatistics plus the quantitative methods of epidemiology used in research. For example, we include commonly used ways to analyze survival data in Chapter 9; illustrations of computer analyses in chapters in which they are appropriate, because researchers today use computers to calculate statistics; and applications of the results of studies to the diagnosis of specific diseases and the care of individual patients, sometimes referred to as medical decision making or evidence-based medicine.

We have added a number of new topics to this edition and have extended our coverage of some others. We have enhanced our discussion of evidence-based medicine and have included the important concept of the number of patients that need to be treated with a given intervention in order to prevent one undesirable outcome (**number needed to treat**). The **likelihood ratio** is now presented in many journal articles that evaluate diagnostic procedures or analyze risk factors; we cover this method in more detail in this edition than we did previously. We have taken advantage of recent developments in computer software to greatly expand the discussion of the number of subjects needed in different types of studies (**power**). It is our impression that an increasing number of research reports use **multivariate** methods, especially **logistic regression** and the **Cox proportional hazard model.** The importance of these methods in medical research is undeniable, even though they are statistically complex. We therefore discuss and illustrate these methods in greater detail, as we also do for the related concepts of **risk** and **odds ratios.** The chapter on survival methods has been expanded, and the discussion of **meta-analysis** and repeated-measures **analysis of variance** has been enhanced.

Our approach deemphasizes calculations and uses computer programs to illustrate the results of statistical tests. In most chapters, we include the calculations of some statistical procedures, mainly because we wish to illustrate the logic behind the tests, not because we believe you need to be able to perform the calculations yourself. Some exercises involve calculations because we have found that some students wish to work through a few problems in detail so as to understand the procedures better. The major focus of the text, however, is on the interpretation and use of research methods.

A word of caution regarding the accuracy of the calculations is in order. Many examples and exercises require several steps. The accuracy of the final answer depends on the number of significant decimal places to which figures are extended at each step of the calculation; we generally extend them to two or three places. Note, however, that a calculator or computer that uses a greater number of significant decimal places at each step yields an answer different from that obtained using only two or three places. The difference usually will be small, but readers should not be concerned if their calculations vary slightly from ours.

The examples used are taken from studies published in the medical literature. Occasionally, we use a subset of the data to illustrate a more complex procedure. In addition, we sometimes focus on only one aspect of the data analyzed in a published study in order to illustrate a concept or statistical test. To explain certain concepts, we often reproduce tables and graphs as they appear in a published study. These reproductions may contain symbols that are not discussed until a later chapter in this book. Simply ignore such symbols for the time being. We chose to work with published studies for two reasons: First, they convince readers of the relevance of statistical methods in medical research; and second, they provide an opportunity to learn about some interesting studies along with the statistics.

We have also made an effort to provide insights into the coherency of statistical methods. We often refer to both previous and upcoming chapters to help tie concepts together and point out connections. This technique requires us to use definitions somewhat differently from many other statistical texts; that is, terms are often used within the context of a discussion without a precise definition. The definition is given later. Several examples appear in the foregoing discussions (eg, vital statistics, means, standard deviations, proportions, rates, validity). We believe that using terms properly within several contexts helps the reader learn complex ideas, and many ideas in statistics become clearer when viewed from different perspectives. Some terms are defined as we go along, but providing definitions for every term would inhibit our ability to point out the connections between ideas. To assist the reader, beginning in Chapter 2 we use boldface for terms (the first few times they are used) that appear in the Glossary of statistical and epidemiologic terms provided at the end of the book.

1.4 THE ORGANIZATION OF THIS BOOK

In addition to the new topics included in this edition, we have reorganized some of the chapters to coincide more closely with the way we think about research. For example, many of the same principles are involved in methods to summarize and display data, so these are now in the same chapter (Chapter 3) and discussed in a more integrated manner. Most biostatistical texts, ours included, divide the methods into chapters, with, for example, a chapter on *t* tests, another chapter on **chi-square tests,** and so forth. In this edition, we have reorganized the methods to relate to the kind of research question being asked. Therefore, there is a chapter on analyzing research questions involving one group of subjects (Chapter 5), another chapter on research questions involving two groups of subjects (Chapter 6), and yet another on research questions involving more than two groups of subjects (Chapter 7). We believe this organization is more logical, and we hope it facilitates the learning process.

Each chapter has an introduction that contains the purpose of the chapter and an **overview** of the ideas discussed. This overview is designed to help the reader organize and visualize the ideas to be discussed. At the conclusion of each chapter is a **summary** that integrates the statistical concepts with the presenting problems used to illustrate them. When flowcharts or diagrams are useful, we include them to help explain how different procedures are related and when they are relevant. The flowcharts are grouped in Appendix C for easy reference.

Patients come to their physicians with various health problems. In describing their patients, physicians commonly say, "The patient presents with . . ." or "The patient's presenting problem is . . . " We use this terminology in this text to emphasize the similarity between medical practice and the research problems discussed in the medical literature. Almost all chapters begin with presenting problems that discuss studies taken directly from the medical literature; these research problems are the reason behind and illustrate the concepts and methods presented in the chapter. In chapters in which statistics are calculated (such as the mean in Chapter 3) or statistical procedures are explained (such as the *t* test in Chapters 5 and 6), data from the presenting problems are used in the calculations. We try to ensure that the medical content of the presenting problems is still valid at the time this text is published. As advances are made in medicine, however, it is possible that some of this content will become outdated; we will attempt to correct that in the next edition.

We have attempted to select presenting problems that represent a broad array of interests, while being sure that the studies use the methods we want to discuss. Beginning with this third edition, we incorporated data from a number of investigators, who generously agreed to share their data with us. Furthermore, many of them agreed to let us publish a subset of their data with this text. This provides us with a number of advantages: We can use real data in the statistical programs, and readers can use the same data to reinforce and extend their knowledge of the methods we discuss. We are very grateful to these authors (who are listed in the acknowledgments). Sometimes we focus on only a small part of the information presented in the article itself, but we usually comment on their findings in the summary of the chapter. We have tried not to misinterpret any of the data or reported findings, and we take responsibility for any errors we may have committed in describing their research. We hope our readers will obtain a copy of the original published article and use it, along with our discussion of the study, to enhance their clinical knowledge as well as their statistical expertise.

Two of the most exciting changes with this edition are the inclusion of actual data and software on the CD-ROM that accompanies this text. The data sets are provided in several different formats to make it easy to use them for statistical analysis.

With this third edition we are very fortunate to have the assistance of Dr. Jerry Hintze, the developer of the Number Cruncher Statistical System (NCSS), a set of statistical procedures, and the Power Analysis Statistical System (PASS), a computer program that estimates the sample sizes needed in a study. NCSS and PASS software is included on the CD that accompanies this text. We have used this software for a number of years and find it comprehensive and easy to use. Many of the illustrations of the statistical procedures in this book were facilitated by using NCSS, and we hope our readers use it to replicate the analyses and to do the exercises. As an added benefit, the procedures included on this version of NCSS can also be used to analyze other data sets. Please refer to the instructions immediately following the Acknowledgments entitled "Using the CD-ROM" for information on finding the documentation for utilizing the programs and data sets on the CD-ROM.

We have established an Internet Web site to provide you with the most up-to-date information and additional resources on biostatistics. The Web site address is

http://www.clinicalbiostatistics.com

We hope you will use the site, and we invite you to send comments or suggestions, including any calculation errors you may find, to us at the e-mail address posted on the Web site.

Some statistical tests are not routinely available on most commercial packages. We have designed a spreadsheet program to analyze these special instances. These files are included in a folder on the CD named Calculations. Again, refer to the instructions immediately following the Acknowledgments entitled "Using the CD-ROM" for more information.

Exercises are provided with all chapters (2–13); answers are given in Appendix B, most with complete solutions. We include different kinds of exercises to meet the different needs of students. Some exercises call for calculating a statistic or a statistical test. Some focus on the presenting problems or other published studies and ask about the design (as in Chapter 2) or about the use of elements such as charts, graphs, tables, and statistical methods. Occasionally, exercises extend a concept discussed in the chapter. This additional development is not critical for all readers to understand, but it provides further insights for those who are interested. Some exercises refer to topics discussed in previous chapters to provide reminders and reinforcements.

Again, we highly recommend that you obtain copies of the original articles and review them in their entirety. If you are using this book in an organized course, we suggest you form small groups to discuss the articles and examine how the concepts covered in the book are dealt with by the various researchers. Finally, in response to a plea from our own students, a collection of multiple-choice questions is given in Chapter 13; these questions provide a useful posttest for students who want to be sure they have mastered the material presented in the text.

The **symbols** used in statistics are sometimes a source of confusion. These symbols are listed on the inside back cover for ready access. When more than one symbol for the same item is encountered in the medical literature, we use the most common one and point out the others. Also, as we mentioned previously, a **glossary** of biostatistical and epidemiologic terms is provided at the end of the book (after Chapter 13).

1.5 ADDITIONAL RESOURCES

We provide a large number of references to other texts and journal articles. With the growth of the Internet, many resources have become easily available for little or no cost. A number of statistical programs and resources are available on the Internet. Some of the programs are freeware, meaning that anyone may use them free of charge; others, called shareware, charge a relatively small fee for their use. Many of the software vendors have free products or software you can download and use for a restricted period of time.

We have listed a few excellent sites for information on biostatistics. Because Internet addresses change periodically, the following sites may be different by the time you try to access them. We will attempt to monitor these sites and will post any changes on our Web site (http://www.clinicalbiostatistics.com).

Statistical Solutions (http://www.statsol.com) has simple programs to find sample sizes for comparing two means or two proportions as well as calculating the statistical tests for comparing two means or two proportions.

The NCSS home page (http://www.ncss.com) has links to a free probability calculator you can use to look up values in statistical distributions (rather than using the tables in Appendix A).

The American Statistical Association (ASA) has a number of sections with a special emphasis, such as Teaching Statistics in the Health Sciences, Biometrics Section, Statistical Education, and others. Many of these Section homepages contain links to statistical resources. The ASA homepage is (http://www.amstat.com); the Teaching Statistics in the Health Sciences homepage is (http://www.bio.ri.ccf.org/ASA_TSHS) and has links to teaching materials.

Dartmouth University (http://www.dartmouth.edu) has links to the impressive Chance Database (http://www.dartmouth.edu/%7Echance/index.html), which contains many teaching resources and, in turn, many useful links to other resources.

The Medical University of South Carolina has links to a large number of evidence-based-medicine sites. Click on *Search* from the homepage (http://www.musc.edu).

Study Designs in Medical Research

2

This chapter introduces the different kinds of studies commonly used in medical research. Many of the illustrations used in this chapter are presenting problems in subsequent chapters, where they are discussed in greater detail. We believe that knowing how a study is designed is important for an understanding of the conclusions that can be drawn and have therefore chosen to devote considerable attention to the topic of study designs. Also, if you are acquainted with this topic, we can describe the type of design used in each presenting problem in this book.

This chapter first describes and illustrates study designs found in the medical literature and then presents the advantages and disadvantages of each design. If you are familiar with the medical literature, you will recognize many of the terms used to describe different study designs. If you are just beginning to read the literature, you should not be dismayed by all the new terminology; the terms are used repeatedly in the following chapters, so there will be ample opportunity to review and become familiar with them. Also, the glossary of terms at the end of the book defines the terms used in the book.

In the final chapter of this book, study designs are discussed once more, within the context of reading journal articles. At that time, pointers are given on how to look for possible biases that can occur in medical studies. A **bias** in a study is an error that leads to an incorrect conclusion. Bias can be due to the ways in which patients are selected, data are collected and analyzed, or the manner in which conclusions are drawn.

2.1 CLASSIFICATION OF STUDY DESIGNS

There are several different schemes for classifying study designs. We have adopted one that divides studies into those in which the subjects were merely observed, sometimes called observational studies, and those in which some intervention was performed, generally called experiments. This approach is simple and reflects the sequence an investigation sometimes takes. With a little practice, you should be able to read medical articles and classify studies according to this outline with no difficulty.

Table 2–1 contains the scheme for classifying pub-

lished research reports. Each design is illustrated in this chapter, using some of the studies that are presenting problems in upcoming chapters. In **observational studies,** one or more groups of patients are observed and characteristics about the patients are recorded for analysis. **Experimental studies** involve an **intervention**—an investigator-controlled maneuver, such as a drug, a procedure, or a treatment—and interest lies in the effect the intervention has on study subjects. Of course, both observational and experimental studies may involve animals or objects, but the vast majority of studies in medicine (and the ones discussed most frequently in this text) involve people.

2.2 OBSERVATIONAL STUDIES

Observational studies are of four main types: **case–series, case–control, cross-sectional** (including **surveys**), and **cohort studies.** When certain characteristics of a group (or series) of patients (or cases) are described in a published report, the result is called a **case–series study.** The simplest design is a set of case reports in which the author describes some interesting or intriguing observations that occurred for a small number of patients.

Case–series studies frequently lead to the generation of hypotheses that are subsequently investigated in a case–control, cross-sectional, or cohort study. These three types of studies are defined by the period of time the study covers and by the direction or focus of the research question. Cohort and case–control studies generally involve an extended period of time defined by the point when the study begins and the point when it ends; some process occurs, and a certain amount of time is required to assess it. For this reason, both cohort and case–control studies are sometimes also called **longitudinal studies.** The major difference between them is the direction of the inquiry or the focus of the research question: Cohort studies are forward-looking, from a risk factor to an outcome, but case–control studies are backward-looking, from an outcome to risk factors. The cross-sectional study analyzes data collected on a group of subjects at one time. Kleinbaum and colleagues (1997) describe a number of hybrids or combinations of these designs if you are interested in greater detail

Table 2–1. Classification of study designs.

I. Observational studies
   A. Descriptive or case–series
   B. Case–control studies (retrospective)
      1. Causes and incidence of disease
      2. Identification of risk factors
   C. Cross-sectional studies, surveys (prevalence)
      1. Disease description
      2. Diagnosis and staging
      3. Disease processes, mechanisms
   D. Cohort studies (prospective)
      1. Causes and incidence of disease
      2. Natural history, prognosis
      3. Identification of risk factors
   E. Historical cohort studies

II. Experimental studies
   A. Controlled trials
      1. Parallel or concurrent controls
         a. Randomized
         b. Not randomized
      2. Sequential controls
         a. Self-controlled
         b. Crossover
      3. External controls (including historical)
   B. Studies with no controls

III. Meta-analyses

than we give in this chapter. If you would like a more detailed discussion of study designs used in medicine, see the companion text on epidemiology by Greenberg and coworkers (1996). A book by Hulley and Cummings (1988) is devoted entirely to designing clinical research. Garb (1996) discusses study design in a book motivated by her experiences in a journal club.

2.2.1 Case–Series Studies

A case–series report is a simple descriptive account of interesting characteristics observed in a group of patients. For example, Alexandrov (1997) presented information on a series of 40 patients who had been referred for evaluation of stroke, transient ischemic attack, or carotid bruit, a presenting problem in Chapter 10. The authors wanted to compare peak systolic velocity with angiographic measurement of carotid stenosis. They were also interested in comparing two methods for the angiographic measurement to see which was the better predictor of peak systolic velocity. The investigators concluded that the relationship between both methods and peak systolic velocity was very strong. It is important to take the complex nature of these relationships into account when data from different centers are compared. A case–series report like this one can point out the need to be cautious in interpreting and comparing results from different laboratories.

Case–series reports generally involve patients seen over a relatively short period of time. Generally case–series studies do not include **control subjects,** persons who do not have the disease or condition being

described. Thus, some investigators would not include case–series in a list of types of studies because they are generally not planned studies and do not involve any research hypotheses. On occasion, however, investigators do include control subjects. Hindmarsh and Brook (1996) reported a study in the *Lancet* involving short normal children who were treated with growth hormone. The eligible subjects were children who were consecutively seen at a growth disorder clinic. Sixteen children received the hormone treatments, but there were seven short children whose parents declined treatment for them. The investigators followed the seven children, and observations on these children were analyzed as controls. We mention case–series studies because of their important descriptive role as a precursor to other studies.

2.2.2 Case–Control Studies

Case–control studies begin with the absence or presence of an outcome and then look backward in time to try to detect possible causes or risk factors that may have been suggested in a case–series report. The *cases* in case–control studies are individuals selected on the basis of some disease or outcome; the *controls* are individuals without the disease or outcome. The history or previous events of both cases and controls are analyzed in an attempt to identify a characteristic or risk factor present in the cases' histories but not in the controls' histories.

Figure 2–1 illustrates that subjects in the study are chosen at the onset of the study after they are known to be either cases with the disease (squares) or controls without the disease (diamonds). The histories of cases and controls are examined over a previous period of time to detect the presence (shaded areas) or absence (unshaded areas) of predisposing characteristics or risk factors, or, if the disease is infectious, whether the subject has been exposed to the presumed infectious agent. In case–control designs, the nature of the inquiry is backward in time, as indicated by the arrows pointing backward in Figure 2–1 to illustrate the backward or retrospective nature of the research process. We can characterize case–control studies as studies that ask "What happened?" In fact, they are sometimes called **retrospective studies** because of their direction of inquiry. Case–control studies are longitudinal as well, because the inquiry covers a period of time.

Kaku and Lowenstein (1990) identified patients between the ages of 15 and 44 who had had a stroke (cases) as well as patients who had not (controls) to investigate the relationship between stroke and recreational drug abuse in young people. A clinical association between drug abuse and stroke was based on the occurrence of stroke symptoms within 6 h of drug administration, positive toxicologic testing in stroke patients admitted in coma, or infectious endocarditis related to intravenous drug abuse. Controls were selected from patients admitted to the hospital with acute medical or surgical conditions for which recre-

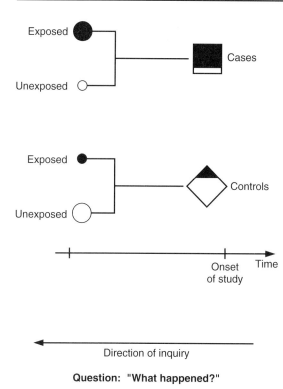

Figure 2–1. Schematic diagram of case–control study design. Shaded areas represent subjects exposed to the antecedent factor; unshaded areas correspond to unexposed subjects. Squares represent subjects with the outcome of interest; diamonds represent subjects without the outcome of interest. (Adapted and reproduced, with permission, from Greenberg RS: Retrospective studies. In Kotz S, Johnson NL [editors]: *Encyclopedia of Statistical Sciences,* Vol 8. Wiley, 1988.)

ational drug abuse has not been shown to be a risk factor. The investigators used **matching** to associate controls with cases on age and sex characteristics. If an investigator feels that such characteristics are so important that an imbalance between the two groups of patients would affect any conclusions, he or she should employ matching. This process ensures that both groups will be similar with respect to important characteristics that may otherwise cloud or confound the conclusions.

Deciding whether a published study is a case–control study or a case–series report is not always easy. Confusion arises because both types of studies are generally conceived and written after the fact rather than having been planned. The easiest way to differentiate between them is to ask yourself whether the author's purpose was to describe a phenomenon or to attempt to explain it by evaluating previous events. If the purpose is simple description, chances are the study is a case–series report.

2.2.3 Cross-Sectional Studies

The third type of observational study goes by all of the following names: cross-sectional studies, surveys, epidemiologic studies, and prevalence studies. We use the term "cross-sectional" because it is descriptive of the time line and does not have the connotation that the terms "surveys" and "prevalence" do. Cross-sectional studies analyze data collected on a group of subjects at one time rather than over a period of time. Cross-sectional studies are designed to determine "What is happening?" right now. Subjects are selected and information is obtained in a short period of time (Figure 2–2; note the short time line). Because they focus on a point in time, they are sometimes also called prevalence studies. Surveys and polls are generally cross-sectional studies, although surveys can be part of a cohort study. Like case–control studies, cross-sectional studies may be designed to address research questions raised by a case–series, or they may be done without a previous descriptive study.

2.2.3.a Diagnosing or Staging a Disease: In a presenting problem in Chapter 10, Soderstrom and his coinvestigators (1997) were interested in learning more about the relationship between demographic measures that might be helpful in identifying trauma patients who have an elevated blood alcohol concentration. They wanted to develop a simple scoring system that could be used to detect these patients when they come to an emergency department. These pa-

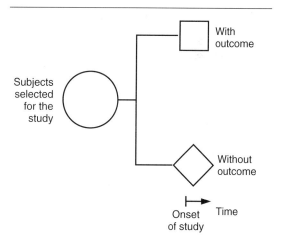

Figure 2–2. Schematic diagram of cross-sectional study design. Squares represent subjects with the outcome of interest; diamonds represent subjects without the outcome of interest.

tients could be targeted for assessment of alcohol abuse and dependence and other possible substance abuse. They chose to look at the time of day (day or night), the day of the week (weekday or weekend), race (white or nonwhite), age (40 years or older versus younger than 40). Using these four simple measures, the investigators were able to construct four models: for men whose injury was intentional, men whose injury was not intentional, women whose injury was intentional, and women whose injury was not intentional.

2.2.3.b Evaluating Different Methods of Doing the Same Thing: A presenting problem in Chapter 5 is a cross-sectional study designed to evaluate two methods for detecting abnormalities of the glenoid labrum (Garneau et al, 1991). The investigators studied the value of magnetic resonance imaging (MRI) in detecting abnormalities in 15 patients with a history of shoulder subluxation and physical examination findings suggesting shoulder instability. All 15 patients underwent arthroscopy or surgery of the shoulder, so that direct visualization of the shoulder joint served as the standard of reference in the evaluation of the MRI images. The investigators compared the diagnosis based on MRI with that directly observed during surgery or arthroscopy. Cross-sectional studies are used in all fields of medicine, but they are especially common in examinations of the usefulness of a new diagnostic procedure.

2.2.3.c Establishing Norms: Knowledge of the range within which most patients fit is very useful to clinicians. Laboratories, of course, establish and then provide the normal limits of most diagnostic tests when they report the results for a given patient. Often these limits are established by testing people who are known to have normal values. We would not, for example, want to use people with diabetes mellitus to establish the norms for serum glucose levels. The results from the people known to have normal values are used to define the range that separates the lowest 2½% of the values and the highest 2½% of the values from the middle 95%. These values are called normal values, or norms.

Outside of the laboratory there are many qualities for which normal ranges have not been established. This was true for two measures of the autoimmune nervous system function. These two measures, heart variation to deep breathing and the Valsalva ratio, are noninvasive tests that can help clinicians evaluate patients with diabetes mellitus and other neuropathic disorders. Gelber and colleagues (1997) analyzed data from subjects recruited from 63 centers throughout North America to develop normative values for these two measurements. The data collected in the process of performing these two tests were analyzed at a single center for taking autonomic nervous system readings. After comparing certain demographic groups, such as males versus females, the investigators established the normative values by finding those

values for heart rate variation to deep breathing and the Valsalva ratio that separated the highest and lowest 2½% from the central 95%.

2.2.3.d Surveys: Surveys are especially useful when the goal is to gain insight into a perplexing topic or to learn how people think and feel about an issue. Surveys are generally cross-sectional in design, but they can be used in case–control and cohort studies as well. A readable text on the use of survey methods in medicine is by Abramson (1999).

Using a questionnaire, Kalichman and Friedman (1992) surveyed over 2000 biomedical trainees about their perceptions on ethical research practices. The questionnaires were distributed through academic departments in basic sciences at a major university. Biomedical trainees were asked about their research training and experience, research plans, and awareness of incidents of scientific misconduct; 27% completed the questionnaires. The results from analyzing the questions indicated that almost one-fourth of the trainees had no ethics training, approximately one-third had observed some type of misconduct, and 15% would consider fudging data themselves. The findings also indicated that prior ethics training was not associated with past or potential unethical behavior.

Interviews are sometimes used in surveys, especially when it is important to probe reasons or explanations more deeply than is possible with a written questionnaire. For example, it has been claimed that the availability of firearms in the home is responsible for the increasing incidence of suicide. To study this issue, Kellerman and coworkers (1992) interviewed a person who had lived in the same residence as a suicide victim as well as a set of control subjects who lived in the same neighborhood. They matched the controls according to the victim's age, sex, and race. Based on their interviews, the researchers found that ready availability of guns was associated with an increase in suicide, and they recommended that gun owners carefully weigh their reasons for wishing to have guns in the home. The use of control subjects and the focus on past availability of firearms indicates this survey is primarily a case–control design.

Increasingly, surveys are performed using existing databases of information. As an illustration, Colquitt and associates (1992) used information from two sources, the National Resident Matching Program and the Association of American Medical Colleges, to examine the relationship between characteristics of medical students and the specialty they select for a residency program. They were able to match data records for U. S. medical school graduates who participated in the 1987 match. The authors also looked at the patterns of change in specialty preference throughout medical school. They found a number of differences in preference for primary care by women compared with men and by underrepresented minority students compared with nonminority students. Differences were also observed on matching rates, with women being most likely and underrepresented minority men being least likely to receive their first choice of specialties.

Many countries and states collect data on a variety of conditions to develop tumor registries and databases of cases of infectious disease. Diermayer and his colleagues (1999) analyzed epidemiologic surveillance data from the State of Oregon and reported an increase in the overall incidence rate of meningococcal disease from 2 cases/100,000 population during 1987–1992 to 4.5 cases/100,000 population in 1994. Epidemiologists from Oregon and the Centers for Disease Control in Atlanta, Georgia, wanted to know if the increased number of cases of meningococcal disease indicated a transition from endemic to epidemic disease. They also sought these other features of an epidemic: the predominance of a single bacterial strain rather than a heterogeneous mix of strains and a shift in age distribution of cases toward older age groups.

2.2.4 Cohort Studies

A cohort is a group of people who have something in common and who remain part of a group over an extended period of time. In medicine, the subjects in **cohort studies** are selected by some defining charac-

teristic (or characteristics) suspected of being a precursor to or risk factor for a disease or health effect. Cohort studies ask the question "What will happen?" and thus, the direction in cohort studies is forward in time. Figure 2–3 illustrates the study design. Researchers select subjects at the onset of the study and then determine whether they have the risk factor or have been exposed. The subjects, both exposed and unexposed, are followed over a certain period of time to observe the effect of these defining characteristics. Because the events of interest transpire after the study is begun, these studies are sometimes called **prospective studies.**

2.2.4.a Typical Cohort Studies: A classical cohort study with which most of you are probably familiar is the Framingham study of cardiovascular disease. This study was begun in 1948 to investigate factors associated with the development of atherosclerotic and hypertensive cardiovascular disease (Gordon and Kannel, 1970). More than 6000 citizens in Framingham, Massachusetts, agreed to participate in this long-term study that involved follow-up interviews and physical examinations every 2 years. Many journal articles have been written about this cohort, and some of the children of the original subjects are now being followed as well.

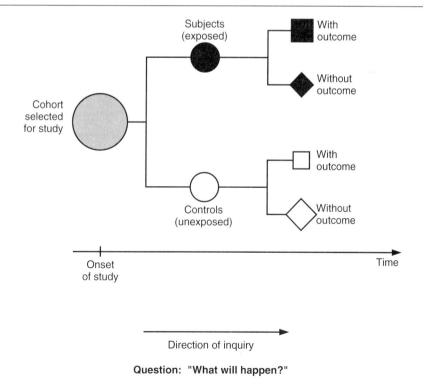

Figure 2–3. Schematic diagram of cohort study design. Shaded areas represent subjects exposed to the antecedent factor; unshaded areas correspond to unexposed subjects. Squares represent subjects with the outcome of interest; diamonds represent subjects without the outcome of interest. (Adapted and reproduced, with permission, from Greenberg RS: Prospective studies. In Kotz S, Johnson NL [editors]: *Encyclopedia of Statistical Sciences,* Vol 7. Wiley, 1986.)

Cohort studies may examine what happens to the disease over time as well as the causes of a disease. Many studies have been done on the Framingham cohort; over 500 journal articles were indexed by **MEDLINE** between 1975 and 2000. Many studies deal with cardiovascular-related conditions for which the study was designed, such as blood pressure response during treadmill testing as a risk for hypertension (Singh et al, 1999) and the association of chronic cough with myocardial infarction (Haider et al, 1999). This very rich source of data is being used to study many other conditions as well, for instance, the association between insulin-like growth factor I and bone mineral density in older women and men (Langlois et al, 1998) and the influence of smoking on the association between body weight and mortality (Sempos et al, 1998).

A presenting problem in Chapters 5 and 10 describes a longitudinal study to determine the course of depression in the elderly (Henderson et al, 1997). The investigators wanted to identify factors associated with the onset or persistence of depressive symptoms and to learn whether depression in the elderly is a risk factor for subsequent dementia or cognitive decline. The study population included 945 community residents and 100 people living in special hostels for the elderly or nursing homes. All were age 70 years or older. These individuals were evaluated in 1990 and reinterviewed 3–6 years later.

Data collected included information on psychologic health, measures of cognitive performance, physical health conditions, social support, recent bereavement, level of daily activities, physician or nurse visits, and apolipoprotein E genotype. Of the 1045 people examined in the initial evaluation, 709 (67.9%) were available for follow-up. The best predictors of the number of depressive symptoms at the follow-up interview included the number of depressive symptoms at the initial visit, deterioration in health and in activities of daily living, poor current health, poor social support, and high levels of use of physician and nurse services. There was no relationship between increasing age and level of depressive symptoms or change in depressive symptoms, nor did symptoms of depression predict subsequent cognitive decline or development of dementia.

2.2.4.b Outcome Assessment: Increasingly, studies that assess medical outcomes are reported in the medical literature. Patient outcomes have always been of interest to health care providers; physicians and others in the health field are interested in how patients respond to different therapies and management regimens. There continues to be a growing focus on the ways in which patients view and value their health, the care they receive, and the results or outcomes of this care. The reasons for the increase in patient-focused health outcomes are complex, and some of the major ones are discussed below. Kane (1997) provides information on reading outcomes research articles.

Interest in outcome assessment was spurred by the Medical Outcomes Study (MOS), designed to determine whether variations in patient outcomes were related to the system of care, clinician specialty, and the technical and interpersonal skill of the clinician (Tarlov et al, 1989). To learn if the variations in outcomes in different geographic locations occurred because of differences in the appropriateness of procedures, Chassin and colleagues (1987) studied three specific procedures (coronary angiography, carotid endarterectomy, and upper gastrointestinal tract endoscopy). They found similar levels of appropriate use in three geographic areas, but the use of some of these procedures varied more than twofold. A similar study revealed variation in resource utilization among different medical specialties and systems of health care, even after controlling for variation in patient mix (Greenfield et al, 1992). Specific focus on the health care organizations reported that poor and elderly patients with chronic illnesses had worse outcomes in health maintenance organizations (HMO) systems compared with fee-for-service systems and recommended that health care plans should carefully monitor patient outcomes (Ware et al, 1995). There are many kinds of patient outcomes: economic, functional status, and satisfaction, among others.

Functional status refers to a person's ability to perform his or her daily activities. Some researchers subdivide functional status into physical, emotional, mental, and social components (Gold et al, 1996). Functional status is related to the level of well-being in patients who have chronic diseases (Stewart et al, 1989). Many instruments used to measure physical functional status have been developed to evaluate the extent of a patient's rehabilitation following injury or illness. These instruments are commonly called measures of activities of daily living (ADL).

Quality of life (QOL) is a broadly defined concept that includes subjective or objective judgments about all aspects of an individual's existence: health, economic status, environmental and spiritual. Interest in measuring QOL was heightened when researchers came to the realization that living a long time does not necessarily imply living a good life. QOL measures can help determine a patient's preferences for different health states and are often used to help decide among alternative approaches to medical management (Wilson and Cleary, 1995).

Patient satisfaction has been discussed for many years. The recent shift to increased awareness and concern with patient satisfaction is being driven by the insurance industry and particularly the managed care organizations (Ware, 1991). One reason for emphasizing patient satisfaction per se is that quantifying the quality of care in medicine is difficult (Kassirer, 1993). It is easier to quantify how patients perceive their medical care, and patients who perceive they are getting good care are more likely to be satisfied with their care (Hall et al, 1993). Patient satisfaction has been shown to be highly associated with whether patients remain with the same physician provider and the degree to which they adhere to their treatment plan (Weingarten et al, 1995).

Another reason that measurement of patient satisfaction has increased is that managed care plans depend on maintaining an adequate enrollment; otherwise, they must cut costs as enrollment declines and services to patients decrease. Patients who are less satisfied leave the organization and enroll in a different plan (Rubin et al, 1993) or request that their employers change to a plan with better services. The insurance industry therefore has a vested interest in determining which factors patients perceive to be important aspects of their care.

Patient satisfaction with their medical care is influenced by a number of factors, not all of which are directly related to quality of care. Examples include time spent in the office waiting for the doctor and waiting for resolution after being seen; ease of access to the doctor, including phone contact; appointment desk activity; parking; building directions; waiting room setting; and friendliness of the staff in general (Lledo et al, 1995).

Patients' perception of physician behavior and attitude is an important aspect of their satisfaction. The physician's attitude has been shown to influence the patient's outcome (O'Connor et al, 1994). Components include the physician's help in resolving the problem and his or her expression of understanding of the problem and caring for the emotional and physical well-being of the patient (Dennis, 1995). In a study focusing on outpatient care, key components were the humanity, efficiency, informativeness, and continuity of communication of the health provider (Avis et al, 1995).

Length of time to event is the length of time to the occurrence or reoccurrence of an event, such as relapse of a disease or readmission to the hospital.

Cost-effectiveness analysis (CEA) is the method used to evaluate economic outcomes of interventions or different modes of treatment. The CEA gives policy makers and health providers critical data needed to make informed judgments about interventions (Gold et al, 1996). The CEA of hospitalized patients typically includes length of hospital stay, procedures, laboratory studies, medications, and so on. Few CEA studies have been done on outpatients other than the Medical Outcomes Studies. Cost of procedures, laboratory and other diagnostic procedures, and medications are obvious economic outcomes to consider. The length of time a patient is disabled or unable to work, however, is a related economic variable that affects the overall cost of health care.

A large number of questionnaires or instruments have been developed to measure outcomes. For quality of life, the most commonly used general purpose instrument is the Medical Outcomes Study MOS 36-Item Short-Form Health Survey (SF-36). Originally developed at the RAND Corporation (Stewart et al, 1988), a refinement of the instrument has been validated and is now used worldwide to provide baseline measures and to monitor the results of medical care. The SF-36 provides a way to collect valid data and does not require very much time to complete. The 36 items are combined to produce a patient profile on eight concepts in addition to summary physical and mental health measures. Another instrument that focuses specifically on QOL is the EuroQol Questionnaire developed and widely used in Europe and the UK (Kind, 1996).

Many instruments are problem-specific. McDowell and Newell (1996) evaluate various scales on general topics in measuring health. Spilker (1996) has edited a volume specifically devoted to quality-of-life instruments, both general purpose and disease-specific.

Some outcome studies address a whole host of topics, and we have used several as presenting problems in upcoming chapters. As efforts continue to contain costs of medical care while maintaining a high level of patient care, we expect to see many additional studies focusing on patient outcomes. A description of outcomes research, including challenges in outcomes research and directions for future research at the Agency for Health Care Policy and Research, is given by Clancy and Eisenberg (1997). The journal *Medical Care* is devoted exclusively to outcome studies.

2.2.4.c Historical Cohort Studies: Many cohort studies are prospective; that is, they begin at a specific time, the presence or absence of the risk factor is determined, and then information about the outcome of interest is collected at some future time, as in the two studies described earlier. One can also undertake a cohort study by using information collected in the past and kept in records or files.

For example, Shipley and his coinvestigators (1999) wanted to assess study outcomes in men with prostate cancer treated with a specific type of radiation therapy. Six medical centers had consistently followed up a group of patients who had previously been treated with this therapy. Shipley used existing records to look at survival and tumor recurrence in 1607 men who were treated between 1988 and 1995 but who had had at least four prostate-specific antigen measurements after radiation. This approach to a study is possible if the records on follow-up are complete and adequately detailed and if the investigators can ascertain the current status of the patients.

Some investigators call this type of study a **historical cohort study** or **retrospective cohort study** because historical information is used; that is, the events being evaluated actually occurred before the onset of the study (Figure 2–4). Note that the direction of the inquiry is still forward in time, from a possible cause or risk factor to an outcome. Studies that merely describe an investigator's experience with a group of patients and attempt to identify features associated with a good

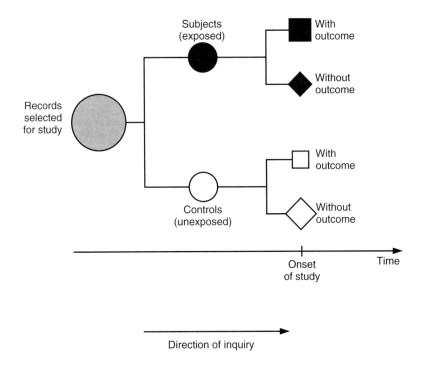

Figure 2–4. Schematic diagram of historical cohort study design. Shaded areas represent subjects exposed to the antecedent factor; unshaded areas correspond to unexposed subjects. Squares represent subjects with the outcome of interest; diamonds represent subjects without the outcome of interest. (Adapted and reproduced, with permission, from Greenberg RS: Retrospective studies. In Kotz S, Johnson NL [editors]: *Encyclopedia of Statistical Sciences,* Vol. 8. Wiley, 1988.)

or bad outcome fall into this category, and many such studies are published in the medical literature.

The time relationship among the different observation study designs is illustrated in Figure 2–5. The figure shows the timing of surveys, which have no direction of inquiry, case–control designs, which look backward in time, and cohort studies, which look forward in time.

2.2.5 Comparison of Case–Control and Cohort Studies

Both case–control and cohort studies evaluate risks and causes of disease, and the design an investigator selects depends in part on the research question.

Consider once more the study by Henderson and colleagues (1997). These investigators undertook a cohort study to look at the risk factors for depression in the elderly. After an initial interview to collect a lot of information on potential risk factors, the investigators reinterviewed the subjects 3–6 years later to reassess their status. The investigators could have designed a case–control study had they asked the research question as follows: "Among elderly people exhibiting dementia or cognitive decline, what are the likely precursors or risk factors?" The investigators would need to have a way to learn what the patients' mental status had been in the past and any other potential reasons that might have been associated with

their present condition. As this illustration shows, a cohort study starts with a risk factor or exposure and looks at consequences; a case–control study takes the outcome as the starting point of the inquiry and looks for precursors or risk factors.

Generally speaking, results from a well-designed cohort study carry more weight in establishing a cause than do results from a case–control study. A large number of possible biasing factors can play a role in case–control studies, and several of them are discussed at greater length in Chapter 13.

The distinction between these two study designs is clearly illustrated in the controversies surrounding the study of tobacco as a risk factor for lung cancer. By the 1950s, many published case–control studies linked lung cancer with prior use of tobacco. The general design of these studies was to begin with a group of patients with lung cancer and a group of control patients without lung cancer and then to compare the smoking histories of both sets of patients. Typically, a greater percentage of those with lung cancer than those without lung cancer had a history of smoking. Some researchers, however, pointed out a possible bias in these studies—the possibility that some factor other than smoking that is common both in smokers and in people who develop lung cancer is responsible for the cancer. Although this point can be made for any case–control study, the tobacco indus-

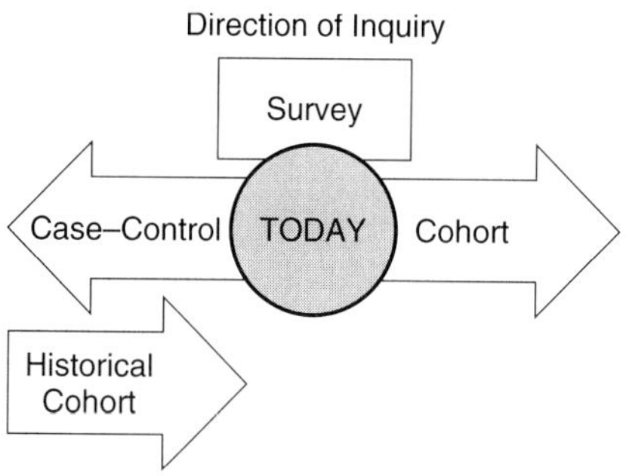

Direction of Inquiry

Figure 2–5. Schematic diagram of the time relationship among different observational study designs. The arrows represent the direction of the inquiry.

try had considerable financial motivation for raising this issue.

To avoid this bias, investigators in England undertook a cohort study of British physicians (Doll and Hill, 1950). They found that physicians who smoked cigarettes had a subsequent mortality rate from lung cancer about ten times greater than physicians who did not smoke. Also striking was the report 26 years later that there had been a 50% decline in cigarette smoking among British physicians since 1950, accompanied by a 40% reduction in mortality from lung cancer. In the general public, however, there was no decrease in smoking or in the number of lung cancer deaths over this period (Doll and Peto, 1976).

The controversy regarding the role of tobacco smoke continues. The focus is now on the risk to nonsmokers who live in the same household (Lash and Aschengrau, 1999) or work in the same environment (eg, airline personnel) as smokers. In spite of their shortcomings with respect to establishing causality, case–control studies are frequently used in medicine and can provide useful insights if well designed. They can be completed in a much shorter time than cohort studies and are correspondingly less expensive to undertake. Case–control studies are especially useful for studying rare conditions or diseases that may not manifest themselves for many years. In addition, they are valuable for testing an original premise; if the results of the case–control study are promising, the investigator can design and undertake a more involved cohort study.

2.3 EXPERIMENTAL STUDIES OR CLINICAL TRIALS

Experimental studies are generally easier to identify than observational studies in the medical literature. Authors of medical journal articles reporting experimental studies tend to state explicitly the type of study design used more often than do authors reporting observational studies. Experimental studies in

medicine that involve humans are called **clinical trials** because their purpose is to draw conclusions about a particular procedure or treatment. Table 2–1 indicates that clinical trials fall into two categories: those with and those without controls.

Controlled trials are studies in which the experimental drug or procedure is compared with another drug or procedure, sometimes a placebo and sometimes the previously accepted treatment. Uncontrolled trials are studies in which the investigators' experience with the experimental drug or procedure is described, but the treatment is not compared with another treatment, at least not formally. Because the purpose of an experiment is to determine whether the intervention (treatment) makes a difference, studies with controls are much more likely than those without controls to detect whether the difference is due to the experimental treatment or to some other factor. Thus, controlled studies are viewed as having far greater validity in medicine than uncontrolled studies. For additional issues regarding clinical trials, consult Matthews and Farewell (1996).

2.3.1 Trials with Independent Concurrent Controls

One way a trial can be controlled is to have two groups of subjects: one that receives the experimental procedure (the experimental group) and the other that receives the placebo or standard procedure (the control group) (Figure 2–6). The experimental and control groups should be treated alike in all ways except for the procedure itself so that any differences between the groups will be due to the procedure and not to other factors. The best way to ensure that the groups are treated similarly is to plan interventions for both groups for the same time period in the same study. In this way, the study achieves **concurrent control.** To reduce the chances that subjects or investigators see what they expect to see, researchers can design **double-blind trials** in which neither subjects nor investigators know whether the subject is in the treatment or the control group. When only the subject is unaware, the study is called a **blind trial.** In some unusual situations, the study design may call for the investigator to be blinded even when the subject cannot be blinded. Blindedness is discussed in detail in Chapter 13. Another issue is how to assign some patients to the experimental condition and others to the control condition; the best method of assignment is random assignment. Methods for randomization are discussed in Chapter 4.

2.3.1.a Randomized Clinical Trials: The randomized clinical trial is the epitome of all research designs because it provides the strongest evidence for concluding causation; it provides the best insurance that the result was due to the intervention.

One of the more noteworthy randomized trials is the Physicians' Health Study (Steering Committee of the Physicians' Health Study Research Group, 1989),

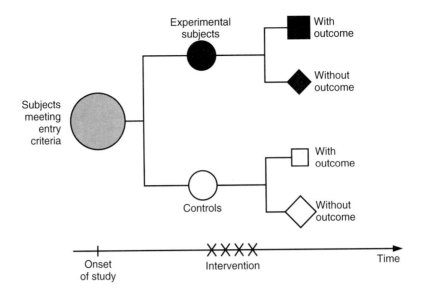

Figure 2–6. Schematic diagram of randomized clinical trial design. Shaded areas represent subjects assigned to the treatment condition; unshaded areas correspond to subjects assigned to the control condition. Squares represent subjects with the outcome of interest; diamonds represent subjects without the outcome of interest.

which investigated the role of aspirin in reducing the risk of cardiovascular disease. (This study is a presenting problem in Chapter 3.) One purpose was to learn whether aspirin in low doses reduces the mortality rate from cardiovascular disease. Participants in this clinical trial were over 22,000 healthy male physicians who were randomly assigned to receive aspirin or placebo and were followed over an average period of 60 months. The investigators found that fewer physicians in the aspirin group experienced a myocardial infarction during the course of the study than did physicians in the group receiving placebo. A subsequent analysis of the effect of this and two other clinical trials of cardiovascular drugs found an increase from 16% to almost 24% in the number of persons using aspirin between 1987 and 1990 (Lamas et al, 1992).

We discuss several randomized trials as presenting problems. For instance, Benson and colleagues (1996) undertook a study of vaginal versus abdominal reconstructive surgery for treatment of pelvic support defects (Chapter 6 presenting problem). They randomly assigned women with cervical prolapse to one surgical approach or the other and found no differences in subsequent morbidity, pain, or length of time in the hospital. The vaginal group had more incontinence, decreased time in the operating room, and lower hospital charges. The investigators found, however, that surgical effectiveness was optimal in twice as many in the abdominal group, 58% compared with 29% in the vaginal group.

2.3.1.b Nonrandomized Trials: Subjects are not always randomized to treatment options. Studies that do not use randomized assignment are generally re-

ferred to as **nonrandomized trials** or simply as clinical trials or comparative studies, with no mention of randomization. Many investigators believe that studies with nonrandomized controls are open to so many sources of bias that their conclusions are highly questionable. Studies using nonrandomized controls are considered to be much weaker because they do nothing to prevent bias in patient assignment. For instance, perhaps it is the stronger patients who receive the more aggressive treatment and the higher-risk patients who are treated conservatively. An example is a nonrandomized study of the use of a paracervical block to diminish cramping and pain associated with cryosurgery for cervical neoplasia (Harper, 1997; Chapter 6 presenting problem). This investigator enrolled the first 40 women who met the inclusion criteria in the group treated in the usual manner (no anesthetic block before cryosurgery) and enrolled the next 45 women in the group receiving the paracervical block. This design is not as subject to bias as a study in which patients are treated without regard to any plan; however, it does not qualify as a randomized study and does present some potential problems in interpretation. Whenever patients are assigned to treatments within big blocks of time, there is always the possibility that an important event occurred between the two time periods, such as a change in the method used for cryotherapy. Although that may not have been true in this study, a randomized design would have been more persuasive.

2.3.2 Trials with Self-Controls

A moderate level of control can be obtained by using the same group of subjects for both experimental and control options. A presenting problem in Chapter 5 describes a study to investigate the influence of humor on how patients with schizophrenia felt about the support they received from the staff (Gelkopf et al, 1994). This was a randomized study in which one group of patients was shown humorous movies over a 3-month period and the other group watched a variety of types of movies. Gelkopf collected information on the patients' perceptions of staff support before beginning the study and again at the completion of the study. Some studies have only one group in which patients are assessed before and after the intervention. This type of study uses patients as their own controls and is called a **self-controlled study.** Studies with self-controls and no other control group are still vulnerable to the well-known Hawthorne effect, described by Roethlisberger and colleagues (1946), in which people change their behavior and sometimes improve simply because they receive special attention by being in a study and not because of the study intervention itself. These studies are similar to cohort studies except for the intervention or treatment that is involved.

The self-controlled study design can be modified to provide a combination of concurrent and self-controls. This design uses two groups of patients: One group is assigned to the experimental treatment, and the second group is assigned to the placebo or control treatment (Figure 2–7). After a period of time, the experimental treatment and placebo are withdrawn from both groups for a "washout" period. During the washout period, the patients generally receive no treatment. The groups are then given the alternative treatment; that is, the first group now receives the placebo, and the second group receives the experimental treatment. This design, called a **crossover study,** is powerful when used appropriately.

2.3.3 Trials with External Controls

The third method for controlling experiments is to use controls external to the study. Sometimes, the result of another investigator's research is used as a comparison. On other occasions, the controls are patients the investigator has previously treated in another manner, called **historical controls.** The study design is illustrated in Figure 2–8.

Historical controls are frequently used to study diseases for which cures do not yet exist. For example, Cooley and colleagues (1990) studied toxicity and clinical response to 2′,3′-dideoxyinosine (ddI) in patients with the acquired immunodeficiency syndrome (AIDS). The investigators compared the responses of 34 patients taking ddI with patients in previous studies of 3′-azido-2′,3′-dideoxythymidine (AZT) and found that ddI appeared to have beneficial qualities similar to AZT but with fewer toxic side effects. They recommended that ddI be studied in controlled clinical trials to provide additional information regarding its efficacy. As with studies of AIDS, historical controls have been commonly used in oncology studies, although more and more oncologic studies use concurrent controls when possible. In

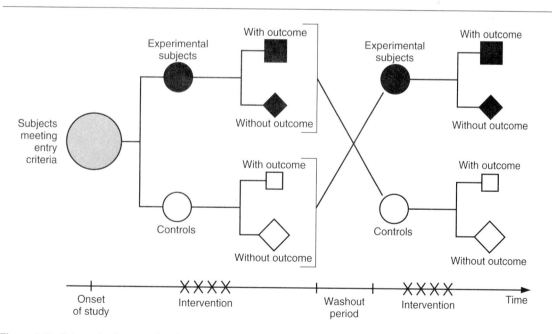

Figure 2–7. Schematic diagram of trial with crossover. Shaded areas represent subjects assigned to the treatment condition; unshaded areas correspond to subjects assigned to the control condition. Squares represent subjects with the outcome of interest; diamonds represent subjects without the outcome of interest.

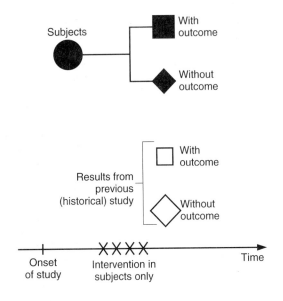

Figure 2–8. Schematic diagram of trial with external controls. Shaded areas represent subjects assigned to the treatment condition; unshaded areas correspond to patients cared for under the control condition. Squares represent subjects with the outcome of interest; diamonds represent subjects without the outcome of interest.

studies involving historical controls, researchers should evaluate whether other factors may have changed since the time the historical controls were treated; if so, any differences may be due to these other factors and not to the treatment.

2.3.4 Uncontrolled Studies

Not all studies involving interventions have controls, and by strict definition they are not really experiments or trials. For example, Crook and associates (1997) (which is a presenting problem in Chapter 9) reported the results of a trial of radiotherapy for prostate carcinoma in which patients were followed for at least 12 and for as long as 70 months. The investigators wanted to determine the length of time a patient had no recurrence of the tumor as well as how long the patients survived. They found some differences in the probability of long-term survival in patients who had different tumor classification scores (scores that measure the severity of the tumor). This study was an **uncontrolled study** because there were no comparisons with patients treated in another manner.

Uncontrolled studies are more likely to be used when the comparison involves a procedure than when it involves a drug. The major shortcoming of such studies is that investigators assume that the procedure used and described is the best one. The history of medicine is filled with examples in which one particular treatment is recommended and then discontinued after a controlled clinical trial is undertaken. The most significant problem with uncontrolled trials is that unproved procedures and therapies can become established, making it very difficult for researchers to undertake subsequent controlled studies.

2.4 META-ANALYSIS & REVIEW PAPERS

A type of study that does not fit specifically in either category of observation studies or experiments is called **meta-analysis ("meta," meaning later and more highly organized)**. Meta-analysis uses published information from other studies and combines the results so as to permit an overall conclusion. Meta-analysis is similar to review articles, but additionally includes a quantitative assessment and summary of the findings. It is possible to do a meta-analysis of observational studies or experiments; however, a meta-analysis should report the findings for these two types of study designs separately. This method is especially appropriate when the studies that have been reported have small numbers of subjects or come to different conclusions.

Veenstra and colleagues (1999) (a presenting problem in Chapter 10) performed a meta-analysis of infection and central venous catheters. The investigators wanted to know whether catheters impregnated with antiseptic were effective in preventing catheter-related bloodstream infection, compared with untreated catheters. They found 12 randomized trials that had addressed this question and combined the results in a statistical manner to reach an overall conclusion about their effectiveness—mainly that the impregnated catheters appear to be effective in reducing the incidence of infection in high-risk patients.

2.5 ADVANTAGES & DISADVANTAGES OF DIFFERENT STUDY DESIGNS

The previous sections introduced the major types of study designs used in medical research, broadly divided into experimental studies, or clinical trials, and observational studies (cohort, case–control, cross-sectional, and case–series designs). Each study design has certain advantages over the others as well as some specific disadvantages. These advantages and disadvantages are discussed in the following sections, beginning with the most powerful study designs, clinical trials, and progressing to the weakest, case–series.

2.5.1 Advantages & Disadvantages of Clinical Trials

The clinical trial is the gold standard, or reference, in medicine—that is, the basic design against which other designs are judged—because it provides the greatest justification for concluding causality and is subject to the least number of problems or biases. Clinical trials are the best type of study to use when the objective is to establish the efficacy of a treatment or a procedure. Clinical trials in which patients are randomly assigned to different treatments, or "arms," are the strongest design of all. One of the treatments is the experimental condition; another is the control condition. The control may be a placebo or a sham procedure; often, it is the treatment or procedure commonly used, called the standard of care or reference standard. For example, patients with coronary artery disease in the Coronary Artery Surgery Study (CASS Principal Investigators and Associates, 1983) (presenting problem in Chapter 4) were randomized to receive either surgical or medical care; no patient was left untreated or given a placebo.

A good argument for using concurrent randomized controls was made by Sacks and colleagues (1982) in an early investigation of the differences in findings in clinical trials utilizing randomized controls. They investigated six therapies that had been studied in 50 randomized clinical trials and 56 trials with historical controls:

1. Surgical shunts versus medical management of cirrhosis with varices
2. Coronary artery surgery
3. Anticoagulants for acute myocardial infarction
4. 5-FU adjuvant drug treatment for colon cancer
5. BCG adjuvant therapy for melanoma
6. DES for managing habitual abortion)

They found that therapy was better than the control regimen in 79% of the historical trials but in only 20% of the trials with concurrent randomized controls. The treated patients had similar outcomes regardless of whether randomized or historical controls were used. The difference between the studies with randomized and historical controls for the same therapy was primarily the result of patients in the historical control groups generally being reported to have worse outcomes than patients in the randomized control groups. Sacks and his colleagues state that "biases in patient selection may irretrievably weight the outcome of historical controlled trials in favor of new therapies." (Biases in patient selection are discussed in detail in Chapter 13.)

The inappropriate use of historical controls has led to serious errors in medicine. For example, Chalmers (1969) describes two erroneous treatments based on studies using historical controls. In one case, patients with peptic ulcers were treated by freezing the gastric area through intubating the patient with a balloon catheter and circulating a coolant in the balloon. In the second case, patients with hepatic failure were treated by using low-protein diets. These treatment methods were abandoned only after studies using concurrent controls showed how ineffective they were.

In some situations, however, historical controls can and should be used. For instance, historical controls may be useful when preliminary studies are needed or when researchers are dealing with late treatment for an intractable disease, such as advanced cancer. Investigators gain some protection against bias when they clearly state a prior hypothesis and when the same investigators treat the historical controls, thereby providing some assurance of similarity between historical controls and current patients. Nevertheless, the biases demonstrated by Sacks and colleagues (1982) should make you wary of trials with historical controls that report in favor of the experimental treatment. Although the differences between studies using concurrent versus historical control may not be as great today, partially because investigators are generally more savvy with respect to designing studies with historical controls and partly because journal editors are more discerning, it would be interesting to replicate the Sacks study on controversial treatments today.

Although clinical trials provide the greatest justification for determining causation, obstacles to using them include their great expense and long duration. For instance, a randomized trial comparing various treatments for carcinoma requires the investigators to follow the subjects for a long time. Another potential obstacle to using clinical trials occurs when certain practices become established and accepted by the medical community, even though they have not been properly justified. For example, Swan-Ganz catheters are used to measure pulmonary artery pressure, but their benefit has never been established by clinical trials. The tremendous increases in medical technology have not been accompanied by changes in the way new approaches are evaluated, according to Robin (1985). As a result, procedures become established that may be harmful to many patients, as evidenced by the controversy over silicone breast implants. As another example, there are many different approaches to managing hypertension, but many of them have never been subjected to a clinical trial that includes the most conservative treatment, diuretics. Researchers subsequently have difficulty obtaining approval to perform properly designed clinical trials from the human subjects committees that oversee the ethics of research in many hospitals and research institutions.

All in all, randomized clinical trials are viewed as the most important way to obtain unbiased data, when it is possible to undertake them. Many investigators feel that the benefits from performing randomized trials are well worth any difficulties they may present.

2.5.2 Advantages & Disadvantages of Cohort Studies

Cohort studies are the design of choice for studying the causes of a condition, the course of a disease, or the risk factors, because they are longitudinal and follow a group of subjects over a period of time. Causation generally cannot be proved with cohort studies because they are observational and do not involve interventions. However, because they follow a cohort of patients forward through time, they possess the correct time sequence to provide strong evidence for possible causes and effects, as in the smoking and lung cancer controversy. In addition, in prospectively designed cohort studies, as opposed to historical cohort studies, investigators can control many sources of bias related to patient selection and recorded measurements.

The length of time required in a cohort study depends on the problem studied. With diseases that develop over a long period of time or with conditions that occur as a result of long-term exposure to some causative agent, many years are needed for study. Extended time periods make such studies costly. They also make it difficult for investigators to argue causation, because other events occurring in the intervening period may have affected the outcome. For example, the long period of time between exposure and effect is one of the reasons it is difficult to study the possible relationship between environmental agents and various carcinomas. Cohort studies that require a long period of time to complete are especially vulnerable to problems associated with patient follow-up, particularly patient attrition (patients stop participating in the study) and patient migration (patients move to other communities). This is one reason that the Framingham study, with its rigorous methods of follow-up, is such a rich source of important information.

2.5.3 Advantages & Disadvantages of Case–Control Studies

Case–control studies are especially appropriate for studying rare diseases or events, for examining conditions that develop over a long time, and for investigating a preliminary hypothesis. They are generally the quickest and least expensive studies to undertake. For example, Kaku and Lowenstein (1990) used a case–control study to investigate the relationship between stroke and recreational drug abuse in young people. With this design, they were able to complete the study in a relatively short time and with relatively small numbers of subjects. Case–control studies are thus ideal for investigators who need to obtain some preliminary data prior to writing a proposal for a more complete, expensive, and time-consuming study; they are also ideal for anyone who needs to complete a clinical research project in a specific amount of time.

The advantages of case–control studies lead to their disadvantages. Of all study methods, they have the largest number of possible biases or errors, and they depend completely on high-quality existing records. Data availability for case–control studies sometimes requires compromises between what researchers wish to study and what they are able to study. One of the authors was involved in a study of elderly burn patients in which the goal was to determine risk factors for survival. The primary investigator wanted to collect data on fluid intake and output. He found, however, that not all of the existing patient records contained this information, and thus it was impossible to study the effect of this factor.

One of the greatest problems in a case–control study is selection of an appropriate control group.

The cases in a case–control study are relatively easy to identify, but deciding on a group of persons who provide a relevant comparison is more difficult. To illustrate the importance (and difficulty) of choosing a proper control group, consider an old case–control study that was designed to examine the relationship between use of tobacco, alcohol, tea, and coffee and incidence of pancreatic cancer (MacMahon et al, 1981). The cases were hospitalized patients who had a histologic diagnosis of pancreatic cancer. For controls, the investigators selected patients who were under the care of the same physician in the same hospital at the same time. Many patients were excluded from consideration as controls: patients with diseases of the pancreas, hepatobiliary tract, or cardiovascular system and patients with diabetes mellitus, respiratory cancer, bladder cancer, or peptic ulcer were all excluded. The results of the study indicated that the cases, patients with pancreatic cancer, had consumed greater amounts of coffee beverages than had the controls.

The problem with the control group in this study is that it included patients with cancer of the stomach and small intestine and patients with nonmalignant gastroenterologic conditions, such as gastritis, enteritis, and colitis; it is quite likely that many of these patients may have discontinued the use of coffee because of their problems. Including these patients in the control group makes it less likely that patients in the control group consumed large amounts of coffee, thereby increasing the chances of an observed relationship between coffee and pancreatic cancer. A better control group would have been patients hospitalized for completely unrelated problems, such as lung cancer. Because of the problems inherent in choosing a control group in a case–control study, some statisticians have recommended the use of two control groups: one control group similar in some ways to the cases (such as having been hospitalized during the same period of time) and another control group of healthy subjects.

2.5.4 Advantages & Disadvantages of Cross-Sectional Studies

Cross-sectional studies are best for determining the status quo of a disease or condition, such as the prevalence of HIV in given populations, and for evaluating diagnostic procedures. Cross-sectional studies are similar to case–control studies in being relatively quick to complete, and they may be relatively inexpensive as well. Their primary disadvantage is that they provide only a "snapshot in time" of the disease or process, which may result in misleading information if the research question is really one of disease process. For example, clinicians used to believe that diastolic blood pressure, unlike systolic pressure, does not increase as patients grow older. This belief was based on cross-sectional studies that had shown mean diastolic blood pressure to be approximately 80 mm Hg in all age groups. In the Framingham cohort study, however, the patients who were followed over a period of several years were observed to have increased diastolic blood pressure as they grew older (Gordon et al, 1959).

This apparent contradiction is easier to understand if we consider what happens in an aging cohort. For example, suppose that the mean diastolic pressure in men aged 40 years is 80 mm Hg, although there is individual variation, with some men having a blood pressure as low as 60 mm Hg and others having a pressure as high as 100 mm Hg. Ten years later there is an increase in diastolic pressure, although it is not an even increase; some men experience a greater increase than others. However, those men who were at the upper end of the **distribution** 10 years earlier and who had experienced a larger increase have died in the intervening period, so they are no longer represented in a cross-sectional study. As a result, the mean diastolic pressure of the men still in the cohort at age 50 is about 80 mm Hg, even though individually their pressures are higher than they were 10 years earlier. Thus, a cohort study, not a cross-sectional study, provides the information leading to a correct understanding of the relationship between normal aging and physiologic processes such as diastolic blood pressure.

Surveys are generally cross-sectional studies. For example, most of the voter preference surveys done prior to an election are one-time samplings of a group of citizens, and different results from week to week are based on different groups of people; that is, the same group of citizens is not followed to determine voting preferences through time. Similarly, consumer-oriented studies on customer satisfaction with automobiles, appliances, health care, and so on are cross-sectional.

A common problem with survey research is obtaining sufficiently large response rates; many people asked to participate in a survey decline because they are busy, not interested, and so forth. The conclusions are therefore based on a subset of people who agree to participate, and these people may not be **representative** of or similar to the entire population. Note that the problem of representative participants is not confined to cross-sectional studies, however; it can be an issue in other studies whenever subjects are selected or asked to participate and decline or drop out. Another issue is the way questions are posed to participants; if questions are asked in a leading or emotionally inflammatory way, the responses may not truly represent the participants' feelings or opinions.

2.5.5 Advantages & Disadvantages of Case–Series Studies

Case–series reports have two advantages: They are easy to write, and the observations may be extremely useful to investigators designing a study to evaluate causes or explanations of the observations. But as we noted previously, case–series studies are susceptible to many possible biases related to subject selection and characteristics observed. In general, you should view them as hypothesis-generating and not as conclusive.

2.6 SUMMARY

This chapter illustrates the study designs most frequently encountered in the medical literature. In medical research, either subjects are observed or experiments are undertaken. Experiments involving humans are called trials. Experimental studies may also use animals and tissue, although we did not discuss them as a separate category; the comments pertaining to clinical trials are relevant to animal and tissue studies as well.

Each type of study discussed has advantages and disadvantages. Randomized, controlled clinical trials are the most powerful designs possible in medical research, but they are often expensive and time-consuming. Well-designed observational studies can provide useful insights on disease causation, even though they do not constitute proof of causes. Cohort studies are best for studying the natural progression of disease or risk factors for disease; case–control studies are much quicker and less expensive. Cross-sectional studies provide a snapshot of a disease or condition at one time, and we must be cautious in inferring disease progression from them. Surveys, if properly done, are useful in obtaining current opinions and practices. Case–series studies should be used only to raise questions for further research.

As much as possible, we have used presenting problems from later chapters to illustrate different study designs. We will point out salient features in the design of the presenting problems as we go along, and we will return to the topic of study design again after all the prerequisites for evaluating the quality of journal articles have been presented.

EXERCISES

Read the descriptions of the following studies and determine the study design used.

1. Kremer and coworkers (1987) designed a study to determine the efficacy of fish oil dietary supplements in treating rheumatoid arthritis. They were particularly interested in the effect of the fish oil on the inhibition of neutrophil leukotriene levels. The study involved a group of 40 patients with class I, II, or III rheumatoid arthritis; each patient was given either a dietary supplement or a placebo for 14 weeks, but the treatment assignment was not randomized. From

weeks 14 to 18, all patients took a placebo for this 4-week period; then they were given the opposite treatment (dietary supplement or placebo) from weeks 1 to 14 for the next 14 weeks.

2. A study of 252 adult day-care providers at six day-care centers and children from three of the centers was undertaken to determine the occupational risk of cytomegalovirus infection among day-care providers (Murphy et al, 1991). This virus is a member of the human herpesvirus group and is the most common cause of viral infections. It has been found in the serum of up to 80% of children at some day-care centers, and the investigators were interested in studying the extent of the disease among day-care providers. All day-care centers in the study accepted children from ages 2 weeks to 5 years. Each center had between 60 and 231 children at the time of the study. After follow-up of 2.5–4.5 years, depending on the center, the investigators reported an overall annual seroconversion rate of 8% among providers; although the rates of conversion varied a great deal among centers, conversion rates appeared to be associated with the level of cytomegalovirus excretion by children at the centers.

3. A study by O'Malley and Fletcher (1987) looked at the efficacy of the breast self-examination (BSE) as a screening test for breast cancer by reviewing studies published on this topic. The authors found the sensitivity of BSE (the percentage of women with breast cancer who have a positive BSE) to be much lower than the sensitivity of a clinical breast examination or mammography. Although training increases the use of BSE and its sensitivity, the number of false-positives (women without breast cancer who have a positive BSE) also increases. The authors suggest the need for a controlled trial on BSE before advocating its use as a screening device.

4. Kilbourne and colleagues (1983) investigated an epidemic in Spain involving multiple organ systems. Patients presented with cough, dyspnea, pleuritic chest pain, headache, fever, and bilateral pulmonary infiltrates. Although an infectious agent was first suspected, a strong association with cooking oil sold as olive oil but containing a high proportion of rapeseed oil was detected. Epidemiologic studies found that virtually all patients had ingested such oil but that unaffected persons had rarely done so.

5. Knutson and associates (1981) treated wound, burn, and ulcer patients using granulated sugar combined with povidone-iodine (PI). The study was undertaken from January 1976 to August 1980, during which time, 759 patients were treated. Of these, 154 were treated with the standard therapy and the remaining 605 were treated with sugar and PI. Uniformity in treatment and

judgment regarding the healing process were enhanced by using three physician-investigators to oversee the process and by documenting wound healing with 35-mm transparencies. The investigators reported that a much lower percentage of patients treated with the sugar and PI mixture required skin grafts than those given the standard treatment; the therapy was painless, and changing the burn dressings was facilitated.

6. Colditz and colleagues (1987) reported on the relationship between menopause and the risk of coronary heart disease in women. Subjects in the study were selected from the Nurses' Health Study originally completed in 1976; the study included 120,000 married female registered nurses, aged 30–55. Colditz and his colleagues identified 116,000 of these women who were premenopausal or who had a known type of menopause and did not have a diagnosis of coronary heart disease at the beginning of the study. The investigators were interested in determining whether the occurrence of menopause alters the risk of coronary heart disease—specifically, whether the influence of menopausal status is altered by the use of postmenopausal estrogen. The original survey provided information on the subjects' age, parental history of myocardial infarction, smoking status, height, weight, use of oral contraceptives or postmenopausal hormones, and history of myocardial infarction or angina pectoris, diabetes, hypertension, or high serum cholesterol levels. Follow-up surveys were done in 1978, 1980, and 1982, and the data were 95.4% complete.

7. Bartle and coworkers (1986) designed a study to examine the association between nonsteroidal antiinflammatory drug use and acute nonvariceal bleeding in the upper gastrointestinal tract. The association between consumption of acetylsalicylic acid and upper gastrointestinal bleeding is well established; however, no information was available on nonacetylsalicylic acid nonsteroidal antiinflammatory drugs. The medical records were reviewed to obtain medication histories of 57 consecutive patients with nonvariceal acute upper gastrointestinal tract hemorrhage presenting at a medical center to compare them with 123 sex-matched and age-matched controls. The investigators found that a larger proportion of patients than of controls had taken nonsteroidal antiinflammatory drugs.

8. Kalman and Laskin (1986) presented information on immunocompetent patients who had been referred to a general hospital with a diagnosis of herpes zoster infection. The investigators wanted to determine the percentage of zosteriform rashes clinically diagnosed as herpes zoster but actually caused by herpes simplex virus. They concluded that physicians should distin-

guish between infections caused by herpes zoster and herpes simplex virus because of the advent of antiviral drugs and the proper use of epidemiologic isolation procedures.

9. Einarsson and colleagues (1985) were interested in learning more about the relationship between bile supersaturation with cholesterol and age. It is known that patients with cholesterol gallstones have higher saturation levels of cholesterol than control populations without gallstones, but it is not known whether saturation levels increase as part of the aging process.

10. **Group Exercise.** The abuse of phenacetin, a common ingredient of analgesic drugs, can lead to kidney disease. There is also evidence that use of salicylate provides protection against cardiovascular disease. How would you design a study to examine the effects of these two drugs on mortality due to different causes and on cardiovascular morbidity?

3

Summarizing Data & Presenting Data in Tables & Graphs

PRESENTING PROBLEMS

Presenting Problem 1. Functional assessment of the autoimmune nervous system is often used to diagnose neuropathic disorders associated with diabetes mellitus and other diseases. Two noninvasive tests used in the assessment of suspected cardiovascular autonomic dysfunction include the measurement of heart rate variation to deep breathing (VAR) and the calculation of the Valsalva ratio (VAL).

Although measurement of VAR and VAL is reliable, or reproducible, normative values have been determined only for small groups of patients. Gelber and colleagues (1997) wanted to establish normative values for VAR and VAL based on data from a large group of normal subjects collected at multiple sites. They also evaluated the effects of various confounding variables, including gender, age, height, weight, blood pressure, and body mass index.

These investigators studied 611 normal healthy subjects from 63 centers over a 15-year period. Heart rate variation measurements were available for 580 patients, and Valsalva ratios were available for 425 patients. The authors wanted to present normal ranges for the two measures for subjects in different age ranges. A random sample of 18 heart rate variation measures is given in Section 3.3.2.a, and the entire data set is in a folder on the CD-ROM entitled "Gelber."

Presenting Problem 2. The aging of the babyboomers is leading to important demographic changes in the population, with significant implications for health care planners. Over the next 30 years in the United States, the proportion of people over the age of 75 years is expected to increase greatly. With the aging of the population, functional decline resulting in disability and morbidity is a major challenge to health care systems.

Hébert and coworkers (1997) designed a study to measure disability and functional changes in a community-dwelling population age 75 years and older over a 2-year period. The study population consisted of 655 residents of a community in Quebec, Canada. Each was interviewed at home by a nurse. The Functional Autonomy Measurement System (SMAF), a 29-item rating scale measuring functional disability in five areas, was administered together with a questionnaire measuring health, cognitive function, and depression. Each individual was interviewed again 1 and 2 years later by the same nurse. The SMAF scale rates each item on a 4-point scale, where 0 is independent and 3 is dependent. Functional decline was defined by an increase of 5 points or more on the questionnaire, improvement as a decrease of 5 points or more, and stability as a change between −4 and +4 points. (The final analysis included 572 subjects, 504 of whom completed both follow-up interviews and 68 of whom died during the study.)

The authors wanted to summarize the data and estimate declines in functional status. They also wanted to examine the relationship between changes in scores over the two 1-year periods. Data are given in Section 3.4 and on the CD-ROM in a folder entitled "Hébert."

Presenting Problem 3. Colorectal cancer is second only to lung cancer as a cause of cancer death in the United States. Approximately 145,000 new cases of colorectal cancer develop in the United States each year. Currently, most colorectal cancers are believed to arise from adenomatous polyps, although only about 1% of these polyps ever become malignant. Environmental factors, particularly diet, appear to be important in the development of this cancer. The Nurses' Health Study demonstrated a positive correlation between a high intake of animal fat and the development of colon cancer.

Five-year survival rates range from greater than 90% in early disease when infiltration of the cancer is no deeper than the submucosa to less than 5% when distant metastases are evident. Overall mortality is about 30 per 100,000 for men and 20 per 100,000 for women. For metastatic disease (stage D), treatment options are palliative surgery and chemotherapy. Patients rarely have a complete response to chemotherapy. For patients with disease extending through the colon wall or with lymph node involvement (stages B2 and C by modified Dukes' classification), adjutant chemotherapy and radiation therapy improve the chances of survival.

The magnitude of the problem has led the American Cancer Society to recommend that asymptomatic persons who have no high-risk factors for colorectal cancer undergo annual digital rectal examination beginning at age 40, annual hemoccult testing of the stool at age 50, and sigmoidoscopy every 3–5 years beginning at age 50. To evaluate progress in the fight against cancer and help determine the need for screening programs, several states and regional cancer centers have developed computerized registries of information about patients who are diagnosed as having cancer. Many of these data sets are available on agency and center Web sites. The data set containing information on all the patients diagnosed with cancer in Illinois from 1991 through 1995 was downloaded from the Illinois Department of Public Health Web site. A random sample of 16,383 patients diagnosed with colorectal cancer during these 5 years is in the folder named "Cancer" on the CD-ROM. In this chapter, we show how information on the age of the patients at the time of diagnosis of colorectal cancer can be displayed in tables and graphs. The results are shown in Section 3.4.2.

Presenting Problem 4. Low doses of aspirin can inhibit cyclooxygenase-dependent platelet enzymes, thereby restricting platelet aggregation. Randomized, controlled trials have shown that aspirin reduces the risk of subsequent MI and ischemic stroke in patients with preexisting cardiovascular disease. Other data also suggest that aspirin reduces the risk of MI in healthy people. The Physicians' Health Study (1989) was undertaken to learn whether aspirin in low doses (325 mg every other day) reduces the mortality from cardiovascular disease. The participants in this clinical trial were 22,071 healthy male physicians who were randomly assigned to receive aspirin or placebo and were evaluated over an average period of 60 months.

Fewer physicians in the aspirin group experienced an MI during the course of the study than did physicians in the group receiving the placebo. Details are given in Section 3.5.1. The investigators wanted to determine the risk for MI in the aspirin group compared with the placebo group.

The use of low-dose aspirin continues to be studied. A meta-analysis of randomized, controlled clinical trials on aspirin usage reported an increased risk of hemorrhagic stroke (He et al, 1998). The authors concluded, however, that the overall benefit of aspirin use in preventing MI and ischemic stroke may outweigh the adverse effects.

Presenting Problem 5. Factor VIII is one of the procoagulants of the intrinsic pathway of coagulation. Hemophilia A, a disease affecting about 1 in 10,000 males, is a hereditary hemorrhagic disorder characterized by deficient or defective factor VIII. Acquired hemophilia is a much rarer hemorrhagic disorder affecting 1 person per million each year and characterized by spontaneous development of an autoantibody directed against factor VIII. Patients often present with ecchymosis, hematomas, hematuria, or compressive neuropathy. The hemorrhagic complications are fatal in 14–22% of patients. Underlying diseases, including autoimmune diseases and malignancies, are often associated with acquired hemophilia.

Optimal treatment is not yet established and because the disease is so rare no randomized, controlled trials of treatment have been undertaken. A retrospective study of 34 patients with acquired hemophilia due to factor VIII inhibitors was conducted along with an extensive literature review to clarify the clinical characteristics of this disease and plan a prospective study of optimal treatment (Bossi et al, 1998). Information from the study is given in Section 3.6. The investigators want to summarize data on some risk factors for men and women separately.

Presenting Problem 6. Premature birth, especially after fewer than 32 weeks of gestation, is associated with a high incidence of respiratory distress syndrome and a form of chronic lung disease known as bronchopulmonary dysplasia. Lung disease is the principal cause of morbidity and mortality in premature infants.

Thyroid hormones stimulate fetal lung development in animals. Little thyroid hormone is transferred from mother to fetus, but thyrotropin-releasing hormone (TRH) given to the mother increases fetal serum concentrations of thyroid hormone. Several studies have shown that the antenatal administration of TRH reduces the incidence and severity of respiratory distress syndrome, chronic lung disease, and death in these high-risk infants. Two other studies showed no benefit from treatment with TRH.

Ballard and her coinvestigators (1998) wanted to reassess the efficacy and safety of antenatal administration of TRH in improving pulmonary outcome in preterm infants. Most of the earlier studies were relatively small, and one had not been blinded. Also, changes in neonatal care implemented in the past decade, particularly the use of surfactant, improved the chances of survival of premature infants.

The study enrolled 996 women in active labor with gestations of at least 24 but fewer than 30 weeks into a randomized, double-blind, placebo-controlled trial of antenatal thyrotropin-releasing hormone. The women receiving active treatment were given four doses of 400 μg of TRH intravenously at 8-h intervals. Those receiving placebo were given normal saline. Both groups received glucocorticoids, and surfactant was given to the infants when clinically indicated. There were 1134 live births (844 single and 290 multiple) and 11 stillbirths.

Infants born at 32 or fewer weeks gestation constituted the group at risk for lung disease; those born at 33 weeks or later were not at risk for lung disease. The primary outcome was infant death on or before the 28th day after delivery or chronic lung disease, defined as the need for oxygen therapy for 21 of the first 28 days of life. Another outcome of the study was the development of respiratory stress syndrome, defined as the need for oxygen and either the need for assisted ventilation for more than 48 h after birth or radiologic findings consistent with respiratory distress syndrome. The authors wanted to find the risk of developing these outcomes in the TRH group compared with the placebo group. Selected results from the study are given in Section 3.7.4.d.

3.1 PURPOSE OF THE CHAPTER

The purpose of this chapter is to introduce the different kinds of data collected in medical research and to demonstrate how to organize and present summaries of them. Regardless of the particular research being done, investigators collect observations and generally want to transform them into tables or graphs or to present summary numbers, such as percentages or means. From a statistical perspective, it does not matter whether the observations are made on people, animals, inanimate objects, or events. What matters is the kind of observations made and the scale on which they are measured. These features determine the statistics used to summarize the data, called **descriptive statistics,** and the types of tables or graphs that best display and communicate the observations.

This chapter discusses measurement scales and how observations are displayed in various kinds of tables and graphs. We present **measures of central tendency** (statistics that describe the location of the center of a distribution of numerical and ordinal measurements) and **measures of dispersion** (statistics that describe the spread of numerical data). **Rates** and **proportions** (the statistics used to summarize nominal data) are also discussed, and some common **vital statistics** rates are defined. Statistics and graphs that describe or illustrate a relationship between two measurements on the same group of subjects are detailed.

Two risk ratios, the **relative risk (RR)** and the **odds ratio (OR)**, are very important measures of the risk in one population compared with that in another. The measures are used to describe the risk of a disease occurring in a population exposed to a known risk factor versus that in a population not exposed to the risk factor. For instance, parents of children in daycare facilities have been reported to be at higher risk of colds and viruses than parents without children in daycare facilities. We will illustrate the use of risk ratios as a measure of the effectiveness of a treatment.

We also define a number of concepts that are becoming increasingly important in the practice of **evidence-based medicine.** Learning these concepts will help you determine, for example, the number of patients that need to be treated with a proposed therapy in order to prevent disease in or to cure one patient.

We use the data from the presenting problems to illustrate the steps involved in calculating the statistics, because we believe that seeing the steps helps most people understand procedures. As we emphasize throughout this book, however, we expect that most people will use a computer to analyze data. In fact, this and following chapters contain numerous illustrations from some commonly used statistical computer programs.

Descriptive statistics and tables are used very frequently in medical journals. Many articles in current journals feature graphs, tables, and simple descriptive statistics. The purpose of this chapter is to help you recognize when these methods are being used and interpreted in a proper manner and to enhance your ability to use them.

3.2 SCALES OF MEASUREMENT

The scale for measuring a characteristic has implications for the way information is displayed and summarized. As we will see in later chapters, the **scale of measurement**—the precision with which a characteristic is measured—also determines the statistical methods for analyzing the data. The measurement scale of a characteristic is therefore an important consideration. The three scales of measurement that occur most often in medicine are nominal, ordinal, and numerical.

3.2.1 Nominal Scales

Nominal scales are used for the simplest level of measurement when data values fit into categories. For example, in Presenting Problem 6 Ballard and colleagues (1998) use the following nominal characteristic to describe the outcome in infants being treated with antenatal TRH: the development of respiratory distress syndrome. (See Section 3.7.4.d.) In this example, the observations are **dichotomous,** or **binary,** that is, the outcome can take on only one of two values: yes or no. Although we talk about nominal data as being on the measurement scale, we do not actually measure nominal data; instead, we count the number of observations with or without the attribute of interest.

Many classifications in medical research are evaluated on a nominal scale. Outcomes of a medical treatment or surgical procedure, as well as the presence of possible risk or exposure factors, are often described as either occurring or not occurring. Outcomes may also be described with more than two categories, such as the classification of anemias as microcytic (including iron deficiency), macrocytic or megaloblastic (including vitamin B_{12} deficiency), and normocytic (often associated with chronic disease).

Data evaluated on a nominal scale are sometimes called **qualitative observations,** because they describe a quality of the person or thing studied, and **categorical observations,** because the values fit into categories. Nominal or qualitative data are generally described in terms of **percentages** or **proportions.** For example, in the study of patients with acquired hemophilia (Bossi et al, 1998), 38% of the patients (13 out of 34) developed hematuria. **Contingency tables** and **bar charts** are most often used to display this type of information and are presented in Section 3.6.

3.2.2 Ordinal Scales

When an inherent order occurs among the categories, the observations are said to be measured on an **ordinal scale.** Observations are still classified, as with nominal scales, but some observations have *more* or are *greater than* other observations. Clinicians often use ordinal scales to determine a patient's amount of risk or the appropriate type of therapy. Tumors, for example, are staged according to their degree of development. The international classification for staging of carcinoma of the cervix is an ordinal scale from 0 to 4, in which stage 0 represents carcinoma in situ and stage 4 represents carcinoma extending beyond the pelvis or involving the mucosa of the bladder and rectum. The inherent order in this ordinal scale is, of course, that the prognosis for stage 4 is worse than that for stage 0.

Classifications based on the extent of disease are sometimes related to a patient's activity level. For example, rheumatoid arthritis is classified, according to the severity of disease, into four classes ranging from normal activity (class 1) to wheelchair-bound (class 4). In Presenting Problem 2 Hébert and coinvestigators (1997) studied the functional activity of elderly people who live in a community. They measured functional activity using the Functional Autonomy Measurement System developed by the World Health Organization. It contains 29 questions that are answered on a scale with 0 = independent, 1 = needs supervision, 2 = needs help, or 3 = dependent.

An important characteristic of ordinal scales is that, although order exists among categories, the difference between two adjacent categories is not the same throughout the scale. To illustrate, consider Apgar scores, which describe the maturity of newborn infants on a scale of 0 to 10, with lower scores indicating depression of cardiorespiratory and neurologic functioning and higher scores indicating good cardiorespiratory and neurologic functioning. The difference between scores of 8 and 9 is probably not of the same clinical magnitude as the difference between scores of 0 and 1.

Some scales consist of scores for multiple factors that are then added to get an overall index. For example, an index frequently used to estimate the cardiac risk in noncardiac surgical procedures was developed by Goldman and his colleagues (1977, 1995). This index assigns points to a variety of risk factors, such as age over 70 years, history of an MI in the past 6 months, specific electrocardiogram abnormalities,

and general physical status. The points are added to get an overall score on the Goldman index from 0 to 53, which is used to indicate the risk of complications or death for different score levels.

Brief mention should be made of a special type of ordered scale called a **rank-order scale,** in which observations are ranked from highest to lowest (or vice versa). For example, health providers could direct their education efforts aimed at the obstetric patient based on ranking the causes of low birthweight in infants, such as malnutrition, drug abuse, and inadequate prenatal care, from most common to least common. Also, the duration of surgical procedures might be converted to a rank scale to obtain one measure of the difficulty of the procedure. In this example, the difference in lengths of time between the first and second procedures is not necessarily the same as that between any two other procedures.

As with nominal scales, percentages and proportions are often used with ordinal scales. The entire set of data measured on an ordinal scale is sometimes summarized by the **median** value, and we will describe how to find the median and what it means. The same types of tables and graphs used to display nominal data may also be used with ordinal data.

3.2.3 Numerical Scales

Observations for which the differences between numbers have meaning on a numerical scale are sometimes called **quantitative observations** because they measure the quantity of something. There are two types of numerical scales: interval,[1] or continuous, scales and discrete scales. A **continuous scale** has values on a continuum (eg, age); a **discrete scale** has values equal to integers (eg, number of fractures).

If the data need not be very precise, continuous data may be reported to the closest integer. Theoretically, however, more precise measurement is possible. For example, Gelber and his colleagues in Presenting Problem 1 examine the heart rate variation to deep breathing in a group of normal subjects (1997). Heart rate variation occurs on a continuum and can be any value between 2.1 and 150.9, based on the Gelber data. In other words, heart rate variation can be specified as precisely as necessary, although the usefulness of using extremely precise data has a practical limit. Age is a continuous measure, and age recorded to the nearest year will generally suffice in studies of adults; however, for young children, age to the nearest month may be preferable. In infants, age

---

[1]Some statisticians differentiate interval scales (with an arbitrary zero point) from ratio scales (with an absolute zero point); examples are temperature on a Celsius scale (interval) and temperature on a Kelvin scale (ratio). Little difference exists, however, in how measures on these two scales are treated statistically, so we call them both simply numerical.

to the nearest hour or even minute may be appropriate, depending on the purpose of the study. Other examples of continuous data include height, weight, length of time of survival, range of joint motion, as well as many laboratory values, such as serum glucose, sodium, potassium, or uric acid levels.

When a numerical observation can take on only integer values, the scale of measurement is discrete. For example, counts of things—number of pregnancies, number of previous operations, number of risk factors—are discrete measures.

In the study by Gelber and colleagues (1997), several subject characteristics were evaluated, including heart rate variation to deep breathing, subject age, and subject gender. The first two characteristics are measured on a continuous numerical scale because they can take on any individual value in the possible range of values. Gender of the subject has a nominal scale with only two values. In the study by Ballard and coworkers (1998), the number of infants who developed respiratory distress syndrome is an example of a discrete numerical scale.

Characteristics measured on a numerical scale are frequently displayed in a variety of tables and graphs. Means and standard deviations are generally used to summarize the values of numerical measures. We next examine ways to summarize and display numerical data and then return to the subject of ordinal and nominal data.

3.3 SUMMARIZING NUMERICAL DATA WITH NUMBERS

When an investigator collects many observations, such as the heart rate variation to deep breathing in normal subjects in Presenting Problem 1, indexes or summary numbers can communicate information about the data.

3.3.1 Measures of the Middle

One of the most useful summary numbers is an index of the center of a distribution of observations, which tells us the middle or average value. The three measures of central tendency used frequently in medicine and epidemiology are the mean, the median, and, to a lesser extent, the mode. All three are used for numerical data, and the median and the mode can be used for ordinal data as well.

3.3.2 Calculating Measures of Central Tendency

3.3.2.a The Mean: Although several means may be mathematically calculated, the arithmetic, or simple, mean is used most frequently in statistics and is the one generally referred to by the term "mean." The **mean** is the arithmetic average of the observations. It is symbolized by $\overline{X}$ (called X-bar) and is calculated as follows:

1. Add the observations to obtain their sum.
2. Divide the sum by the number of observations.

The formula for the mean is written $\Sigma X/n$, where Σ (Greek letter sigma) means to add, X represents the individual observations, and n is the number of observations.

Table 3–1 gives data for 18 subjects in a study of the cardiovascular autonomic nervous system (Gelber et al, 1997). We randomly selected these values from the entire data set to simplify our illustrations. (We will learn about random sampling in Chapter 4.) The mean heart rate variation to deep breathing value for these 18 subjects is

$$\overline{X} = \frac{\Sigma X}{n} = \frac{19.2 + 51.9 + 33.1 + \cdots + 43.6}{18}$$

$$= \frac{877.8}{18} = 48.8$$

The mean is used when the numbers can be added (ie, when the characteristics are measured on a numerical scale); it should not be used with ordinal data because of the arbitrary nature of an ordinal scale. The mean is sensitive to extreme values in a set of observations, especially when the sample size is fairly small. For example, the values of 86.7 and 85.7 for subjects 4 and 15 are relatively high compared with the values for other subjects in this group. If these values were not present, the mean would be 44.1 instead of 48.8.

If the original observations are not available, the mean can be estimated from a frequency table. A **weighted average** is formed by multiplying each

Table 3–1. Heart rate variation to deep breathing in a random sample of 18 patients.

Subject ID	Variation in Heart Rate
1	19.2
2	51.9
3	33.1
4	86.7
5	29.1
6	45.3
7	14.4
8	67.1
9	64.8
10	15.9
11	75.8
12	42.6
13	74.2
14	41.4
15	85.7
16	22.1
17	64.9
18	43.6

Source: Data, used with permission of the author and publisher, from Gelber DA, Pfeifer M, Dawson B, Schumer M: Cardiovascular autonomic nervous system tests: Determination of normative values and effect of confounding variables. *J Auton Nerv Syst* 1997;**62**:40–44. Table produced with NCSS; used with permission.

data value by the number of observations that have that value, adding the products, and dividing the sum by the number of observations. We have formed a frequency table of heart rate variation data in Table 3–2, and we can use it to estimate the mean heart rate variation for all subjects in the study who had this measurement recorded. The weighted-average estimate of the mean, using the number of subjects and the midpoints in each interval, is

$$\frac{(11 \times 46) + (25 \times 70) + \cdots + (85 \times 29) + (100 \times 33)}{580}$$
$$= \frac{28,471}{580} = 49.09$$

Note that we used 100 as the midpoint of the category ">90"; this was a somewhat arbitrary choice based on clinical knowledge. Another selection, such as 95 or 110, could also be justified. Based on this calculation, the mean heart rate variation for the 580 subjects is 49.09. The value of the mean calculated from a frequency table is not always the same as the value obtained with raw numbers. In fact, the mean heart rate variation for these 580 subjects calculated from the raw numbers is 49.7, fairly close to the one calculated from the frequency table in this example. Investigators who calculate the mean for presentation in a paper or talk have the original observations, of course, and should use the exact formula. The formula for use with a frequency table is helpful when we as readers of an article do not have access to the raw data but want an estimate of the mean.

3.3.2.b The Median: The **median** is the middle observation, that is, the point at which half the observations are smaller and half are larger. The median is sometimes symbolized by *M* or *Md*, but it has no conventional symbol. The procedure for calculating the median is as follows:

1. Arrange the observations from smallest to largest (or vice versa).

2. Count in to find the middle value. The median is the middle value for an odd number of observations; it is defined as the mean of the two middle values for an *even* number of observations.

For example, in rank order (from lowest to highest), the heart rate variation to deep breathing observations in Table 3–1 are as follows:

14.4, 15.9, 19.2, 22.1, 29.1, 33.1, 41.4, 42.6, 43.6, 45.3, 51.9, 64.8, 64.9, 67.1, 74.2, 75.8, 85.7, 86.7

For 18 observations, the median is the mean of the ninth and tenth values (43.6 and 45.3), or 44.45. The median tells us that half the heart rate variation values in this group of subjects are less than 44.45 and half are greater than 44.45. We will learn later in this chapter that the median is easy to determine from a **stem-and-leaf plot** of the observations.

The median is less sensitive to extreme values than is the mean. For example, if the two largest observations, 85.7 and 86.7, were excluded from the sample, the median would be the average of 42.6 and 43.6, or 43.1, which is not very different from 44.45. Another useful feature of the median is that it can be used with ordinal observations because its calculation does not use actual values of the observations.

The median, like the mean, may also be estimated from a frequency table. Because this procedure is rarely needed and the formula is complicated, we will not describe it.

3.3.2.c The Mode: The **mode** is the value that occurs most frequently. It is commonly used for a large number of observations when the researcher wants to designate the value that occurs most often. No single observation occurs most frequently among the heart rate data in Table 3–1. When a set of data has two modes, it is called *bimodal*. For frequency tables or a small number of observations, the mode is sometimes estimated by the **modal class,** which is the interval having the largest number of observa-

Table 3–2. Heart rate variation to deep breathing in 10-point intervals.

Interval	Frequency	Valid Percent	Cumulative Percent
2–20	46	7.9	7.9
21–30	70	12.1	20.0
31–40	108	18.6	38.6
41–50	106	18.3	56.9
51–60	74	12.8	69.7
61–70	72	12.4	82.1
71–80	42	7.2	89.3
81–90	29	5.0	94.3
>90	33	5.7	100.0
Total	580	100.0	

Source: Data, used with permission of the author and publisher, from Gelber DA, Pfeifer M, Dawson B, Schumer M: Cardiovascular autonomic nervous system tests: Determination of normative values and effect of confounding variables. *J Auton Nerv Syst* 1997;**62**:40–44. Table produced with SPSS; used with permission.

tions. For the heart rate variation data in Table 3–2, the modal class is 31–40 because this category has the largest number of subjects, 108.

3.3.2.d The Geometric Mean: Another measure of central tendency is the geometric mean; however, it is not used as often as the arithmetic mean or the median. The **geometric mean,** sometimes symbolized as *GM* or *G,* is defined as the *n*th root of the product of the *n* observations. In symbolic form, for *n* observations $X_1, X_2, X_3, \ldots, X_n$, the geometric mean is

$$GM = \sqrt[n]{(X_1)(X_2)(X_3) \cdots (X_n)}$$

The geometric mean is generally used with data measured on a logarithmic scale, such as titers of antineutrophil immunoglobulin G. Note that if we take the logarithm of both sides of the preceding equation, we obtain

$$\log GM = \sum \frac{\log X}{n}$$

That is, the logarithm of the geometric mean is equal to the mean of the logarithms of the observations.

Use the CD-ROM and find the mean, median, and mode for heart rate variation to deep breathing for all of the subjects in the study by Gelber and colleagues (1997). Repeat for men and for women separately. Do you think Gelber was justified in combining the samples, based on the measures of central tendency?

3.3.2.e Using Measures of Central Tendency: An investigator may naturally ask which measure of central tendency is best with a particular set of observations. Two factors are important in making this decision: the scale of measurement (ordinal or numerical) and the shape of the distribution of observations. Although distributions are discussed in more detail in Chapter 4, we can consider here the notion of whether a distribution is symmetric about the mean or is skewed to the left or the right of the mean. This information helps us decide which measure of central tendency is best.

If outlying observations occur in only one direction—either a few small values or a few large ones—the distribution is said to be a **skewed distribution.** If the outlying values are small, the distribution is skewed to the left, or negatively skewed; if the outlying values are large, the distribution is skewed to the right, or positively skewed. A **symmetric distribution** has the same shape on both sides of the mean. Figure 3–1 gives examples of negatively skewed, positively skewed, and symmetric distributions.

The following points help a reader know the shape of a distribution without actually seeing it.

1. If the mean and the median are equal, the distri-

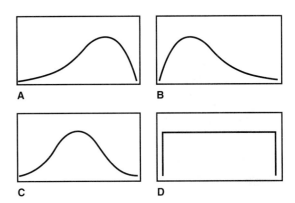

Figure 3–1. Shapes of common distributions of observations. **A:** Negatively skewed. **B:** Positively skewed. **C** and **D:** Symmetric.

bution of observations is generally symmetric, as in Figures 3–1C and 3–1D.

2. If the mean is larger than the median, the distribution is skewed to the right, as in Figure 3–1B.

3. If the mean is smaller than the median, the distribution is skewed to the left, as in Figure 3–1A.

In a study of the relationship between indebtedness and choice of medical specialty in medical students, Kassebaum and Szenas (1992) reported the median level of debt for graduating students. The investigators stated that the median rather than the mean was appropriate because only a relatively small number of students had extremely high debts, which caused the mean to be an overestimate. The following guidelines help an investigator to decide which measure of central tendency is best with a given set of data.

1. The mean is used for numerical data and for symmetric (not skewed) distributions.

2. The median is used for ordinal data or for numerical data if the distribution is skewed.

3. The mode is used primarily for bimodal distributions.

4. The geometric mean is used primarily for observations measured on a logarithmic scale.

3.3.3 Measures of Spread

Suppose all you know about the 18 randomly selected subjects in Presenting Problem 1 is that the mean heart rate variation to deep breathing is 48.8. The mean is useful information, but to have a better idea of the distribution of heart rate values in these subjects, you also need to know something about the spread, or the variation, of the observations. Several statistics are used to describe the dispersion of data: range, standard deviation, coefficient of variation, percentile rank, and interquartile range. All are described in the following sections.

3.3.4 Calculating Measures of Spread

3.3.4.a The Range: The **range** is the difference between the largest and the smallest observation. It is easy to determine once the data have been arranged in rank order. For example, the lowest heart rate value among the 18 subjects is 14.4, and the highest is 86.7; thus, the range is 86.7 minus 14.4, or 72.3. Many authors give minimum and maximum values instead of the range, and in some ways these values are more useful. The precise range cannot always be determined from data presented in a frequency table, but a close estimate is possible.

3.3.4.b The Standard Deviation: The standard deviation is the most commonly used measure of dispersion with medical and health data. Although its meaning and computation are somewhat complex, it is definitely worth knowing about. The standard deviation is used to describe how observations cluster around the mean, and it is very important in statistical inference. Undoubtedly, most of you will use a computer to determine the standard deviation, but we present the steps involved in its calculation because it will allow you a greater understanding of the meaning of this statistic.

The **standard deviation** is a measure of the spread of data about their mean. Before we present the formula, however, let us briefly discuss an approach that may at first seem ideal for calculating an index of deviation. If we need to measure how observations are dispersed about the mean, an average, or mean, deviation seems like a good idea. For example, we can compute the deviation of each observation from the mean, add these deviations, and divide the sum by n to form an analogy to the mean itself. In symbols, the mean deviation is

$$\frac{\Sigma\,(X - \overline{X})}{n}$$

The problem with this index is that the sum of deviations of observations from their mean is always zero, and the value of the index will be zero in all cases (see Exercise 1). This problem can be solved in two ways: by summing the absolute values of the deviations or by squaring the deviations before they are added. The **absolute value** of a number ignores the sign of the number and is denoted by vertical bars on each side of the number. For example, the absolute value of 5, |5|, is 5, and the absolute value of –5, |–5|, is also 5. For the absolute value approach, the mean deviation is

$$\frac{\Sigma\,|X - \overline{X}|}{n}$$

Although there is nothing wrong with this approach conceptually, it lacks some important statistical prop-erties, and so is not used. The second approach of squaring deviations is therefore used instead—with two slight modifications: $n - 1$ replaces n in the denominator, and the square root is taken to express the value in the original scale of measurement of the observations. The standard deviation can be symbolized as *SD, sd,* or simply s (in this text we use *SD*), and its formula is then

$$SD = \sqrt{\frac{\Sigma(X - \overline{X})^2}{n - 1}}$$

The name of the statistic before the square root is taken is the **variance,** but the standard deviation is the statistic of primary interest.

The reason for using $n - 1$ instead of n in the standard deviation is complicated. We simply mention that $n - 1$ in the denominator produces a more accurate estimate of the true population standard deviation and has desirable mathematical properties for statistical inferences. A more precise explanation involves restrictions imposed on the data by the definition of standard deviation; that is, the quantities squared and then summed are deviations from the mean of the data. If there are n observations, there are also n deviations from the mean. However, because the sum of the deviations equals zero, once $n - 1$ of the deviations are specified, the last deviation is already determined as the value that causes the sum of the deviations to be zero (see Exercise 4). Hence, the denominator uses the number of quantities that are free to vary, called the **degrees of freedom.**[2]

The preceding formula for standard deviation, called the **definitional formula,** is not usually presented in introductory textbooks as the best one for calculating that value. Another formula, the **computational formula,** is generally used instead. Assuming that most of you will not actually need to compute a standard deviation very often, the illustrations in this text use the more meaningful but computationally less efficient definitional formula for calculations. For the curious, the computational formula is given in Exercise 7.

Now let us try a calculation. The observations on heart rate variation for the 18 subjects (see Table 3–1) are repeated in Table 3–3, which also shows the computations needed. The steps follow:

1. Let X be the change in heart rate variation for each subject, and find the mean change: the mean is 48.77, as we calculated earlier. (The calculations are carried to two places to minimize round-off error when the square root is taken.)

2. Subtract the mean, 48.77, from each observation to form the deviations X – mean (see column 3 in Table 3–3).

---

[2]We cover the concept of degrees of freedom in succeeding chapters on statistical tests.

Table 3–3. Calculations for standard deviation of heart rate variation to deep breathing in a random sample of 18 patients.

Patient	X	X – X̄	(X – X̄)²
1	19.20	–29.57	874.19
2	51.90	3.13	9.82
3	33.10	–15.67	245.44
4	86.70	37.93	1438.94
5	29.10	–19.67	386.78
6	45.30	–3.47	12.02
7	14.40	–34.37	1181.07
8	67.10	18.33	336.11
9	64.80	16.03	257.07
10	15.90	–32.87	1080.22
11	75.80	27.03	730.80
12	42.60	–6.17	38.03
13	74.20	25.43	646.85
14	41.40	–7.37	54.27
15	85.70	36.93	1364.07
16	22.10	–26.67	711.11
17	64.90	16.13	260.28
18	43.60	–5.17	26.69
Sum	877.80		9653.76
Mean	48.77		

Source: Data, used with permission of the author and publisher, from Gelber DA, Pfeifer M, Dawson B, Schumer M: Cardiovascular autonomic nervous system tests: Determination of normative values and effect of confounding variables. *J Auton Nerv Syst* 1997;**62**:40–44. Table produced with NCSS; used with permission.

3. Square each deviation to form $(X - \text{mean})^2$.

4. Add the squared deviations to obtain the sum.

5. Divide the result in step 4 by $n - 1$; we get 567.87. This value is the variance.

6. Take the square root of the answer in step 5; we get 23.83. This value is the standard deviation

The standard deviation of the heart rate variation in breathing is 23.83. But note the relatively large squared deviations for 86.7 and 85.7 for subjects 4 and 15 in Table 3–3. These two observations contribute substantially to the variation in the data. The standard deviation of the remaining 16 subjects (after eliminating subjects 4 and 15) is smaller, 20.82, demonstrating the effect that outlying observations can have on the value of the standard deviation. The effect would be even greater if one of the values was even larger, such as 150.

The standard deviation, like the mean, requires numerical data. Also, like the mean, the standard deviation is a very important statistic. First, it is an essential part of many **statistical tests** (which are discussed in detail in later chapters). Second, the standard deviation is very useful in describing the spread of the observations about the mean value. The following two rules of thumb are important when using the standard deviation follow.

1. Regardless of how the observations are distributed, at least 75% of the values *always* lie between

these two numbers: the *mean minus 2 standard deviations* and the *mean plus 2 standard deviations*. In the heart rate variation example, the mean change is 48.8 and the standard deviation is 23.8; therefore, at least 75% of the 18 observations are guaranteed to be between 48.8 – 2(23.8) and 48.8 + 2(23.8), or between 1.2 and 96.4. In this example, all of the 18 observations fall between these limits.

2. If the distribution of observations is **bell-shaped,** then even more can be said about the percentage of observations that lie between the mean and ± 2 standard deviations. For a bell-shaped distribution, approximately:

67% of the observations lie between

$$\bar{X} - 1 \ SD \quad \text{and} \quad \bar{X} + 1 \ SD$$

95% of the observations lie between

$$\bar{X} - 2 \ SD \quad \text{and} \quad \bar{X} + 2 \ SD$$

99.7% of the observations lie between

$$\bar{X} - 3 \ SD \quad \text{and} \quad \bar{X} + 3 \ SD$$

For further discussion on the use of the mean and standard deviation with a bell-shaped distribution, see Chapter 4.

Use the CD-ROM, and find the range and standard deviation for heart rate variation to deep breathing for all of the subjects in the Gelber and colleagues study (1997). Repeat for men and for women separately. Do you think Gelber and colleagues were justified in combining the samples, based on the measures of variability?

3.3.4.c The Coefficient of Variation: The coefficient of variation (*CV*) is a useful measure of *relative* spread in data and is used frequently in the biologic sciences. For example, suppose Gelber and his colleagues (1997) wanted to compare the variability in heart rate variation with the variability in the Valsalva ratio in the subjects in their study. The mean and the standard deviation of heart rate variation in the total sample, are 49.7 and 23.4, respectively; for the Valsalva ratio, they are 1.97 and 0.43, respectively. A comparison of the standard deviations, 23.4 and 0.43, makes no sense because heart rate variation and Valsalva ratio are measured on much different scales. The coefficient of variation adjusts the scales so that a sensible comparison can be made.

The coefficient of variation is defined as the standard deviation divided by the mean times 100%. It produces a measure of relative variation—variation that is relative to the size of the mean. The formula for the **coefficient of variation** is

$$CV = \frac{SD}{\overline{X}}(100\%)$$

From this formula, the *CV* for heart rate variation is (23.4/49.7)(100%) = 47.08%, and the *CV* for Valsalva ratio is (0.43/1.97)(100%) = 21.83%. We can therefore conclude that the relative variation in heart rate is more than twice the variation in Valsalva ratio. A frequent application of the coefficient of variation in the health field is in laboratory testing and quality control procedures.

Use the CD-ROM and find the coefficient of variation for heart rate variation to deep breathing for men and women separately in Gelber and colleagues' study. What is your final conclusion about the appropriateness of combining the men and women to find norms?

3.3.4.d Percentiles: A **percentile** is the percentage of a distribution that is equal to or below a particular number. For example, consider the standard physical growth chart for girls from birth to 36 months old given in Figure 3–2. For girls 21 months of age, the 95th percentile of weight is 12 kg, as noted by the arrow in the chart. This percentile means that among 21-month-old girls, 95% weigh 12 kg or less and only 5% weigh more than 12 kg. The 50th percentile is, of course, the same value as the median; for 21-month-old girls, the median or 50th percentile weight is approximately 10.6 kg.

Percentiles are often used to compare an individual value with a norm. They are extensively used to develop and interpret physical growth charts and measurements of ability and intelligence. They also determine normal ranges of laboratory values; the normal limits of many laboratory values are set by the 2½ and 97½ percentiles, so that the normal limits contain the central 95% of the distribution. This approach was taken by Gelber and colleagues (1997) when they developed norms for mean heart variation to breathing and Valsalva ratio (see Exercise 2).

3.3.4.e Interquartile Range: A measure of variation that makes use of percentiles is the **interquartile range,** defined as the difference between the 25th and 75th percentiles, also called the **first** and **third quartiles,** respectively. The interquartile range contains the central 50% of observations. For example, the interquartile range of weights of girls who are 9 months of age (see Figure 3–2) is the difference between 7.5 kg (the 75th percentile) and 6.5 kg (the 25th percentile); that is, 50% of infant girls weigh between 6.5 and 7.5 kg at 9 months of age.

3.3.4.f Using Different Measures of Dispersion: The following guidelines help investigators decide which measure of dispersion is most appropriate for a given set of data.

1. The standard deviation is used when the mean is used—that is, with symmetric (not skewed) numerical data.

2. Percentiles and the interquartile range are used in two situations:

a. When the median is used (ie, with ordinal data or with skewed numerical data).

b. When the mean is used but the objective is to compare individual observations with a set of norms.

3. The interquartile range is used to describe the central 50% of a distribution, regardless of its shape.

4. The range is used with numerical data when the purpose is to emphasize extreme values.

5. The coefficient of variation is used when the intent is to compare numerical distributions measured on different scales.

3.4 DISPLAYING NUMERICAL DATA IN TABLES & GRAPHS

We all know the saying, "A picture is worth 1000 words," and researchers in the health field certainly make frequent use of graphic and pictorial displays of data. Numerical data may be presented in a variety of ways, and we will use the data from the study by Hébert and colleagues (1997) on functional decline in the elderly (Presenting Problem 2) to illustrate some of the more common methods. The subjects in this study were 75 years of age or older. We use a subset of their data, the 72 patients age 85 years or older who completed the Functional Autonomy Measurement System (SMAF). The total score on the SMAF for these subjects in year 1, year 3, and the differences in score between year 3 and year 1 in are given in Table 3–4.

3.4.1 Stem-and-Leaf Plots

Stem-and-leaf plots are graphs developed in 1977 by Tukey, a statistician interested in meaningful ways to communicate by visual display. They provide a convenient means of tallying the observations and can be used as a direct display of data or as a preliminary step in constructing a frequency table.

The observations in Table 3–4 show that many of the differences in total scores are small, but also that some people have large positive scores, indicating large declines in function. The data are not easy to understand, however, by simply looking at a list of the raw numbers. The first step in organizing data for a stem-and-leaf plot is to decide on the number of subdivisions, called classes or intervals (it should generally be between 6 and 14; more details on this decision are given in Section 3.4.2). Ini-

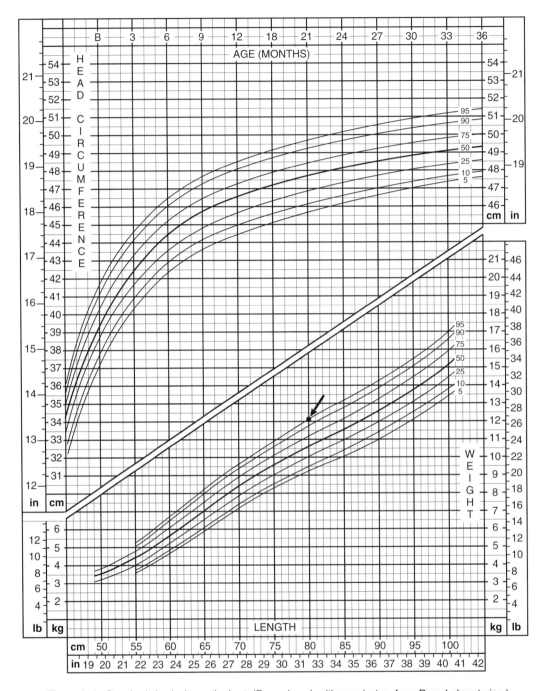

Figure 3–2. Standard physical growth chart. (Reproduced, with permission, from Ross Laboratories.)

tially, we categorize observations by 5s, from –9 to –5, –4 to 0, 1 to 5, 6 to 10, 11 to 15, 16 to 20, and so on.

To form a **stem-and-leaf plot,** draw a vertical line, and place the first digits of each class—called the stem—on the left side of the line, as in Table 3–5. The numbers on the right side of the vertical line rep-

resent the second digit of each observation; they are the leaves. The steps in building a stem-and-leaf plot are as follows:

1. Take the score of the first person, –8, and write the second digit, 8, or leaf, on the *right* side of the vertical line, opposite the first digit, or stem, corresponding to –9 to –5.

Table 3–4. Difference in total score on the Functional Autonomy Measurement System for patients age 85 years or older. Positive differences indicate a decline.

Age	Sex	SMAF at Time 1	SMAF at Time 3	Difference (Time 3 − Time 1)
90	F	28	20	−8
88	F	8	11	3
88	F	6	9	3
90	F	22	18	−4
88	M	6	7	1
86	F	9	9	0
86	M	23	15	−8
85	F	12	40	28
88	F	9	30	21
86	F	5	15	10
95	F	20	16	−4
88	F	3	26	23
87	F	22	24	2
86	F	20	20	0
86	M	0	1	1
93	F	30	34	4
87	F	13	23	10
94	F	47	52	5
86	F	1	20	19
85	F	3	50	47
87	M	4	57	53
89	F	12	14	2
87	F	1	4	3
87	F	13	16	3
85	F	1	1	0
85	F	35	30	−5
88	F	22	19	−3
88	M	1	1	0
86	F	2	17	15
88	M	3	3	0
86	F	21	39	18
85	F	2	2	0
85	M	7	8	1
88	M	8	10	2
85	F	7	5	−2
89	F	11	20	9
87	F	1	0	−1
88	F	12	19	7
87	F	19	56	37
94	F	21	16	−5
86	M	17	26	9
85	F	27	21	−6
85	M	4	2	−2
85	F	9	5	−4
85	M	7	34	27
87	F	38	34	−4
85	F	13	22	9
85	F	4	4	0
85	F	17	27	10
90	F	23	27	4
86	M	12	13	1
88	M	30	29	−1
85	M	27	26	−1
87	F	26	47	21
86	M	44	46	2
85	F	21	23	2
86	M	17	57	40
88	M	10	19	9
85	F	15	22	7
86	F	4	6	2
88	F	10	12	2
88	M	18	22	4

(continued)

Table 3–4. Difference in total score on the Functional Autonomy Measurement System for patients age 85 years or older. Positive differences indicate a decline. (continued)

Age	Sex	SMAF at Time 1	SMAF at Time 3	Difference (Time 3 – Time 1)
87	M	12	20	8
85	M	37	47	10
85	F	17	14	–3
89	F	14	19	5
85	F	11	14	3
87	F	4	6	2
86	F	16	26	10
90	F	5	6	1
85	F	48	51	3
88	M	9	17	8

Source: Data, used with permission of the author and the publisher, from Hébert R, Brayne C, Spiegelhalter D: Incidence of functional decline and improvement in a community-dwelling very elderly population. *Am J Epidemiol* 1997;**145**:935–944.

2. For the second person, write the 3 (leaf) on the right side of the vertical line opposite 1 to 5 (stem).

3. For the third person, write the 3 (leaf) opposite 1 to 5 (stem) next to the previous score of 3.

4. For the fourth person, write the –4 (leaf) opposite –4 to 0 (stem); and so on.

5. When the observation is only one digit, such as for subjects 1 through 7 in Table 3–4, that digit is the leaf.

6. When the observation is two digits, however, such as the score of 28 for subject 8, only the second digit, or 8 in this case, is written.

The leaves for the first ten people are given in Table 3–5. The complete stem-and-leaf plot for the score changes of all the subjects is given in Table 3–6. The plot both provides a tally of observations and shows how the changes in scores are distributed. The choice of class widths of 5 points is reasonable, although we usually prefer to avoid having the many

Table 3–5. Constructing a stem-and-leaf plot of change in total function scores using 5-point categories: Observations for the first 10 subjects.

Stem	Leaves
–9 to –5	8 8
–4 to 0	4 0
+1 to +5	3 3 1
+6 to +10	0
+11 to +15	
+16 to +20	
+21 to +25	1
+26 to +30	8
+31 to +35	
+36 to +40	
+41 to +45	
+46 to +50	
+51 to +55	
+56 to +60	

Source: Data, used with permission of the author and the publisher, from Hébert R, Brayne C, Spiegelhalter D: Incidence of functional decline and improvement in a community-dwelling very elderly population. *Am J Epidemiol* 1997; **145**:935–44.

empty classes at the high end of the scale. It is generally preferred to have equal class widths and to avoid open-ended intervals, such as 30 or higher, although some might choose to combine the higher classes in the final plot.

Usually the leaves are reordered from lowest to highest within each class. A stem-and-leaf plot for these data, again using class widths of 5 years and reordering within each class, is given in Table 3–7. After the reordering, it is easy to locate the median of the distribution by simply counting in from either end. With 72 observations, the middle is halfway between the 36th and 37th observations. A caret (^) has been placed at the median in Table 3–7, and the plus (+) signs denote the 25th and 75th percentile values. For these 72 elderly citizens 85 years of age or older, the median change in functional score is 2.0, indicating that 50% of them declined less than 2.0 points and 50% declined more than 2.0 points. The 25th and 75th percentiles are 0 and 9, respectively, giving an interquartile range of 9 points. From this information we know that half of the score changes fell between 0 and 9 points.

Use the CD-ROM and the routine for generating stem-and-leaf plots using the data on heart rate variation to deep breathing for men and for women separately in the Gelber and colleagues study (1997).

3.4.2 Frequency Tables

Scientific journals often present information in frequency distributions or frequency tables. Tables are more difficult to construct for numerical data than for nominal data because the scale of the observations must first be divided into classes, as in stem-and-leaf plots. The observations in each class are then counted. The steps for constructing a frequency table are as follows:

1. Identify the largest and smallest observations.

2. Subtract the smallest observation from the largest to obtain the **range** of the data.

3. Determine the number of classes. Several rules are available for calculating the number of classes,

Table 3–6. Stem-and-leaf plot of change in total function scores using 5-point categories.

Stem	Leaves
−9 to −5	8 8 5 5 6
−4 to 0	4 0 4 0 0 3 0 0 0 2 1 2 4 4 0 1 1 3
+1 to +5	3 3 1 2 1 4 5 2 3 3 1 2 4 1 2 2 2 2 4 5 3 2 1 3
+6 to +10	0 0 9 7 9 9 0 9 7 8 0 8 0
+11 to +15	5
+16 to +20	9 8
+21 to +25	1 3 1
+26 to +30	8 7
+31 to +35	
+36 to +40	7 0
+41 to +45	7
+46 to +50	
+51 to +55	3
+56 to +60	

Source: Data, used with permission of the author and the publisher, from Hébert R, Brayne C, Spiegelhalter D: Incidence of functional decline and improvement in a community-dwelling very elderly population. *Am J Epidemiol* 1997; **145**:935–944.

but common sense is usually adequate for making this decision. The following guidelines are suggested.

a. Between 6 and 14 classes is generally adequate to provide enough information without being overly detailed.

b. There should be enough classes to demonstrate the shape of the distribution but not so many that minor fluctuations are noticeable.

4. Divide the range of observations by the number of classes to obtain the width of the classes. For some applications, deciding on the class width first may make more sense; then use the class width to determine the number of classes. The following are some guidelines for determining class width.

a. **Class limits** (beginning and ending numbers) must not overlap. For example, they must be stated as "40–49" or "40 up to 50," not as "40–50" or "50–60." Otherwise, you cannot tell the class to which an observation of 50 belongs.

b. If possible, class widths should be equal. Unequal class widths present graphing problems and

should be used only when large gaps occur in the data.

c. If possible, open-ended classes at the upper or lower end of the range should be avoided because they do not accurately communicate the range of the observations. Examples of open-ended classes are 49 years or less and the >90 category for heart rate variation we used in Table 3–2.

d. If possible, class limits should be chosen so that most of the observations in the class are closer to the midpoint of the class than to either end of the class. Doing so results in a better estimate of the raw data mean when the weighted mean is calculated from a frequency table (see Section 3.3.2.a and Exercise 3).

5. Tally the number of observations in each class. If you are constructing a stem-and-leaf plot, the actual value of the observation is noted. If you are constructing a frequency table, you need use only the number of observations that fall within the class.

Table 3–8 is a frequency table of the ages of patients diagnosed with colorectal cancer from Present-

Table 3–7. Final stem-and-leaf plot of change in total function scores using 5-point categories.

Stem	Leaves
−9 to −5	8 8 6 5 5
−4 to 0	4 4 4 4 3 3 2 2 1 1 1 0 0 0 0 0 0 0
+1 to +5	1 1 1 1 1 2 2 2 2 2 2 2 2 3 3 3 3 3 4 4 4 5 5
+6 to +10	7 7 8 8 9 9 9 9 0 0 0 0 0
+11 to +15	5
+16 to +20	8 9
+21 to +25	1 1 3
+26 to +30	7 8
+31 to +35	
+36 to +40	0 7
+41 to +45	7
+46 to +50	
+51 to +55	3
+56 to +60	

Source: Data, used with permission of the author and the publisher, from Hébert R, Brayne C, Spiegelhalter D: Incidence of functional decline and improvement in a community-dwelling very elderly population. *Am J Epidemiol* 1997;**145**:935–944.

Table 3–8. Frequency table for ages of patients diagnosed with colorectal cancer.

Age Group	Frequency	Percent	Cumulative Percent
15–34	17	0.7	0.7
35–44	56	2.4	3.1
45–54	159	6.9	10.0
55–64	407	17.6	27.6
65–74	742	32.0	59.6
≥75	937	40.4	100.0
Total	2318	100.0	

Source: Public data set for incidence of cancer for the years 1992–1996 from the Illinois Department of Public Health Web site (random sample). (http://www.idph.state.il.us/about/epi/intropds.htm)

ing Problem 3. We did not form the class intervals for age, because the data set provided by the state of Illinois contains the age of subjects already collapsed into these categories. This practice is not one we generally recommend because it is always possible to collapse raw data into intervals, but it is impossible to reverse the process and create intervals from collapsed data. Table 3–8 illustrates the situation in which we must use the weighted means formula for frequency tables to determine the mean age of patients with colorectal cancer.

Note that computer programs will list every value that occurs, along with its frequency. Users of the programs must generally designate the class limits if they want to form frequency tables for values in specific intervals, such as in Table 3–8. An easy way to do this is to compute a new variable and then recode the values into classes.

Some tables present only frequencies (number of patients or subjects); others present percentages as well. **Percentages** are found by dividing the number of observations in a given class, n_i, by the total number of observations, n, and then multiplying by 100. For example, for the age class from 55 to 64 years of age, the percentage is

$$\frac{n_i}{n} \times 100 = \frac{407}{2318} \times 100 = 0.176 \times 100, \text{ or } 17.6\%$$

For some applications, cumulative frequencies, or percentages, are desirable. The **cumulative frequency** is the percentage of observations for a given value plus that for all lower values. The cumulative value in the last column of Table 3–8, for instance, shows that 27.6% of patients diagnosed with colorectal cancer in Illinois between 1991 and 1995 were younger than 65.

Frequency tables may also be constructed for data measured on an ordinal scale. For example, if we want to examine the number of patients diagnosed at each stage of disease, we can use the stages as classes and tally the number of patients in each stage.

Use the random sample on the CD-ROM of patients with cancer to generate a frequency distribution for patients with cancer at different sites.

3.4.3 Histograms, Box Plots, & Frequency Polygons

Graphs are used extensively in medicine—in journals in the health field, in slides for presentations at professional meetings, and in advertising literature directed at health professionals. Three graphic devices especially useful in medicine are histograms, box plots, and frequency polygons (or line graphs). The first step in constructing any of these graphs is to create a stem-and-leaf plot or a frequency table, as illustrated in the previous two sections.

3.4.3.a Histograms: A histogram of the changes in scores for elderly subjects in the Hébert and coworkers' (1997) study of functional stability is shown in Figure 3–3. **Histograms** usually present the measurement of interest along the X-axis and the number or percentage of observations along the Y-axis, although some computer programs do the opposite. Whether numbers or percentages are used depends on the purpose of the histogram. For example, percentages are needed when two histograms based on different numbers of subjects are compared.

You may notice that the numbers of patients in each class are different from the numbers we found when creating the stem-and-leaf plots. This incongruity occurs because the Statistical Package for the Social Sciences (SPSS) computer program determines the class limits automatically.

Note that the area of each bar is proportionate to the percentage of observations in that interval; for example, the 9 observations in the –5 interval (which contains values between –7.5 and –2.5) account for 9/72, or 12.5%, of the area covered by this histogram. A histogram therefore communicates information about *area*. The area concept is one reason the width of classes should be equal; otherwise the heights of columns in the histogram must be appropriately mod-

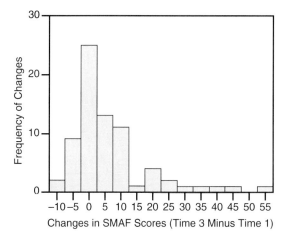

Figure 3–3. Histogram of change in total function scores using 5-point categories. (Data, used with permission, from Hébert R, Brayne C, Spiegelhalter D: Incidence of functional decline and improvement in a community-dwelling very elderly population. *Am J Epidemiol* 1997;**145**:935–944. Graph produced with SPSS, a registered trademark of SPSS, Inc.; used with permission.)

ified to maintain the correct area. For example, in Figure 3–3, if the lowest class were 10 score points wide (from –12.5 to –2.5) and all other classes remained 5 score points wide, 11 observations would fall in the interval. The height of the column for that interval would be only 5.5 units, however (instead of 11 units), to compensate for its doubled width.

3.4.3.b Box Plots: A **box plot,** sometimes called a **box-and-whisker plot,** is another way to display information when the objective is to illustrate certain locations in the distribution (Tukey, 1977). It is constructed from the information in a stem-and-leaf plot. A stem-and-leaf plot for patients 85 years of age or older is given in Table 3–9. The median and the first and third quartiles of the distribution are used in constructing box plots. Computer programs do not routinely denote the mean and 75th and 25th quartiles with stem-and-leaf plots, but it is easy to request this information, as illustrated in Table 3–9. The median change in SMAF score is 2.5, the 75th percentile is 9, and the 25th percentile is 0.

Note that the values for the stem in Table 3–9 are different from the ones we used. This incongruity occurs because NCSS determines the stem values. In Table 3–9, there is a stem value for every two values of change in SMAF score. Although it is not very obvious, the stem values represent class sizes of 2 and are interpreted as follows:

* represents numbers ending in 0 and 1.

T represents numbers ending in 2 and 3.

F represents numbers ending in 4 and 5.

S represents numbers ending in 6 and 7.

● represents numbers ending in 8 and 9.

The depth is the cumulative number of leaves, counting in from the nearest end.

A box plot of the changes in SMAF scores for patients 85 years of age or older is given in Figure 3–4.[3] A box is drawn with the top of the box at the third quartile and the bottom at the first quartile; quartiles are sometimes referred to as *hinges* in box plots. The length of the box is a visual representation of the interquartile range; that is, the box represents the middle 50% of the data. The width of the box is not important. The location of the midpoint or median of the distribution is indicated with a horizontal line in the box. Finally, straight lines, or *whiskers,* extend 1.5 times the interquartile range above and below the 75th and 25th percentiles. Any values above or below the whiskers are called outliers.

Box plots communicate a great deal of information; for example, we can easily see from Figure 3–4 that the score changes range from about –10 to about 55 (actually, from –8 to 53, as we know from the stem-and-leaf plot). Half of the score changes were between about 0 and 8, and the median is a little larger than 0. There are four outlying values; four patients had score changes greater than 35 points, one of which was greater than 50 points.

Use the CD-ROM to generate box plots for heart rate variation to deep breathing for men and women separately in the Gelber and colleagues study (1997). Do these graphs enhance your understanding of the distributions?

3.4.3.c Frequency Polygons: Frequency polygons are line graphs similar to histograms and are especially useful when comparing two distributions on the same graph. As a first step in constructing a frequency polygon, a stem-and-leaf plot or frequency table is generated. Table 3–10 contains the frequencies of men and women who had different levels of heart rate variation to deep breathing.

Figure 3–5 is a histogram based on the frequencies for men with a frequency polygon superimposed on it. It demonstrates that frequency polygons are constructed by connecting the midpoints of the columns of a histogram. The same guidelines therefore hold for constructing frequency tables and histograms as for constructing frequency polygons. Note that the line extends from the midpoint of the first and last columns to the X-axis in order to close up both ends of the distribution and indicate zero frequency of any values beyond the extremes. Because a frequency polygon is based on a histogram, approximately the

---

[3]For this analysis, we selected the following patients: ≥ 85 years, score on the total SMAF at 3 ≥ –1.

Table 3–9. Descriptive information and stem-and-leaf plot of SMAF score changes for subjects 85 years old or older.

Quartile Section of SMAF Score Changes

Parameter	10th Percentile	25th Percentile	50th Percentile	75th Percentile	90th Percentile
Value	−4	0	2.5	9	22.4
95% LCL	−6	−3	1	5	10
95% UCL	−2	1	4	18	40

Stem-and-Leaf Section of SMAF Score Changes

Depth	Stem	Leaves
2	•	88
3	S	6
9	F	554444
13	T	3322
19	−0*	111000
28	0*	000011111
(14)	T	22222222333333
30	F	44455
25	S	77
23	•	889999
17	1*	00000
12	T	
12	F	5
11	S	
11	•	89
9	2*	11
High		23, 27, 28, 37, 40, 47, 53

Unit = 1   Example: 1 | 2 Represents   12

Source: Data, used with permission of the author and the publisher, from Hébert R, Brayne C, Spiegelhalter D: Incidence of functional decline and improvement in a community-dwelling very elderly population. *Am J Epidemiol* 1997;**145**:935–944. Plot produced with NCSS; used by permission.

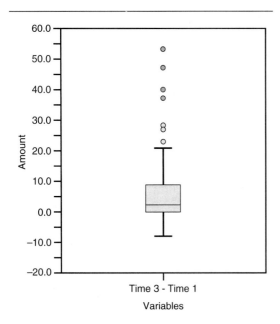

Figure 3–4. Box plot of SMAF score changes for subjects 85 years old or older. (Data, used with permission, from Hébert R, Brayne C, Spiegelhalter D: Incidence of functional decline and improvement in a community-dwelling very elderly population. *Am J Epidemiol* 1997;**145**:935–944. Plot produced with NCSS; used by permission.)

same area is under the line as is in the histogram. Thus, frequency polygons also portray area.

3.4.3.d Graphs Comparing Two or More Groups: Table 3–10 contains the heart rate variation to deep breathing for women as well as men. Merely looking at the numbers in the table is insufficient for deciding if the distributions are similar. The following methods are useful for comparing distributions.

Box plots are very effective when there is more than one group. For example, box plots of the distribution of variation in heart rate for men and women is given in Figure 3–6. It is easy to see that distributions of heart rate variation for men and women are very similar. The box plots illustrate the soundness of Gelber and colleagues' decision to combine men and women to generate normal values rather than producing norms for the sexes separately.

Percentage polygons are also useful for comparing two frequency distributions. Percentage polygons for heart rate variation in both men and women are shown in Figure 3–7. Frequencies must be converted to percentages when the two distributions being compared have an unequal number of observations, and this conversion has been made for Figure 3–7. Examination of the polygons indicates that the distribution of heart rate variation does not appear to be very different for men and women; most of the area in one polygon is overlapped by that in the other. Thus, the

Table 3–10. Frequency table for heart rate variation to deep breathing.

A. Heart Rate Variation in Men

Category	Count	Cumulative Count	Percent	Cumulative Percent
≤20	18	18	8.14	8.14
21–30	22	40	9.95	18.10
31–40	45	85	20.36	38.46
41–50	35	120	15.84	54.30
51–60	28	148	12.67	66.97
61–70	31	179	14.03	81.00
71–80	17	196	7.69	88.69
81–90	12	208	5.43	94.12
>90	13	221	5.88	100.00

B. Heart Rate Variation in Women

Category	Count	Cumulative Count	Percent	Cumulative Percent
≤20	11	11	5.34	5.34
21–30	28	39	13.59	18.93
31–40	31	70	15.05	33.98
41–50	38	108	18.45	52.43
51–60	31	139	15.05	67.48
61–70	25	164	12.14	79.61
71–80	17	181	8.25	87.86
81–90	13	194	6.31	94.17
>90	12	206	5.83	100.00

Source: Data, used with permission of the author and publisher, from Gelber DA, Pfeifer M, Dawson B, Schumer M: Cardiovascular autonomic nervous system tests: Determination of normative values and effect of confounding variables. *J Auton Nerv Syst* 1997;**62**:40–44.

visual message of box plots and frequency polygons is consistent.

Another type of graph often used in the medical literature is an error bar plot. Figure 3–8 contains error bars for men and women. The circle designates the mean, and the bars illustrate the standard deviation, although some authors use the mean and standard error (a value smaller than the standard devia-

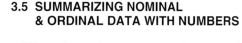

Figure 3–5. Frequency polygon of heart rate variation to deep breathing for men. (Data, used with permission, from Gelber DA, Pfeifer M, Dawson B, Schumer M: Cardiovascular autonomic nervous system tests: Determination of normative values and effect of confounding variables. *J Auton Nerv Syst* 1997;**62**:40–44. Plot produced with NCSS; used by permission.)

tion, discussed in Chapter 4). We recommend using standard deviations and discuss this issue further in Chapter 4. The graphs indicate the similarity of the distributions, just as the percentage polygons and the box plots do.

3.5 SUMMARIZING NOMINAL & ORDINAL DATA WITH NUMBERS

When observations are measured on a **nominal,** or **categoric,** scale, the methods just discussed for describing the middle and the spread of a distribution will not work. Characteristics measured on a nominal scale do not have numerical values but are counts or frequencies of occurrence. Presenting Problem 4 involves two characteristics of the group of physicians who participated in the Physicians' Aspirin Study: (1) method of treatment—whether physician subjects were given aspirin or placebo, and (2) outcome—whether they had an MI during the study. Both characteristics are **dichotomous,** or **binary,** meaning that only two categories are possible. In this section, we examine measures that can be used with such observations.

3.5.1 Ways to Describe Nominal Data

Nominal data can be measured using several methods: proportions, percentages, ratios, and rates. To illustrate these measures, we will use the numbers of physicians who did and those who did not have an

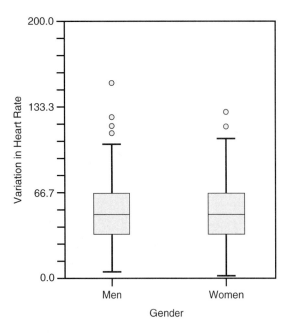

Figure 3–6. Box plot of heart rate variation to deep breathing for men and women. (Data, used with permission, from Gelber DA, Pfeifer M, Dawson B, Schumer M: Cardiovascular autonomic nervous system tests: Determination of normative values and effect of confounding variables. *J Auton Nerv Syst* 1997;**62**:40–44. Plot produced with NCSS; used by permission.)

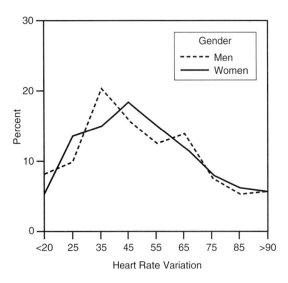

Figure 3–7. Frequency polygon of heart rate variation to deep breathing for men and women. (Data, used with permission, from Gelber DA, Pfeifer M, Dawson B, Schumer M: Cardiovascular autonomic nervous system tests: Determination of normative values and effect of confounding variables. *J Auton Nerv Syst* 1997;**62**: 40–44. Graph produced with SPSS, a registered trademark of SPSS, Inc.; used with permission.)

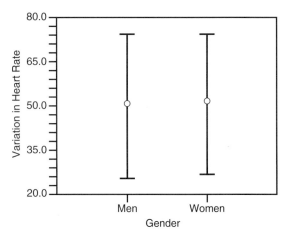

Figure 3–8. Error bar charts of heart rate variation to deep breathing for men and women. (Data, used with permission, from Gelber DA, Pfeifer M, Dawson B, Schumer M: Cardiovascular autonomic nervous system tests: Determination of normative values and effect of confounding variables. *J Auton Nerv Syst* 1997;**62**:40–44. Graph produced with SPSS, a registered trademark of SPSS, Inc.; used with permission.)

MI while taking aspirin or a placebo (Presenting Problem 4); the data are given in Table 3–11.

3.5.1.a Proportions and Percentages: A proportion is the number, *a,* of observations with a given characteristic (such as those who had an MI) divided by the total number of observations, *a* + *b,* in a given group (such as those who took aspirin). That is,

$$\text{Proportion} = \frac{a}{a + b}$$

A proportion is always defined as a *part* divided by the *whole* and is useful for ordinal and numerical data as well as nominal data, especially when the observations have been placed in a frequency table. In the aspirin study, the proportion of physicians taking aspirin who had an MI is 139/11,037 = 0.0126, and the proportion taking the placebo who had an MI is 239/11,034 = 0.0217.

Note that the proportion is really a special case of the mean in which the observations with the given characteristic (eg, physicians who had an MI) are assigned the value 1; observations without the characteristic (eg, physicians who had no MI) are assigned the value 0. Then the ΣX in the numerator of the formula for the mean is simply the sum of the zeroes and ones (and is equal to *a*); the denominator is still *n*. A **percentage** is the proportion multiplied by 100%.

3.5.1.b Ratios and Rates: A **ratio** is the number, *a,* of observations in a given group with a given

Table 3–11. Confirmed cardiovascular end points in the aspirin component of the Physicians' Health Study, according to treatment group.

	Aspirin Group	Placebo Group
Number of patients	11,037	11,034
End Point		
Myocardial infarction		
Fatal	10	26
Nonfatal	129	213
Total	139	239
Person-years of observation	54,560.0	54,355.7
Stroke		
Fatal	9	6
Nonfatal	110	92
Total	119	98
Person-years of observation	54,650.3	54,635.8

Source: Adapted and reproduced, with permission, from Steering Committee of the Physicians' Health Study Research Group: Final report on the aspirin component of the ongoing Physicians' Health Study. *N Engl J Med* 1989; **321:**129–135.

characteristic divided by the number, *b,* of observations without the given characteristic:

$$Ratio = \frac{a}{b}$$

A ratio is always defined as a *part* divided by another *part.* For example, among physicians taking aspirin, the ratio of those who had an MI to those who did not is 139/10,898 = 0.0128. In the placebo group, the ratio of MI to no MI is 239/10,795 = 0.0221.

Rates are similar to proportions except that a multiplier (eg, 1000, 10,000, or 100,000) is used, and they are computed over a specified period of time. The multiplier is called the **base,** and the formula is

$$Rate = \frac{a}{a + b} \times Base$$

For example, if the aspirin study had lasted exactly 1 year, the rate of MI *per 10,000 physicians* taking aspirin per year would be (139/11,037) × (10,000), or 0.0126 × 10,000, or 126 per 10,000 physicians per year.

3.5.2 Vital Statistics Rates

Rates are very important in epidemiology and evidence-based medicine; they are the basis of the calculation of vital statistics, which describe the health status of populations. Some of the most commonly used rates are briefly defined in the following sections.

3.5.2.a Mortality Rates: Mortality rates provide a standard way to compare numbers of deaths occurring in different populations, deaths due to different diseases in the same population, or deaths at different periods of time. The numerator in a mortality rate is the number of people who died during a given period of time, and the denominator is the number of people who were at risk of dying during the same period. Because the denominator is often difficult to obtain, the number of people alive in the population halfway through the time period is frequently used as an estimate. Table 3–12 gives death data from *Vital Statistics of the United States.*

A crude rate is a rate computed over all individuals in a given population. For example, the crude annual mortality rate in the entire population from Table 3–12 is 872.5 per 100,000 in 1996. The **sex-specific mortality rate** for males is 896.4 during that same year, and for females it is 849.7 per 100,000. Comparing the sex-specific mortality rates across the years given in Table 3–12, the mortality rate appears to have increased for women. Does this make sense, or could there be another explanation? Consider that a larger number of older women may have been living in 1996 than in previous years. This hypothesis can be examined by adjusting the mortality rates for the age of people at risk. When age-adjusted rates are examined in Table 3–12, we see that the rates have been declining as we would expect. We talk more about adjusting rates in Section 3.5.4.

Cause-specific mortality rates measure deaths in a population from a specific disease or adverse event. Comparing cause-specific mortality rates over a period of time helps epidemiologists to determine possible predisposing factors in the development of disease as well as to make projections about future trends. For example, Figure 3–9 presents annual mortality rates from a group of diseases in the population of England and Wales between 1900 and 1983. Barker (1989) uses the patterns of increasing mortality rates followed by decreasing mortality rates to suggest that changes in hygiene, diet, and other environmental factors in childhood are important in determining risk for these diseases in later life.

Other commonly used mortality rates are infant mortality rate and case fatality rate. The infant mortality rate, which is sometimes used as an indicator of the level of general health care in a population, is the number of infants who die before 1 year of age per 1000 live births. The case fatality rate is the number of deaths from a specific disease occurring in a given period divided by the number of individuals with the specified disease during the same period.

3.5.2.b Morbidity Rates: Morbidity rates are similar to mortality rates, but many epidemiologists think morbidity rates provide a more direct measure of health status in a population. The **morbidity rate** is the number of individuals who develop a disease in a given period of time divided by the number of people in the population at risk.

Prevalence and incidence are measures of morbidity frequently used in epidemiology as the basis for planning and evaluating health programs. **Prevalence**

Table 3–12. Number of deaths, death rates, and age-adjusted death rates, by race and sex: United States 1987–1996[a]

Number of Deaths in the United States: 1987–1996

	All Races			White			Black		
Year	Both Sexes	Male	Female	Both Sexes	Male	Female	Both Sexes	Male	Female
1996	2,314,690	1,163,569	1,151,121	1,992,966	991,984	1,000,982	282,089	149,472	132,617
1995	2,312,132	1,172,959	1,139,173	1,987,437	997,277	990,160	286,401	154,175	132,226
1994	2,278,994	1,162,747	1,116,247	1,959,875	988,823	971,052	282,379	153,019	129,360
1993	2,268,553	1,161,797	1,106,756	1,951,437	988,329	963,108	282,151	153,502	128,649
1992	2,175,613	1,122,336	1,053,277	1,873,781	956,957	916,824	269,219	146,630	122,589
1991	2,169,518	1,121,665	1,047,853	1,868,904	956,497	912,407	269,525	147,331	122,194
1990	2,148,463	1,113,417	1,035,046	1,853,254	950,812	902,442	265,498	145,359	120,139
1989	2,150,466	1,114,190	1,036,276	1,853,841	950,852	902,989	267,642	146,393	121,249
1988	2,167,999	1,125,540	1,042,459	1,876,906	965,419	911,487	264,019	144,228	119,791
1987	2,123,323	1,107,958	1,015,365	1,843,067	953,382	889,685	254,814	139,551	115,263

Death Rates in the United States per 100,000: 1987–1996

	All Races			White			Black		
1996	872.5	896.4	849.7	906.9	918.1	896.2	842.0	939.9	753.5
1995	880.0	914.1	847.3	911.3	932.1	891.3	864.2	980.7	759.0
1994	875.4	915.0	837.6	905.4	931.6	880.1	864.3	987.8	752.9
1993	880.0	923.5	838.6	908.5	938.8	879.4	876.8	1,006.3	760.1
1992	852.9	901.6	806.5	880.0	917.2	844.3	850.5	977.5	736.2
1991	860.3	912.1	811.0	886.2	926.2	847.7	864.9	998.7	744.5
1990	863.8	918.4	812.0	888.0	930.9	846.9	871.0	1,008.0	747.9
1989	871.3	926.3	818.9	893.2	936.5	851.8	887.9	1,026.7	763.2
1988	886.7	945.1	831.2	910.5	957.9	865.3	888.3	1,026.1	764.6
1987	876.4	939.3	816.7	900.1	952.7	849.8	868.9	1,006.2	745.7

Age-Adjusted Death Rates in the United States per 100,000: 1987–1996

	All Races			White			Black		
1996	491.6	623.7	381.0	466.8	591.4	361.9	738.3	967.0	561.0
1995	503.9	646.3	385.2	476.9	610.5	364.9	765.7	1,016.7	571.0
1994	507.4	654.6	385.2	479.8	617.9	364.9	772.1	1,029.9	572.0
1993	513.3	664.9	388.3	485.1	627.5	367.7	785.2	1,052.2	578.8
1992	504.5	656.0	380.3	477.5	620.9	359.9	767.5	1,026.9	568.4
1991	513.7	669.9	386.5	486.8	634.4	366.3	780.7	1,048.9	575.1
1990	520.2	680.2	390.6	492.8	644.3	369.9	789.2	1,061.3	581.6
1989	528.0	689.3	397.3	499.6	652.2	376.0	805.9	1,082.8	594.3
1988	539.9	706.1	406.1	512.8	671.3	385.3	809.7	1,083.0	601.0
1987	539.2	706.8	404.6	513.7	674.2	384.8	796.4	1,063.6	592.4

[a]Crude rates on an annual basis per 100,000 population in specified group; age-adjusted rates per 100,000 U.S. standard million population. Rates are based on populations enumerated as of April 1 for census years and estimated as of July 1 for all other years. Excludes deaths of nonresidents of the United States.
Source: Adapted, with permission, from Peters KD, Kochanek KD, Murphy SL: Deaths: Final data for 1996. *National Vital Statistics Report;* Vol. 47, no. 9, p. 16. National Center for Health Statistics, 1998.

is defined as the number of individuals with a given disease at a given point in time divided by the population at risk for that disease at that time. **Incidence** is defined as the number of new cases that have occurred during a given interval of time divided by the population at risk at the beginning of the time interval. (Because prevalence does not involve a period of time, it is actually a proportion, but it is often mistakenly termed a rate.) The term "incidence" is frequently used erroneously in the literature when the term "prevalence" is meant. One way to distinguish between them is to look for units: An incidence rate should always be expressed in terms of a unit of time.

We can draw an analogy between prevalence and incidence and two of the study designs discussed in Chapter 2. Prevalence is like a snapshot in time, as is a cross-sectional study. In fact, some cross-sectional studies are called prevalence studies by epidemiologists. Incidence, on the other hand, requires a period of time to transpire, similar to cohort studies. Recall that cohort studies begin at a given time and continue to examine outcomes over the specified length of the study.

Epidemiologists use prevalence and incidence rates to evaluate disease patterns and make future projections. For example, diabetes mellitus has an increasing prevalence even though the annual incidence rate of approximately 230 cases per 100,000 has remained relatively stable over the past several years. The reason for the difference is that once this disease occurs, an individual continues to have diabetes the remainder of his or her life; but advances in care of

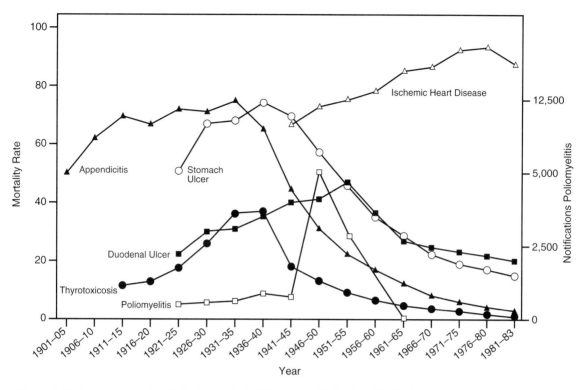

Figure 3–9. Average annual mortality from selected diseases in England and Wales from 1901, and number of notifications of poliomyelitis in 5-year periods. (Reproduced, with permission, from Barker DJP: Rise and fall of Western diseases. *Nature* 1989;**338**:371–372.)

diabetic patients have led to greater longevity for these patients. In contrast, for diseases with a short duration (eg, influenza) or with an early mortality (eg, pancreatic cancer), the incidence rate is generally larger than the prevalence.

3.5.3 Adjusting Rates

We can use crude rates to make comparisons between two different populations only if the populations are similar in all characteristics that might affect the rate. For example, if the populations are different or **confounded** by factors such as age, gender, or race, then age-, gender-, or race-specific rates must be used, or the crude rates must be adjusted; otherwise, comparisons will not be valid.

Rates in medicine are commonly adjusted for age. Often, two populations of interest have different age distributions; yet many characteristics studied in medicine are affected by age, becoming either more or less frequent as individuals grow older. If the two populations are to be compared, the rates must be adjusted to reflect what they would be had their age distributions been similar.

3.5.3.a Direct Method of Adjusting Rates:
As an illustration, suppose a researcher compares the infant mortality rates from a developed country

with those from a developing country and concludes that the mortality rate in the developing country is almost twice as high as the rate in the developed country. Is this conclusion misleading; are possible confounding factors affecting the infant mortality that might distribute it differently in the two countries? A relationship between birthweight and mortality certainly exists, and in this example, a valid comparison of mortality rates requires that the distribution of birthweights be similar in the two countries. Hypothetical data are given in Table 3–13.

The crude infant mortality rate for the developed country is 12.0 per 1000 infants; for the developing country, it is 23.9 per 1000. The specific rates for the developing country are higher in all birthweight categories. However, the two distributions of birthweights are not the same: The percentage of low-birthweight infants (<2500 g) is more than twice as high in the developing country as in the developed country. Because birthweight of infants and infant mortality are related, we cannot determine how much of the difference in crude mortality rates between the countries is due to differences in weight-specific mortality and how much is due to the developing country's higher proportion of low-birthweight ba-

Table 3–13. Infant mortality rate adjustment: Direct method.

	Developed Country				Developing Country			
	Infants Born		Deaths		Infants Born		Deaths	
Birthweight	*N* (in 1000s)	%	No.	Rate	*N* (in 1000s)	%	No.	Rate
< 1500 g	20	10	870	43.5	30	21	1860	62.0
1500–2499 g	30	15	480	16.0	45	32	900	20.0
≥ 2500 g	150	75	1050	7.0	65	47	585	9.0
Total	200		2400	12.0	140		3345	23.9

bies. In this case, the mortality rates must be standardized or adjusted so that they are independent of the distribution of birthweight.[4]

Determining an **adjusted rate** is a relatively simple process when information such as that in Table 3–13 is available. For each population, we must know the specific rates. Note that the crude rate in each country is actually a *weighted average* of the specific rates, with the *number of infants* born in each birthweight category used as the *weights*. For example, the crude mortality rate in the developed country is 2400/200,000 = 0.012, or 12 per 1000, and is equal to

$$\frac{\Sigma \,(\text{Rate} \times N)}{\text{Total } N} = \frac{(43.5 \times 20) + (16.0 \times 30) + (7.0 \times 150)}{20 + 30 + 150}$$

$$= \frac{2400}{200}, \text{ or } 12 \text{ per } 1000$$

Because the goal of adjusting rates is to have them reflect similar distributions, the numbers in each category from one population, called the *reference* population, are used as the weights to form weighted averages for both populations. Which population is chosen as the standard does not matter; in fact, a set of frequencies corresponding to a totally separate reference population may be used. The point is that the same set of numbers must be applied to both populations.

For example, if the numbers of infants born in each birthweight category in the developed country are used as the standard and applied to the specific rates in the developing country, we obtain

$$\text{Adjusted rate} = \frac{\Sigma \,(\text{Rate} \times N \text{ in standard})}{\text{Total } N \text{ in standard}}$$

$$= \frac{(62.0 \times 20) + (20.0 \times 30) + (9.0 \times 150)}{20 + 30 + 150}$$

$$= \frac{3190}{200}, \text{ or } 15.95 \text{ per } 1000$$

The crude mortality rate in the developing country would therefore be 15.95 per 1000 (rather than 23.9 per 1000) if the proportions of infant birthweights were distributed as they are in the developed country.

To use this method of adjusting rates, you must know the specific rates for each category in the populations to be adjusted and the frequencies in the reference population for the factor being adjusted. This method is known as the **direct method of rate standardization.**

3.5.3.b Indirect Method of Adjusting Rates: Sometimes specific rates are not available in one or both of the populations being compared. If the frequencies of the adjusting factor, such as age or birthweight, are known for each population, and any set of specific rates (either for one of the populations being compared or for still another population) is available, an indirect method may be used to adjust rates. The indirect method results in the **standardized mortality ratio,** defined as the number of observed deaths divided by the number of expected deaths.

To illustrate, suppose the distribution of birthweights is available for both the developed and the developing countries, but we have specific death rates only for another population, denoted the *Standard Population* in Table 3–14. The expected number of deaths is calculated in *each* population by using the specific rates from the standard population. For the developed country, the expected number of deaths is

$$(50.0 \times 20) + (20.0 \times 30) + (10.0 \times 150) = 3100$$

Table 3–14. Infant mortality rate adjustment: Indirect method.

	Number of Infants Born (in 100s)		Specific Death Rates per 1000 in Standard Population
Birthweight	Developed Country	Developing Country	
< 1500	20	30	50.0
1500–2499 g	30	45	20.0
≥ 2500 g	150	65	10.0
Number of Deaths	2400	3345	

---

[4]Of course factors other than birthweight may affect mortality, and it is important to remember that correcting for one factor may not correct for others.

In the developing country, the expected number of deaths is

$$(50.0 \times 30) + (20.0 \times 45) + (10.0 \times 65) = 3050$$

The standard mortality ratio (the observed number of deaths divided by the expected number) for the developed country is 2400/3100 = 0.77. For the developing country, the standard mortality ratio is 3345/3050 = 1.1. If the standard mortality ratio is greater than 1, as in the developing country, the population of interest has a mortality rate greater than that of the standard population. If the standard mortality rate is less than 1, as in the developed country, the mortality rate is less than that of the standard population. Thus, the indirect method allows us to make a relative comparison; in contrast, the direct method allows us to make a direct comparison. If rates for one of the populations of interest are known, these rates may be used; then the standardized mortality ratio for this population is 1.0.

3.6 TABLES & GRAPHS FOR NOMINAL & ORDINAL DATA

Tables and graphs are useful for summarizing and communicating information about nominal and ordinal data, and we describe some of the more common methods in this section.

To illustrate how to construct tables for nominal data, consider the observations on sepsis and catheter culture given in Table 3–15 for the 34 patients with acquired hemophilia (Bossi, 1998) in Presenting Problem 5. The simplest way to present nominal data (or ordinal data, if there are not too many points on the scale) is to list the categories in one column of the table and the **frequency** (counts) or percentage of observations in another column. Table 3–16 shows a simple way of presenting data for the number of patients who did or did not have hematuria at the time of diagnosis of their hemophilia.

When two characteristics on a nominal scale are examined, a common way to display the data is in a

Table 3–15. Data on 34 patients with acquired hemophilia due to factor VIII.

ID	Age	Sex	Ecchymoses	Hematoma	Hematuria	Factor VIII	RBC Units >5
1	70	Men	Yes	No	Yes	5.0	Yes
2	70	Women	Yes	Yes	Yes	0.0	No
3	75	Women	Yes	Yes	No	1.0	Yes
4	93	Women	Yes	Yes	No	5.0	No
5	69	Men	No	No	Yes	5.0	No
6	85	Men	Yes	Yes	No	6.0	Yes
7	80	Women	No	No	No	1.0	No
8	26	Women	Yes	Yes	Yes	2.5	No
9	33	Women	Yes	Yes	Yes	3.5	Yes
10	81	Men	Yes	Yes	No	1.3	No
11	42	Women	Yes	Yes	No	30.0	No
12	74	Men	Yes	Yes	Yes	0.0	Yes
13	55	Men	Yes	Yes	Yes	3.0	Yes
14	86	Women	Yes	Yes	Yes	3.0	No
15	71	Men	Yes	Yes	No	6.0	No
16	89	Men	Yes	Yes	No	5.0	Yes
17	81	Women	Yes	Yes	No	0.0	Yes
18	82	Women	Yes	Yes	Yes	1.0	No
19	82	Women	Yes	Yes	No	3.0	No
20	71	Women	Yes	Yes	Yes	1.0	Yes
21	32	Women	Yes	Yes	Yes	2.0	Yes
22	30	Women	Yes	Yes	No	2.0	Yes
23	29	Women	Yes	Yes	No	0.0	No
24	78	Men	Yes	Yes	No	13.0	No
25	58	Men	Yes	Yes	Yes	1.0	No
26	26	Women	Yes	Yes	No	0.0	Yes
27	51	Men	Yes	Yes	No	3.0	No
28	69	Men	Yes	Yes	No	0.0	Yes
29	67	Men	Yes	Yes	No	1.0	No
30	44	Men	Yes	Yes	No	3.0	No
31	59	Women	Yes	Yes	No	3.0	Yes
32	59	Women	Yes	Yes	No	6.0	No
33	40	Men	Yes	Yes	Yes	3.0	Yes
34	22	Women	Yes	Yes	No	1.0	No

Source: Data, used with permission, from Bossi P, Cabane J, Ninet J, et al: Acquired hemophilia due to factor VIII inhibitors in 34 patients. *Am J Med* 1998;**105:**400–408.

Table 3–16. Contingency table for frequency of hematuria in patients with acquired hemophilia.

Hematuria	Number of Patients
Yes	13
No	21

Source: Data, used with permission, from Bossi R, Cabane J, Ninet J, et al: Acquired hemophilia due to factor VIII inhibitors in 34 patients. *Am J Med* 1998;**105**:400–408.

Table 3–18. Contingency table for men and for women with and without hematuria.

Sex	No Hematuria	Hematuria
Men	9	6
Women	12	7

Source: Data, used with permission, from Bossi R, Cabane J, Ninet J, et al: Acquired hemophilia due to factor VIII inhibitors in 34 patients. *Am J Med* 1998;**105**:400–408.

contingency table, in which observations are classified according to several dimensions. Contingency tables are easy to construct and interpret. Suppose we want to know the number of men and women who had hematuria at the time of diagnosis. The first step is to list the categories to appear in the table: men with and without hematuria and women with and without hematuria. The four categories for our example are shown in Table 3–17. Tallies are then placed for each patient who meets the criteria. Patient 1 has a tally in the cell "Men with hematuria"; patient 2 has a tally in the cell "Women with hematuria"; and so on. Tallies for the first seven patients are listed in Table 3–17.

The sum of the tallies in each cell is then used to construct a contingency table such as Table 3–18, which contains cell counts for all 34 patients in the study. Percentages are often given along with the cell counts.

For a graphic display of nominal or ordinal data, bar charts are most commonly used. In a **bar chart,** counts or percentages of the characteristic in different categories are shown as bars. The investigators in this example could have used a bar chart to present the number of patients with and without hematuria, as illustrated in Figure 3–10. The categories of hematuria (yes or no) are placed along the horizontal, or *X*-axis, and the number of patients along the vertical, or *Y*-axis. Bar charts may also be rotated 90° to have the categories along the vertical axis and the numbers along the horizontal axis.

Other graphic devices such as pie charts and pictographs are often used in newspapers, magazines, and advertising brochures. They are used in the health field to display such resource information as the portion of the gross national product devoted to health expenditures or the geographic distribution of primary-care physicians. Look, for example, at the occurrence of tuberculosis. Tuberculosis is a chronic infectious disease caused by mycobacteria, mainly *Mycobacterium tuberculosis*. During the Industrial Revolution it was the leading cause of death in young people around the world, and it is still a major medical problem in developing countries. In the United States the number of reported cases had been declining by 5% per year from 1953 to 1984, but an increase in reported cases occurred in 1986 and again in 1989, leading to concern about the resurgence of tuberculosis, in part because of its association with human immunodeficiency virus (HIV) infection.

Table 3–17. Step 1 in constructing contingency table for men and for women with and without hematuria.

Category	Tally
Men with hematuria	//
Men without hematuria	/
Women with hematuria	/
Women without hematuria	///

Source: Data, used with permission, from Bossi R, Cabane J, Ninet J, et al: Acquired hemophilia due to factor VIII inhibitors in 34 patients. *Am J Med* 1998;**105**:400–408.

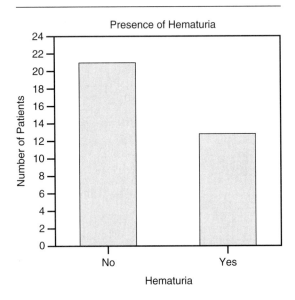

Figure 3–10. Illustration of a bar chart. (Data, used with permission, from Bossi P, Cabane J, Ninet J, et al: Acquired hemophilia due to factor VIII inhibitors in 34 patients. *Am J Med* 1998;**105**:400–408. Graph produced with SPSS, a registered trademark of SPSS, Inc.; used with permission.)

In a review of tuberculosis, Dowling (1991) provided important information on the epidemiology of the disease. In the white population tuberculosis is primarily a disease of the elderly, but among the non-white population the disease is concentrated among young adults. Other groups at high risk include nursing home residents, the homeless, substance abusers, and people with HIV infection. The author chose a pie chart to illustrate the distribution of tuberculosis according to race and ethnicity. Figure 3–11 shows that more persons with tuberculosis (37.1%) are non-Hispanic blacks than any other ethnic group. Pie charts are used to display the parts of a whole. They are effective communication devises and easy to produce, especially with the graphics packages available for computers today.

3.7 DESCRIBING RELATIONSHIPS BETWEEN TWO CHARACTERISTICS

The measures discussed thus far are appropriate for summarizing observations on only one characteristic. Much of the research in medicine, however, concerns the relationship between two or more characteristics. The following discussion focuses on examining the relationship between two variables measured on the same scale when both are numerical, both are ordinal, or both are nominal.

3.7.1 The Relationship between Two Numerical Characteristics

In Presenting Problem 2, Hébert and colleagues (1997) wanted to estimate the relationship between two numerical measures: the scores patients had at the first administration of the Functional Autonomy Measurement System (SMAF) and their score at the second and third administrations. The **correlation coefficient** (sometimes called the Pearson product moment correlation coefficient, named for the statistician who defined it) is one measure of the relationship between two numerical characteristics, symbolized by X and Y. The formula for the correlation coefficient, symbolized by r, is

$$r = \frac{\Sigma\,(X - \overline{X})(Y - \overline{Y})}{\sqrt{\Sigma\,(X - \overline{X})^2\,\Sigma\,(Y - \overline{Y})^2}}$$

Table 3–19 gives the information needed to calculate the correlation between the mental function scores at baseline and at the end of 2 years for women 85 years old and older for the 51 subjects who had both of these measures.

As with the standard deviation, we give the formula and computation for illustration purposes only and, for that reason, use the definitional rather than the computational formula. Using the data from Table 3–19, we obtain a correlation of

$$r = \frac{\Sigma\,(X - \overline{X})(Y - \overline{Y})}{\sqrt{\Sigma\,(X - \overline{X})^2\,\Sigma\,(Y - \overline{Y})^2}}$$
$$= \frac{179.0588}{\sqrt{(220.3529)(428.5098)}}$$
$$= \frac{179.0588}{307.2839} = 0.5827$$

3.7.2 Interpreting Correlation Coefficients

Now we define the meaning of the correlation (0.58) between mental functioning at time 1 and 2 years later. (In this text, we will follow the generally accepted procedure of reporting correlations to two decimal places.) Chapter 8 discusses methods used by investigators to tell whether a statistically significant relationship exists; for now, we will discuss a few characteristics of the correlation coefficient that will help us to interpret its numerical value and describe a relationship.

The correlation coefficient always ranges from –1 to +1, with –1 describing a perfect negative linear (straight-line) relationship and +1 describing a perfect positive linear relationship. A correlation of 0 means no linear relationship exists between the two variables.

Sometimes the correlation is squared (r^2) to form a useful statistic called the **coefficient of determination.** For the mental functioning data, the coefficient

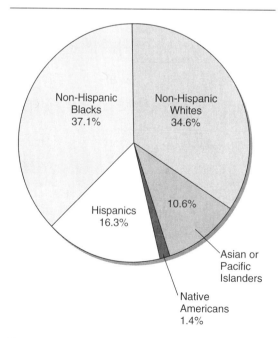

Figure 3–11. Pie chart for distribution of tuberculosis. (Reproduced, with permission, from Figure 1 in Dowling PT: Return of tuberculosis: Screening and preventive therapy. *Am Fam Pract* 1991;**43**:457–467.)

Table 3–19. Calculation for correlation coefficient between mental ability at time 1 (X) and time 3 (Y) for women patients 85 years of age or older.[a]

Patient	X	Y	$(X-\bar{X})$	$(Y-\bar{Y})$	$(X-\bar{X})^2$	$(Y-\bar{Y})^2$	$(X-\bar{X})(Y-\bar{Y})$
1	6.0000	4.0000	4.4118	1.9020	19.4640	3.6176	8.3912
2	0.0000	0.0000	−1.5882	−2.0980	2.5224	4.4016	3.3320
3	1.0000	0.0000	−0.5882	−2.0980	0.3460	4.4016	1.2340
22	2.0000	3.0000	0.4118	0.9020	0.1696	0.8136	0.3714
24	1.0000	0.0000	−0.5882	−2.0980	0.3460	4.4016	1.2340
42	2.0000	8.0000	0.4118	5.9020	0.1696	34.8336	2.4304
72	3.0000	4.0000	1.4118	1.9020	1.9932	3.6176	2.6852
103	1.0000	1.0000	−0.5882	−1.0980	0.3460	1.2056	0.6458
114	2.0000	0.0000	0.4118	−2.0980	0.1696	4.4016	−0.8640
121	0.0000	2.0000	−1.5882	−0.0980	2.5224	0.0096	0.1556
122	2.0000	3.0000	0.4118	0.9020	0.1696	0.8136	0.3714
123	1.0000	0.0000	−0.5882	−2.0980	0.3460	4.4016	1.2340
132	0.0000	4.0000	−1.5882	1.9020	2.5224	3.6176	−3.0208
151	0.0000	0.0000	−1.5882	−2.0980	2.5224	4.4016	3.3320
159	8.0000	9.0000	6.4118	6.9020	41.1112	47.6376	44.2542
161	0.0000	0.0000	−1.5882	−2.0980	2.5224	4.4016	3.3320
162	0.0000	7.0000	−1.5882	4.9020	2.5224	24.0296	−7.7854
173	0.0000	0.0000	−1.5882	−2.0980	2.5224	4.4016	3.3320
183	0.0000	0.0000	−1.5882	−2.0980	2.5224	4.4016	3.3320
188	0.0000	0.0000	−1.5882	−2.0980	2.5224	4.4016	3.3320
220	0.0000	1.0000	−1.5882	−1.0980	2.5224	1.2056	1.7438
237	7.0000	1.0000	5.4118	−1.0980	29.2876	1.2056	−5.9422
241	3.0000	2.0000	1.4118	−0.0980	1.9932	0.0096	−0.1384
251	0.0000	2.0000	−1.5882	−0.0980	2.5224	0.0096	0.1556
266	3.0000	5.0000	1.4118	2.9020	1.9932	8.4216	4.0970
273	0.0000	0.0000	−1.5882	−2.0980	2.5224	4.4016	3.3320
332	1.0000	0.0000	−0.5882	−2.0980	0.3460	4.4016	1.2340
347	0.0000	1.0000	−1.5882	−1.0980	2.5224	1.2056	1.7438
348	0.0000	0.0000	−1.5882	−2.0980	2.5224	4.4016	3.3320
376	0.0000	0.0000	−1.5882	−2.0980	2.5224	4.4016	3.3320
377	3.0000	12.0000	1.4118	9.9020	1.9932	98.0496	13.9796
396	0.0000	0.0000	−1.5882	−2.0980	2.5224	4.4016	3.3320
425	5.0000	4.0000	3.4118	1.9020	11.6404	3.6176	6.4892
472	1.0000	1.0000	−0.5882	−1.0980	0.3460	1.2056	0.6458
501	3.0000	1.0000	1.4118	−1.0980	1.9932	1.2056	−1.5502
518	1.0000	3.0000	−0.5882	0.9020	0.3460	0.8136	−0.5306
526	1.0000	0.0000	−0.5882	−2.0980	0.3460	4.4016	1.2340
527	1.0000	1.0000	−0.5882	−1.0980	0.3460	1.2056	0.6458
531	2.0000	0.0000	0.4118	−2.0980	0.1696	4.4016	−0.8640
592	8.0000	11.0000	6.4118	8.9020	41.1112	79.2456	57.0778
604	3.0000	1.0000	1.4118	−1.0980	1.9932	1.2056	−1.5502
628	1.0000	1.0000	−0.5882	−1.0980	0.3460	1.2056	0.6458
634	0.0000	0.0000	−1.5882	−2.0980	2.5224	4.4016	3.3320
638	1.0000	1.0000	−0.5882	−1.0980	0.3460	1.2056	0.6458
706	4.0000	3.0000	2.4118	0.9020	5.8168	0.8136	2.1754
714	0.0000	1.0000	−1.5882	−1.0980	2.5224	1.2056	1.7438
722	0.0000	0.0000	−1.5882	−2.0980	2.5224	4.4016	3.3320
748	0.0000	1.0000	−1.5882	−1.0980	2.5224	1.2056	1.7438
755	1.0000	6.0000	−0.5882	3.9020	0.3460	15.2256	−2.2952
792	0.0000	0.0000	−1.5882	−2.0980	2.5224	4.4016	3.3320
793	3.0000	3.0000	1.4118	0.9020	1.9932	0.8136	1.2734
Sum	81.0000	107.0000	0.0018	0.002	220.3529	428.5098	179.0588

[a]Values are reported to four decimal places to minimize round-off error.
Source: Data, used with permission of the author and the publisher, from Hébert R, Brayne C, Spiegelhalter D: Incidence of functional decline and improvement in a community-dwelling very elderly population. *Am J Epidemiol* 1997;**145**:935–944. Table produced with NCSS; used with permission.

of determination is $(0.58)^2$, or 0.34. This means that 34% of the variability in one of the measures, such as mental functioning at 2 years, may be accounted for (or predicted) by knowing the value of the other measure, mental functioning at baseline. Stated another way, if we know the value of an elderly woman's score on the mental functioning part of the SMAF and take that into consideration when examining the score 2 years later, the variance (standard deviation squared, from Section 3.3.4.b) of the score after 2 years would be reduced by 34%, or about one-third.

Several other characteristics of the correlation coefficient deserve mention. The value of the correlation coefficient is independent of the particular units used to measure the variables. For example, suppose two medical students measure the heights and weights of a group of preschool children to determine the correlation between height and weight. They measure the children's height in centimeters and record their weight in kilograms, and they calculate a correlation coefficient equal to 0.70. What would the correlation be if they had used inches and pounds instead? It would, of course, still be 0.70, because the denominator in the formula for the correlation coefficient adjusts for the scale of the units.

The value of the correlation coefficient is markedly influenced by outlying values, just as the standard deviation is. The correlation does not therefore describe the relationship between two variables well when the distribution of either variable is skewed or contains outlying values. In this situation, a **transformation** of the data that changes the scale of measurement and moderates the effect of outliers (eg, rank or logarithmic transformation, discussed in Chapter 5) should be done before the correlation is computed.

Students first learning about the correlation coefficient often ask, "How large should a correlation be?" The answer depends on the application. For example, when physical characteristics are measured and good measuring devices are available, as in many physical sciences, fairly high correlations are possible. Measurement in the biologic sciences, however, often involves characteristics that are less well defined and measuring devices that are imprecise; in such cases, lower correlations may occur. Colton (1974) gives the following crude rule of thumb for interpreting the size of correlations:

> Correlations from 0 to 0.25 (or –0.25) indicate little or no relationship; those from 0.25 to 0.50 (or –0.25 to –0.50) indicate a fair degree of relationship; those from 0.50 to 0.75 (or –0.50 to –0.75) a moderate to good relationship; and those greater than 0.75 (or –0.75) a very good to excellent relationship.

Colton also cautions against correlations of 0.95 or higher in the biologic sciences because of the inherent variability in most biologic characteristics. When you encounter a correlation with this value, you should ask whether it is an error or an artifact. An artifact occurs, for instance, when the number of pounds lost by patients in the first week of a diet program is correlated with the number of pounds they lost during the entire 2-month program. In this case, the number of pounds lost during the first week is included in the number of pounds lost during the 2-month period and results in a spuriously high correlation. The correct comparison is between the number of pounds lost in week 1 and the number of pounds lost in weeks 2 through 8.

Two final reminders are worth mention. First, the correlation coefficient measures only a straight-line relationship; two characteristics may, in fact, have a strong curvilinear relationship, even though the correlation is quite small. Therefore, when you analyze relationships between two characteristics, always plot the data as we do in Section 3.8 (or have a computer do so), and calculate a correlation coefficient. A graph will also help you detect outliers and skewed distributions. The second reminder is the adage that "correlation does not imply causation." The statement that one characteristic causes another must be justified on the basis of experimental observations or logical argument, not solely because of a correlation coefficient.

Use the CD-ROM and find the correlation between heart rate variation to deep breathing and the Valsalva ratio using Gelber and colleagues' study (1997). Interpret the correlation using the guidelines just described.

3.7.3 The Relationship Between Two Ordinal Characteristics

The **Spearman rank correlation,** sometimes called Spearman's rho (also named for the statistician who defined it), is frequently used to describe the relationship between two ordinal (or one ordinal and one numerical) characteristics. It is also the appropriate statistic to use with numerical variables when their distributions are skewed and outlying observations occur. The calculation of the Spearman rank correlation, symbolized as r_s, involves rank-ordering the values on each of the characteristics from lowest to highest; the ranks are then treated as though they were the actual values themselves. Although the formula is simple when no ties occur in the values, the computation is quite tedious. Because the calculation is available on many computer programs, we postpone its illustration until Chapter 8, where it is discussed in greater detail.

The Spearman rank correlation may range from –1 to +1, like the Pearson correlation coefficient; but +1 or –1 indicates perfect agreement between the *ranks* of the values rather than between the values themselves. Otherwise, its interpretation is similar to that for the Pearson *r*. An example of its application is a study in which a pediatrician wishes to investigate the relationship between Apgar score and birthweight in a group of premature infants. Because Apgar scores are measured on an ordinal scale, the Spearman rank correlation is appropriate for measuring the relationship.

3.7.4 The Relationship Between Two Nominal Characteristics

In many studies involving two characteristics, both measured on a nominal scale, the primary interest is often in determining whether a significant relationship exists between the two, rather than in describing the magnitude of the relationship. These studies are the subject of Chapter 6. Sometimes, however, simply describing the strength of the relationship between two nominal measures is of interest, such as the occurrence of a given outcome relative to whether a risk or predisposing factor is present. Two ratios used to estimate risk are the **relative risk** and the **odds ratio,** both often referred to as **risk ratios.** For example, in Presenting Problem 4, the investigators may have wished to learn whether aspirin reduces the risk for MI by examining the risk among physicians taking aspirin relative to that for physicians taking the placebo.

In the context of this discussion, we introduce some of the important concepts and terms that are increasingly used in the medical and health literature, including the useful notion of the number of patients who need to be treated in order to observe one positive outcome.

3.7.4.a Experimental and Control Event Rates: A building block in the computation of the measures of risk is called the event rate. Using the notation in Table 3–20, we are interested in the event of a disease occurring. The experimental event rate (EER) is the number of people with the risk factor who have or develop the disease, or $A/(A + B)$. The control event rate (CER) is the number of people without the risk factor who have or develop the disease, or $C/(C + D)$.

3.7.4.b The Relative Risk: The **relative risk,** or risk ratio, of a disease, symbolized by RR, is the ratio of the incidence in people with the risk factor (exposed persons) to the incidence in people without the risk factor (nonexposed persons). It can therefore be found by dividing the EER by the CER. Table 3–11 gives data on MI for physicians taking aspirin and physicians taking a placebo (Presenting Problem 4). In this study, taking aspirin assumes the role of the risk factor. Physicians taking aspirin and those taking the placebo were followed to learn the number in each group who had an MI. The EER is the incidence of MI in physicians who took aspirin, or $139/11,037 = 0.0126$; the CER is the incidence of MI in those who took a placebo, or $239/11,034 = 0.0217$. The relative risk of MI with aspirin, compared with MI with placebo, is therefore

$$RR = \frac{EER}{CER} = \frac{A/(A + B)}{C/(C + D)} = \frac{139/11,037}{239/11,034}$$
$$= \frac{0.0126}{0.0217} = 0.581$$

Table 3–20. Table arrangement and formulas for several important measures of risk.

	Disease	No Disease	
Risk factor present	A	B	B + B
Risk factor absent	C	D	C + D
	A + C	B + D	

Experimental event rate (EER) $= \dfrac{A}{(A + B)}$

Control event rate (CER) $= \dfrac{C}{(C + D)}$

Absolute risk reduction (ARR) $= |\,EER - CER\,|$

Number needed to treat (NNT) $= \dfrac{1}{ARR}$

Relative risk reduction (RRR) $= \dfrac{|\,EER - CER\,|}{CER} = ARR/CER$

Relative risk (RR) $= \dfrac{EER}{CER} = \dfrac{A/(A + B)}{C/(C + D)}$

Odds ratio (OR) $= \dfrac{[A/(A + C)]/[C/(A + C)]}{[B/(B + D)]/[D/(B + D)]} = \dfrac{A/C}{B/D} = \dfrac{AD}{BC}$

Because fewer MIs occurred among the group taking aspirin than those taking the placebo, the relative risk is less than 1. If we take the reciprocal and look at the relative risk of having an MI for physicians in the placebo group, the relative risk is $1/0.58 = 1.72$. Thus, physicians in the placebo group were 1.7 times more likely to have an MI than physicians in the aspirin group.

The relative risk can be calculated only from a cohort study or a clinical trial in which a group of subjects with the risk factor and a group without it are first identified and then followed through time to determine which persons develop the outcome of interest. In this situation, the investigator determines the number of subjects in each group.

3.7.4.c Absolute Risk Reduction and Number Needed to Treat:

As we saw earlier, the relative risk compares the risk in one group to the risk in another. The **absolute risk reduction (ARR)** provides a way to appraise the reduction in risk compared with the baseline risk itself. Based on the physician aspirin study data in Table 3–11, the experimental event rate for an MI from any cause was 139/11,037, or 0.0126, in the aspirin group, and the control event rate was 239/11,034, or 0.0217, in the placebo group. The ARR is the absolute value of the difference between these two groups:

$$ARR = |EER - CER| = |0.0126 - 0.0217|$$
$$= |-0.0091| = 0.0091$$

A good way to interpret these numbers is to think about them in terms of events per 10,000 people. Then the risk of MI is 126 in a group taking aspirin and 217 in a group taking placebo, and the absolute risk reduction is 91 per 10,000 people.

An added advantage of interpreting risk data in terms of absolute risk reduction is that its reciprocal, 1/ARR, is the **number needed to treat (NNT)** in order to prevent one event. The number of people that need to be treated to avoid one MI is then 1/0.0091, or 109.9 (about 110 people). This type of information helps clinicians evaluate the relative risks and benefits of a particular treatment. Based on the risks associated with taking aspirin, do you think it is a good idea to prescribe aspirin for 110 people in order to prevent one of them from having an MI? The articles by Glasziou and coworkers (1998) and Sackett and associates (1998) contain excellent discussions of this topic.

Some treatments or procedures increase the risk for a serious undesirable side effect or outcome. In this situation, the (absolute value of the) difference between the EER and the CER is termed the **absolute risk increase (ARI)**. He and colleagues (1998), in their report of a meta-analysis of randomized trials of aspirin use, found an absolute risk reduction in MI of 137 per 10,000 persons, a result even larger than in the physician aspirin study. They also looked at the outcome of stroke and reported an absolute risk reduction in ischemic stroke of 39 in 10,000. Based on their results, the NNT for the prevention of MI is 1/0.0137, or 72.99 (about 73), and the NNT for the prevention of ischemic stroke is 1/0.0039, or 256.41 (about 257). At the same time, aspirin therapy resulted in an absolute risk increase in hemorrhagic stroke of 12 in every 10,000 persons. The reciprocal of the absolute risk increase, 1/ARI, is called the **number needed to harm (NNH)**. Based on the report by He and colleagues, for hemorrhagic stroke the number needed to harm is 1/0.0012, or 833. Based on these numbers, the authors concluded that the overall benefits from aspirin therapy outweigh the risk for hemorrhagic stroke.

We should mention a related concept, called the **relative risk reduction (RRR)**, because it is often presented in the literature. This measure gives the amount of risk reduction relative to the baseline risk; that is, the EER minus the CER all divided by the control (baseline) event rate, CER. The RRR in the physician aspirin study is

$$RRR = \frac{|EER - CER|}{CER}$$
$$= \frac{0.0091}{0.0217} = 0.4194$$

or approximately 42%. The relative risk reduction tells us that, relative to the baseline risk of 217 MIs in 10,000 people, giving aspirin reduces the risk by 42%.

Many clinicians feel that the absolute risk reduction is a more valuable index than the relative risk reduction since its reciprocal is the number needed to treat. If a journal article gives only the relative risk reduction, it can (fairly easily) be converted to the absolute risk reduction by multiplying by the control event rate, a value that is almost always given in an article. For instance, 0.4194×0.0217 is 0.0091, the same value for the ARR that we found at the beginning of this section.

3.7.4.d The Odds Ratio:

The odds ratio provides a way to look at risk in case-control studies. To discuss the odds ratio, recall the study by Ballard and coworkers (1998)[5] in which the use of antenatal thyrotropin-releasing hormone was studied. Data from

---

[5]The authors could have presented the relative risk because the study was a clinical trial, but they chose to give the odds ratio as well. At one time, use of the odds ratio was generally reserved for case–control studies. One of the statistical methods used increasingly in medicine, **logistic regression,** can be interpreted in terms of odds ratios. We discuss this method in detail in Chapter 10. We discuss the issue of statistical significance and risk ratios in Chapter 8.

this study are given in Table 3–21. The **odds ratio** (**OR**) is the odds that a person with an adverse outcome was exposed or at risk divided by the odds that a person without an adverse outcome was not exposed or at risk. The odds ratio is easy to calculate when the observations are given in a 2×2 table. The numbers of infants developing respiratory distress syndrome in Table 3–21 are rearranged and given in Table 3–22.

In this study, the odds that an infant with respiratory distress syndrome was exposed to TRH are

$$\frac{(260/504)}{(244/504)} = \frac{260}{244} = 1.0656$$

and the odds that an infant without respiratory distress syndrome was exposed to TRH are

$$\frac{(132/265)}{(133/265)} = \frac{132}{133} = 0.9925$$

Putting these two odds together to obtain the odds ratio gives

$$\frac{1.0656}{0.9925} = 1.0737, \text{ or approximately 1.1}$$

An odds ratio of 1.1 means that an infant in the TRH group is 1.1 times more likely to develop respiratory distress syndrome than an infant in the placebo group. This risk does not appear to be much greater, and Ballard and coworkers (1998) reported that the odds ratio was not statistically significant.

The odds ratio is also called the cross-product ratio because it can be defined as the ratio of the product of the diagonals in a 2×2 table:

$$\frac{(260)\,(133)}{(244)\,(132)} = 1.0737$$

In case–control studies, the investigator decides how many subjects with and without the disease will be studied. This is the opposite from cohort studies and clinical trials, in which the investigator decides the number of subjects with and without the risk factor. The odds ratio should therefore be used with case–control studies.

Readers interested in more detail are referred to the very readable elementary text on epidemiology by Fletcher and colleagues (1988). Information on other measures of risk used in epidemiology, such as the attributable risk percent and the rate ratio, and the odds ratio for matched designs, can be found in Greenberg (1996).

3.8 GRAPHS FOR TWO CHARACTERISTICS

Most studies in medicine involve more than one characteristic, and graphs displaying the relationship between two characteristics are common in the literature. No graphs are commonly used for displaying a relationship between two characteristics when both are measured on a nominal scale; the numbers are simply presented in contingency tables. When one of the characteristics is nominal and the other is numerical, the data can be displayed in box plots like the one in Figure 3–6. Alternatively, both frequency distributions can be displayed in error plots, as in Figure 3–8. The center of each frequency distribution is often denoted in some manner; in Figure 3–8, a circle has been drawn at the center, but an X or some other symbol could be used instead.

Also common in medicine is the use of **bivariate plots** (also called **scatterplots** or scatter diagrams) to illustrate the relationship between two characteristics when both are measured on a numerical scale. In the study by Hébert and colleagues (1997), information was collected on the mental functioning of each patient at three times, each 1 year apart. Box 3–1 contains a scatterplot of mental functioning scores at times 1 and 3 for women age 85 or older. A scatterplot is constructed by drawing X- and Y-axes; the

Table 3–21. Outcomes of infants in the thyrotropin-releasing hormone and placebo groups.

	Infants at Risk			Infants Not at Risk		
Outcome	TRH ($N = 392$)	Placebo ($N = 377$)	Odds Ratio (95% CI)	TRH ($N = 171$)	Placebo ($N = 194$)	Odds Ratio (95% CI)
Respiratory distress syndrome	260	244	1.1 (0.8–1.5)	5	13	0.4 (0.1–1.3)
Death ≤ 28 days after delivery	43	42	1.0 (0.6–1.6)	2	1	2.3 (0.1–135)
Chronic lung disease or death ≤ 28 days after delivery	175	157	1.1 (0.8–1.3)	3	2	1.7 (0.2–20.7)

Source: Data, used with permission, from Table 2 in Ballard RA, Ballard PL, Chaan A, et al: Antenatal thyrotropin-releasing hormone to prevent lung disease in preterm infants. *N Engl J Med* 1998;**338**:493–498.

Table 3–22. Data for odds ratio for infants at 32 weeks or fewer of gestation.

Group	With Respiratory Distress	Without Respiratory Distress	Total
TRH	260	132	392
Placebo	244	133	377
Total	**504**	**265**	

Source: Data, used with permission, from Table 2 in Ballard RA, Ballard PL, Chaan A, et al: Antenatal thyrotropin-releasing hormone to prevent lung disease in preterm infants. *N Engl J Med* 1998;**338**:493–498.

characteristic hypothesized to explain or predict or the one that occurs first (sometimes called the risk factor) is placed on the *X*-axis. The characteristic or outcome to be explained or predicted or the one that occurs second is placed on the *Y*-axis. In applications in which a noncausal relationship is hypothesized, placement for the *X*- and *Y*-axes does not matter. Each observation is represented by a small circle; for example, the circle in the lower right in the graph in Box 3–1 represents subject 237, who had a score of 7 at baseline and a score of 1 two years later. More information on interpreting scatterplots is presented in Chapter 8, but we see here that the data in Box 3–1

suggest the possibility of a positive relationship between the two scores. At this point, we cannot say whether the relationship is significant or one that simply occurs by chance; this topic is covered in Chapter 8.

Some of you may notice that fewer data points occur in Box 3–1 than in Table 3–19. This results when several data points have the same value. Both NCSS and SPSS have an option for using so-called sunflowers, in which each sunflower petal stands for one observation. Use the CD-ROM to produce a scatter plot, and choose the sunflower option. Do you think this is helpful in interpreting the plot?

As a final note, there is a correspondence between the size of the correlation coefficient and a **scatterplot** of the observations. We also included in Box 3–1 the output from NCSS giving the correlation coefficient. Recall that a correlation of 0.58 indicates a moderate to good relationship between the two mental functioning scores. When the correlation is near 0, the shape of the pattern of observations is more or less circular. As the value of the correlation gets closer to +1 or –1, the shape becomes more elliptical, until, at +1 and –1, the observations fall directly on a straight line. With a correlation of 0.58, we expect a scatter plot of the data to be somewhat oval-shaped, as it is in Box 3–1.

3.9 EXAMPLES OF MISLEADING CHARTS & GRAPHS

The quality of charts and graphs published in the medical literature is higher than that in similar displays in the popular press. The most significant problem with graphs (and tables as well) in medical journal articles is their complexity. Many authors attempt to present too much information in a single graphic display, and it may take the reader a long time to decipher it. In these situations, many of us give up and consequently miss or misinterpret important information.

Before illustrating misleading displays, we wish to emphasize that the purpose of tables and graphs is to present information (often based on large numbers of observations) in a concise way so that the reader can comprehend and remember it more easily. The following cardinal rules therefore apply to graphic displays: (1) Charts, tables, and graphs should be simple and easily understood by the reader, and (2) concise but complete labels and legends should accompany them.

Knowing about common errors helps you correctly interpret information in articles and presentations, provides a hint about the research skills of the investigators, and helps you design your own charts and graphs. We illustrate four errors we have seen with sufficient frequency to warrant their discussion. We use hypo-

Box 3–1. Illustration of a scatterplot.

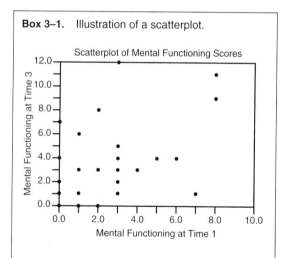

Scatterplot of Mental Functioning Scores

Pearson Correlations Study

	Time 1	Time 3
Time 1	1.000000	0.582715
Time 3	0.582715	1.000000

Data, used with permission, from Hébert R, Brayne C, Spiegelhalter D: Incidence of functional decline and improvement in a community-dwelling very elderly population. *Am J Epidemiol* 1997;**145**:935–944. Plot produced with NCSS; used by permission.

thetical examples to illustrate these errors and do not imply that they necessarily occurred in the presenting problems used in this text. An interesting and entertaining report by Wainer (1984) draws on published tables and graphs from various nonmedical sources and is recommended if you would like more information on misleading graphs. If you are interested in learning more about table and graph construction, a discussion by Wainer (1992) makes recommendations for designing tables for data, and the book by Cleveland (1985), especially the first two chapters, illustrates different graphs. Spirer and colleagues (1998) provide an entertaining discussion of graphs. Briscoe (1996) has suggestions for improving all types of presentations and posters, as well as publications.

A researcher can easily make a change appear more or less dramatic by selecting a starting time for a graph, either before or after the change begins. Figure 3–12A shows the decrease in annual mortality from a disease, beginning in 1950. The major decrease in mortality from this disease occurred in the 1960s. Although not incorrect, a graph that begins in 1970 (Figure 3–12B) deemphasizes the decrease and implies that the change has been small.

If the values on the Y-axis are large, the entire scale cannot be drawn. For example, suppose an investigator wants to illustrate the number of deaths from cancer, beginning in 1960 (when there were 200,000 deaths) to the year 2010 (when 600,000 deaths are projected). Even if the vertical scale is in thousands of deaths, it must range from 200 to 600. If the Y-axis is not interrupted, the implied message is inaccurate; a misunderstanding of the scale makes the change appear larger than it really is. This error, called **suppression of zero,** is common in histograms and line graphs. Figure 3–13A illustrates the effect of suppression of zero on the number of deaths from cancer per year; Figure 3–13B illustrates the correct construction. The error of suppression of zero is more serious on the Y-axis than on the X-axis, because the scale on the Y-axis represents the magnitude of the characteristic of interest. Many researchers today use computer programs to generate their graphics. Some programs make it difficult or impossible to control the scale of the Y-axis (and the X-axis as well). As readers, we therefore need to be vigilant and not be unintentionally mislead by this practice.

The magnitude of change can also be enhanced or minimized by the choice of scale on the vertical axis. For example, suppose a researcher wishes to compare the ages at death in a group of men and a group of women. Figure 3–14A, by suppressing the scale, indicates that the ages of men and women at death are

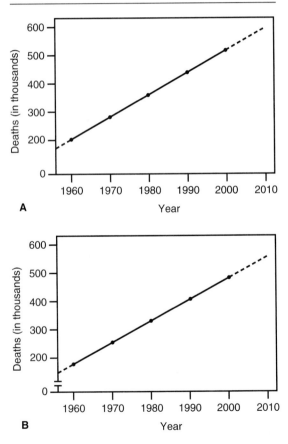

A

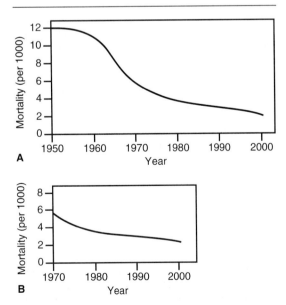

Figure 3–12. Illustration of effect of portraying change at two different times. **A:** Mortality from a disease since 1950. **B:** Mortality from a disease since 1970.

Figure 3–13. Illustration of effect of suppression of zero on Y-axis in graphs showing deaths from cancer. **A:** No break in the line on Y-axis. **B:** Break in the line correctly placed on Y-axis.

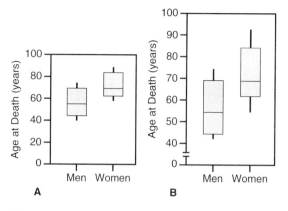

Figure 3–14. Illustration of effect of suppressing or stretching the scale in plots showing age at death. **A:** Suppressing the scale. **B:** Stretching the scale.

Table 3–23. Effect of calculating column percentages versus row percentages for study of compliance with medication versus insurance coverage.

A. Percentages Based on Level of Compliance (Column %)

Insurance Coverage	Level of Compliance with Medication		
	Low	Medium	High
Medicaid	30	20	15
Medicare	20	25	30
Medicaid and Medicare	5	5	5
Other insurance	10	30	40
No insurance	35	20	10

B. Percentages Based on Insurance Coverage (Row %)

Insurance Coverage	Level of Compliance with Medication		
	Low	Medium	High
Medicaid	45	30	25
Medicare	25	35	40
Medicaid and Medicare	33	33	33
Other insurance	15	35	50
No insurance	55	30	15

similar; Figure 3–14B, by stretching the scale, magnifies the differences in age at death between men and women.

Our final example is a table that gives irrelevant percentages, a somewhat common error. Suppose that the investigators are interested in the relationship between levels of patient compliance and their type of insurance coverage. When two or more measures are of interest, the purpose of the study generally determines which measure is viewed within the context of the other. Table 3–23A shows the percentage of patients with different types of insurance coverage within three levels of patient compliance, so the percentages in each column total 100%. The percentages in Table 3–23A make sense if the investigator wishes to compare the type of insurance coverage of patients who have specific levels of compliance; it is possible to conclude, for example, that 35% of patients with low levels of compliance have no insurance.

Contrast this interpretation with that obtained if percentages are calculated within insurance status, as in Table 3–23B, in which percentages in each row total 100%. From Table 3–23B, one can conclude that 55% of patients with no insurance coverage have a low level of compliance. In other words, the format of the table should reflect the questions asked in the study. If one measure is examined to see whether it explains another measure, such as insurance status explaining compliance, investigators should present percentages within the explanatory measure (insurance status, in our example).

3.10 COMPUTER PROGRAMS

As you have already seen, we give examples of output from **computer packages** especially designed to analyze statistical data. We briefly note here the various packages illustrated in this text. As much as possible, we reproduce the actual output obtained in analyzing observations from the presenting problems, even though the output frequently contains statistics not yet discussed. We discuss the important aspects of the output, and, for the time being, you can simply ignore unfamiliar information on the printout; in subsequent chapters, we will explain many of the statistics. Statistical computer programs are designed to meet the needs of researchers in many different fields, so some of the statistics in the printouts may rarely be used in medical studies and hence are not included in this book. If you would like more detail on this topic, Altman (1991a) also describes uses of computers for medical research.

We use the output from several comprehensive statistical programs in this text, including NCSS, SPSS, SYSTAT, MINITAB, and JMP. For the most part, we concentrate on the first two packages. In later chapters we also use specialized programs for estimating the sample size needed for a study.

3.11 SUMMARY

This chapter presents two important biostatistical concepts: the different scales of measurement used in medicine and appropriate methods for summarizing and displaying information, depending on the measurement scale. We used data from the presenting problems to demonstrate different methods of summarizing and displaying data so as to communicate pertinent information easily. Some of the summary measures we introduce in this chapter form the basis of statistical tests illustrated in subsequent chapters.

The simplest level of measurement is a nominal scale, also called a categorical, or qualitative, scale. Nominal scales measure characteristics that can be classified into categories; the number of observations in each category is counted. Examples include gender, race, and type of disease. Dichotomous, or binary, characteristics have only two values. Proportions, ratios, and percentages are commonly used to summarize categorical data. Nominal characteristics are displayed in contingency tables and in bar charts.

The next level of measurement is an ordinal scale, which is used for characteristics that have an underlying order. The differences between values on the scale are not equal throughout the scale, however; the numbers are arbitrary and have no inherent meaning. Examples are Apgar scores, which range from 0 to 10, and many cancer staging schemes, which have four or five categories corresponding to the severity and invasiveness of the tumor. Medians, percentiles, and ranges are the summary measures of choice because they are less affected by outlying measurements. Ordinal characteristics, like nominal characteristics, are displayed in contingency tables and bar charts. When the number of ordered categories is large, methods appropriate for numerical scales are sometimes used as well.

Numerical scales are the highest level of measurement; they are also called interval, or quantitative, scales. Characteristics measured on a numerical scale can be continuous (taking on any value on the number line) or discrete (taking on only integer values).

We recommend that the mean—a measure of the middle of a distribution—be used with observations that have a symmetric distribution. The median, also a measure of the middle, is used with ordinal observations or numerical observations that have a skewed distribution. When the mean is appropriate for describing the middle, the standard deviation is appropriate for describing the spread, or variation, of the observations. The value of the standard deviation is affected by outlying or skewed values, so percentiles or the interquartile range should be used with observations for which the median is appropriate. The range gives information on the extreme values, but it does not provide any insight into how the observations themselves are distributed. The geometric mean is sometimes used with extremely skewed data, such as observations measured on a logarithmic scale.

An easy way to determine whether the distribution of observations is symmetric or skewed is to create a histogram or box plot. This is only one of the several graphic devices that can be used to present numerical observations. Others include frequency polygons or line graphs, and error plots. Although each method provides information on the distribution of the observations, box plots are especially useful as concise displays because they show at a glance the distribution of the values. Stem-and-leaf plots combine features of frequency tables and histograms; they show the frequencies as well as the shape of the distribution. Frequency tables summarize numerical observations; the scale is divided into classes, and the number of observations in each class is counted. Both frequencies and percentages are commonly used in frequency tables.

When measurements consist of one nominal and one numerical characteristic, frequency polygons, box plots, and error plots illustrate the distribution of numerical observations for each value of the nominal characteristic.

Practitioners often wish to describe the relationship between two measurements made on the same group of individuals. The correlation coefficient indicates the degree of the relationship between the two measurements. Spearman's rank correlation is used with skewed or ordinal observations, that is, in the same situations for which medians are appropriate. When the characteristics are measured on a nominal scale and proportions are calculated to describe them, the relative risk or the odds ratio may be used to measure the relationship between two characteristics.

The study by Gelber and colleagues (1997) in Presenting Problem 1 used data from a large group of normal subjects to establish normative values for heart rate variation to deep breathing (VAR) and the calculation of the Valsalva ratio (VAL). The 95% range for normative values was determined for both VAR and VAL. No gender effect was apparent for either measurement. VAR correlated inversely with age and mean arterial pressure, however, whereas VAL correlated inversely with age and body mass index. We used data from this study to illustrate the calculation of common statistics for summarizing data, such as the mean, median, and standard deviation, and to provide some useful ways of displaying data in graphs

Hébert and colleagues (1997) in Presenting Problem 2 focused on disability and functional changes in the elderly. We used observations on subjects 85 years of age or older to illustrate stem-and-leaf plots and box plots. In the article, Hébert and colleagues reported that baseline SMAF scores indicated that women were significantly more disabled than men for activities of daily living, mobility, and mental function. Women were more independent in instrumental activities of daily living (housekeeping, meal preparation, shopping, medication use, budgeting). Generally, subjects showed significant declines in all areas of functioning between baseline interview and the second interview 1 year later. Functional decline was associated with age, but not with sex. Interestingly, the functional score declines were not significant (except for a slight decline in instrumental activities of daily living) between the second and third interviews. The authors proposed three explanations to account for this phenomenon: floor effect, survival effect, and regression toward the mean—topics discussed later in this text. The annual incidence of functional decline was 11.9% among previously stable subjects age 75 and older. The risk of functional decline doubles every 5 years. Disability is one of the important outcome measures in studies of the elderly population. We also examined the relationship between SMAF scores at baseline and 2 years later in this study and found a moderate to good relationship between these measures.

The results of the study on aspirin versus placebo in preventing MI (Presenting Problem 4) were used to illustrate that proportions and percentages can be used interchangeably to describe the relationship of a part to the whole; ratios relate the two parts themselves. When a proportion is calculated over a period of time, the result is called a rate. Some of the rates commonly used in medicine were defined and illustrated. For comparison of rates from two different populations, the populations must be similar with respect to characteristics that might affect the rate; adjusted rates are necessary when these characteristics differ between the populations. In medicine, rates are frequently adjusted for disparities in age. Contingency tables display two nominal characteristics measured on the same set of subjects. Bar and pie charts are common ways to illustrate nominal data.

There is a vast array of public health information and vital statistics available via the Internet. The Centers for Disease Control, the National Institutes of Health, and the National Center for Health Statistics all have an impressive number of resources available to health providers, researchers, patients, and the general public. Using publicly available data, our analysis of colorectal cancer in Illinois (Presenting Problem 3) found that 72.4% of patients are 65 years of age or older when their cancer is diagnosed. Furthermore, only 0.7% are younger than 35 years, and only 3.1% are younger than 45.

Acquired hemophilia is a rare, life-threatening disease caused by development of autoantibodies directed against factor VIII. It is often associated with an underlying disease. In Presenting Problem 5 Bossi and colleagues (1998) studied the characteristics and outcomes of 34 patients who had this disease. The results from their study help clinicians understand the presentation and clinical course of acquired hemophilia. Treatments have included administration of porcine factor VIII, immunosuppressive drugs, and intravenous immunoglobulins. These researchers point out the need for randomized, controlled studies of treatment.

The study by Ballard and coworkers (1998) found that the antenatal administration of thyrotropin-releasing hormone had no effect on the pulmonary outcome in these premature infants. No significant differences occurred between the treatment and placebo groups in the incidence of respiratory distress syndrome, death, or chronic lung disease. We used the data to illustrate the odds ratio for the development of respiratory distress, and our results (not significant) agreed with those of the authors. The investigators concluded that treatment with thyrotropin-releasing hormone is not indicated for women at risk of delivering a premature infant.

EXERCISES

1. Show that the sum of the deviations from the mean is equal to 0. Demonstrate this fact by finding the sum of the deviations for heart rate variation in Table 3–3.
2. Normal limits of many laboratory values are set by the 2½ and 97½ percentiles, so that the normal limits contain the central 95% of the distribution. This approach was taken by Gelber and colleagues (1997) when they developed norms for mean heart variation to breathing and the Valsalva ratio. Find the normal limits for heart rate variation.
3. Generate a frequency table of mean, median, minimum, and maximum heart rate variation for patients in age categories. Use the age category column in the data set and the Descriptives procedure in NCSS. There are 490 patients for whom both age and heart rate variation are available. Your table should look like Table 3–24. Estimate the overall mean age of the patients. Estimate the overall mean variation to heart rate. Compare each to the mean calculated with NCSS. Which is more accurate? Why?
4. To illustrate that only $n - 1$ deviations from the mean are free to vary, consider the ages of five patients seen in the clinic on a given afternoon. The mean age has been determined and subtracted from each patient's age in Table 3–25.
    a. What is X – the mean for patient 5?
    b. If the mean age of the patients is 40, what are the ages of the five patients?
5. What is the most likely shape of the distribution of observations in the following studies?
    a. The age of subjects in a study of patients with Crohn's disease.
    b. The number of babies delivered by all physicians who delivered babies in a large city during the past year.
    c. The number of patients transferred to a tertiary care hospital by other hospitals in the region.
6. Draw frequency polygons to compare men and women SMAF scores on mental functioning at time 1 in the study by Hébert and coworkers (1997). Repeat for time 2. What do you conclude?
7. The computational formula for the standard deviation is

$$SD = \sqrt{\frac{\Sigma X^2 - \frac{(\Sigma X)^2}{n}}{n - 1}}$$

Table 3–24. Frequency table showing mean heart rate variation to deep breathing broken down by 10-year age groups.

Age	Count	Heart Rate Variation			
		Mean	**Median**	**Minimum**	**Maximum**
11–20	52	63.0	57.6	24.0	150.9
21–30	162	57.6	56.1	13.3	124.4
31–40	144	51.1	48.3	14.0	128.9
41–50	78	39.6	37.6	9.4	105.5
51–60	20	34.0	32.3	7.2	85.7
61–70	23	29.1	23.5	3.3	70.9
> 70	11	16.8	17.3	2.1	28.3
Total	490				

Source: Data, used with permission of the author and publisher, from Gelber DA, Pfeifer M, Dawson B, Shumer M: Cardiovascular autonomic nervous system tests: Determination of normative values and effect of confounding variables. J *Auton Nerv Syst* 1997;**62**:40–44. Table produced with NCSS; used with permission.

Illustrate that the value of the standard deviation calculated from this formula is equivalent to that found with the definitional formula using heart rate variation data in Table 3–3. From Section 3.3.4.b, the value of the standard deviation of heart rate variation using the definitional formula is 28.83. (Use the sums in Table 3–3 to save some calculations.)

8. The following questions give brief descriptions of some studies; you may wish to refer to the articles for more information.

   a. Kremer and associates (1987) examined the relationship between decreases in neutrophil leukotriene B_4 production and decreases in the number of tender joints in patients with rheumatoid arthritis who were given fish oil dietary supplements. What graphic device best illustrates this information?

   b. During their investigation of an unusual new illness involving multiple-organ systems, Kilbourne and coworkers (1983) reviewed the medical records of 121 patients in a severely affected town near Madrid. The epidemiologic investigation linked the occurrence of illness with ingestion of an unlabeled, illegally marketed cooking oil. The illness was self-limited in many patients and could not be determined in some, but severe neuromuscular manifestations occurred late in the disease in 23% of the patients. The investigators suspect that onset of illness early in the epidemic is associated with progression to muscular illness and wish to display this relationship graphically. What type(s) of graphic display should they use?

   c. In the study of nonsteroidal antiinflammatory drug use and acute nonvariceal upper gastrointestinal bleeding, Bartle and colleagues (1986) had the following information to present to readers:

   Of the 57 patients with acute nonvariceal upper GI bleeding, 14 had taken acetylsalicylic acid and 10 had taken NSAIDs. Among the 123 control subjects, the numbers were 16 and 7, respectively.

   What is the best way to display this information in a table?

9. What measures of central tendency and dispersion are the most appropriate to use with the following sets of data?

   a. Salaries of 125 physicians in a clinic
   b. The test scores of all medical students taking USLME Step I of the National Board Examination in a given year
   c. Serum sodium levels of healthy individuals
   d. Number of tender joints in 30 joints evaluated on a standard examination for disease activity in rheumatoid arthritis patients
   e. Presence of diarrhea in a group of infants
   f. The disease stages for a group of patients with Reye's syndrome (six stages, ranging from 0 = alert wakefulness to 5 = unarousable, flaccid paralysis, areflexia, pupils unresponsive)
   g. The age at onset of breast cancer in females
   h. The number of pills left in subjects' medicine bottles when investigators in a study counted the pills to evaluate compliance in taking medication

Table 3–25. Illustrating that only $n - 1$ deviations exist.

Patient	Age in Deviations from Mean Age $(X - \bar{X})$
1	10
2	−7
3	−5
4	3
5	

10. Graphs can also illustrate relationships when more than two characteristics are of interest. In a study of the risk of coronary heart disease in women, Willett and associates (1987) used three-dimensional histograms; Figure 3–15 shows the rate of coronary heart disease (CHD) by age and number of cigarettes smoked per day. What conclusions are possible from this graph?

11. Examine the pattern of distribution of mean heart rate variation for different age groups in Table 3–24 (Gelber et al, 1997). What do you observe? How would you learn whether or not your hunch is correct?

12. The correlation between age and heart rate variation is –0.45 (Gelber et al, 1997). How do you interpret this value? What are the implications for norms for heart rate variation?

13. Refer to Figure 3–2 to answer the following questions:
  a. What is the mean weight of girls 24 months old?
  b. What is the 90th percentile for head circumference for 12-month-old girls?
  c. What is the fifth percentile in weight for 12-month-old girls?

14. Find the coefficient of variation of mean change in red blood cell units for men and for women using the data from Bossi and colleagues (1998). Does one sex have greater relative variation in the number of red blood cells?

15. Refer to Presenting Problem 4, the Physicians' Health Study (Steering Committee of the Physi-cians' Health Study Research Group, 1989) to answer the following questions:
  a. The authors used person-years of observation to calculate the odds ratio. Calculate the odds ratio using person-years of observation and compare its value to the value we obtained. Give some reasons for their similarity in magnitude. Under what circumstances could they differ?
  b. The authors also calculated the odds ratio adjusted for age and use of beta-carotene. What do they mean by this statement?
  c. How could the healthy volunteer effect contribute to the finding of no difference in total mortality from cardiovascular causes between the aspirin and placebo group?

16. From their own experiences in an urban public hospital, Kaku and Lowenstein (1990) noted that stroke related to recreational drug use was occurring more frequently in young people. To investigate the problem, they identified all patients between 15 and 44 years of age admitted to a given hospital and selected sex- and age-matched controls from patients admitted to the hospital with acute medical or surgical conditions for which recreational drug abuse has not been shown to be a risk factor. Data are given in Table 3–26. What is the odds ratio?

17. Group Exercise. Obtain a copy of the study by Moore and colleagues (1991) from your medical library, and answer the following questions:
  a. What was the purpose of this study?
  b. What was the study design?
  c. Why were two groups of patients used in the study?
  d. Examine the box plots in the article's Figure 1. What conclusions are possible from the plots?
  e. Examine the box plots in the article's Figure 2. What do these plots tell you about pH levels in normal healthy men?

18. Group Exercise. It is important that scales recommended to physicians for use in assessing risk or making management decisions be shown to be reliable and valid. Select an area of interest, and consult some journal articles that de-

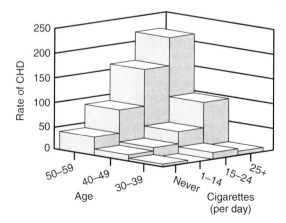

Figure 3–15. Three-dimensional histogram of rates of coronary heart disease (CHD). (Modified and reproduced, with permission, from Willett WC et al: Relative and absolute excess risks of coronary heart disease among women who smoke cigarettes. *N Engl J Med* 1987;**317**:1303–1309.)

Table 3–26. Data for odds ratio for stroke with history of drug abuse.

	Stroke	Control
Drug Abuse	73	18
No Drug Abuse	141	196
Total	214	214

Source: Reproduced, with permission, from Kaku DA, Lowenstein DH: Emergency of recreational drug abuse as a major risk factor for stroke in young adults. *Ann Intern Med* 1990:**113**:821–827.

scribe scales or decision rules. Evaluate whether the authors presented adequate evidence for the reproducibility and validity of these scales. What kind of reproducibility was established? What type of validity? Are these sufficient to warrant the use of the scale? (For example, if you are in-terested in assessing surgical risk for noncardiac surgery, you can consult the articles on an index of cardiac risk by Goldman [1995] and Goldman and associates [1977], as well as a follow-up re-port of an index developed by Detsky and col-leagues [1986].)

Probability & Related Topics for Making Inferences about Data

4

PRESENTING PROBLEMS

Presenting Problem 1. *Neisseria meningitidis,* a gram-negative diplococcus, has as its natural reservoir the human posterior nasopharynx where it can be cultured from 2% to 15% of healthy individuals during nonepidemic periods. The bacterial organism can be typed into at least 13 serogroups based on capsular antigens. These serogroups can be further subdivided by antibodies to specific subcapsular membrane proteins. In the United States, serogroups B and C have accounted for 90% of meningococcal meningitis cases in recent decades. The major manifestations of meningococcal disease are acute septicemia and purulent meningitis. The age-specific attack rate is greatest for children under 5 years of age.

Epidemiologic surveillance data from the state of Oregon detected an increase in the overall incidence rate of meningococcal disease from 2 cases per 100,000 population during 1987–1992 to 4.5 cases per 100,000 population in 1994 (Diermayer et al, 1999). Epidemiologists from Oregon and the Centers for Disease Control wanted to know if the increased numbers of cases of meningococcal disease were indications of a transition from endemic to epidemic disease. The investigators found a significant rise in serogroup B disease; they also discovered that most of the isolates belonged to the ET-5 clonal strain of this serogroup. In addition, a shift toward disease in older age groups, especially 15- through 19-year-olds, was observed.

Information from the study is given in Section 4.2.1. We use these data to illustrate basic concepts of probability and to demonstrate the relationship between time period during the epidemic and site of infection.

Presenting Problem 2. A local blood bank was asked to provide information on the distribution of blood types among males and females. This information is useful in illustrating some basic principles in probability theory. The results are given in Section 4.2.1.

Presenting Problem 3. What do former U. S. Senator and presidential candidate Bob Dole and General Norman Schwartzkopf have in common? They both have been diagnosed with prostate cancer

and talked publicly about it to heighten awareness. In the United States, prostate cancer is the second leading cause of death among men who die of neoplasia, accounting for 12.3% of cancer deaths.

Controversial management issues include when to treat a patient with radical prostatectomy and when to use definitive radiation therapy. Radical prostatectomy is associated with a high incidence of impotence and occasional urinary incontinence. Radiation therapy produces less impotence but can cause radiation cystitis, proctitis, and dermatitis. Prostate specific antigen (PSA) evaluation, available since 1988, leads to early detection of prostate cancer and of recurrence following treatment and may be a valuable prognostic indicator and measure of tumor control after treatment.

Although radical radiation therapy is used to treat prostate cancer in about 60,000 men each year, only a small number of these men from any single institution have had a follow-up of more than 5 years during the era when the PSA test has been available. Shipley and colleagues (1999) wanted to assess the cancer control rates for men treated with external beam radiation therapy alone by pooling data on 1765 men with clinically localized prostate cancer treated at six institutions. The PSA value, along with the Gleason score (a histologic scoring system in which a low score indicates well-differentiated tumor and a high score poorly differentiated tumor) and tumor palpation state, was used to assess pretreatment prognostic factors in the retrospective, nonrandomized, multiinstitutional pooled analysis. A primary treatment outcome was the measurement of survival free from biochemical recurrence. Biochemical recurrence was defined as three consecutive rises in PSA values or any rise great enough to trigger additional treatment with androgen suppression.

Prognostic indicators including pretreatment PSA values indicate the probability of success of treatment with external beam radiation therapy for subsets of patients with prostate cancer. The probabilities of 5-year survival in men with given levels of pretreatment PSA are given in Section 4.5. We use these rates to illustrate the binomial probability distribution.

Presenting Problem 4. The Coronary Artery Surgery Study (CASS, 1983) was a prospective, randomized, multicenter collaborative trial of medical and surgical therapy in subsets of patients with stable ischemic heart disease. This classic study established that the 10-year survival rate in this group of patients was equally good in the medically treated and surgically (coronary revascularization) treated groups (Alderman et al, 1990). A second part of the study compared the effects of medical and surgical treatment on the quality of life.

Over a 5-year period, 780 patients with stable ischemic heart disease were subdivided into three clinical subsets (groups A, B, and C). Patients within each subset were randomly assigned to either medical or surgical treatment. All patients enrolled had 50% or greater stenosis of the left main coronary artery or 70% or greater stenosis of the other operable vessels. In addition, Group A had mild angina and an ejection fraction of at least 50%; group B had mild angina and an ejection fraction less than 50%; group C had no angina after myocardial infarction. History, examination, and treadmill testing were done at 6, 18, and 60 months; a follow-up questionnaire was completed at 6-month intervals. Quality of life was evaluated by assessing chest pain status; heart failure; activity limitation; employment status; recreational status; drug therapy; number of hospitalizations; and risk factor alteration, such as smoking status, blood pressure control, and cholesterol level. Data on number of hospitalizations after mean follow-up of 11 years will be used to illustrate the Poisson probability distribution (Rogers et al, 1990).

Presenting Problem 5. An individual's blood pressure has important health implications; hypertension is among the most commonly treated chronic medical problems. To establish the factors that influence blood pressure and determine what constitutes an abnormal level, the Society of Actuaries (1980) presented data from a study of systolic and diastolic blood pressures in men and women age 15–69 years. The results are summarized in Section 4.4.3.c.

For men and women between the ages of 20 and 39, mean systolic pressure is approximately 120 mm Hg. Standard deviations were approximately 10 for systolic pressure and approximately 8 for diastolic pressure. We use this information to calculate probabilities of patients' having blood pressures at different levels.

4.1 PURPOSE OF THE CHAPTER

The previous chapter presented methods for summarizing information from studies: graphs, plots, and summary statistics. A major reason for performing clinical research, however, is to generalize the findings from the set of observations on one group of subjects to others who are similar to those subjects.

For example, in Presenting Problem 3, Shipley and colleagues (1999) concluded that the initial level of PSA can be used to estimate freedom from biochemical recurrence of tumor. This conclusion was based on their study and follow-up for at least 5 years of 448 men from six institutions. Studying all patients in the world with T1b, T1c, or T2 tumors (but unknown nodal status) is neither possible nor desirable; therefore, the investigators made **inferences** to a larger **population** of patients on the basis of their study of a **sample** of patients. They indicated these data could be used for evidence-based counseling of prostate cancer patients about radiation treatment. They cannot be sure that men with a specific level of pretreatment PSA will respond to treatment as the average man did in this study, but they can use the data to find the **probability** of a positive response.

This chapter discusses concepts that allow investigators to make statements about the probability of possible outcomes, such as long-term survival. First, probability is defined and discussed, and elementary rules for calculating probabilities are given. Methods for selecting a random sample of subjects to be included in a study are then illustrated. **Probability** and **sampling distributions** are introduced, along with examples of how they are used to draw conclusions.

Some people find the concepts presented in this chapter difficult; however, they really are important for an understanding of what statistical inference means—or what investigators mean when they make statements like the following:

> The difference between treatment and control groups was tested by using a *t* test and found to be significantly greater than zero.
> An α value of 0.01 was used for all statistical tests.
> The sample sizes were determined to give 90% power of detecting a difference of 30% between treatment and control groups.

Our experience indicates that the concepts underlying statistical inference are not easily absorbed in a first reading. We suggest the following approach: Read this chapter and become acquainted with the basic concepts. Then, after completing Chapters 5 through 9, read this chapter again. It should be easier to understand the basic ideas of inference using this approach.

4.2 THE MEANING OF THE TERM "PROBABILITY"

Assume that an experiment can be repeated many times, with each replication (repetition) called a **trial;** and assume that one or more outcomes can result from each trial. Then, the **probability** of a given outcome is the number of times that outcome occurs divided by the total number of trials. If the outcome is sure to occur, it has a probability of 1; if an outcome cannot occur, its probability is 0.

An estimate of probability may be determined empirically, or it may be based on a theoretical model. To use a familiar example, we all know that the probability of flipping a fair coin and getting tails is 0.50, or 50%. If a coin is flipped 10 times, there is no guarantee, of course, that exactly 5 tails will be observed; the proportion of tails can range from 0 to 1, although in most cases we expect it to be closer to 0.50 than to 0 or 1. If the coin is flipped 100 times, the chances are even better that the proportion of tails will be close to 0.50, and with 1000 flips, the chances are better still. As the number of flips becomes larger, the proportion of coin flips that result in tails approaches 0.50; therefore, the probability of tails on any one flip is 0.50.

Our definition of probability is sometimes called objective probability, as opposed to **subjective probability,** which reflects a person's opinion, hunch, or best guess about whether an outcome will occur. Subjective probabilities are important in medicine because they form the basis of a physician's opinion about whether a patient has a specific disease. In Chapter 11, we will discuss how this estimate, based on information gained in the history and physical examination, changes as the result of diagnostic procedures.

4.2.1 Basic Definitions & Rules of Probability

Probability concepts are helpful for understanding and interpreting data presented in tables and graphs in published articles. In addition, the concept of probability lets us make statements about how much confidence we have in such estimates as means, proportions, or relative risks (introduced in the previous chapter). Understanding probability is essential for understanding the meaning of P values given in journal articles.

We will use two examples to illustrate some definitions and rules for determining probabilities: Presenting Problem 1 on meningococcal disease (Table 4–1) and the information given in Table 4–2 on gender and blood type. All illustrations of probability assume the observation has been randomly selected from a population of observations. We discuss these concepts in more detail in the next section.

In probability, an **experiment** is defined as any planned process of data collection. For Presenting Problem 1, the experiment is the process of determining the site of infection in patients with meningococcal disease. An experiment consists of a number of independent **trials** (replications) under the same conditions; in this example, a trial consists of determining the site of infection for an individual person. Each trial can result in one of four outcomes: sepsis, meningitis, both sepsis and meningitis, or unknown.

The probability of a particular outcome, say outcome A, is written $P(A)$. The data from Table 4–1 have been condensed into a table on the site of infection with total numbers and are given in Table 4–3. For example, in Table 4–3, if outcome A is sepsis, the probability that a randomly selected person from the study has meningitis without sepsis as the site of infection is

$$P(\text{meningitis alone}) = \frac{110}{408} = 0.27$$

In Presenting Problem 2, the probabilities of different outcomes are already computed. The outcomes of

Table 4–1. Characteristics of serogroup B cases, Oregon, 1987–1996.[a]

		Time Period					
		Preepidemic 1987–1992		Early Epidemic 1993–1994		Recent Epidemic 1995–1996	
		Count	Column %	Count	Column %	Count	Column %
Sex	Men	75	50	59	50	75	53
	Women	75	50	58	50	66	47
Race	White	120	80	94	80	110	78
	African American	5	3	0	0	1	1
	Hispanic	2	1	10	9	11	8
	Native American	2	1	2	2	0	0
	Asian	0	0	0	0	2	1
	Unknown	21	14	11	9	17	12
Site of infection	Sepsis	66	44	45	38	40	28
	Meningitis	39	26	32	27	39	28
	Both	39	26	32	27	34	24
	Unknown	6	4	8	7	28	20
Died during epidemic	No	141	94	108	92	132	94
	Yes	9	6	9	8	9	6

[a]Data are presented as numbers and percentages.
Source: Adapted, with permission, from Diermayer M, Hedberg K, Hoesly F, et al: Epidemic serogroup B meningococcal disease in Oregon. *JAMA* 1999;**281:**1493–1497. Produced with SPSS; used with permission.

Table 4–2. Distribution of blood type by gender.

Blood Type	Probabilities		
	Males	Females	Total
O	0.21	0.21	0.42
A	0.215	0.215	0.43
B	0.055	0.055	0.11
AB	0.02	0.02	0.04
Total	0.50	0.50	1.00

each trial to determine blood type are O, A, B, and AB. From Table 4–2, the probability that a randomly selected person has type A blood is

$$P(\text{type A}) = 0.43$$

The blood type data illustrate two important features of probability:

1. The probability of each outcome (blood type) is greater than or equal to 0.

2. The sum of the probabilities of the various outcomes is 1.

Events may be defined either as single outcomes or as a set of outcomes. For example, the outcomes for the site of infection in the meningitis study are sepsis, meningitis, both, or unknown, but we may wish to define an event as having known meningitis versus not having known meningitis. The event of known meningitis contains the two outcomes of meningitis alone plus both (meningitis and sepsis), and the event of not having known meningitis also contains two outcomes (sepsis and unknown).

Sometimes, we want to know the probability that an event will not happen; an event opposite to the event of interest is called a **complementary event.** For example, the complementary event to "having known meningitis" is "not having known meningitis." The probability of the complement is

$$
\begin{aligned}
P(\text{complement} \\
\text{of known meningitis}) &= P(\text{not known meningitis}) \\
&= P(\text{sepsis or unknown}) \\
&= \frac{151 + 42}{408} = 0.473
\end{aligned}
$$

Note that the probability of a complementary event may also be found as 1 minus the probability of the event itself, and this calculation may be easier in some situations. To illustrate,

$$
\begin{aligned}
P(\text{complement} \\
\text{of known meningitis}) &= 1 - P(\text{known meningitis}) \\
&= 1 - \frac{110 + 105}{408}
\end{aligned}
$$

4.2.2 Mutually Exclusive Events & the Addition Rule

Two or more events are **mutually exclusive** if the occurrence of one precludes the occurrence of the others. For example, a person cannot have both blood type O and blood type A. By definition, all complementary events are also mutually exclusive; however, events can be mutually exclusive without being complementary if three or more events are possible.

As we indicated earlier, what constitutes an event is a matter of definition. Let us define the experiment in Presenting Problem 2 so that each outcome (blood type O, A, B, or AB) is a separate event. The probability of two mutually exclusive events occurring is the probability that either one event occurs *or* the other event occurs. This probability is found by adding the probabilities of the two events, which is called the **addition rule** for probabilities. For example, the probability that a randomly selected person has either blood type O or blood type A is

$$
\begin{aligned}
P(\text{O or A}) &= P(\text{O}) + P(\text{A}) \\
&= 0.42 + 0.43 = 0.85
\end{aligned}
$$

Does the addition rule work for more than two events? The answer is yes, as long as they are all mutually exclusive. We discuss the approach to use with nonmutually exclusive events in Section 4.2.5.

4.2.3 Independent Events & the Multiplication Rule

Two different events are **independent events** if the outcome of one event has no effect on the outcome of the second. Using the blood type example, let us also define a second event as the gender of the

Table 4–3. Site of infection for serogroup B cases, Oregon, 1987–1996.

		Time Period			
		Preepidemic 1987–1992	Early Epidemic 1993–1994	Recent Epidemic 1995–1996	Total
Site of infection	Sepsis	66	45	40	151
	Meningitis	39	32	39	110
	Both	39	32	34	105
	Unknown	6	8	28	42
Total		150	117	141	408

Source: Adapted, with permission, from Diermayer M, Hedberg K, Hoesly F, et al: Epidemic serogroup B meningococcal disease in Oregon. *JAMA* 1999;**281**:1493–1497. Produced with SPSS; used with permission.

person; this event consists of the outcomes male and female. In this example, gender and blood type are independent events; the sex of a person does not affect the person's blood type, and vice versa. The probability of two independent events is the probability that both events occur. This probability is found by multiplying the probabilities of the two events, which is called the **multiplication rule** for probabilities. For example, the probability of being male and of having blood type O is

$$P(\text{male and blood type O}) = P(\text{male}) \times P(\text{blood type O})$$
$$= 0.50 \times 0.42 = 0.21$$

The probability of being male, 0.50, and the probability of having blood type O, 0.42, are both called **marginal probabilities;** that is, they appear on the margins of a probability table. The probability of being male and of having blood type O, 0.21, is called a **joint probability;** it is the probability of both male and type O occurring jointly.

Is having an unknown site of infection independent from the time period of the epidemic in Presenting Problem 1? Table 4–3 gives the data we need to determine the answer to this question. If two events are independent, the product of the marginal probabilities will equal the joint probability in all instances. To show that two events are not independent, we need demonstrate only one instance in which the product of the marginal probabilities is not equal to the joint probability. For example, to show that having an unknown site of infection and preepidemic period are not independent, find the joint probability of a randomly selected person having an unknown site and being diagnosed in the preepidemic period. Table 4–3 shows that

$$P(\text{unknown site and preepidemic}) = \frac{6}{408} = 0.015$$

However, the product of the marginal probabilities does not yield the same result; that is,

$$P(\text{unknown site}) \times P(\text{preepidemic}) = \frac{42}{408} \times \frac{150}{408}$$
$$= 0.103 \times 0.368$$
$$= 0.038$$

We could show that the product of the marginal probabilities is not equal to the joint probability for any of the combinations in this example, but we need show only one instance to prove that two events are not independent.

4.2.4 Nonindependent Events & the Modified Multiplication Rule

Finding the joint probability of two events when they are not independent is a bit more complex than simply multiplying the two marginal probabilities.

When two events are not independent, the occurrence of one event depends on whether the other event has occurred. Let A stand for the event "known meningitis" and B for the event "recent epidemic" (in which known meningitis is having either meningitis alone or meningitis with sepsis). We want to know the probability of event A given event B, written $P(A \mid B)$ where the vertical line, |, is read as "given." In other words, we want to know the probability of event A, assuming that event B has happened. From the data in Table 4–3, the probability of known meningitis, given that the period of interest is the recent epidemic, is

$$P(\text{known meningitis} \mid \text{recent epidemic}) = \frac{39 + 34}{141}$$
$$= 0.518$$

This probability, called a **conditional probability,** is the probability of one event given that another event has occurred. Put another way, the probability of a patient having known meningitis is conditional on the period of the epidemic; it is substituted for $P(\text{known meningitis})$ in the multiplication rule. If we put these expressions together, we can find the joint probability of having known meningitis *and* contracting the disease in the recent epidemic:

$$P(\text{known meningitis and recent epidemic}) = P(\text{known meningitis} \mid \text{recent epidemic})$$
$$\times P(\text{recent epidemic})$$
$$= \frac{39 + 34}{141} \times \frac{141}{408}$$
$$= 0.518 \times 0.346$$
$$= 0.179$$

The probability of having known meningitis during the recent epidemic can also be determined by finding the conditional probability of contracting the disease during the recent epidemic period, given known meningitis, and substituting that expression in the multiplication rule for $P(\text{recent epidemic})$. To illustrate,

$$P(\text{known meningitis and recent epidemic}) = P(\text{recent epidemic and known meningitis})$$
$$= P(\text{recent epidemic} \mid \text{known meningitis})$$
$$\times P(\text{known meningitis})$$
$$= \frac{39 + 34}{110 + 105} \times \frac{110 + 105}{408}$$
$$= 0.340 \times 0.527$$
$$= 0.179$$

4.2.5 Nonmutually Exclusive Events & the Modified Addition Rule

Remember that two or more mutually exclusive events cannot occur together, and the addition rule applies for the calculation of the probability that one or another of the events occurs. Now we find the probability that either of two events occurs when they are not mutually exclusive. For example, gender and blood type O are **nonmutually exclusive events** because the occurrence of one does not preclude the occurrence of the other. The addition rule must be modified in this situation; otherwise, the probability that both events occur will be added into the calculation twice.

In Table 4–2, the probability of being male is 0.50 and the probability of blood type O is 0.42. The probability of being male *or* of having blood type O is not 0.50 + 0.42, however, because in this sum, males with type O blood have been counted twice. The joint probability of being male *and* having blood type O, 0.21, must therefore be subtracted. The calculation is

P(male or
type O) = P(male) + P(type O) − P(male and type O)
    = 0.50 + 0.42 − 0.21
    = 0.71

Of course, if we do not know that P(male *and* type O) = 0.21, we must use the multiplication rule (for independent events, in this case) to determine this probability.

4.2.6 Summary of Rules & an Extension

Let us summarize the rules presented thus far so we can extend them to obtain a particularly useful rule for combining probabilities called **Bayes' theorem.** Remember that questions about mutual exclusiveness use the word "or" and the addition rule; questions about independence use the word "and" and the multiplication rule. We use letters to represent events; A, B, C, and D are four different events with probability $P(A)$, $P(B)$, $P(C)$, and $P(D)$.

The **addition rule** for the occurrence of either of two or more events is as follows: If A, B, and C are mutually exclusive, then

$$P(A \text{ or } B \text{ or } C) = P(A) + P(B) + P(C)$$

If two events such as A and D are not mutually exclusive, then

$$P(A \text{ or } D) = P(A) + P(D) − P(A \text{ and } D)[1]$$

The **multiplication rule** for the occurrence of both of two or more events is as follows: If A, B, and C are independent, then

$$P(A \text{ and } B \text{ and } C) = P(A) \times P(B) \times P(C)$$

---

[1]The probability of three or more events that are not mutually exclusive or not independent involves complex calculations beyond the scope of this book. Interested readers can consult any introductory book on probability.

If two events such as B and D are not independent, then

$$P(B \text{ and } D) = P(B \mid D) \times P(D)$$
or
$$P(D \text{ and } B) = P(D \mid B) \times P(B)$$

The multiplication rule for probabilities when events are not independent can be used to derive one form of an important formula called Bayes' theorem. Because $P(B \text{ and } D)$ equals both $P(B \mid D) \times P(D)$ and $P(B) \times P(D \mid B)$, these latter two expressions are equal. Assuming $P(B)$ and $P(D)$ are not equal to zero, we can solve for one in terms of the other, as follows:

$$P(B \mid D) \times P(D) = P(D \mid B) \times P(B)$$

Then

$$P(B \mid D) = \frac{P(D \mid B) \times P(B)}{P(D)}$$

which is found by dividing both sides of the equation by $P(D)$. Similarly,

$$P(D \mid B) = \frac{P(B \mid D) \times P(D)}{P(B)}$$

In the equation for $P(B \mid D)$, $P(B)$ in the right-hand side of the equation is sometimes called the **prior probability,** because its value is known prior to the calculation; $P(B \mid D)$ is called the **posterior probability,** because its value is known only after the calculation.

The two formulas of Bayes' theorem are important because investigators frequently know only one of the pertinent probabilities and must determine the other. Examples are diagnosis and management, discussed in detail in Chapters 11 and 12.

4.2.7 A Comment on Terminology

Although in everyday use the terms **probability, odds,** and **likelihood** are sometimes used synonymously, mathematicians do not use them that way. **Odds** can best be thought of as the probability that an event occurs divided by the probability that the event does not occur—or as the probability of an event divided by the probability of its complement. For example, the odds that a person has blood type O are 0.42/(1 − 0.42) = 0.72 to 1, but "to 1" is not always stated explicitly. This interpretation is consistent with the meaning of the odds ratio, discussed in Chapter 3. It is also consistent with the use of odds in gaming events such as football games and horse races.

Likelihood may be related to Bayes' theorem for conditional probabilities. Suppose a physician is trying to determine which of three likely diseases a patient has: myocardial infarction, pneumonia, or reflux esophagitis. Chest pain can appear with any one of these three diseases; and the physician needs to know the probability that chest pain occurs with myocardial infarction, the probability that chest pain occurs with pneumonia, and the probability that chest pain occurs with reflux esophagitis. The probabilities of a given outcome (chest pain) when evaluated under different hypotheses (myocardial infarction, pneumonia, and reflux esophagitis) are called likelihoods of the hypotheses (or diseases).

4.3 POPULATIONS & SAMPLES

A major purpose of doing research is to infer, or generalize, from a sample to a larger population. This process of **inference** is accomplished by using statistical methods based on probability. **Population** is the term statisticians use to describe a large set or collection of items that have something in common. In the health field, population generally refers to patients or other living organisms, but the term can also be used to denote collections of inanimate objects, such as sets of autopsy reports, hospital charges, or birth certificates. A **sample** is a subset of the population, selected so as to be representative of the larger population.

There are many good reasons for studying a sample instead of an entire population, and the four commonly used methods for selecting a sample are discussed in this section. Before turning to those topics, however, we note that the term "population" is frequently misused to describe what is, in fact, a sample. For example, researchers sometimes refer to the "population of patients in this study." After you have read this book, you will be able to spot such errors when you see them in the medical literature. If you want more information, Levy and Lemeshow (1999) provide a comprehensive treatment of sampling.

4.3.1 Reasons for Sampling

There are at least six reasons to study samples instead of populations:

1. Samples can be studied *more quickly* than populations. Speed can be important if a physician needs to determine something quickly, such as a vaccine or treatment for a new disease.

2. A study of a sample is *less expensive* than studying an entire population, because a smaller number of items or subjects are examined. This consideration is especially important in the design of large studies that require a lengthy follow-up.

3. A study of an entire population (census) is *impossible* in most situations. Sometimes, the process of the study destroys or depletes the item being studied. For example, in a study of cartilage healing in limbs of rats after 6 weeks of limb immobilization, the animals may be sacrificed in order to perform histologic studies. On other occasions, the desire is to

infer to future events, such as the study of men with prostate cancer. In these cases, a study of a population is impossible.

4. Sample results are often *more accurate* than results based on a population. For samples, more time and resources can be spent on training the people who perform observations and collect data. In addition, more expensive procedures that improve accuracy can be used for a sample because fewer procedures are required.

5. If samples are properly selected, probability methods can be used to *estimate the error* in the resulting statistics. It is this aspect of sampling that permits investigators to make probability statements about observations in a study.

6. Samples can be selected to *reduce heterogeneity*. For example, systemic lupus erythematosus (SLE) has many clinical manifestations, resulting in a heterogeneous population. A sample of the population with specified characteristics is more appropriate than the entire population for the study of certain aspects of the disease.

To summarize, bigger does not always mean better in terms of sample sizes. Thus, investigators must plan the sample size appropriate for their study prior to beginning research. This process is called determining the **power** of a study and is discussed in detail in later chapters. See Abramson (1999) for an introductory discussion of sampling.

4.3.2 Methods of Sampling

The best way to ensure that a sample will lead to reliable and valid inferences is to use **probability samples,** in which the probability of being included in the sample is known for each subject in the population. Four commonly used probability sampling methods in medicine are simple random sampling, systematic sampling, stratified sampling, and cluster sampling, all of which use random processes.

The following example illustrates each method: Consider a physician applying for a grant for a study that involves measuring the tracheal diameter on radiographs. The physician wants to convince the granting agency that these measurements are reliable. To estimate **intrarater** reliability, the physician will select a sample of chest x-ray films from those performed during the previous year, remeasure the tracheal diameter, and compare the new measurement with the original one on file in the patient's chart. The physician has a population of 3400 radiographs, and we assume that the physician has learned that a sample of 200 films is sufficient to provide an accurate estimate of intrarater reliability. Now the physician must select the sample for the reliability study.

4.3.2.a Simple Random Sampling: A **simple random sample** is one in which every subject (every film in the example) has an equal probability of being selected for the study. The recommended way to select a simple random sample is to use a table of random numbers or a computer-generated list of random numbers. For this approach, each x-ray film must have an identification (ID) number, and a list of ID numbers, called a **sampling frame,** must be available. For the sake of simplicity, assume that the radiographs are numbered from 1 to 3400. Using a random number table, after first identifying a starting place in the table at random, the physician can select the first 200 digits between 1 and 3400. The x-ray films with the ID numbers corresponding to 200 random numbers make up the simple random sample. If a computer-generated list of random numbers is available, the physician can request 200 numbers between 1 and 3400. To illustrate the process with a random number table, a portion of Table A–1 in Appendix A is reproduced as Table 4–4. One way to select a starting point is by tossing a die to select a row and a column at random. Tossing a die twice determines, first, which block of *rows* and, second, which individual row within the block contains our number. For example, if we throw a 2 and a 3, we begin in the second block down, third row, beginning with the number 83. (If, on our second throw, we had thrown a 6, we would toss the die again, because there are only five rows.) Now, we must select a beginning *column* at random, again by tossing the die twice to select a block and a column within the block. For example, if we toss a 3 and a 1, we use the third block (across) of columns and the first column, headed by the number 1. The starting point in this example is therefore located where the row beginning with 83 and the column beginning with 1 intersect at the number 6 (underlined in Table 4–4).

Because there are 3400 radiographs, we must read four-digit numbers; the first ten numbers are 6221,

7678, 9781, 2624, 8060, 7562, 5288, 1071, 3988, and 8549. The numbers less than 3401 are the IDs of the films to be used in the sample. In the first ten numbers selected, only two are less than 3401; so we use films with the ID numbers 2624 and 1071. This procedure continues until we have selected 200 radiographs. When the number in the bottom row (7819) is reached, we go to the top of that same column and move one digit to the right for numbers 6811, 1465, 3226, and so on.

If a number less than 3401 occurs twice, the x-ray film with that ID number can be selected for the sample and used in the study a second time (called sampling with replacement). In this case, the final sample of 200 will be 200 measurements rather than 200 radiographs. Frequently, however, when a number occurs twice, it is ignored the second time and the next eligible number is used instead (called sampling without replacement). The differences between these two procedures are negligible when we sample from a large population.

4.3.2.b Systematic Sampling: A **systematic random sample** is one in which every kth item is selected; k is determined by dividing the number of items in the sampling frame by the desired sample size. For example, 3400 radiographs divided by 200 is 17, so every 17th x-ray film is sampled. In this approach, we must select a number randomly between 1 and 17 first, and we then select every 17th film. Suppose we randomly select the number 12 from a random number table. Then, the systematic sample consists of radiographs with ID numbers 12, 29, 46, 63, 80, and so on; each subsequent number is determined by adding 17 to the last ID number.

Systematic sampling should not be used when a cyclic repetition is inherent in the sampling frame.

Table 4–4. Random numbers.

927415	956121	168117	169280	326569	266541
926937	515107	014658	159944	821115	317592
867169	388342	832261	993050	639410	698969
867169	542747	032683	131188	926198	371071
512500	843384	085361	398488	774767	383837
062454	423050	670884	840940	845839	979662
806702	881309	772977	367506	729850	457758
837815	163631	622143	938278	231305	219737
926839	453853	767825	284716	916182	467113
854813	731620	978100	589512	147694	389180
851595	452454	262448	688990	461777	647487
449353	556695	806050	123754	722070	935916
169116	586865	756231	469281	258737	989450
139470	358095	528858	660128	342072	681203
433775	761861	107191	515960	759056	150336
221922	232624	398839	495004	881970	792001
740207	078048	854928	875559	246288	000144
525873	755998	866034	444933	785944	018016
734185	499711	254256	616625	243045	251938
773112	463857	781983	078184	380752	492215

For example, systemic sampling is not appropriate for selecting months of the year in a study of the frequency of different types of accidents, because some accidents occur more often at certain times of the year. For instance, skiing injuries and automobile accidents most often occur in cold-weather months, whereas swimming injuries and farming accidents most often occur in warm-weather months.

4.3.2.c Stratified Sampling: A **stratified random sample** is one in which the population is first divided into relevant strata (subgroups), and a random sample is then selected from each stratum. In the radiograph example, the physician may wish to stratify on the age of patients, because the trachea varies in size with age and measuring the diameter accurately in young patients may be difficult. The population of radiographs may be divided into infants younger than 1 year old, children from 1 year old to less than 6 years old, children from 6 to younger than 16 years old, and subjects 16 years of age or older; a random sample is then selected from each age stratum. Other commonly used strata in medicine besides age include gender of patient, severity or stage of disease, and duration of disease. Characteristics used to stratify should be related to the measurement of interest, in which case stratified random sampling is the most efficient, meaning that it requires the smallest sample size.

4.3.2.d Cluster Sampling: A **cluster random sample** results from a two-stage process in which the population is divided into clusters and a subset of the clusters is randomly selected. Clusters are commonly based on geographic areas or districts, so this approach is used more often in epidemiologic research than in clinical studies. For example, the sample for a household survey taken in a city may be selected by using city blocks as clusters; a random sample of city blocks is selected, and all households (or a random sample of households) within the selected city blocks are surveyed. In multicenter trials, the institutions selected to participate in the study constitute the clusters; patients from each institution can be selected using another random-sampling procedure. Cluster sampling is somewhat less efficient than the other sampling methods, because it requires a larger sample size, but in some situations, such as in multicenter trials, it is the method of choice for obtaining adequate numbers of patients.

4.3.2.e Nonprobability Sampling: The sampling methods just discussed are all based on probability, but nonprobability sampling methods also exist, such as convenience samples or quota samples. **Nonprobability samples** are those in which the probability that a subject is selected is unknown. Nonprobability samples often reflect selection biases of the person doing the study and do not fulfill the requirements of randomness needed to estimate sampling errors. When we use the term "sample" in the context of observational studies, we will assume that the sample has been randomly selected in an appropriate way.

4.3.2.f Random Assignment: Random sampling methods are used when a sample of subjects is selected from a population of possible subjects in observational studies, such as cohort, case–control, and cross-sectional studies. In experimental studies such as randomized clinical trials, subjects are first selected for inclusion in the study on the basis of appropriate criteria; they are then assigned to different treatment modalities. If the assignment of subjects to treatments is done by using random methods, the process is called **random assignment.** Random assignment may also occur by randomly assigning treatments to subjects. In either case, random assignment helps ensure that the groups receiving the different treatment modalities are as similar as possible. Thus, any differences in outcome at the conclusion of the study are more likely to be the result of differences in the treatments used in the study rather than differences in the compositions of the groups.

Random assignment is best carried out by using random numbers. As an example, consider the CASS study (1983), in which patients meeting the entry criteria were divided into clinical subsets and then randomly assigned to either medical or surgical treatment. Random assignment in this study could have been accomplished by using a list of random numbers (obtained from a computer or a random number table) and assigning the random numbers to patients as they entered the trial. If a study involves several investigators at different sites, such as in a multicenter trial, the investigator preparing to enter an eligible patient in the study may call a central office to learn which treatment assignment is next. As an alternative, separately randomized lists may be generated for each site. Of course, in **double-blind** studies, someone other than the investigator must keep the list of random assignments.

Suppose investigators in the CASS study wanted an equal number of patients at each site participating in the study. For this design, the assignment of random numbers might have been balanced within blocks of patients of a predetermined size. For example, balancing patients within blocks of 12 would guarantee that every time 12 patients entered the study at a given site, 6 patients received the medical treatment and 6 received the surgical treatment. Within the block of 12 patients, however, assignment would be random until 6 patients were assigned to one or the other of the treatments.

A study design may match subjects on important characteristics, such as gender, age group, or severity of disease, and then make the random assignment. This stratified assignment controls for possible confounding effects of the characteristic(s); it is equivalent to stratified random sampling in observational studies.

Many types of biases may result in studies in which patients are not randomly assigned to treatment modalities. For instance, early studies comparing medical and surgical treatment for coronary artery disease did not randomly assign patients to treatments and were criticized as a result. Some critics claimed that sicker patients were not candidates for surgery, and thus, the group receiving surgery was biased by having healthier subjects. Other critics stated that the healthier patients were given medical treatment because their disease was not as serious as that of the sicker patients. In nonrandomized studies, the problem is determining which biases are operating and which conclusions are appropriate; in fact, the CASS study was designed partly in response to these criticisms. A description of different kinds of biases that threaten the validity of studies is given in Chapter 13.

4.3.2.g Using and Interpreting Random Samples:

In actual clinical studies, patients are not always randomly selected from the population from which the investigator wishes to infer. Instead, the clinical researcher often uses all patients at hand who meet the entry criteria for the study. This practical procedure is used especially when studies involve rather uncommon conditions. Colton (1974) makes a useful distinction between the target population and the sampled population. The **target population** is the population to which the investigator wishes to generalize; the **sampled population** is the population from which the sample was actually drawn. Figure 4–1 presents a scheme of these concepts.

For example, Shipley and colleagues (1999) in Presenting Problem 3 clearly wished to generalize their findings about survival to all men with localized prostate cancer, such as patients who live in other locations and perhaps even patients who do not yet have the disease. The sample was the set of patients at six medical centers with T1b, T1c, and T2 tumors treated between 1988 and 1995 using external beam radiation. Statistical inference permits generalization from the sample to the population sampled. In order to make inferences from the population sampled to the target population, we must ask whether the population sampled is representative of the target population. A **population** (or sample) is **representative** of the target population if the distribution of important characteristics in the sampled population is the same as that in the target population. This judgment is clinical, not statistical. It points to the importance of always reading the Method section of journal articles to learn what population was actually sampled so that you can determine the representativeness of that population.

4.3.3 Population Parameters & Sample Statistics

Statisticians use precise language to describe characteristics of populations and samples. Measures of central tendency and variation, such as the mean and the standard deviation, are fixed and invariant charac-

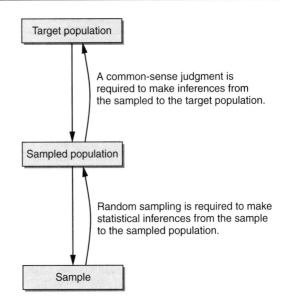

Figure 4–1. Target and sampled populations.

teristics in populations and are called **parameters.** In samples, however, the observed mean or standard deviation calculated on the basis of the sample information is actually an estimate of the population mean or standard deviation; these estimates are called **statistics.** Statisticians customarily use Greek letters for population parameters and Roman letters for sample statistics. Some of the frequently encountered symbols used in this text are summarized in Table 4–5.

4.4 RANDOM VARIABLES & PROBABILITY DISTRIBUTIONS

The characteristic of interest in a study is called a **variable.** Diermayer and colleagues (1999) examined several variables for the study described in Presenting Problem 1, such as sex, race, site of infection, and period in the epidemic during which the patient contracted the disease. The term "variable" makes sense because the value of the characteristic varies from one subject to another. This variation results from in-

Table 4–5. Commonly used symbols for parameters and statistics.

Characteristic	Parameter Symbol	Statistical Symbol
Mean	μ	$\bar{X}$
Standard deviation	σ	SD
Variance	σ^2	s^2
Correlation	ρ	r
Proportion	π	p

herent biologic variation among individuals and from errors, called measurement errors, made in measuring and recording a subject's value on a characteristic. A **random variable** is a variable in a study in which subjects are randomly selected. If the subjects in Presenting Problem 1 are a random sample selected from a larger population of citizens, then sex, race, and site of infection are examples of random variables.

Just as values of characteristics, such as site of infection or PSA level, can be summarized in frequency distributions, values of a random variable can be summarized in a frequency distribution called a **probability distribution.** For example, if X is a random variable defined as the PSA level prior to treatment in Presenting Problem 3, X can take on any value between 0.1 and 2500; and we can determine the probability that the random variable X has any given value or range of values. For instance, from Box 4–1, the probability that $X < 10$ is 130/799, or

0.163 (or about 1 in 6). In some applications, a formula or rule will adequately describe a distribution; the formula can then be used to calculate the probability of interest. In other situations, a theoretical probability distribution provides a good fit to the distribution of the variable of interest.

Several theoretical probability distributions are important in statistics, and we shall examine three that are useful in medicine. Both the binomial and the Poisson are *discrete* probability distributions; that is, the associated random variable takes only integer values, 0, 1, 2,..., n. The normal (gaussian) distribution is a *continuous* probability distribution; that is, the associated random variable has values measured on a continuous scale. We will examine the binomial and Poisson distributions briefly, using examples from the presenting problems to illustrate each; then we will discuss the normal distribution in greater detail.

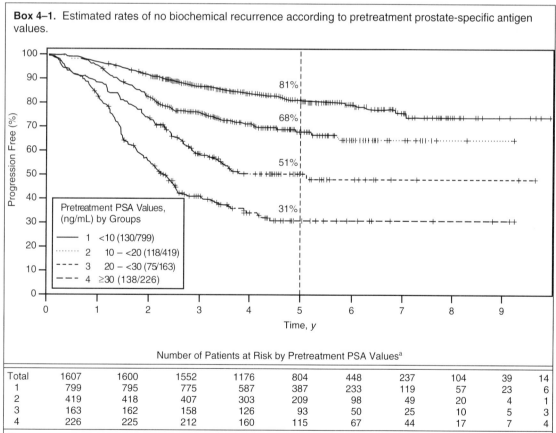

Box 4–1. Estimated rates of no biochemical recurrence according to pretreatment prostate-specific antigen values.

Pretreatment PSA Values, (ng/mL) by Groups
— 1   <10 (130/799)
······ 2   10 – <20 (118/419)
---- 3   20 – <30 (75/163)
--- 4   ≥30 (138/226)

Number of Patients at Risk by Pretreatment PSA Values[a]

Total	1607	1600	1552	1176	804	448	237	104	39	14
1	799	795	775	587	387	233	119	57	23	6
2	419	418	407	303	209	98	49	20	4	1
3	163	162	158	126	93	50	25	10	5	3
4	226	225	212	160	115	67	44	17	7	4

[a]Data represent 1607 patients with stage T1b, T1c, T2, and NX tumors; $P < 0.001$ for all groups. PSA = prostate-specific antigen. Reproduced, with permission, from Shipley WU et al: Radiation therapy for clinically localized prostate cancer: A multiinstitutional pooled analysis. *JAMA* 1999;**281**:1598–1604.

4.4.1 The Binomial Distribution

Suppose an event can have only binary outcomes (eg, yes and no, or positive and negative), denoted A and B. The probability of A is denoted by π, or $P(A) = \pi$, and this probability stays the same each time the event occurs. The probability of B must therefore be $1 - \pi$, because B occurs if A does not. If an experiment involving this event is repeated n times and the outcome is independent from one trial to another, what is the probability that outcome A occurs exactly X times? Or equivalently, what proportion of the n outcomes will be A? These questions frequently are of interest, especially in basic science research, and they can be answered with the binomial distribution.

Basic principles of the binomial distribution were developed by the 17th century Swiss mathematician Jakob Bernoulli, who made many contributions to probability theory. He was the author of what is generally acknowledged as the first book devoted to probability, published in 1713. In fact, in his honor, each trial involving a binomial probability is sometimes called a Bernoulli trial, and a sequence of trials is called a Bernoulli process. The **binomial distribution** gives the probability that a specified outcome occurs in a given number of independent trials. The binomial distribution can be used to model the inheritability of a particular trait in genetics, to estimate the occurrence of a specific reaction (eg, the single packet, or quantal release, of acetylcholine at the neuromuscular junction), or to estimate the death of a cancer cell in an in vitro test of a new chemotherapeutic agent.

We use the information collected by Shipley and colleagues (1999) in Presenting Problem 3 to illustrate the binomial distribution. Assume, for a moment, that the entire population of men with a localized prostate tumor and a pretreatment PSA < 10 has been studied, and the probability of 5-year survival is equal to 0.8 (we use 0.8 for computational convenience, rather than 0.81 as reported in the study). Let S represent the event of 5-year survival and D represent death before 5 years; then, $\pi = P(S) = 0.8$ and $1 - \pi = P(D) = 0.2$. Consider a group of $n = 2$ men with a localized prostate tumor and a pretreatment PSA < 10. What is the probability that exactly two men live 5 years? That exactly one lives 5 years? That none lives 5 years? These probabilities are found by using the multiplication and addition rules outlined earlier in this chapter.

The probability that exactly two men live 5 years is found by using the multiplication rule for independent events. We know that $P(S) = 0.8$ for patient 1 and $P(S) = 0.8$ for patient 2. Because the survival of one patient is independent from (has no effect on) the survival of the other patient, the probability of *both* surviving is

$$P(S \text{ for patient 1 and } S \text{ for patient 2}) = P(S) \, P(S)$$
$$= (0.8)(0.8) = 0.64$$

The event of exactly one patient living 5 years can occur in two ways: patient 1 survives 5 years and patient 2 does not, or patient 2 survives 5 years and patient 1 does not. These two events are mutually exclusive; therefore, after using the multiplication rule to obtain the probability of each event, we can use the addition rule for mutually exclusive events to combine the probabilities as follows:

$$P(S \text{ for patient 1 and } D \text{ for patient 2}) = P(S) \, P(D)$$
$$= (0.8)(0.2)$$
$$= 0.16$$

and

$$P(D \text{ for patient 1 and } S \text{ for patient 2}) = P(D) \, P(S)$$
$$= (0.2)(0.8)$$
$$= 0.16$$

Therefore,

$$P(\text{event 1 or event 2}) = 0.16 + 0.16$$
$$= 0.32$$

Finally, the probability that neither lives 5 years is

$$P(D \text{ for patient 1 and } D \text{ for patient 2}) = P(D) \, P(D)$$
$$= (0.2)(0.2)$$
$$= 0.04$$

These computational steps are summarized in Table 4–6. Note that the total probability is

$$(0.8)^2 + 2(0.8)(0.2) + (0.2)^2 = 1.0$$

which you may recognize as the binomial formula, $(a + b)^2 = a^2 + 2ab + b^2$.

The same process can be applied for a group of patients of any size or for any number of trials, but it becomes quite tedious. An easier technique is to use the formula for the binomial distribution, which follows. The probability of X outcomes in a group of size n, if each outcome has probability π and is independent from all other outcomes, is given by

$$P(X) = \frac{n!}{X!(n - X)!} \, \pi^X (1 - \pi)^{n - X}$$

where ! is the symbol for factorial; $n!$ is called n factorial and is equal to the product $n(n-1)(n-2)\cdots(3)(2)(1)$.

Table 4–6. Summary of probabilities for two patients.

Outcome		Number of Ways to Occur	Probability
First Patient	Second Patient		
S	S	1	$0.8 \times 0.8 = 0.64$
D	S	} 2	$2 \times 0.8 \times 0.2 = 0.32$
S	D		
D	D	1	$0.2 \times 0.2 = 0.04$

For example, $4! = (4)(3)(2)(1) = 24$. The number $0!$ is defined as 1. The symbol π^X indicates that the probability is raised to the power X, and $(1 - \pi)^{n-X}$ means that 1 minus the probability is raised to the power $n - X$. The expression $n!/[X!(n - X)!]$ is sometimes referred to as the formula for **combinations** because it gives the number of combinations (or assortments) of X items possible among the n items in the group.

To verify that the probability that exactly $X = 1$ of $n = 2$ patients survives 5 years is 0.32, we use the formula:

$$P(1) = \frac{2!}{1!(2 - 1)!} (0.8)^1 (1 - 0.8)^{2-1}$$

$$= \frac{(2)(1)}{1(1)} (0.8)(0.2)$$

$$= 2(0.8)(0.2)$$

$$= 0.32$$

To summarize, the binomial distribution is useful for answering questions about the probability of X number of occurrences in n independent trials when there is a constant probability π of success on each trial. For example, suppose a new series of men with prostate tumors is begun with ten patients. We can use the binomial distribution to calculate the probability that any particular number of them will survive 5 years. For instance, the probability that all ten will survive 5 years is

$$P(10) = \frac{10!}{10!(10 - 10)!} (0.8)^{10} (1 - 0.8)^{10-10}$$

$$= \frac{10!}{(10!)(0!)} (0.8)^{10} (0.2)^0$$

$$= (1)(0.8)^{10}(1)$$

$$= 0.107$$

Similarly, the probability that exactly eight patients will survive 5 years is

$$P(8) = \frac{10!}{8!(10 - 8)!} (0.8)^8 (1 - 0.8)^{10-8}$$

$$= \frac{10(9)(8!)}{(8!)(2!)} (0.8)^8 (0.2)^2$$

$$= \frac{10(9)}{(2)(1)} (0.168)(0.04)$$

$$= (45)(0.168)(0.04)$$

$$= 0.302$$

Table 4–7 lists the probabilities for $X = 0, 1, 2, 3, \ldots,$ 10; a plot of the binomial distribution when $n = 10$ and $\pi = 0.8$ is given in Figure 4–2. The mean of the binomial distribution is $n\pi$; so $(10)(0.8) = 8$ is the mean number of patients surviving 10 years in this example. The standard deviation is

$$\sqrt{n\pi(1 - \pi)}$$

which for this example is

$$\sqrt{10(0.8)(0.2)} = 1.265$$

Table 4–7. Probabilities for binomial distribution with $n = 10$ and $\pi = 0.8$

Number of Patients Surviving	$\dfrac{n!}{X!(n - X)!}$	π^X	$(1 - \pi)^{n-x}$	$P(X)^a$
0	1	1	0.0000001	0
1	10	0.8	0.0000005	0
2	45	0.64	0.0000026	0.0001
3	120	0.512	0.0000128	0.0008
4	210	0.410	0.000064	0.0055
5	252	0.328	0.00032	0.0264
6	210	0.262	0.0016	0.0881
7	120	0.210	0.008	0.2013
8	45	0.168	0.04	0.3020
9	10	0.134	0.2	0.2684
10	1	0.107	1	0.1074

^{a}Rounded to four decimal places.

Thus, the only two pieces of information needed to define a binomial distribution are n and π, which are called the parameters of the binomial distribution. Studies involving dichotomous, or binary, variables often use a proportion rather than a number (eg, the proportion of patients surviving a given length of time rather than the number of patients). When a proportion is used instead of a number of successes, the same two pieces of information (n and π) are needed. Because the proportion is found by dividing X by n, however, the mean of the distribution of the proportion becomes π, and the standard deviation becomes

$$\sqrt{\frac{\pi(1 - \pi)}{n}}$$

Even using the formula for the binomial distribution becomes time-consuming, especially if the numbers are large. Also, the formula gives the probability of observing exactly X successes, and interest fre-

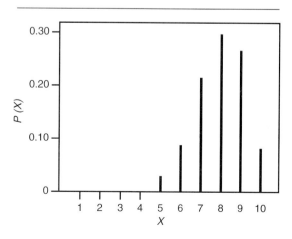

Figure 4–2. Binomial distribution for $n = 10$ and $\pi = 0.8$.

quently lies in knowing the probability of X or more successes or of X or less successes. For example, to find the probability that eight or more patients will survive 5 or more years, we must use the formula to find the separate probabilities that eight will survive, nine will survive, and ten will survive and then sum these results; from Table 4–7, we obtain $P(X \geq 8) = P(X = 8) + P(X = 9) + P(X = 10) = 0.3020 + 0.2684 + 0.1074 = 0.6778$. Tables giving probabilities for the binomial distribution are presented in many elementary texts. Much research in the health field is conducted with samples sizes large enough to use an approximation to the binomial distribution; this approximation is discussed in Chapter 5.

4.4.2 The Poisson Distribution

The Poisson distribution is named for the French mathematician who derived it, Siméon D. Poisson. Like the binomial, the Poisson distribution is a discrete distribution applicable when the outcome is the number of times an event occurs. The **Poisson distribution** can be used to determine the probability of rare events; that is, it gives the probability that an outcome occurs a specified number of times when the number of trials is large and the probability of any one occurrence is small. For instance, the Poisson distribution is used to plan the number of beds a hospital needs in its intensive care unit, the number of ambulances needed on call, or the number of operators needed on a switchboard to ensure that an adequate number of resources is available. It can also be used to model the number of cells in a given volume of fluid, the number of bacterial colonies growing in a certain amount of medium, or the emission of radioactive particles from a specified amount of radioactive material.

Consider a random variable representing the number of times an event occurs in a given time or space interval. Then the probability of exactly X occurrences is given by the formula:

$$P(X) = \frac{\lambda^X e^{-\lambda}}{X!}$$

in which λ (the lowercase Greek letter lambda) is the value of both the mean and the variance of the Poisson distribution, and e is the base of the natural logarithms, equal to 2.718. The term λ is called the parameter of the Poisson distribution, just as n and π are the parameters of the binomial distribution. Only one piece of information, λ, is therefore needed to characterize any given Poisson distribution.

A random variable having a Poisson distribution was used in the Coronary Artery Surgery Study (Rogers et al, 1990) summarized in Presenting Problem 4. The number of hospitalizations for each group of patients (medical and surgical) followed Poisson distributions. This model is appropriate because the chance that a patient goes into the hospital during any one time interval is small and can be assumed to be independent from patient to patient. After mean follow-up of 11 years, the 390 patients randomized to the medical group were hospitalized a total of 1256 times; the 390 patients randomized to the surgical group were hospitalized a total of 1487 times. The mean number of hospitalizations for medical patients is $1256/390 = 3.22$, and the mean for the surgical patients is $1487/390 = 3.81$. We can use this information and the formula for the Poisson model to calculate probabilities of numbers of hospitalizations. For example, the probability that a patient in the medical group has zero hospitalizations is

$$\begin{aligned} P(X = 0) &= \frac{3.22^0 e^{-3.22}}{0!} \\ &= \frac{(1)(0.04)}{1} \\ &= 0.04 \end{aligned}$$

The probability that a patient has exactly one hospitalization is

$$\begin{aligned} P(X = 1) &= \frac{3.22^1 e^{-3.22}}{1!} \\ &= \frac{(3.22)(0.04)}{1} \\ &= 0.129 \end{aligned}$$

The calculations for the Poisson distribution when $\lambda = 3.22$ and $X = 0, 1, 2, \ldots, 7$ are given in Table 4–8.

Figure 4–3 is a graph of the Poisson distribution for $\lambda = 3.22$. The mean of the distribution is between 3 and 4 (actually, it is 3.22). Note the slight positive skew of the Poisson distribution; the skew becomes more pronounced as λ becomes smaller.

4.4.3 The Normal (Gaussian) Distribution

We now turn to the most famous probability distribution in statistics, called the normal, or gaussian, distribution (or bell-shaped curve). The normal curve was first discovered by French mathematician Abraham de Moivre and published in 1733. Two

Table 4–8. Probabilities for Poisson distribution with $\lambda = 3.22$.

Number of Hospitalizations	3.22^a	$e^{-3.22}$	$X!$	$P(X)^a$
0	1	0.040	0	0.040
1	3.22	0.040	1	0.129
2	10.37	0.040	2	0.207
3	33.39	0.040	6	0.223
4	107.50	0.040	24	0.179
5	346.16	0.040	120	0.115
6	1114.64	0.040	720	0.062
7	3589.15	0.040	5040	0.028

[a]Rounded to three decimal places.

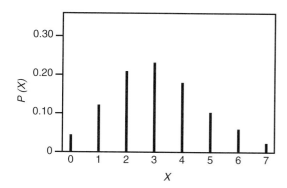

Figure 4–3. Poisson distribution for $\lambda = 3.22$.

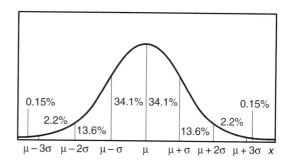

Figure 4–4. Normal distribution and percentage of area under the curve.

mathematician-astronomers, however, Pierre-Simon Laplace from France and Karl Friedrich Gauss from Germany, were responsible for establishing the scientific principles of the normal distribution. Many consider Laplace to have made the greatest contributions to probability theory, but Gauss' name was given to the distribution after he applied it to the theory of the motions of heavenly bodies. Some statisticians prefer to use the term *gaussian* instead of "normal" because the latter term has the unfortunate (and incorrect) connotation that the normal curve describes the way characteristics are distributed in populations composed of "normal"—as opposed to sick—individuals. We use the term "normal" in this text, however, because it is more frequently used in the medical literature.

4.4.3.a Describing the Normal Distribution: The normal distribution is continuous, so it can take on any value (not just integers, as do the binomial and Poisson distributions). It is a smooth, bell-shaped curve and is symmetric about the mean of the distribution, symbolized by μ (Greek letter mu). The curve is shown in Figure 4–4. The standard deviation of the distribution is symbolized by σ (Greek letter sigma); σ is the horizontal distance between the mean and the point of inflection on the curve. The point of inflection is the point where the curve changes from convex to concave. The mean and the standard deviation (or variance) are the two parameters of the normal distribution and completely determine the location on the number line and the shape of a normal curve. Thus, many different normal curves are possible, one each for every value of the mean and the standard deviation. Because the normal distribution is a probability distribution, the area under the curve is equal to 1. (Recall that one of the properties of probability is that the sum of the probabilities for any given set of events is equal to 1.) Because it is a **symmetric distribution,** half the area is on the left of the mean and half is on the right.

Given a random variable X that can take on any value between negative and positive infinity ($-\infty$ and

$+\infty$), (∞ represents infinity), the formula for the normal distribution is as follows:

$$\int_{-\infty}^{+\infty} \frac{1}{\sqrt{2\pi\sigma^2}} \exp\left[-\frac{1}{2}\left(\frac{X-\mu}{\sigma}\right)^2\right]$$

where exp stands for the base e of the natural logarithm and $\pi = 3.1416$. The function depends only on the mean μ and standard deviation σ because they are the only components that vary.

Because the area under the curve is equal to 1, we can use the curve for calculating probabilities. For example, to find the probability that an observation falls between a and b on the curve in Figure 4–5, we integrate the preceding equation between a and b, where $-\infty$ is given the value a and $+\infty$ is given the value b. (Integration is a mathematical technique in calculus used to find area under a curve.)

4.4.3.b The Standard Normal (z) Distribution: Fortunately, there is no need to integrate this function because tables for it are available. So that we do not need a different table for every value of μ and σ, however, we use the **standard normal curve (distribution)**, which has a mean of 0 and a standard deviation of 1, as shown in Figure 4–6. This curve is also called the z **distribution.** Table A–2 (see Appendix A)

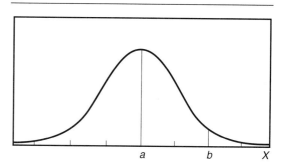

Figure 4–5. Area under a normal curve between a and b.

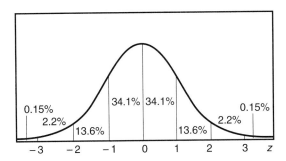

Figure 4–6. Standard normal (*z*) distribution.

gives the area under the curve between −*z* and +*z*, the sum of the areas to the left of −*z* and the right of +*z*, and the area to either the left of −*z* or the right of +*z*.

Before we use Table A–2, look at the standard normal distribution in Figure 4–6 and estimate the proportion (or percentage) of these areas:

1. Above 1
2. Below −1
3. Above 2
4. Below −2
5. Between −1 and 1
6. Between −2 and 2

Now turn to Table A–2 and find the designated areas. The answers follow.

1. 0.159 of the area is to the right of 1 (from the fourth column in Table A–2).

2. Table A–2 does not list values for *z* less than 0; however, because the distribution is symmetric about 0, the area below −1 is the same as the area to the right of 1, which is 0.159.

3. 0.023 of the area is to the right of 2 (from the fourth column in Table A–2).

4. The same reasoning as in answer 2 applies here; so 0.023 of the area is to the left of −2.

5. 0.683 of the area is between −1 and 1 (from the second column in Table A–2).

6. 0.954 of the area is between −2 and 2 (from the second column in Table A–2).

When the mean of a gaussian distribution is not 0 and the standard deviation is not 1, a simple transformation, called the *z* transformation, must be made so that we can use the standard normal table. The *z* transformation expresses the deviation from the mean in standard deviation units. That is, any normal distribution can be transformed to the standard normal distribution by using the following steps:

1. Move the distribution up or down the number line so that the mean is 0. This step is accomplished by subtracting the mean μ from the value for *X*.

2. Make the distribution either narrower or wider so that the standard deviation is equal to 1. This step is accomplished by dividing by σ.

To summarize, the transformed value is

$$z = \frac{X - \mu}{\sigma}$$

and is variously called a *z* **score,** a normal deviate, a standard score, or a **critical ratio.**

4.4.3.c Examples Using the Standard Normal Distribution: To illustrate the standard normal distribution, we consider Presenting Problem 5, assuming systolic blood pressure (BP) in normal healthy individuals is normally distributed with μ = 120 and σ = 10 mm Hg (Table 4–9). Make the appropriate transformations to answer the following questions. (*Hint:* Make sketches of the distribution to be sure you are finding the correct area.)

1. What area of the curve is above 130 mm Hg?
2. What area of the curve is above 140 mm Hg?
3. What area of the curve is between 100 and 140 mm Hg?
4. What area of the curve is above 150 mm Hg?
5. What area of the curve is either below 90 mm Hg or above 150 mm Hg?
6. What is the value of the systolic blood pressure that divides the area under the curve into the lower 95% and the upper 5%?
7. What is the value of the systolic blood pressure that divides the area under the curve into the lower 97.5% and the upper 2.5%?

The answers, referring to the sketches in Figure 4–7, are shown in the following list.

1. *z* = (130 − 120)/10 = 1.00, and the area above 1.00 is 0.159. So 15.9% of normal healthy individuals have a systolic blood pressure above 1 standard deviation (>130 mm Hg).

2. *z* = (140 − 120)/10 = 2.00, and the area above 2.00 is 0.023. So 2.3% have a systolic blood pressure above 2 standard deviations (>140 mm Hg).

3. z_1 = (100 − 120)/10 = −2.00, and z_2 = (140 − 120)/10 = 2.00; the area between −2 and +2 is 0.954. So 95.4% have a systolic blood pressure between −2 and +2 standard deviations (between 100 and 140 mm Hg).

4. *z* = (150 − 120)/10 = 3.00, and the area above 3.00 is 0.001. So only 0.1% have a systolic blood pressure above 3 standard deviations (>150 mm Hg).

5. z_1 = (90 − 120)/10 = −3.00, and z_2 = 3.00; the area below −3 and above +3 is 0.003. So only 0.3%

Table 4–9. Mean blood pressures.

	Men		Women	
Ages	Systolic	Diastolic	Systolic	Diastolic
16	115	70	112	69
19	119	71	114	70
24	122	73	115	71
29	122	75	116	72
39	123	76	118	74
49	125	78	123	76
59	128	79	128	79
69	132	79	134	80

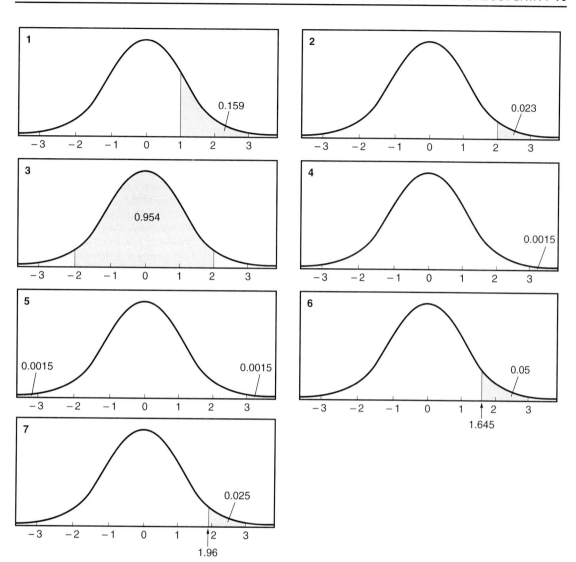

Figure 4–7. Finding areas under a curve using normal distribution.

have a systolic blood pressure either below or above 3 standard deviations (<90 or >150 mm Hg).

6. This problem is a bit more difficult and must be worked backward. The value of z, obtained from Table A–2, that divides the lower 0.95 of the area from the upper 0.05 is 1.645. Substituting this value for z in the formula and solving for X yields

$$z = \frac{X - \mu}{\sigma}$$

$$1.645 = \frac{X - 120}{10}$$

$$10 \times 1.645 = X - 120$$

$$136.45 = X$$

A systolic blood pressure of 136.45 mm Hg is therefore at the 95th percentile (a more specific blood pressure measurement than is generally made). So 95% of normal, healthy people have a systolic blood pressure of 136.45 mm Hg or lower.

7. Working backward again, we obtain the value 1.96 for z. Substituting and solving for X yields

$$1.96 = \frac{X - 120}{10}$$

$$19.6 = X - 120$$

$$139.6 = X$$

Thus, a systolic blood pressure of 139.6 mm Hg divides the distribution of normal, healthy individuals into the lower 97.5% and the upper 2.5%.

From the results of the previous exercises, we can state some important guidelines for using the normal distribution. As mentioned in Chapter 3, the normal distribution has the following distinguishing features:

1. The mean ±1 standard deviation contains approximately 66.7% of the area under the normal curve.

2. The mean ±2 standard deviations contains approximately 95% of the area under the normal curve.

3. The mean ±3 standard deviations contains approximately 99.7% of the area under the normal curve.

Although these features indicate that the normal distribution is a valuable tool in statistics, its value goes beyond merely describing distributions. In actuality, few characteristics are normally distributed. The systolic blood pressure data in Presenting Problem 5 surely are not exactly normally distributed in the population at large. In some populations, data are positively skewed: More people are found with systolic pressures above 120 mm Hg than below. Elveback and coworkers (1970) showed that many common laboratory values are not normally distributed; consequently, using the mean ±2 standard deviations may cause substantially more or less than 5% of the population to lie outside 2 standard deviations. Used judiciously, however, the three guidelines are good rules of thumb about characteristics that have approximately normal distributions.

The major importance of the normal distribution is in the role it plays in statistical inference. In the next section, we show that the normal distribution forms the basis for making statistical inferences even when the population is not normally distributed. The following point is very important and will be made several times: Statistical inference generally involves mean values of a population, not values related to individuals. The examples we just discussed deal with individuals and, if we are to make probability statements about individuals using the mean and standard deviation rules, the distribution of the characteristic of interest must be approximately normally distributed.

4.5 SAMPLING DISTRIBUTIONS

We just learned that the binomial, Poisson, and normal distributions can be used to determine how likely it is that any specific measurement is in the population. Now we turn to another type of distribution, called a **sampling distribution,** that is very important in statistics. Understanding sampling distributions is essential for grasping the logic underlying the prototypical statements from the literature. After we have a basic comprehension of sampling distributions, we will have the tools to learn about **estimation** and **hypothesis testing,** methods that permit investigators to generalize study results to the population that the sample represents. Throughout, we assume that the sample has been selected using one of the proper methods of random sampling discussed in Section 4.3.

The distribution of individual observations is very different from the distribution of means, which is called a **sampling distribution.** In Chapter 3, Gelber and colleagues (1997) collected data on heart rate variation to deep breathing and the Valsalva ratio in order to establish population norms. A national sample of 490 subjects was the basis of establishing norm values for heart rate variation, but clearly the authors wished to generalize from this sample to all healthy adults. If another sample of 490 healthy individuals were evaluated, it is unlikely that exactly this distribution would be observed.

Although the focus in this study was on the normal range, defined by the central 95% of the observed distribution, the researchers were also interested in the mean heart rate variation. The mean in another sample is likely to be less (or more) than the 50.17 observed in their sample, and they might wish to know how much the mean can be expected to differ. To find out, they could randomly select many samples from the target population of patients, compute the mean in each sample, and then examine the distribution of means to estimate the amount of variation that can be expected from one sample to another. This distribution of means is called the **sampling distribution of the mean.** It would be very tedious, however, to have to take many samples in order to estimate the variability of the mean. The sampling distribution of the mean has several desirable characteristics, not the least of which is that it permits us to answer questions about a mean with only one sample.

In the following section, we use a simple hypothetical example to illustrate how a sampling distribution can be generated. Then we show that we need not generate a sampling distribution in practice; instead, we can use statistical theory to answer questions about a single observed mean.

4.5.1 The Sampling Distribution of the Mean

Four features define a sampling distribution. The first is the statistic of interest, for example, the mean, standard deviation, or proportion. Because the sampling distribution of the mean plays such a key role in statistics, we use it to illustrate the concept. The second defining feature is a random selection of the sample. The third—and very important—feature is the size of the random sample. The fourth feature is specification of the population being sampled.

To illustrate, suppose a physician is trying to decide whether to begin mailing reminders to patients who have waited more than a year to schedule their annual examination. The physician reviews the files of all patients who came in for an annual checkup during the past month and determines how many months had passed since their previous visit. To keep calculations simple, we use a very small population size of five patients. Table 4–10 lists the number of months since the last examination for the five patients in this population. The following discussion presents details about generating and using a sampling distribution for this example.

4.5.1.a Generating a Sampling Distribution: To generate a sampling distribution from the population of five patients, we select all possible samples of two patients per sample and calculate the mean number of months since the last examination for each sample. For a population of five, 25 different possible samples of two can be selected. That is, patient 1 (12 months since last checkup) can be selected as the first observation and returned to the sample; then, patient 1 (12 months), or patient 2 (13 months), or patient 3 (14 months), and so on, can be selected as the second observation. The 25 different possible samples and the mean number of months since the patient's last visit for each sample are given in Table 4–11.

4.5.1.b Comparing the Population Distribution with the Sampling Distribution: Figure 4–8 is a graph of the population of patients and the number of months since their last examination. The probability distribution in this population is *uniform,* because every length of time has the same (or uniform) probability of occurrence; because of its shape, this distribution is also referred to as *rectangular.* The mean in this population is 14 months, and the standard deviation is 1.41 months (see Exercise 8).

Figure 4–9 is a graph of the sampling distribution of the mean number of months since the last visit for a sample of size 2. The sampling distribution of means is certainly not uniform; it is shaped somewhat like a pyramid. The following are three important characteristics of this sampling distribution:

1. The mean of the 25 separate means is 14 months, the same as the mean in the population.

2. The variability in the sampling distribution of means is less than the variability in the original population. The standard deviation in the population is 1.41; the standard deviation of the means is 1.00.

3. The shape of the sampling distribution of means, even for a sample of size 2, is beginning to

Table 4–11. Twenty-five samples of size 2 patients each.

Sample	Patients Selected	Number of Months for Each	Mean
1	1, 1	12, 12	12.0
2	1, 2	12, 13	12.5
3	1, 3	12, 14	13.0
4	1, 4	12, 15	13.5
5	1, 5	12, 16	14.0
6	2, 1	13, 12	12.5
7	2, 2	13, 13	13.0
8	2, 3	13, 14	13.5
9	2, 4	13, 15	14.0
10	2, 5	13, 16	14.5
11	3, 1	14, 12	13.0
12	3, 2	14, 13	13.5
13	3, 3	14, 14	14.0
14	3, 4	14, 15	14.5
15	3, 5	14, 16	15.0
16	4, 1	15, 12	13.5
17	4, 2	15, 13	14.0
18	4, 3	15, 14	14.5
19	4, 4	15, 15	15.0
20	4, 5	15, 16	15.5
21	5, 1	16, 12	14.0
22	5, 2	16, 13	14.5
23	5, 3	16, 14	15.0
24	5, 4	16, 15	15.5
25	5, 5	16, 16	16.0

"approach" the shape of the normal distribution, although the shape of the population distribution is rectangular, not normal.

4.5.1.c Using the Sampling Distribution: The sampling distribution of the mean is extremely useful because it allows us to make statements about the probability that specific observations will occur. For example, using the sampling distribution in Figure 4–9, we can ask questions such as "If the mean number of months since the previous checkup is really 14, how likely is a random sample of $n = 2$ patients in which the mean is 15 or more months?" From the sampling distribution, we see that a mean of 15 or more can occur 6 times out of 25, or 24% of the time. A random sample with a mean of 15 or more is therefore not all that unusual.

In medical studies, the sampling distribution of the mean can answer questions such as "If there really is no difference between the therapies, how often would

Table 4–10. Population of months since last examination.

Patient	Number of Months Since Last Examination
1	12
2	13
3	14
4	15
5	16

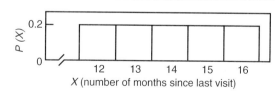

Figure 4–8. Distribution of population values of number of months since last office visit (data from Table 4–10).

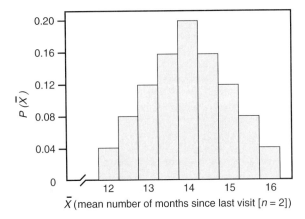

Figure 4–9. Distribution of mean number of months since last office visit for $n = 2$ (data from Table 4–11).

the observed outcome (or something more extreme) occur simply by chance?"

4.5.2 The Central Limit Theorem

Generating the sampling distribution for the mean each time an investigator wants to ask a statistical question would be too time-consuming, but this process is not necessary. Instead, statistical theory can be used to determine the sampling distribution of the mean in any particular situation. These properties of the sampling distribution are the basis for one of the most important theorems in statistics, called the central limit theorem. A mathematical proof of the central limit theorem is not possible in this text, but we will advance some empirical arguments that hopefully convince you that the theory is valid. The following list details the features of the **central limit theorem.**

Given a population with mean μ and standard deviation σ, the sampling distribution of the mean based on repeated random samples of size n has the following properties:

1. The mean of the sampling distribution, or the mean of the means, is equal to the population mean μ based on the individual observations.

2. The standard deviation in the sampling distribution of the mean is equal to $\sigma/\sqrt{n}$. This quantity, called the **standard error of the mean,** plays an important role in many of the statistical procedures discussed in several later chapters. The standard error of the mean is variously written as

$$\sigma_{\bar{X}}, \; SD_{\bar{X}}, \; SE_{\bar{X}}, \; SEM$$

or sometimes simply *SE,* if it is clear the mean is being referred to.

3. If the distribution in the population is normal, then the sampling distribution of the mean is also

normal. More importantly, for sufficiently large sample sizes, the sampling distribution of the mean is approximately normally distributed, *regardless* of the shape of the original population distribution.

The central limit theorem is illustrated for four different population distributions in Figure 4–10. In row A, the shape of the population distribution is uniform, or rectangular, as in our example of the number of months since a previous physical examination. Row B is a bimodal distribution in which extreme values of the random variable are more likely to occur than middle values. Results from opinion polls in which people rate their agreement with political issues sometimes have this distribution, especially if the issue polarizes people. Bimodal distributions also occur in biology when two populations are mixed, as they are for ages of people who have Crohn's disease. Modal ages for these populations are mid-20s and late 40s to early 50s. In row C, the distribution is negatively skewed because of some small outlying values. This distribution can model a random variable, such as age of patients diagnosed with breast cancer. Finally, row D is similar to the normal distribution.

The second column of distributions in Figure 4–10 illustrates the sampling distributions of the mean when samples of size 2 are randomly selected from the parent populations. In row A, the pyramid shape is the same as in the example on months since a patient's last examination. Note that, even for the bimodal population distribution in row B, the sampling distribution of means begins to approach the shape of the normal distribution. This bell shape is more evident in the third column of Figure 4–10, in which the sampling distributions are based on sample sizes of 10. Finally, in the fourth row, for sample sizes of 30, all sampling distributions resemble the normal distribution.

A sample of 30 is commonly used as a cutoff value because sampling distributions of the mean based on sample sizes of 30 or more are considered to be normally distributed. A sample this large is not always needed, however. If the parent population is normally distributed, the *means of samples of any size* will be normally distributed. In nonnormal parent populations, large sample sizes are required with extremely skewed population distributions; smaller sample sizes can be used with moderately skewed distributions. Fortunately, guidelines about sample sizes have been developed, and they will be pointed out as they arise in our discussion.

In Figure 4–10, also note that in every case the mean of the sampling distributions is the same as the mean of the parent population distribution. The variability of the means decreases as the sample size increases, however, so the standard error of the mean decreases as well. Another feature to note is that the relationship between sample size and standard error of the mean is not linear; it is based on the square root of the sample size, not the sample size itself. It is therefore necessary to quadruple, not double, the

Distribution in the Population

Sampling Distribution of the Mean, $\bar{X}$

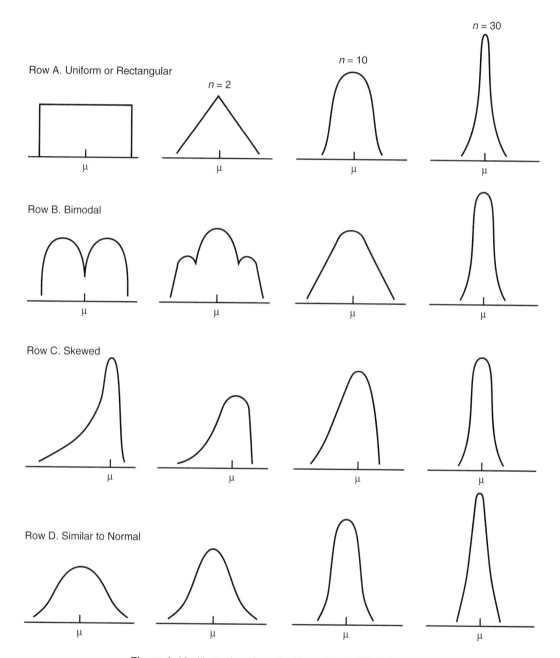

Figure 4–10. Illustration of ramifications of central limit theorem.

sample size in order to reduce the standard error by half.

4.5.3 Points to Remember

Several points deserve reemphasis. In practice, selecting repeated samples of size n and generating a sampling distribution for the mean is not necessary. Instead, only one sample is selected, the sample mean is calculated (as an estimate of the population mean), and, if the sample size is 30 or more, the central limit theorem is invoked to argue that the sampling distribution of the mean is known and does not need to be generated. Then, because the mean has a known distribution, statistical questions can be addressed.

4.5.3.a Standard Deviation versus Standard Error:
The value σ measures the standard deviation in the population and is based on measurements of individuals. That is, the standard deviation tells us how much variability can be expected among *individuals.* The standard error of the mean, however, is the standard deviation of the means in a sampling distribution; it tells us how much variability can be expected among *means* in future samples.

For example, earlier in this chapter we used the fact that systolic blood pressure is approximately normally distributed in normal healthy populations, with mean 120 mm Hg and standard deviation 10, to illustrate how areas under the curve are related to probabilities. We also demonstrated that the interval defined by the mean ±2 *SD* contains approximately 95% of the individual observations when the observations have a normal distribution. Because the central limit theorem tells us that a sample mean is normally distributed (when the sample size is 30 or more), we can use these same properties to relate areas under the normal curve to probabilities when the sample mean instead of an individual value is of interest. Also, we will soon see that the interval defined by the sample mean ±2 *SE* generally contains about 95% of the *means* (not the individuals) that would be observed if samples of the same size were repeatedly selected.

4.5.3.b The Use of the Standard Deviation in Research Reports:
Authors of research reports sometimes present data in terms of the mean and standard deviation. At other times, authors report the mean and standard error of the mean. This practice is especially prominent in graphs. Although some journal editors now require authors to use the standard deviation (Bartko, 1985), many articles still use the standard error of the mean. There are two reasons for increasing use of the standard deviation instead of the standard error. First, the standard error is a function of the sample size, so it can be made smaller simply by increasing n. Second, the interval (mean ±2 *SE*) will contain approximately 95% of the *means* of samples, but it will never contain 95% of the observations on *individuals;* in the latter situation, the mean ±2 *SD* is needed. By definition, the standard error pertains to means, not to individuals. When physicians consider applying research results, they generally wish to apply them to individuals in their practice, not to groups of individuals. The standard deviation is therefore generally the more appropriate measure to report.

4.5.3.c Other Sampling Distributions:
Statistics other than the mean, such as standard deviations, medians, proportions, and correlations, also have sampling distributions. In each case, the statistical issue is the same: How can the statistic of interest be expected to vary across different samples of the same size?

Although the sampling distribution of the mean is approximately normally distributed, the sampling distributions of most other statistics are not. In fact, the sampling distribution of the mean assumes that the value of the population standard deviation σ is known. In actuality, it is rarely known; therefore, the population standard deviation is estimated by the sample standard deviation *SD,* and the *SD* is used in place of the population value in the calculation of the standard error; that is, the standard error in the population is estimated by

$$SE_{\bar{x}} = \frac{SD}{\sqrt{n}}$$

When the *SD* is used, the sampling distribution of the mean actually follows a *t* **distribution** instead of the normal distribution. This important distribution is similar to the normal distribution and is discussed in detail in Chapters 5 and 6.

As other examples, the sampling distribution of the ratio of two variances (squared standard deviations) follows an *F* **distribution,** a theoretical distribution presented in Chapters 6 and 7. The proportion, which is based on the binomial distribution, is normally distributed under certain circumstances, as we shall see in Chapter 5. For the correlation to follow the normal distribution, a transformation must be applied, as illustrated in Chapter 8. Nevertheless, one property that all sampling distributions have in common is having a standard error, and the variation of the statistic in its sampling distribution is called the standard error of the statistic. Thus, the standard error of the mean is just one of many standard errors, albeit the one most commonly used in medical research.

4.5.4 Applications Using the Sampling Distribution of the Mean

Let us turn to some applications of the concepts introduced so far in this chapter. Recall that the **critical ratio** (or *z* score) transforms a normally distributed random variable with mean μ and standard deviation σ to the standard normal (*z*) distribution with mean 0 and standard deviation 1 by subtracting the mean and dividing by the standard deviation:

$$z = \frac{X - \mu}{\sigma}$$

When we are interested in the mean rather than individual observations, the mean itself is the entity transformed. According to the central limit theorem, the mean of the sampling distribution is still μ, but the standard deviation of the mean is the standard error of the mean. The critical ratio that transforms a mean to have distribution with mean 0 and standard deviation 1 is therefore

$$z = \frac{\overline{X} - \mu}{\sigma/\sqrt{n}}$$

The use of the critical ratio is illustrated in the following examples.

Example 1: Suppose a health care provider studies a randomly selected group of 25 men and women between 20 and 39 years of age and finds that their mean systolic blood pressure (BP) is 124 mm Hg. How often would a sample of 25 patients have a mean systolic BP this high or higher? Using the data from Presenting Problem 5 on mean blood pressure (Society of Actuaries, 1980) as a guide (see Table 4–9), we assume that systolic BP is a normally distributed random variable with a known mean of 120 mm Hg and a standard deviation of 10 mm Hg in the population of normal healthy adults. The provider's question is equivalent to asking: If repeated samples of 25 individuals are randomly selected from the population, what proportion of samples will have *mean* values greater than 124 mm Hg?

Solution: The sampling distribution of the mean is normal because the population of blood pressures is normally distributed. The mean is 120 mm Hg, and the *SE* (based on the known standard deviation) is equal to $\overline{X} = 10/5 = 2$. Therefore, the critical ratio is

$$z = \frac{124 - 120}{10/\sqrt{25}} = \frac{4}{2} = 2.0$$

From column 4 of Table A–2 (Appendix A) for the normal curve, the proportion of the z distribution area above 2.0 is 0.023; therefore, 2.3% of random samples with $n = 25$ can be expected to have a mean systolic BP of 124 mm Hg or higher. Figure 4–11A illustrates how the distribution of means is transformed to the critical ratio.

Example 2: Suppose a health care provider wants to detect adverse effects on systolic BP in a random sample of 25 patients using a drug that causes vasoconstriction. The provider decides that a mean systolic BP in the upper 5% of the distribution is cause

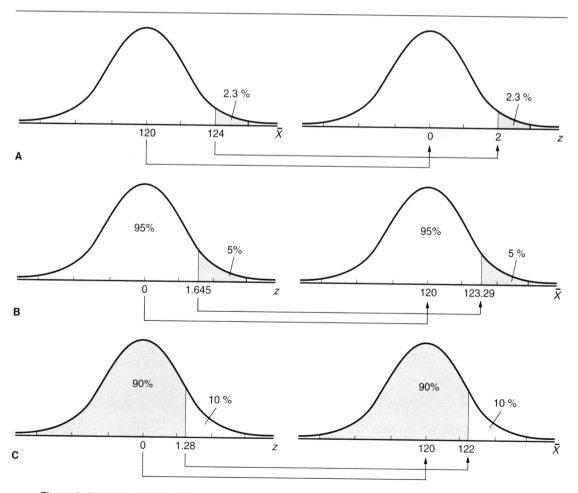

Figure 4–11. Using normal distribution to draw conclusions about systolic blood pressure in healthy adults.

for alarm; therefore, the provider must determine the value that divides the upper 5% of the sampling distribution from the lower 95%.

Solution: The solution to this example requires working backward from the area under the standard normal curve to find the value of the mean. The value of z that divides the area into the lower 95% and the upper 5% is 1.645 (we find 0.05 in column 4 of Table A–2 and read 1.645 in column 1). Substituting this value for z in the critical ratio and then solving for the mean yields

$$1.645 = \frac{(\bar{X} - 120)}{10/\sqrt{25}} = \frac{\bar{X} - 120}{2}$$
$$\text{and} \quad (1.645)(2) + 120 = \bar{X}$$
$$\text{or} \quad \bar{X} = 123.29$$

A mean systolic BP of 123.29 is the value that divides the sampling distribution into the lower 95% and the upper 5%. So, there is cause for alarm if the mean in the sample of 25 patients surpasses this value (see Figure 4–11B).

Example 3: Continuing with Examples 1 and 2, suppose the health care provider does not know how many patients should be included in a study of the drug's effect. After some consideration, the provider decides that, 90% of the time, the mean systolic blood pressure in the sample of patients must not rise above 122 mm Hg. How large a random sample is required so that 90% of the means in samples of this size will be 122 mm Hg or less?

Solution: The answer to this question requires determining n so that only 10% of the sample means exceed $\mu = 120$ by 2 or more, that is, $X - \mu = 2$. The value of z in Table A–2 that divides the area into the lower 90% and the upper 10% is 1.28. Using $z = 1.28$ and solving for n yields

$$1.28 = \frac{122 - 120}{10/\sqrt{n}} = \frac{(2)(\sqrt{n})}{10}$$

Therefore,

$$\frac{(1.28)(10)}{2} = \sqrt{n} \quad \text{or} \quad \sqrt{n} = 6.40$$
$$\text{and} \quad n = 6.40^2 = 40.96$$

Thus, a random sample of 41 individuals is needed for a sampling distribution of means in which no more than 10% of the mean systolic BPs are above 122 mm Hg (see Figure 4–11C).

Example 4: Presenting Problem 1 in Chapter 3 is a study by Gelber and colleagues (1997) in which they found a mean heart rate variation of 49.7 ng/mL with a standard deviation of 23.4 in 580 normal healthy subjects. What proportion of *individuals* can be expected to have a heart rate variation between 27 and 73, assuming a normal distribution?

Solution: This question involves individuals, and the critical ratio for individual values of X must be used. To simplify calculations, we round off the mean to 50 and the standard deviation to 23. The transformed values of the z distribution for $X = 27$ and $X = 73$ are

$$z = \frac{X - \mu}{\sigma} = \frac{27 - 50}{23} = \frac{-23}{23} = -1.00$$
$$\text{and} \quad z = \frac{X - \mu}{\sigma} = \frac{73 - 50}{23} = \frac{23}{23} = 1.00$$

The proportion of area under the normal curve between -1 and $+1$, from Table A–2, column 2, is 0.683. Therefore, 68.3% of normal healthy individuals can be expected to have a heart rate variation between 27 and 73 (Figure 4–12A).

Example 5: If repeated samples of six healthy individuals are randomly selected, what proportion will have a *mean* Po_2 between 27 and 73 ng/mL?

Solution: This question concerns means, not individuals, so the critical ratio for means must be used to find appropriate areas under the curve. For $\bar{X} = 27$,

$$z = \frac{\bar{X} - \mu}{\sigma/\sqrt{n}}$$
$$= \frac{27 - 50}{23/\sqrt{6}}$$
$$= \frac{-23}{23/2.5}$$
$$= -2.5$$

Similarly, for $\bar{X} = 73$, $z = +2.5$. We must therefore find the area between -2.5 and $+2.5$. From Table A–2, the area is 0.988. Therefore, 98.8% of the area lies between ± 2.5, and 98.8% of the mean heart rate variation values in samples with six subjects will fall between 27 and 73 ng/mL (see Figure 4–12B).

Examples 4 and 5 illustrate the contrast between drawing conclusions about individuals and drawing conclusions about means.

Example 6: For 100 healthy individuals in repeated samples, what proportion of the samples will have mean values between 27 and 73 ng/mL?

Solution: We will not do computations for this example; from the previous calculations, we can see that the proportion of means is very large. (The z values are ± 10, which go beyond the scale of Table A–2.)

Example 7: What mean value of heart rate variation divides the sampling distribution for 16 individuals into the central 95% and the upper and lower 2.5%?

Solution: The value of z is ± 1.96 from Table A–2. First we substitute -1.96 in the critical ratio to get

$$-1.96 = \frac{\bar{X} - 50}{23/\sqrt{16}} \quad \text{and} \quad -1.96\left(\frac{23}{4}\right)$$
$$+ 50 = 38.73 = \bar{X}$$

Similarly, using $+1.96$ gives $X = 61.27$. Thus, 61.27 ng/mL divides the upper 2.5% of the sampling distri-

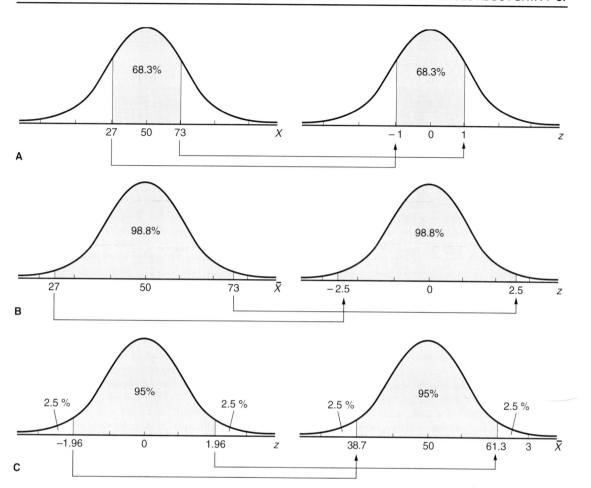

Figure 4–12. Using normal distribution to draw conclusions about levels of Po_2 in healthy adults.

bution of heart rate variation from the remainder of the distribution, and 38.73 ng/mL divides the lower 2.5% from the remainder (see Figure 4-12C).

Example 8: What size sample is needed to ensure that 95% of the sample means for heart rate variation will be within 3 ng/mL of the population mean?

Solution: To obtain the central 95% of any normal distribution, we use $z = 1.96$, as in Example 7. Substituting 1.96 into the formula for z and solving for n yields

$$1.96 = \frac{3}{23/\sqrt{n}} \quad \text{or} \quad \sqrt{n} = \frac{(1.96)(23)}{3} = 15.03$$

$$\text{and} \quad n = (15.03)^2 = 225.8, \text{ or } 226$$

Thus, a sample of 226 individuals is needed to ensure that 95% of the sample means are within 3 ng/mL of the population mean. Note that sample sizes are always rounded up to the next whole number.

These examples illustrate how the normal distribution can be used to draw conclusions about distribu-

tions of individuals and of means. Although some questions were deliberately contrived to illustrate the concepts, the important point is to understand the logic involved in these solutions. The exercises provide additional practice in solving problems of these types.

4.6 ESTIMATION & HYPOTHESIS TESTING

We discussed the process of making inferences from data in this chapter, and now we can begin to illustrate the inference process itself. There are two approaches to statistical inference: estimating parameters and testing hypotheses.

4.6.1 The Need for Estimates

Suppose we wish to evaluate the relationship between toxic reactions to drugs and fractures resulting from falls among elderly patients. For logistic and economic reasons, we cannot study the entire population of elderly patients to determine the proportion who have toxic drug reactions and fractures. Instead, we conduct a cohort study with a random sample of elderly patients followed for a specified period. The proportion of patients in the sample who experience drug reactions and fractures can be determined and used as an estimate of the proportion of drug reactions and fractures in the population; that is, the sample proportion is an estimate of the population proportion π.

In another study, we may be interested in the mean rather than the proportion, so the mean in the sample is used as an estimate of the mean population μ. For example, in a study of a low-calorie diet for weight loss, suppose the mean weight loss in a random sample of patients is 20 lb; this value is an estimate of the mean weight loss in the population of subjects represented by the sample.

Both the sample proportion and the sample mean are called **point estimates** because they involve a specific number rather than an interval or a range. Other point estimates are the sample standard deviation SD as an estimate of σ and the sample correlation r as an estimate of the population correlation ρ.

4.6.2 Properties of Good Estimates

A good estimate should have certain properties; one is that it should be **unbiased,** meaning that systematic error does not occur. Recall that when we developed a sampling distribution for the mean, we found that the mean of the mean values in the sampling distribution is equal to the population mean. Thus, the mean of a sampling distribution of means is an unbiased estimate. Both the mean and the median are unbiased estimates of the population mean μ. However, the sample standard deviation SD is not an unbiased estimate of the population standard deviation σ if n is used in the denominator. Recall that the formula for SD uses $n - 1$ in the denominator (see Chapter 3). Using n in the denominator of SD produces an estimate of σ that is systematically too small; using $n - 1$ makes the SD an unbiased estimate of σ.

Another property of a good estimate is small variability from one sample to another; this property is called **minimum variance.** One reason the mean is used more often than the median as a measure of central tendency is that the standard error of the median is approximately 25% larger than the standard error of the mean when the distribution of observations is approximately normal. Thus, the median has greater variability from one sample to another, and the chances are greater, in any one sample, of obtaining a median value that is farther away from the population mean than the sample mean is. For this reason, the mean is the recommended statistic when the distribution of observations follows a normal distribution. (If the distribution of observations is quite skewed, however, the median is the better statistic, as we discussed in Chapter 3, because the median has minimum variance in skewed distributions.)

4.6.3 Confidence Intervals and Confidence Limits

Sometimes, instead of giving a simple point estimate, investigators wish to indicate the variability the estimate would have in other samples. To indicate this variability, they use interval estimates. A shortcoming of point estimates, such as a mean weight loss of 20 lb, is that they do not have an associated probability indicating how likely the value is. In contrast, we can associate a probability with interval estimates, such as the interval from, say, 15 to 25 lb. Interval estimates are called **confidence intervals;** they define an upper limit (25 lb) and a lower limit (15 lb) with an associated probability. The ends of the confidence interval (15 and 25 lb) are called the **confidence limits.**

Confidence intervals can be established for any population parameter. You may commonly encounter confidence intervals for the mean, proportion, relative risk, odds ratio, and correlation, as well as for the difference between two means, two proportions, and so on. Confidence intervals for these parameters will be introduced in subsequent chapters.

4.6.4 Hypothesis Testing

As with estimation and confidence limits, the purpose of a **hypothesis test** is to permit generalizations from a sample to the population from which it came. Both statistical hypothesis testing and estimation make certain assumptions about the population and then use probabilities to estimate the likelihood of the results obtained in the sample, given the assumptions about the population. Again, both assume a random sample has been properly selected.

Statistical hypothesis testing involves stating a null hypothesis and an alternative hypothesis and then doing a statistical test to see which hypothesis should be concluded. Generally the goal is to disprove the null hypothesis and accept the alternative. Like the term "probability," the term "hypothesis" has a more precise meaning in statistics than in everyday use, as we will see in the following chapters.

The next several chapters will help clarify the ideas presented in this chapter, because we shall reiterate the concepts and illustrate the process of estimation and hypothesis testing using a variety of published studies. Although these concepts are difficult to understand, they become easier with practice.

4.7 SUMMARY

This chapter focused on several concepts that explain why the results of one study involving a certain set of subjects can be used to draw conclusions about other similar subjects. These concepts include probability, sampling, probability distributions, and sampling distributions. We began with examples to illustrate how the rules for calculating probabilities can help us determine the distribution of characteristics in samples of people (eg, the distribution of blood types in men and women; the distribution of heart rate variation).

The addition rule, multiplication rule, and modifications of these rules for nonmutually exclusive and nonindependent events were also illustrated. The addition rule is used to add the probabilities of two or more mutually exclusive events. If the events are not mutually exclusive, the probability of their joint occurrence must be subtracted from the sum. The multiplication rule is used to multiply the probabilities of two or more independent events. If the events are not independent, they are said to be conditional; Bayes' theorem is used to obtain the probability of conditional events. Application of the multiplication rule allowed us to conclude that gender and blood type are independently distributed in humans. The site of infection, however, was not independent from the time during an epidemic at which an individual contracted serogroup B meningococcal disease.

The advantages and disadvantages of different methods of random sampling were illustrated for a study involving the measurement of tracheal diameters. A simple random sample was obtained by randomly selecting radiographs corresponding to random numbers taken from a random number table. Systematic sampling was illustrated by selecting each 17th x-ray film. We noted that systematic sampling is easy to use and is appropriate as long as there is no cyclical component to the data. Radiographs from different age groups were used to illustrate stratified random sampling. Stratified sampling is the most efficient method and is therefore used in many large studies. In clinical trials, investigators must randomly assign patients to experimental and control conditions (rather than randomly select patients) so that biases threatening the validity of the study conclusions are minimized.

Three important probability distributions were presented: binomial, Poisson, and normal (gaussian). The binomial distribution is used to model events that have a binary outcome (ie, either the outcome occurs or it does not) and to determine the probability of outcomes of interest. We used the binomial distribution to obtain the probabilities that a specified number of men with localized prostate tumor survive at least 5 years.

The Poisson distribution is used to determine probabilities for rare events. In the CASS study of coronary artery disease, hospitalization of patients during the 10-year follow-up period was relatively rare. We calculated the probability of hospitalization for patients randomly assigned to medical treatment. Exercise 5 asks for calculations for similar probabilities for the surgical group.

The normal distribution is used to determine the probability of characteristics measured on a continuous numerical scale. When the distribution of the characteristics is approximately bell-shaped, the normal distribution can be used to show how representative or extreme an observation is. We used the normal distribution to determine percentages of the population expected to have systolic blood pressures above and below certain levels. We also found the level of systolic blood pressure that divides the population of normal, healthy adults into the lower 95% and the upper 5%.

We emphasized the importance of the normal distribution in making inferences to other samples and discussed the sampling distribution of the mean. If we know the sampling distribution of the mean, we can observe and measure only one random sample, draw conclusions from that sample, and generalize the conclusions to what would happen if we had observed many similar samples. Relying on sampling theory saves time and effort and allows research to proceed.

We presented the central limit theorem, which says that the distribution of the *mean* follows a normal distribution, regardless of the shape of the parent population, as long as the sample sizes are large enough. Generally, a sample of 30 observations or more is large enough. We used the values of heart rate variation from a presenting problem in Chapter 3 and values of blood pressure from the Society of Actuaries (1980) to illustrate use of the normal distribution as the sampling distribution of the mean.

Estimation and hypothesis testing are two methods for making inferences about a value in a population of subjects by using observations from a random sample of subjects. In subsequent chapters, we illustrate both confidence intervals and hypothesis tests. We also demonstrate the consistency of conclusions drawn regardless of the approach used.

EXERCISES

1. **a.** Show that gender and blood type are independent; that is, that the joint probability is the product of the two marginal probabilities for each cell in Table 4–2.

   b. What happens if you use the multiplication rule with conditional probability when two events are independent? Use the gender and blood type data for males, type O, to illustrate this point.

2. The term "aplastic anemia" refers to a severe pancytopenia (anemia, neutropenia, thrombocytopenia) resulting from an acellular or markedly hypocellular bone marrow. Patients with severe disease have a high risk of dying from bleeding or infections. Allogeneic bone marrow trans-

plantation is probably the treatment of choice for patients under 40 years of age with severe disease who have a human leukocyte antigen (HLA)-matched donor.

Researchers reported results of bone marrow transplantation into 50 patients with severe aplastic anemia who did not receive a transfusion of blood products until just before the marrow transplantation (Anasetti et al, 1986). The probability of 10-year survival in this group of nontransfused patients was 82%; the survival rate was 43–50% for patients studied earlier who had received multiple transfusions. Table 4–12 gives the incidence of acute graft-versus-host disease, chronic graft-versus-host disease, and death in subgroups of patients defined according to serum titers of antibodies to cytomegalovirus from this study. Use the table to answer the following questions.

  a. What is the probability of chronic graft-versus-host disease?
  b. What is the probability of acute graft-versus-host disease?
  c. If a patient seroconverts, what is the probability that the patient has acute graft-versus-host disease?
  d. How likely is it that a patient who died was seropositive?
  e. What proportion of patients were seronegative? If this value were the actual proportion in the population, how likely would it be for 4 of 8 new patients to be seronegative?

Table 4–12. Incidence of graft-versus-host disease.

Condition	Sero-Negative[a]	Sero-Converters[b]	Sero-Positive[c]
Acute graft-versus-host disease	6/17	2/18	2/12
Chronic graft-versus-host disease	7/14	3/18	2/10
Death	3/7	3/18	2/12

[a]Patients who had titers of less than 1:8 before transplant and never showed consistent titer increases. One patient received marrow from a cytomegalovirus seropositive donor and 16 patients, from seronegative donors.
[b]Initially seronegative patients who became seropositive within 100 days after transplant. Six patients received marrow from cytomegalovirus seropositive donors and 10 from cytomegalovirus seronegative donors. Serum titers in 2 donors were not determined for antibodies to cytomegalovirus.
[c]Patients with titers of more than 1:8 before transplant. Within this group, seven patients had fourfold increases in serum titers of antibodies to cytomegalovirus and one other patient showed cultures of virus within 3 months of transplantation. Two of the eight patients developed acute graft-versus-host disease, one had chronic graft-versus-host disease, and one died.
Source: Adapted and reproduced, with permission, from Anasetti C et al: Marrow transplantation for severe aplastic anemia. *Ann Intern Med* 1986;**104**:461–466.

3. Refer to Table 4–1 on the 150 patients in the preepidemic time period for the development of serogroup B meningococcal disease. Assume a patient is selected at random from the patients in this study.
  a. What is the probability a patient selected at random had sepsis as the only site of infection?
  b. What is the probability a patient selected at random had sepsis as one of the sites of infection?
  c. If race and sex are independent, how many of the white patients can be expected to be male?
4. A plastic surgeon wants to compare the number of successful skin grafts in her series of burn patients with the number in other burn patients. A literature survey indicates that approximately 30% of the grafts become infected but that 80% survive. She has had 7 of 8 skin grafts survive in her series of patients and has had one infection.
  a. How likely is only 1 out of 8 infections?
  b. How likely is survival in 7 of 8 grafts?
5. Use the Poisson distribution to estimate the probability that a surgical patient in the CASS study would have five hospitalizations in the 10 years of follow-up reported by Rogers and coworkers (1990). (Recall that the 390 surgical patients had a total of 1487 hospitalizations.) Compare this estimate to that for patients treated medically.
6. The values of serum sodium in healthy adults approximately follow a normal distribution with a mean of 141 mEq/L and a standard deviation of 3 mEq/L.
  a. What is the probability that a normal healthy adult will have a serum sodium value above 147 mEq/L?
  b. What is the probability that a normal healthy adult will have a serum sodium value below 130 mEq/L?
  c. What is the probability that a normal healthy adult will have a serum sodium value between 132 and 150 mEq/L?
  d. What serum sodium level is necessary to put someone in the top 1% of the distribution?
  e. What serum sodium level is necessary to put someone in the bottom 10% of the distribution?
7. Calculate the binomial distribution for each set of parameters: $n = 6$, $\pi = 0.1$; $n = 6$, $\pi = 0.3$; $n = 6$, $\pi = 0.5$. Draw a graph of each distribution, and state your conclusions about the shapes.
8. a. Calculate the mean and the standard deviation of the number of months since a patient's last office visit from Table 4–10.
  b. Calculate the mean and the standard deviation of the sampling distribution of the mean number of months from Table 4–11. Verify

that the standard deviation in the sampling distribution of means (*SE*) is equal to the standard deviation in the population (found in part A) divided by the square root of the sample size, 2.

9. Assume that serum chloride has a mean of 100 mEq/L and a standard deviation of 3 in normal healthy populations.

   a. What proportion of the population has serum chloride levels greater than 103 and less than 97 mEq/L?

   b. If repeated samples of 36 were selected, what proportion of them would have means less than 99 and greater than 101 mEq/L?

10. The relationship between alcohol consumption and psoriasis is unclear. Some studies have suggested that psoriasis is more common among people who are heavy alcohol drinkers, but this opinion is not universally accepted. To clarify the nature of the association between alcohol intake and psoriasis, Poikolainen and colleagues (1990) undertook a case–control study of patients between the ages of 19 and 50 who were seen in outpatient clinics. Cases were men who had psoriasis, and controls were men who had other skin diseases. Subjects completed questionnaires assessing their life styles and alcohol consumption for the 12 months before the onset of disease and for the 12 months immediately before the study. Use the information in Table

Table 4–13. Alcohol intake (g/day) and frequency of intoxication (times/year) before onset of skin disease among patients with psoriasis and controls.

	Mean	SEM	Number of Cases	P value[a]
Alcohol intake:				
Patients with psoriasis	42.9	7.2	142	0.004
Controls	21.0	2.1	265	
Frequency of intoxication				
Patients with psoriasis	61.6	6.2	131	0.007
Controls	42.6	3.3	247	

[a]Two sided *t*-test; separate variance estimate.
Source: Reproduced with permission from Table III in Poikolainen K et al: Alcohol intake: A risk factor for psoriasis in young and middle-aged men? *Br Med J* 1990;**300**:780–783.

4–13 on the frequency of intoxication among patients with psoriasis.

   a. What is the probability a patient selected at random from the group of 131 will be intoxicated more than twice a week, assuming the standard deviation is the actual population value σ? *Hint:* Remember to convert the standard error to the standard deviation.

   b. How many times a year would a patient need to be intoxicated in order to be in the top 5% of all patients?

Research Questions about One Group

PRESENTING PROBLEMS

Presenting Problem 1. Barbara Dennison and her colleagues (1997) asked an intriguing question relating to nutrition in young children: How does fruit juice consumption affect growth parameters during early childhood? Several observations in the medical literature are relevant to this question. Fruit juice consumption by infants and young children has increased in recent years. The American Academy of Pediatrics has warned that excessive use of fruit juice may cause gastrointestinal symptoms, including diarrhea, pain, and bloating caused by fructose malabsorption and the presence of the nonabsorbable sugar alcohol, sorbitol. Excessive fruit juice consumption has been reported as a contributing factor in failure to thrive.

These investigators designed a cross-sectional study including 116 two-year-old children and 107 five-year-old children selected from a primary care, pediatric practice. The children's parents were asked to complete a 7-day dietary record that included the child's daily consumption of beverage—milk, fruit juice, soda pop, and other drinks. Height was measured to the nearest 0.1 cm and weight to the nearest 0.25 lb. Excess fruit juice consumption was defined as ≥ 12 fl oz/day. Both the body mass index (BMI) and the ponderal index were used as measures of obesity.

They found that the dietary energy intake of the children in their study population, 1245 kcal for the 2-year-olds and 1549 kcal for the 5-year-olds, was remarkably similar to that reported in the National Health and Nutrition Examination Survey (NHANES) taken from a nationally representative sample of white children. Children drinking excess fruit juice did not have a statistically higher total energy intake in either the 2-year-old or the 5-year-old age group. The children drinking excess juice, however, consumed a much higher percentage of total calories as simple carbohydrates than children drinking less juice. The prevalence of short stature and obesity was higher among children consuming excess fruit juice. Forty-two percent of children drinking ≥ 12 fl oz/day of fruit juice were short compared with 14% of children drinking <12 fl oz/day. For obesity the percentages were 53% and 32%, respectively.

The authors suggest that their findings linking excess fruit juice consumption to short stature and obesity should be evaluated in other populations, but until proven otherwise, parents should limit fruit juice consumption by young children to <12 fl oz/day.

In this chapter, we focus on the appropriate statistical procedures for evaluating the mean in one group, using the observations on the group of 2-year-old children (Section 5.2.1), and find that the t distribution and t test are appropriate. The entire data set, including information on 5-year-olds as well, is available in the folder entitled "Dennison" on the CD-ROM.

Presenting Problem 2. Prevention of deep venous thrombosis (DVT) is a critical issue in patients undergoing total hip replacement surgery. Pulmonary embolism, a well-known complication of a proximal DVT, is the most common cause of death after an elective total hip replacement. Orthopedic surgeons recognize the importance of prophylactic measures in the treatment of their patients but do not agree on an optimal method. Intermittent pneumatic compression (IPC) of the lower extremities is a simple and inexpensive technique that is not associated with increased bleeding, and thus is preferable to anticoagulants if it were shown to be effective.

Woolson and Watt (1991) performed a prospective, randomized study of the effectiveness of intraoperative and postoperative IPC alone and in combination with either aspirin or low dosages of warfarin. The study included 196 patients who underwent 217 total hip arthroplasties, each randomized to one of three groups: IPC alone (group I), IPC and aspirin 650 mg twice daily (group II), or IPC and warfarin 7.5 or 10 mg given as the initial dose and adjusted daily thereafter (group III). The compression was started at the beginning of the operation rather than in the recovery room as in may other studies of IPC.

Patients were studied by B-mode venous ultrasound scans alone or with venography approximately 7 days after the operation. The overall occurrence of proximal DVT in this study (10%) was lower than the 20–50% observed in untreated patients in other studies (historical controls). A proximal DVT was found in 12% of the patients treated with IPC alone, 10% of those treated with IPC and aspirin, and 9% of those treated with IPC and warfarin. The investigators want to know if IPC reduces the rate of DVT compared with historical controls and whether the relative frequency of proximal DVT is different after total hip replacement using one of the three prophylactic measures. We will see that the z test based on the standard normal distribution can be used to answer research questions about a proportion (or percentage). The observations are summarized in Section 5.4; the data sets are in a folder called "Woolson" on the CD-ROM.

Presenting Problem 3. Schizophrenia is a chronic and devastating brain disorder that affects approximately 1% of the world population and is characterized by hallucinations and delusions as well as emotional and social dysfunction. Many patients are institutionally confined because of their severe thought disorders and lack of appropriate social behavior. Gelkopf and his colleagues (1994) evaluated the use of humor as a means of improving the development of social networks in institutionalized schizophrenic patients. They cite data supporting the value of humor as a powerful social facilitator. They note that "shared laughter can promote a sense of intimacy, belonging, warmth and friendliness and acts as a natural tension reducer" (Gelkopf et al, 1994, p. 177). In short, it can help establish group membership.

They studied 34 patients diagnosed with chronic schizophrenia who had spent at least 3 years of residence in the same psychiatric ward. Two wards consisting of 17 patients each were shown two different movies twice daily (four presentations per day), 5 days a week for 3 months. The experimental group was shown only comedies. In the control group an assortment of different films was shown, but only 15% were comedies.

A social support questionnaire was administered before and after the completion of the study. Part of the questionnaire asked the patients to list the people who supplied emotional or instrumental support. Emotional support was defined as encouragement, caring and loving, and support in times of need; instrumental support included behaviors such as helping patients with their laundry, taking them out of the institution to run errands, or bringing patients things they needed. Section 5.5.2 gives some information about the groups, including the numbers of supportive family and staff the patients listed before and after the experiment; and the data sets are in a folder on the CD-ROM called "Gelkopf." We use the data from this study to illustrate before and after study designs with a numerical variable and learn that the t distribution and t test are appropriate in this situation as well.

Presenting Problem 4. The glenoid labrum is a circular rim of fibrocartilaginous tissue that attaches on the circumference of the glenoid fossa. Labral tears are considered to be a source of shoulder pain by many orthopedic surgeons, but opinion is divided about the relative importance of the glenoid labrum in providing stability to the shoulder. Garneau and his colleagues (1991) studied the value of magnetic resonance imaging (MRI) in detecting abnormalities of the glenoid labrum in 15 patients with a history of shoulder subluxation and physical examination findings suggesting shoulder instability. All 15 patients underwent arthroscopy or surgery of the shoulder so that direct visualization of the shoulder joint served as the standard of reference in the evaluation of the MRIs, and 9 patients had tears of the glenoid labrum. Nine volunteers with no history of shoulder problems also had MRIs of the shoulder.

Two radiologists interpreted the MRIs of the patients and volunteers without knowledge of the clinical history. Six months later the two radiologists again evaluated the images without knowledge of the previous conclusions. The ability to identify correctly the presence of a tear of the labrum and to grade its severity was poor. Radiologist A identified six patients with and nine patients without labral tears, and radiologist B identified nine patients with and six without; however, they agreed on only three patients with and three patients without labral tears. See the data in Section 5.6.1 and the file entitled "Garneau" on the CD-ROM. The authors wish to describe the level of agreement between the two radiologists, and we will illustrate the use of a statistic called kappa as the best way to measure agreement between two people on a binary variable.

Presenting Problem 5. Symptoms of depression in the elderly may be more subtle than in younger patients. Elderly patients are often reluctant to complain about mental symptoms and may initially focus on somatic complaints instead. In addition, depression is a common complication of serious medical illness, such as coronary artery disease, cancer, and stroke—problems encountered more often in the elderly. Recognition of depression in the elderly is important because it can be treated.

Henderson and colleagues in Australia designed a study to gain further insight into depression in the elderly (1997). They wished to investigate the outcome of depressive states 3–4 years after initial diagnosis to identify factors associated with the persistence of depressive symptoms and to test the hypothesis that depressive symptoms in the elderly are a risk factor for dementia or cognitive decline.

The study population included 945 community residents and 100 people living in special hostels for the elderly or nursing homes. All were age 70 years or older. These individuals were evaluated in 1990 and reinterviewed 3–6 years later using the Canberra Interview for the Elderly (CIE). The CIE measures depressive symptoms and cognitive performance. Data included information on psychologic health, measures of cognitive performance, physical health conditions, social support, recent bereavement, level of daily activities, physician or nurse visits, and apolipoprotein E genotype. Information also included the person's current marital status: married, single, widowed, divorced, separated.

Of the 1045 people examined in the initial evaluation, 709 (67.9%) were available for follow-up (227 had died, 22 could not be contacted, and 87 refused to participate). Depression was diagnosed in 30 of the participants at the initial evaluation and in 24 patients at the follow-up. Only 4 of these 24 had been diagnosed with depression at the outset of the study.

We have data on the 595 people who completed the interview on both occasions. The data set is in the folder entitled "Henderson" on the CD-ROM. We recode the data as married versus not married in Section 5.6.2 and use the McNemar statistic to see if the proportion of married people is different at the end of the study.

5.1 PURPOSE OF THE CHAPTER

The methods we discussed in Chapter 3 are called **descriptive statistics,** not surprisingly, because they help investigators describe and summarize data. Chapter 4 provided the basic tools we need to evaluate data using statistical methods. The probability concepts introduced in that chapter are very important for making decisions about data and applying the results. Without probability theory, we could not make statements about populations without studying everyone in the population—clearly an undesirable and often impossible task. In this chapter we begin the study of **inferential statistics;** these are the statistical methods we use to draw conclusions from a sample and make inferences to the entire population. In all the presenting problems in this and future chapters dealing with inferential methods, we assume the investigators selected a random sample of individuals to study from a larger population to which they wanted to generalize.

In this chapter, we focus specifically on research questions that involve *one group of subjects* who are measured on one or two occasions. In statistics, as in most other fields, we often find more than one right way to approach a problem, and the one we use may depend on the way we pose the research question and the assumptions we are willing to make. On some occasions, researchers want to know the amount of variation they can expect in another group. For example, Dennison and colleagues (1997) wanted to estimate how much the mean quantity of fruit juice consumed might be expected to vary from the specific value observed in their findings if the study were repeated elsewhere. When researchers pose their questions in this manner, they generally use **confidence intervals** to help evaluate the amount of expected variation. On other occasions, researchers want to compare one group to a norm. For example, Woolson and Watt (1991) wanted to compare a proportion of patients treated with IPC who had a DVT with the proportion observed in other studies. When researchers pose questions about differences in this manner, they are **testing a hypothesis.**

In this chapter we present the logic and methods for both confidence intervals and hypothesis tests. Specifically, we look at two kinds of studies that involve a single group of subjects. First are studies involving a single group measured one time in which the goal is to

1. Estimate or test the mean value of a numerical variable, such as the mean juice consumption and energy intake in 2-year-old children. We use the *t* **distribution** to find confidence intervals and to test hypotheses in Section 5.2.

2. Estimate the proportion of subjects who have a specific characteristic, such as the presence or absence of DVT. We use the standard normal, or *z,* **distribution** introduced in Chapter 4 to find confidence intervals and to test hypotheses in Section 5.4.

3. Estimate or test the median value of an ordinal variable or a numerical variable that is not normally distributed. If energy intake is not normally distributed, we can use a **nonparametric test** called the **sign test** to test hypotheses, as we illustrate in Section 5.7.

The second kind of study occurs when a single group of subjects is evaluated before and after an intervention or event to learn if a change takes place. In these studies, the goal is to

4. Determine whether the mean in a single group has changed as a result of a treatment or intervention, such as number of staff viewed as supportive by schizophrenic patients. We can use the *t* distribution to form confidence intervals or perform the **paired *t*** test, as shown in Section 5.5.

5. Determine whether a proportion has changed, such as the proportion of elderly who were married at the beginning of the study compared with 3–4 years later. Or to compare the proportions observed by two different researchers, such as the MRIs of labral tears evaluated by radiologists on two separate occasions. We use the **McNemar test** or the **kappa statistic κ,** respectively, for these situations, illustrated in Section 5.6.

6. Determine whether the median in a single group has changed as a result of a treatment or intervention. For example, if we find that change in the number of supportive staff is not normally distributed, we can use a **nonparametric test** called the **Wilcoxon signed rank** test, discussed in Section 5.8.

We spend a lot of time on confidence intervals and hypothesis testing in this chapter in order to introduce the logic behind these two approaches. We also discuss some of the traditional topics associated with hypothesis testing, such as the errors that can be made, and we explain what *P* values mean. In subsequent chapters we streamline the presentation of the procedures, but we believe it is worthwhile to emphasize all the details in this chapter to help reinforce the concepts.

When observations are not normally distributed, investigators sometimes **transform** them and then use the same methods as used with normally distributed variables; we illustrate some of the more common transformations used in medicine. Finally, we summarize the issues researchers need to consider when they decide how large a sample size is needed for studies involving one group, and we show some statistical programs that can be used to estimate sample size.

Surveys of statistical methods used in journals indicate that the *t* test and the chi-square test discussed in the next chapter are the two most commonly used statistical methods. The percentages of articles that use the *t* test range from 10% to more than 60%. For specific journals, see the reports by Emerson and Colditz (1983) for the *New England Journal of Medicine;* Reznick, Dawson-Saunders, and Folse (1987) for surgery journals; Hokanson and coworkers (1987a; 1987b) for otolaryngology and pathology journals; Hokanson and associates (1986b) for psychiatry; Hokanson, Luttman, and Weiss (1986a) for oncology; Fromm and Snyder (1986) for family practice; Welch and Gabbe (1996) for obstetrics and gynecology, and Williams and colleagues (1997) for articles in circulatory physiology. In addition, the nonparametric procedures we introduce in this chapter are used in 3–18% of the articles in the same journals. Furthermore, Williams and colleagues (1997) noted a number of problems in using the *t* test, including a lack of discussion of assumptions in more than 85% of the articles, and Welch and Gabbe (1996) found a number of errors in using the *t* test when a nonparametric procedure is called for. Thus, being able to evaluate the use of tests comparing means—whether they are used properly and how to interpret the results—is an important skill for medical practitioners.

We depart from some of the traditional texts and present formulas in terms of sample statistics rather than population parameters. We also use the formulas that best reflect the concepts rather than the ones that are easiest to calculate, for the very reason that calculations are not the important issue.

5.2 A MEAN IN ONE GROUP WHEN THE OBSERVATIONS ARE NORMALLY DISTRIBUTED

5.2.1 Introduction to Questions About Means

Dennison and her colleagues (1997) wanted to estimate the average consumption of various beverages in 2- and 5-year-old children and to determine whether nutritional intake in the children in their study differed from that reported in a national study

of nutrition (NHANES III). Some of their findings are given in Table 5–1. Focusing specifically on the 2-year-olds, we can state their research questions in two ways: (1) How confident can we be that the observed mean fruit juice consumption is 5.97 oz/day? and, (2) Is the mean energy intake (1242 kcal) in their study of 2-year-olds significantly different from 1286 kcal, the value reported in NHANES III? Stated differently, do the measurements of energy intake in their study of 2-year-old children come from the same population as the measurements in NHANES III? We will use the *t* **distribution** to form confidence limits and perform statistical tests to answer these kinds of research questions.

Before we discuss research questions involving means, let us take a moment and think about what it takes to convince us that a mean in a study is significantly different from a norm or a population mean. Suppose we want to determine whether the mean energy intake in 2-year-old children in our practice is different from the mean in a national nutrition study. What evidence must we have to conclude that energy intake is really different in our group and not just a random occurrence? If the mean energy intake is much larger or smaller than the mean in the national nutrition study, such as the situation in Figure 5–1A, we will probably conclude that the difference is real. What if the difference is relatively moderate, as is the situation in Figure 5–1B?

What other factors can help us decide whether the difference is real? Figure 5–1B gives a clue: The sample values vary substantially, compared with Figure 5–1A, in which there is less variation. This means the standard deviation is smaller in the sample in Figure 5–1A, which may convince you that the difference is real, even though it is relatively small, if the observations do not vary much. For the variability to be small, subjects must be relatively similar (homogeneous) and the method of measurement must be relatively precise. In contrast, if the characteristic measured varies widely from one person to another or if the measuring device is relatively crude, the standard deviations will be greater. If the variation is great, we will need to observe a greater difference to be convinced that the difference is real and not just a random occurrence.

A final important factor is the number of patients included in the sample. Most of us have greater intuitive confidence in findings that are based on a larger rather than a smaller sample, and we will demonstrate the sound statistical reasons for this confidence.

To summarize, three factors play a role in deciding whether an observed mean is different from a norm: (1) the difference between the observed mean and the norm, (2) the amount of variability among subjects, and (3) the number of subjects in the study. We will see later in this chapter that the first two factors are important when we want to estimate the needed sample size before beginning a study.

Table 5–1. Data on average consumption in 2-year-old children.

Row	ID	Weight	Height	Juice	Soda	Energy
1	1.00	31.00	91.10	1.29	2.00	1361.23
2	2.00	43.00	107.50	0.57	2.29	1919.29
3	3.00	30.75	92.90	2.00	1.14	754.38
4	4.00	42.25	111.80	0.00	0.86	1721.98
5	5.00	29.80	90.80	5.34	0.00	1184.59
6	6.00	26.25	91.60	3.07	4.36	984.12
7	7.00	24.00	87.70	14.00	0.00	1115.39
8	8.00	30.00	93.00	7.43	1.29	1458.32
9	10.00	34.50	92.70	9.71	0.57	1676.85
10	11.00	25.00	81.60	16.43	0.00	923.18
11	12.00	34.00	88.40	0.21	2.36	1360.29
12	13.00	30.00	83.10	1.43	0.86	1035.34
13	14.00	32.75	91.40	8.43	0.21	804.94
14	15.00	31.00	87.60	8.57	0.00	1785.38
15	18.00	32.00	92.60	10.07	1.07	1074.43
16	19.00	27.00	86.30	3.14	2.00	1293.83
17	21.00	35.50	99.40	2.14	1.86	1636.00
18	23.00	24.50	84.70	5.33	0.00	944.83
19	25.00	44.00	118.10	10.57	1.14	1763.84
20	26.00	46.25	117.80	1.43	1.29	1268.58
21	27.00	34.50	94.20	0.00	0.00	1379.75
22	28.00	29.25	93.10	8.86	1.14	1595.82
23	29.00	41.00	108.90	9.21	0.00	1670.65
24	30.00	36.50	104.30	4.86	0.71	1521.40
25	32.00	39.00	108.50	3.36	1.14	1496.36
26	33.00	27.00	87.50	3.57	2.00	930.92
27	34.00	42.50	109.40	0.00	0.43	1875.67
28	35.00	31.00	86.30	8.79	0.00	1530.82
29	36.00	30.50	91.50	10.14	0.21	1249.01
30	37.00	30.00	91.20	2.36	0.71	1317.63
31	39.00	28.75	92.90	2.10	0.00	1287.97
32	41.00	26.00	86.10	8.39	4.00	1627.34
33	42.00	57.75	126.10	3.06	1.53	1621.34
34	44.00	27.50	86.00	8.64	1.43	1510.70
35	45.00	43.00	112.40	7.43	0.00	1402.42
36	46.00	47.75	119.70	3.57	0.00	1475.16
37	47.00	47.00	112.90	6.86	3.43	1661.32
38	48.00	53.80	123.90	4.29	4.57	1627.36
39	50.00	42.50	113.60	1.71	8.50	1988.63
40	51.00	29.50	91.30	9.43	1.14	1192.12
41	52.00	57.00	112.00	1.57	1.71	1462.08
42	53.00	41.66	112.90	2.29	0.00	1261.34
43	54.00	46.50	112.40	0.14	3.43	1595.22
44	56.00	47.20	114.40	3.71	2.00	1681.05
45	57.00	36.25	100.00	4.79	0.86	1122.28
46	58.00	35.25	95.30	1.57	2.86	1433.81
47	60.00	52.75	121.20	5.57	0.86	1263.42
48	61.00	35.00	97.20	1.86	0.00	1376.19
49	63.00	41.20	109.80	10.93	2.43	1941.62
50	65.00	30.00	93.90	0.86	0.00	1348.54
51	66.00	25.25	88.70	0.64	1.50	947.55
52	67.00	32.30	90.50	6.29	0.00	1192.35
53	69.00	38.25	99.80	5.50	2.14	1727.23
54	70.00	31.50	91.80	8.71	2.57	1448.06
55	71.00	28.00	84.80	0.00	1.71	1138.43
56	72.00	23.50	82.80	1.07	0.00	1009.83
57	73.00	33.50	94.90	2.57	1.14	1494.85
58	74.00	47.50	115.70	1.71	0.00	1489.22
59	75.00	25.50	92.00	1.14	3.14	1366.55
60	76.00	26.25	89.00	0.00	0.00	1029.15
61	77.00	42.80	111.30	0.00	1.14	1311.75
62	78.00	47.90	114.70	6.86	2.71	1295.58
63	79.00	50.25	117.70	0.29	0.00	1542.93
64	80.00	49.00	119.00	1.14	2.29	1446.17
65	81.00	45.50	108.90	15.43	3.86	1653.05
66	82.00	26.00	76.70	14.36	0.00	1087.06
67	83.00	39.00	110.50	4.64	4.71	1960.26
68	85.00	34.20	92.50	5.57	0.86	1108.74

(continued)

Table 5–1. Data on average consumption in 2-year-old children. (continued)

Row	ID	Weight	Height	Juice	Soda	Energy
69	87.00	26.75	88.90	20.04	2.00	1191.05
70	88.00	28.50	84.60	4.86	0.00	992.09
71	89.00	29.50	87.00	4.36	0.00	1173.30
72	90.00	27.50	90.20	2.70	0.64	1140.86
73	91.00	60.00	121.70	0.86	4.43	1312.97
74	92.00	24.75	84.00	6.43	2.57	1337.60
75	93.00	27.25	94.00	3.36	0.43	1175.76
76	94.00	31.00	93.50	2.21	0.00	990.46
77	95.00	41.00	108.10	7.71	5.71	1580.54
78	97.00	49.50	116.70	0.00	6.61	1579.71
79	98.00	31.25	89.00	3.64	0.90	1395.66
80	99.00	36.25	104.60	2.29	1.14	1725.28
81	100.00	36.50	94.30	22.30	0.00	1860.29
82	101.00	35.25	95.20	5.14	1.71	1788.58
83	105.00	26.00	84.90	4.79	1.71	1502.42
84	106.00	30.00	88.40	1.13	0.11	1098.76
85	108.00	27.75	87.80	1.71	0.29	1192.69
86	109.00	31.50	90.20	6.00	5.36	1741.91
87	110.00	26.00	86.10	0.00	1.00	871.25
88	111.00	29.25	92.80	0.21	0.00	784.07
89	112.00	33.75	97.10	3.71	0.00	1037.19
90	114.00	47.00	114.10	5.93	7.43	1685.25
91	121.00	39.25	108.10	5.79	1.64	1729.69
92	124.00	41.00	108.10	5.14	4.86	1496.74
93	125.00	26.50	85.90	13.14	2.86	1553.70
94	127.00	29.25	91.10	10.43	0.29	1156.89
95	128.00	46.25	109.70	0.00	0.00	1368.98
96	129.00	28.00	87.00	12.07	8.86	1437.98
97	130.00	45.75	112.10	6.00	1.86	1448.43
98	131.00	48.25	111.70	0.86	1.29	1703.80
99	132.00	33.50	97.80	0.00	1.50	1213.32
100	133.00	39.25	110.60	0.00	1.43	1353.61
101	134.00	24.75	83.10	3.43	3.14	1110.85
102	135.00	31.25	93.10	0.00	0.86	1415.58
103	137.00	45.50	110.30	4.57	5.14	1604.54
104	138.00	32.00	85.50	12.57	1.14	1271.83
105	140.00	40.00	106.20	10.86	0.40	1408.57
106	142.00	30.75	87.40	12.50	0.00	1308.86
107	143.00	31.00	85.50	1.71	0.57	1321.53
108	144.00	41.75	111.30	4.71	3.57	2206.71
109	145.00	35.50	104.50	2.86	1.14	1686.05
110	146.00	23.75	81.10	9.36	0.00	1110.32
111	147.00	51.00	115.80	4.43	0.43	1442.08
112	148.00	28.00	85.90	10.71	0.00	1253.14
113	149.00	40.25	110.80	11.04	0.86	1513.10
114	152.00	43.75	111.70	7.71	4.00	2490.33
115	155.00	30.75	88.50	8.29	2.57	1142.86
116	157.00	34.50	108.60	7.36	0.43	1207.96
117	159.00	40.00	110.30	7.93	2.29	1302.36
118	161.00	30.50	89.50	1.29	0.00	1353.41
119	162.00	28.50	87.80	3.91	4.14	1653.48
120	163.00	29.25	90.70	4.43	0.00	1229.13
121	164.00	34.25	100.20	7.13	1.29	1088.53
122	165.00	43.00	105.30	1.93	0.21	951.13
123	166.00	29.75	86.40	4.57	0.43	880.52
124	168.00	29.25	86.20	12.86	1.14	2154.31
125	169.00	37.00	104.30	1.14	1.50	1432.49
126	171.00	24.50	80.70	4.07	5.21	846.47
127	174.00	28.75	85.10	2.14	0.21	1285.44
128	175.00	44.50	114.70	8.86	3.14	1434.79
129	176.00	25.50	87.30	13.71	2.86	1177.24
130	177.00	40.50	104.80	8.57	4.00	2285.65
131	178.00	25.00	82.80	1.69	1.26	1290.07
132	179.00	28.50	88.40	14.43	1.07	1500.29
133	180.00	38.25	112.10	1.07	1.29	1487.11
134	181.00	42.25	114.10	5.29	2.00	1439.99
135	182.00	63.00	116.70	4.29	5.29	1594.05
136	183.00	34.50	94.10	13.57	0.57	1258.85

(continued)

Table 5–1. Data on average consumption in 2-year-old children. (continued)

Row	ID	Weight	Height	Juice	Soda	Energy
137	184.00	47.25	114.60	8.29	2.29	1443.55
138	185.00	38.50	107.60	6.00	0.00	1552.84
139	186.00	40.25	111.60	3.50	1.29	1431.74
140	187.00	43.50	109.40	0.57	2.00	1412.87
141	188.00	44.50	109.20	7.43	0.00	1330.37
142	189.00	38.50	113.00	6.00	1.00	726.72
143	192.00	26.00	84.50	4.19	1.29	906.89
144	196.00	32.50	97.30	10.57	1.00	1133.09
145	197.00	32.75	88.80	15.43	0.00	1401.53
146	198.00	40.00	105.80	2.29	3.14	1877.10
147	199.00	24.50	88.20	7.14	2.57	1241.20
148	201.00	38.00	107.60	19.14	0.43	1762.36
149	202.00	40.25	105.00	3.00	1.71	1296.83
150	203.00	42.25	107.10	6.00	1.14	1769.47
151	204.00	42.50	111.40	8.43	0.00	1408.37
152	205.00	45.00	110.70	2.00	1.29	1616.60
153	206.00	27.00	81.70	14.71	0.29	1259.94
154	207.00	23.00	80.70	14.71	0.29	1060.85
155	208.00	26.75	90.80	3.57	1.57	907.95
156	209.00	28.50	87.10	1.00	0.00	930.37
157	213.00	39.25	105.60	0.86	2.14	1873.10
158	214.00	31.00	94.50	3.61	0.64	1565.48
159	216.00	23.25	86.20	4.79	0.00	1096.98
160	220.00	55.50	108.00	13.00	3.43	1652.53
161	221.00	41.50	112.50	0.00	2.14	1391.93
162	227.00	43.75	112.60	4.71	6.21	1289.40
163	229.00	27.75	87.00	7.00	0.43	1248.31
164	230.00	25.25	85.00	0.00	0.00	1235.56
165	231.00	29.75	88.00	5.71	0.00	1194.34
166	232.00	39.75	107.40	5.00	1.71	1879.66
167	233.00	35.00	88.30	5.14	0.57	1054.41
168	237.00	25.50	83.80	10.36	1.14	909.58

Variables	Count	Mean	Median	Standard Deviation
Weight	168	35.59887	34.1	8.593439
Height	168	98.675	94.25	12.03473
Juice	168	5.5295	4.6785	4.61938
Soda	168	1.575435	1.143	1.748458
Energy	168	1383.249	1367.767	310.3222

Source: Data, used with permission, from Dennison BA, Rockwell HL, Baker SL: Excess fruit juice consumption by preschool-aged children is associated with short stature and obesity. *Pediatrics* 1997;**99**:15–22. Table produced with NCSS; used with permission.

5.2.2 Introduction to the *t* Distribution

The *t* test is used a great deal in all areas of science. The *t* distribution is similar in shape to the *z* distribution introduced in the previous chapter, and one of its major uses is to answer research questions about means. Because we use the *t* distribution and the *t* test in several chapters, it is necessary to develop a basic understanding of *t*.

You might be interested in knowing that the *t* test is sometimes called "Student's *t* test" after the person who first studied the distribution of means from small samples in 1890. Student was really a mathematician named William Gosset who worked for the Guiness Brewery; he was forced to use the pseudonym Student because of company policy prohibiting employees from publishing their work. Gosset discovered that when observations come from a normal distribution, the means are normally distributed *only if the true stan-*

dard deviation in the population is known. When the true standard deviation is not known and researchers have to use the sample standard deviation in its place, however, the means are no longer normally distributed. Gosset named the distribution of means when the sample standard deviation is used the *t* distribution.

If you think about it, you will recognize that we almost always use samples instead of populations in medical research. As a result, we seldom know the true standard deviation and almost always use the sample standard deviation. Our conclusions are therefore more likely to be accurate if we use the *t* distribution rather than the normal distribution, although the difference between *t* and *z* becomes very small when *n* is greater than 30.

The formula (or critical ratio) for the *t* test has the observed mean (X) minus the hypothesized value of the population mean (μ) in the numerator, and the standard error of the mean in the denominator. The symbol μ stands for the true mean in the population;

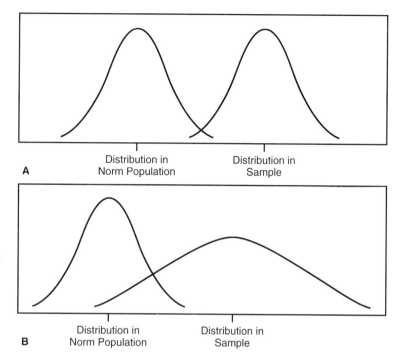

A Distribution in Norm Population   Distribution in Sample

B Distribution in Norm Population   Distribution in Sample

Figure 5–1. Comparison of distributions.

it is the Greek letter mu, pronounced "mew." The formula for the *t* test is

$$t = \frac{\overline{X} - \mu}{SD/\sqrt{n}}$$

$$= \frac{\overline{X} - \mu}{SE}$$

We know the standard normal, or *z*, distribution is symmetric with a mean of 0 and a standard deviation of 1. The *t* distribution is also symmetric and has a mean of 0, but its standard deviation is larger than 1. The precise size of the standard deviation depends on a complex concept related to the sample size, called **degrees of freedom (df)**, which is beyond the scope of this book. When we use the *t* distribution to answer questions about one group, it has *n* − 1 degrees of freedom.

The *t* distribution has a larger standard deviation, so it is wider and its tails are higher than those for the *z* distribution. As the sample size increases, however, the degrees of freedom also increase, and the *t* distribution becomes almost the same as the standard normal distribution. Remember that when the sample size is 30 or more, the two curves are, for all practical purposes, so close that either *t* or *z* can be used. It is generally the case, however, that the *t* distribution is used in medicine, even when the sample size is 30 or greater, and we will follow that practice in this book. Computer programs, such as Visual Statistics

(module on continuous distributions), ConStats, or Conceptual Statistics, that allow for the plotting of different distributions can be used to generate *t* distributions for different sample sizes in order to compare them. We did that in Figure 5–2.

When using the *t* distribution to answer research questions, we have to find the area under the curve, just as with the *z* distribution. The area can be found by using calculus to integrate a mathematical function, but fortunately we do not need to do so. Formerly, statisticians used tables (as we do when illustrating some points in this book), but today most of us use computer programs. Table A–3 in Appendix A gives the critical values for the *t* distribution corresponding to areas in the tail of the distribution equal to 0.10, 0.05, 0.02, 0.01, and 0.001 for two-tailed tests (half that size for one-tailed tests).

We must assume that the observations are normally distributed in order to use the *t* distribution. We discuss this assumption in detail in Section 5.2.5. When the observations are not normally distributed, a nonparametric statistical test, called the sign test, is used instead; we show how to use the sign test in Section 5.7.

5.2.3 The *t* Distribution and Confidence Intervals about the Mean in One Group

Confidence intervals are used increasingly in medical journals, so it is important to be able to interpret them properly. We learned in Chapter 4 that the *z* test

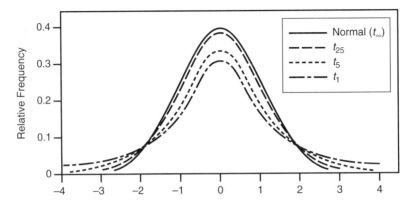

Figure 5–2. t Distribution with 1, 5, and 25 degrees of freedom and standard normal (z) distribution.

can be used to analyze questions involving means if the *population standard deviation* is known. This, however, is rarely the case in applied research. So researchers typically use the t test to analyze research questions involving means. The general format for confidence intervals for one mean is

Observed mean ± (**Confidence coefficient**)
× A measure of variability of the mean

The **confidence coefficient** is a number related to the level of confidence we want; typical values are 90%, 95%, and 99%, with 95% being by far the most common. Refer to the t distribution values in Table A–3 to find the confidence coefficients. For example, for 95% confidence, we want the value that separates the central 95% of the distribution from the 5% in the two tails; with 10 degrees of freedom this value is 2.228. As the sample size becomes very large, the confidence coefficient for a 95% confidence interval is the same as the z distribution, 1.96, as shown in the bottom line of Table A–3.

Recall from Chapter 4 that the standard error of the mean, *SE*, is used to estimate how much the mean can be expected to vary from one sample to another. It is the standard deviation divided by the square root of the sample size.

Using $\overline{X}$ as the observed (sample) mean, the formula for a 95% confidence interval for the true mean is

$$\overline{X} \pm t \frac{SD}{\sqrt{n}} = \overline{X} \pm t \times SE$$

where t stands for the confidence coefficient (critical value from the t distribution), which, as we saw earlier, depends on the degrees of freedom (which in turn depend on the sample size).

We use the data from Dennison and coworkers (1997) to illustrate confidence limits for the mean

fruit juice consumption in 2-year-old children. From data in Table 5–1, the mean is 5.97 oz/day and the standard deviation is 4.77. The degrees of freedom for testing the mean in a single group is $n − 1$, or 94 − 1 = 93 in our example. In Table A–3, the value corresponding to 95% confidence limits is about halfway between 2.00 for 60 degrees of freedom and 1.98 for 120 degrees of freedom, so we use 1.99. Using these numbers in the preceding formula, we get

$$\overline{X} \pm t \frac{SD}{\sqrt{n}}$$
$$= 5.97 \pm 1.99 \left(\frac{4.77}{\sqrt{94}} \right)$$
$$= 5.97 \pm 1.99(0.49)$$
$$= 5.97 \pm 0.98$$

or approximately 4.99–6.95 oz/day. We interpret this confidence interval as follows. In other samples of 2-year-old children, Dennison and coworkers (or other researchers) would almost always observe a mean juice consumption different from the one in this study. They would not know the true mean, of course. If they calculated a 95% confidence interval for each mean, however, 95% of these confidence intervals would contain the true mean. They can therefore have 95% confidence that the interval from 4.99 to 6.95 oz/day contains the actual mean juice consumption in 2-year-old children. Medical researchers often use error graphs to illustrate means and confidence intervals. Box 5–1 shows an error graph of the mean fruit juice consumption among 2-year-old children, along with the 95% confidence limits. You can replicate this analysis using the Dennison file and the SPSS Explore procedure.

There is nothing sacred about 95% confidence intervals; they simply are the ones most often reported in the medical literature. If researchers want to be more confident that the interval contains the true mean, they can use a 99% confidence interval. Will this interval be wider or narrower than the interval corresponding to 95% confidence?

5.2.4 The *t* Distribution and Testing Hypotheses about the Mean in One Group

Some investigators test hypotheses instead of finding and reporting confidence intervals. The conclusions are the *same,* regardless of which method is used. More and more, statisticians recommend confidence intervals because they actually provide more information than hypothesis tests. Some researchers still prefer hypothesis tests, however, possibly because tests have been used traditionally. We will return to this point after we illustrate the procedure for testing a hypothesis concerning the mean in a single sample.

As with estimation and confidence limits, the purpose of a **hypothesis test** is to permit generalizations from a sample to the population from which the sample came. Both statistical hypothesis testing and estimation make certain assumptions about the population and then use probabilities to estimate the likelihood of the results obtained in the sample, given these assumptions.

To illustrate the concepts of hypothesis testing, we use the energy intake data from Dennison and coworkers (1997) in Table 5–1. We use these observations to test whether the mean energy intake in 2-year-olds in this study is different from the mean energy intake in the NHANES III data shown in Table 5–2, assuming the latter is the norm. Another way to state the research question is: On average, do 2-year-old children in the sample studied by Dennison and coworkers have the same energy intake as 2-year-olds in the NHANES III study?

Statistical hypothesis testing seems to be the reverse of our nonstatistical thinking. We first assume that the mean energy intake is the same as in NHANES III (1286 kcal), and then we find the probability of observing mean energy intake equal to 1242 kcal in a sample of 94 children, given this assumption. If the probability is large, we conclude that the assumption is justified and the mean energy intake in the study is not statistically different from that reported by NHANES III. If the probability is small, however—such as 1 out

---

Box 5–1. 95% Confidence interval and error graph for the mean fruit juice consumption in 2-year-old children.

One-Sample Test

Test value = 0

| | *t* | *df* | Significance (2-tailed) | Mean Difference | 95% Confidence Interval of the Difference | |
					Lower	Upper
Juice	12.129	93	.000	5.9714	4.9938	6.9490

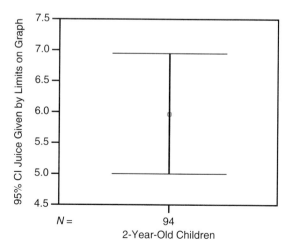

Data, used with permission, from Dennison BA, Rockwell HL, Baker SL, et al: Excess fruit juice consumption by preschool-aged children is associated with short stature and obesity. *Pediatrics* 1997;**99**:15–22. Table produced with SPSS; used with permission.

Table 5-2. Children's energy and macronutrient intake.

Dietary Variable	Our Study 2.0–2.9 years (n = 94)	NHANES III[a] 1.0–2.9 years (n = 424)	Our Study 5.0–5.9 years (n = 74)	NHANES III[a] 3.0–5.0 years (n = 425)
Energy (kcal)	1242 ± 30[b]	1286 ± 22	1549 ± 34	1573 ± 28
Protein (g)	43 ± 1.3	47 ± 0.9	53 ± 1.6	55 ± 1.2
(% kcal)	14.0 ± 0.2	14.7 ± 0.2	13.7 ± 0.2	14.1 ± 0.21
Carbohydrate (g)	169 ± 4.6	171 ± 3.3	211 ± 5.1	215 ± 4.0
(% kcal)	54.4 ± 0.6	53.9 ± 0.6	54.7 ± 0.6	55.3 ± 0.5
Total fat (g)	46 ± 1.3	49 ± 1.1	57 ± 1.6	58 ± 1.4
(% kcal)	33.2 ± 0.5	33.5 ± 0.4	33.0 ± 0.5	32.7 ± 0.4
Saturated fat (g)	19 ± 0.6	20 ± 0.5	23 ± 0.7	22 ± 0.6
(% kcal)	13.7 ± 0.3	13.8 ± 0.2	13.2 ± 0.3	12.5 ± 0.2
Cholesterol	155 ± 6.7	168 ± 70	173 ± 7.2	175 ± 7.2
(mg/1000 kcal)	126 ± 5.1	131[c]	111 ± 4.1	111[c]

[a]Non-Hispanic White.
[b]Mean ± standard error of the mean.
[c]Calculated from NHANES III data; no standard deviation or standard error of the mean available.
Source: Reproduced from Table 2, with permission from the author and publisher, from Dennison BA, Rockwell HL, Baker SL: Excess fruit juice consumption by preschool-aged children is associated with short stature and obesity. *Pediatrics* 1997;**99**:15–22.

of 20 (0.05) or 1 out of 100 (0.01)—we conclude that the assumption is not justified and that there really is a difference; that is, 2-year-old children in the Dennison and coworkers study have a mean energy intake different from those in NHANES III. Following a brief discussion of the assumptions we make when using the *t* distribution, we will use the Dennison and coworkers study to illustrate the steps in hypothesis testing.

5.2.5 Assumptions in Using the *t* Test

For the *t* distribution or the *t* test to be used, observations should be normally distributed. Many computer programs, such as NCSS and SPSS, overlay a plot of the normal distribution on a histogram of the data. Often it is possible to look at a histogram or a box-and-whisker plot and make a judgment call. Sometimes we know the distribution of the data from past research, and we can decide whether or not the assumption of normality is reasonable. This assumption can be tested empirically by plotting the observations on a normal probability graph, called a Lilliefors graph (Iman, 1982), or by using the chi-square test for goodness of fit discussed in Chapter 6. The NCSS computer program produces a normal probability plot as part of the Descriptive Statistics Report, which we illustrate in Section 5.8.2 (see Box 5–2). It is always a good idea to plot data before beginning the analysis, just in case some strange values are present that need to be investigated.

You may wonder why it matters. What happens if the *t* distribution is used for observations that are not normally distributed? Consider these two cases: 30 or more observations are made versus fewer than 30 observations. With 30 or more observations, the central limit theorem (see Chapter 4) tells us that means are normally distributed, regardless of the distribution of the original observations. So, for research questions con-

cerning the mean, the central limit theorem basically says that we do not need to worry about the underlying distribution with reasonable sample sizes. However, using the *t* distribution with observations that are not normally distributed and when the sample size is fewer than 30 can lead to confidence intervals that are too narrow. In this situation, we erroneously conclude that the true mean falls in a narrower range than is really the case. If the observations deviate from the normal distribution in only minor ways, the *t* distribution can be used anyway, because it is **robust** for nonnormal data. (Robustness means we can draw the proper conclusion even when all our assumptions are not met.)

5.3 HYPOTHESIS TESTING

We now illustrate the steps in testing a hypothesis and discuss some related concepts using data from the study by Dennison and coworkers.

5.3.1 Steps in Hypothesis Testing

A statistical hypothesis is a statement of belief about population parameters. Like the term "probability," the term "hypothesis" has a more precise meaning in statistics than in everyday use.

Step 1: State the research question in terms of statistical hypotheses. The **null hypothesis**, symbolized by H_0, is a statement claiming that there is no difference between the assumed or hypothesized value and the population mean; that is, **null** means "no difference." The **alternative hypothesis**, which we symbolize by H_1 (some textbooks use H_A) is a statement that disagrees with the null hypothesis.

If the null hypothesis is rejected as a result of sample evidence, then the alternative hypothesis is concluded. If the evidence is insufficient to reject the

Box 5–2. Sign test of changes in the number of staff listed as supportive before and after an intervention. (See page 124 for discussion.)

Tests of Assumptions Section

Assumption	Value	Probability	Decision (5%)
Skewness Normality	3.9352	0.000083	Reject normality
Kurtosis Normality	2.9243	0.003453	Reject normality
Omnibus Normality	24.0371	0.000006	Reject normality

Nonparametric Tests Section

Quantile (Sign) Test

Hypothesized Value	Quantile	Number Lower	Number Higher	Probability Lower	Probability Higher	Probability Both
0	0.5	3	11	0.028687	0.028687	0.057373

Wilcoxon Signed Rank Test for Difference in Medians

W Sum Ranks	Mean of W	Standard Deviation of W	Number of Zeros	Number Sets of Ties	Multiplicity Factor
313	192.5	51.92422	20	3	366

Alternative Hypothesis	Approximation without Continuity Correction			Approximation with Continuity Correction		
	z-Value	Probability Level	Decision (5%)	z-Value	Probability Level	Decision (5%)
Median < > 0	2.32	0.020	Reject H_0	2.31	0.021	Reject H_0

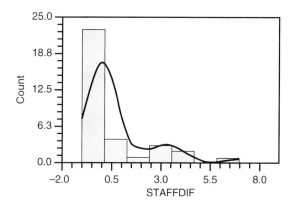

Data, used with permission, from Gelkopf M, Sigal M, Kramer R: Therapeutic use of humor to improve social support in an institutionalized schizophrenic inpatient community. *J Soc Psychol* 1994;**134**(2):175–182. Analyzed with NCSS 97, a registered trademark of the Number Cruncher Statistical System; used with permission.

null hypothesis, it is retained but *not* accepted per se. Scientists distinguish between not rejecting and accepting the null hypothesis; they argue that a better study may be designed in which the null hypothesis will be rejected. Traditionally, we therefore do not accept the null hypothesis from current evidence; we merely state that it cannot be rejected.

For the Dennison and coworkers study, the null and alternative hypotheses are as follows:

H_0: The mean energy intake in 2-year-old children in the study, μ_1, is not different from the norm (mean in NHANES III), μ_0, sometimes written $\mu_1 = \mu_0$.

H_1: The mean energy intake in 2-year-old children in the Dennison and coworkers study, μ_1, is different from the norm (mean in NHANES III), μ_0, sometimes written $\mu_1 \neq \mu_0$.

Recall that μ stands for the true mean in the population.

These hypotheses are for a **two-tailed** (or nondirectional) test: The null hypothesis will be rejected if mean energy intake is sufficiently greater than 1286 kcal or if it is sufficiently less than 1286 kcal. A two-tailed test is appropriate when investigators do not have an a priori expectation for the value in the sample; they want to know if the sample mean differs from the population mean in either direction.

A one-tailed (or directional) test can be used when investigators have an expectation about the sample value, and they want to test only whether it is larger or smaller than the mean in the population. Examples of an alternative hypothesis are

H_1: The mean energy intake in 2-year-old children in the Dennison and coworkers study, μ_1, is larger than the norm (mean in NHANES III), μ_0, sometimes written $\mu_1 > \mu_0$

or

H_1: The mean energy intake in 2-year-old children in the Dennison and coworkers study, μ_1, is *not* larger than the norm (mean in NHANES III), μ_0, sometimes written as $\mu_1 \leq \mu_0$.

A one-tailed test has the advantage over a two-tailed test of obtaining statistical significance with a smaller departure from the hypothesized value, because there is interest in only one direction. Whenever a one-tailed test is used, it should therefore make sense that the investigators really were interested in a departure in only one direction before the data were examined. The disadvantage of a one-tailed test is

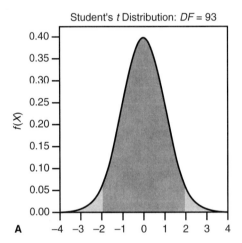

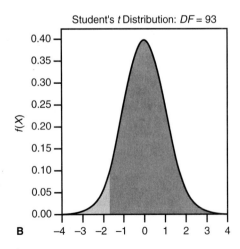

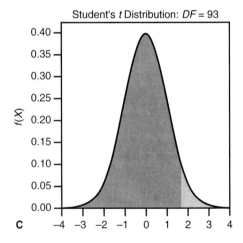

Figure 5–3. Defining areas of acceptance and rejection in hypothesis testing using $\alpha = 0.05$. **A:** Two-tailed or nondirectional. **B:** One tailed or directional lower tail. **C:** One-tailed or directional upper tail. (Data, used with permission, from Dennison BA, Rockwell HL, Baker SL: Excess fruit juice consumption by preschool-aged children is associated with short stature and obesity. *Pediatrics* 1997;**99**:15–22. Graphs produced using the Visualizing Continuous Distributions module in Visual Statistics, a program published by McGraw-Hill Companies; used with permission.)

that once investigators commit themselves to this approach, they are obligated to test only in the hypothesized direction. If, for some unexpected reason, the sample mean departs from the population mean in the opposite direction, the investigators cannot rightly claim the departure as significant. Medical researchers often need to be able to test for possible unexpected adverse effects as well as the anticipated positive effects, so they most frequently choose a two-tailed hypothesis even though they have an expectation about the direction of the departure. A graphic representation of a one-tailed and a two-tailed test is given in Figure 5–3.

Step 2: Decide on the appropriate test statistic. Some texts use the term "critical ratio" to refer to **test statistics.** Choosing the right test statistic is a major topic in statistics, and subsequent chapters focus on which test statistics are appropriate for answering specific kinds of research questions.

We decide on the appropriate statistic as follows. Each test statistic has a probability distribution. In this example, the appropriate test statistic is based on the t distribution because we want to make inferences about a mean, and we have to use the sample standard deviation because the population standard deviation is unknown. The t test is the test statistic for testing one mean; it is the difference between the sample mean and the hypothesized mean divided by the standard error.

$$t = \frac{\bar{X} - \mu}{SD/\sqrt{n}}$$
$$= \frac{\bar{X} - \mu}{SE}$$

Step 3: Select the level of significance for the statistical test. The **level of significance,** when chosen before the statistical test is performed, is called the **alpha value,** denoted by α (Greek letter alpha); it gives the probability of incorrectly rejecting the null hypothesis when it is actually true. This probability should be small, because we do not want to reject the null hypothesis when it is true. Traditional values used for α are 0.05, 0.01, and 0.001. We will use this approach and choose $\alpha = 0.05$.

Step 4: Determine the value the test statistic must attain to be declared significant. This significant value is also called the **critical value** of the test statistic. Determining the critical value is simple (we already found it when we calculated a 95% confidence interval), but detailing the reasoning behind the process is instructive. Each test statistic has a distribution; the distribution of the test statistic is divided into an area of (hypothesis) acceptance and an area of (hypothesis) rejection. The critical value is the dividing line between the areas.

An illustration should help clarify the idea. The test statistic in our example follows the t dis-

tribution; α is 0.05; and a two-tailed test was specified. Thus, the area of acceptance is the central 95% of the t distribution, and the areas of rejection are the 2½% areas in each tail (see Figure 5–3). From Table A–3, the value of t (with $n - 1$ or $94 - 1 = 93$ degrees of freedom) that defines the central 95% area is between -1.99 and 1.99, as we found for the 95% confidence interval. Thus, the portion of the curve below -1.99 contains the lower 2½% of the area of the t distribution with 93 degrees of freedom, and the portion above $+1.99$ contains the upper 2½% of the area. The null hypothesis (that the mean energy intake of the group studied by Dennison and coworkers is equal to 1286 kcal as reported in the NHANES III study) will therefore be rejected if the critical value of the test statistic is less than -1.99 or if it is greater than $+1.99$.

In practice, however, almost everyone uses computers to do their statistical analyses. As a result, researchers do not usually look up the critical value before doing a statistical test. Although researchers need to decide beforehand the alpha level they will use to conclude significance, in practice they wait and see the more exact ***P* value** calculated by the computer program. We discuss the P value in the following sections.

Step 5: Perform the calculation. To summarize, the mean energy intake among the 94 two-year-old children studied by Dennison and coworkers was 1242 kcal with standard deviation 256 and standard error 26.4.[1] We compare this value with the assumed population value of 1286 kcal. Substituting these values in the test statistic yields

$$t = \frac{\bar{X} - \mu}{SD/\sqrt{n}}$$
$$= \frac{1242 - 1286}{256/\sqrt{94}}$$
$$= \frac{-44}{26.4}$$
$$= -1.67$$

Step 6: Draw and state the conclusion. Stating the conclusion in words is important because, in our experience, people learning statistics sometimes focus on the mechanics of hypothesis testing but have difficulty applying the concepts. In our example, the observed value for t is -1.67. Referring to Figure 5–3, we can see that -1.67 falls within the acceptance

---

[1]Where does the value of 26.4 come from? Recall from Chapter 4 that the standard error of the mean, *SE,* is the standard deviation of the mean, not the standard deviation of the original observations. We calculate the standard error of the mean by dividing the standard deviation by the square root of the sample size:

$$SE = \frac{SD}{\sqrt{n}}$$

area of the distribution. The decision is therefore not to reject the null hypothesis that the mean energy intake in the 2-year-old children in the sample studied by Dennison and coworkers differs from that reported in the NHANES III study. Another way to state the conclusion is that we do not reject the hypothesis that the sample of energy intake values could come from a population with mean energy intake of 1286 kcal. This means that, on average, the energy intake values observed in 2-year-olds by Dennison and her colleagues are not statistically significantly different from those in the NHANES III. The probability of observing a mean energy intake of 1242 kcal in a random sample of 94 two-year-olds, if the true mean is actually 1286 kcal, is greater than 0.05, the alpha value chosen for the test.

Use the CD-ROM to confirm our calculations. Then use the t test with the data on 5-year-old children, and compare the mean to 1573 in the NHANES III study.

5.3.2 Equivalence of Confidence Intervals and Hypothesis Tests

Now, let us review the result of the hypothesis test and ask what it implies about a confidence interval for the mean energy level. The results from the hypothesis test lead us to conclude that the mean energy intake in the 2-year-old children studied by Dennison and coworkers is not different from the mean in the NHANES III study (1286 kcal), using a P value of 0.05. Although we did not illustrate the calculations, the 95% confidence interval for mean energy intake is 1189–1295 kcal, meaning that we are 95% confident that this interval contains the true mean energy intake among 2-year-old children. Note that 1286, the value from the NHANES III study, is contained within the interval; therefore, we can conclude that the mean in Dennison and coworkers' study could well be 1286 kcal, even though the observed mean intake was 1242 kcal. When we compare the two approaches, we see that the degrees of freedom, $94 - 1 = 93$, are the same, the critical value of t is the same, ±1.99, and the conclusions are the same. The only difference is that the confidence interval gives us an idea of the range within which the mean could occur by chance. In other words, confidence intervals give more information than hy-

pothesis tests yet are no more costly in terms of work; thus we get more for our money, so to speak.

There is every indication that more and more results will be presented using confidence intervals. For example, the *British Medical Journal* established the policy of having its authors use confidence intervals instead of hypothesis tests if confidence intervals are appropriate to their study (Gardner and Altman, 1986; 1989). To provide practice with both approaches to statistical inference, we will use both hypothesis tests and confidence intervals throughout the remaining chapters.

The possibility of using confidence intervals to report weather forecasts and political poll results was raised in a newspaper article (see Exercise 13). Replicate our findings using the CD-ROM. Also find the 99% confidence interval. Is it narrower or wider? Why?

5.3.3 Errors in Hypothesis Tests

Two errors can be made in testing a hypothesis. In step 3, we tacitly referred to one of these errors—rejecting the null hypothesis when it is true—as a consideration when selecting the significance level α for the test. This error results in our concluding a difference when none exists. Another error is possible: *not* rejecting the null hypothesis when it is actually false, that is, not accepting the alternative hypothesis when it is true. This error results in our concluding that *no* difference exists when one really does. Table 5–3 summarizes these errors. The situation marked by I, called a **type I error** (see the upper right box), is rejecting the null hypothesis when it is really true; α is the probability of making a type I error. In the study of children's mean energy intake, a type I error would be concluding that the mean energy intake in the sample studied by Dennison and coworkers is different from the mean in NHANES III (rejecting the null hypothesis) when, in fact, the sample mean is not different from that in NHANES III.

A **type II error** occurs in the situation marked by II (see lower left box in Table 5–3); this error is failing to reject the null hypothesis when it is false (or not rejecting the null hypothesis when the alternative hypothesis is true). The probability of a type II error is denoted by β (Greek letter beta). In the energy intake example, a type II error would be concluding that the mean energy

Table 5–3. Correct decisions and errors in hypothesis testing.

		True Situation	
		Difference Exists (H₁)	No Difference (H₀)
Conclusion from hypothesis test	Difference Exists (Reject H₀)	* (Power or $1 - \beta$)	I (Type I error, or α error)
	No Difference (Do not reject H₀)	II (Type II error, or β error)	*

intake in the Dennison and coworkers study is not different from that in NHANES III (not rejecting the null hypothesis) if Dennison and coworkers' study mean level of energy intake was, in fact, actually different from that in NHANES III.

The situations marked by the asterisk (*) are correct decisions. The upper left box in Table 5–3 correctly rejects the null hypothesis when a difference exists; this situation is also called the power of the test, a concept we will discuss in the next section. Finally, the lower right box is the situation in which we correctly retain the null hypothesis when there is no difference.

5.3.4 Power

Power is important in hypothesis testing. **Power** is the probability of rejecting the null hypothesis when it is indeed false or, equivalently, concluding that the alternative hypothesis is true when it really is true. Some people think of power as the ability of a study to detect a true difference. Obviously, high power is a valuable attribute for a study, because all investigators want to detect a significant result if it really is present. Power is calculated as $(1 - \beta)$ or $(1 - a$ type II error) and is intimately related to the sample size used in the study. The importance of addressing the issue of the power of a study cannot be overemphasized; we discuss it in more detail in the following sections where we illustrate programs for estimating sample sizes and in subsequent chapters.

5.3.5 *P* Values

Another vital concept related to significance and to the α level is the *P* **value,** commonly reported in medical journals. The *P* value is always related to a hypothesis test; it is the probability of obtaining a result as extreme as (or more extreme than) the one observed, *if* the null hypothesis is true. Some people like to think of the *P* value as the probability that the observed result is due to chance alone. The *P* value is calculated *after* the statistical test has been performed; if the *P* value is less than α, the null hypothesis is rejected.

Referring to the data from Dennison and coworkers once more, the *P* value for this test cannot be precisely obtained from Table A–3. The value of the *t* statistic was −1.67. Looking at the values for 60 and 120 degrees of freedom (recall that 94 − 1 = 93 degrees of freedom were reported in the illustration), we see that the value for $\alpha = 0.10$ is between 1.671 and 1.658, or approximately 1.665. In the lower part of the distribution, the value would be −1.665, slightly less than the value of −1.67 we found. We could therefore report the *P* value as $P > 0.10$ or $P > 0.05$ to indicate that the significance level is more than 0.10 or 0.05, respectively. It is easier and more precise to use a computer program to do this calculation, however. Using the program for the one-group *t* test, we found the reported two-tailed significance to be 0.101, consistent with the conclusion that $P > 0.10$.

Some authors report that the *P* value is less than some traditional value such as 0.05 or 0.01; however, more authors now report the precise *P* value produced by computer programs. The practice of reporting values less than some traditional value was established prior to the availability of computers, when statistical tables such as those in Appendix A were the only source of probabilities. Reporting the actual *P* value communicates the significance of the findings more precisely. We prefer this practice; using the arbitrary traditional values may lead an investigator (or reader of a journal article) to conclude that a result is significant when $P = 0.05$ but is not significant when $P = 0.06$, a dubious distinction.

5.3.6 Analogies to Hypothesis Testing

Analogies often help us better understand new or complex topics. Certain features of diagnostic testing, such as sensitivity and specificity, provide a straightforward analogy to hypothesis testing. A type I error, incorrectly concluding significance when the result is not significant, is similar to a false-positive test that incorrectly indicates the presence of a disease when it is absent. Similarly, a type II error, incorrectly concluding no significance when the result is significant, is analogous to a false-negative test that incorrectly indicates the absence of disease when it is present. The power of a statistical test, the ability to detect significance when a result is significant, corresponds to the sensitivity of a diagnostic test: the test's ability to detect a disease that is present. We may say we want the statistical test to be sensitive to detecting significance when it should be detected. We illustrate diagnostic testing concepts in detail in Chapters 11 and 12.

Consider an analogy to the U. S. legal system. Assuming that the null hypothesis is true until proven false is like assuming that a person is innocent until proven guilty. Just as it is the responsibility of the prosecution to present evidence that the accused person is guilty, the investigator must provide evidence that the null hypothesis is false. In the legal system, in order to avoid a type I error of convicting an innocent person, the prosecution must provide evidence to convince jurors "beyond a reasonable doubt" that the accused is guilty before the null hypothesis of innocence can be rejected. In research, the evidence for a false null hypothesis must be so strong that the probability of incorrectly rejecting the null hypothesis is very small, typically, but not always, less than 0.05.

The U. S. legal system opts to err in the direction of setting a guilty person free rather than unfairly convicting an innocent person. In scientific inquiry, the tradition is to prefer the error of missing a significant difference (arguing, perhaps, that others will come along and design a better study) to the error of incorrectly concluding significance when a result is not significant. These two errors are, of course, related to each other. If a society decides to reduce the number of guilty people that go free, it must increase the chances that innocent people will be convicted. Similarly, an investigator who wishes to decrease the probability of missing a significant difference by decreasing β necessarily increases the probability α of falsely concluding a difference. The way the legal system can simultaneously reduce both types of errors is by requiring more evidence for a decision. Likewise, the way simultaneously to reduce both type I and type II errors in scientific research is by increasing the sample size n. When that is not possible—because the study is exploratory, the problem studied is rare, or the costs are too high—the investigator must carefully evaluate the values for α and β and make a judicious decision.

5.4 RESEARCH QUESTIONS ABOUT A PROPORTION IN ONE GROUP

When a study uses nominal or binary (yes/no) data, the results are generally reported as proportions or percentages (see Chapter 3). In medicine we sometimes observe a single group and want to compare the proportion of subjects having a certain characteristic with some well-accepted standard or norm. For example, Woolson and Watt (1991) in Presenting Problem 2 wanted to examine the efficacy of IPC during and after total hip replacement to prevent a proximal DVT. They could use the procedure with a sample of patients and determine the proportion of hip replacement procedures in which the patient develops DVT. Findings from this study are given in Table 5–4.

The binomial distribution introduced in Chapter 4 can be used to determine confidence limits or to test hypotheses about the observed proportion. Recall that the **binomial distribution** is appropriate when a specific number of independent trials is conducted (symbolized by n), each with the same probability of success (symbolized by the Greek letter π, pronounced "pie"), and this probability can be interpreted as the proportion of people with or without the characteristic we are interested in. Applied to the data in this study, each hip replacement surgery ($n = 217$) is considered a trial, and the probability of developing DVT is estimated by the proportion of people who developed DVT (proportion $= 22/217 = 0.101$).

The binomial distribution has some interesting features, and we can take advantage of these. Figure 5–4 shows the binomial distribution when the population proportion π is 0.2 and 0.4 for sample sizes of 5, 10, and 25. It is easy to see how the distribution becomes more bell-shaped as the sample size increases and as the proportion approaches 0.5. This result should not be surprising because a proportion is actually a special case of a mean in which successes equal 1 and failures equal 0. Recall from Chapter 4 that the central limit theorem states that the sampling distribution of means for large samples resembles the normal distribution. These observations lead naturally to the idea of using the standard normal, or z, distribution as an approximation to the binomial distribution.

5.4.1 A Proportion of Subjects with a Given Attribute

In the Woolson and Watt study (1991), the proportion of people who developed DVT was 0.101. Of course, 0.101 is only an estimate of the unknown true proportion in the entire population of patients at risk for DVT. How much do you think the proportion of patients who develop DVT would vary from one sample to another? We can use the sampling distribution for proportions from large samples to help us answer this question. Recall from Chapter 4 that, in order to use a sampling distribution, we need to know the mean and standard error. For a proportion, the mean is simply the proportion itself (symbolized as π in the population and lower case p in the sample), and the standard error is the square root of $\pi(1 - \pi)$ divided by n in the population or $p(1 - p)$ divided by n in the sample; that is, the standard error is

$$\sqrt{\frac{\pi(1 - \pi)}{n}} \quad \text{or} \quad \sqrt{\frac{p(1 - p)}{n}}$$

Then the 95% confidence limits for the true population proportion π are given by

$$\text{Observed proportion} \pm 1.96 \times \text{Standard error}$$
of the observed proportion
or
$$p \pm 1.96 \times \sqrt{\frac{p(1 - p)}{n}}$$

Where did 1.96 come from? From Appendix A–2, we find that 1.96 is the value that separates the central

Table 5–4. Outcomes from using intermittent pneumatic compression during and following total hip replacement surgery.

	Group I (IPC[a] Alone)	Group II (IPC and Aspirin)	Group III (IPC and Warfarin)
Number of hip surgeries	76	72	69
Number of hip surgeries complicated by proximal DVT[a]	9 (12%)	7 (10%)	6 (9%)

[a]Abbreviations: IPC = intermittent pneumatic compression; DVT = deep venous thrombosis.
Source: Adapted and reproduced from Table IV, with permission from the author and publisher, from Woolson ST, Watt JM: Intermittent pneumatic compression to prevent proximal deep venous thrombosis during and after total hip replacement. *J Bone Joint Surg* 1991;73–A:507–511.

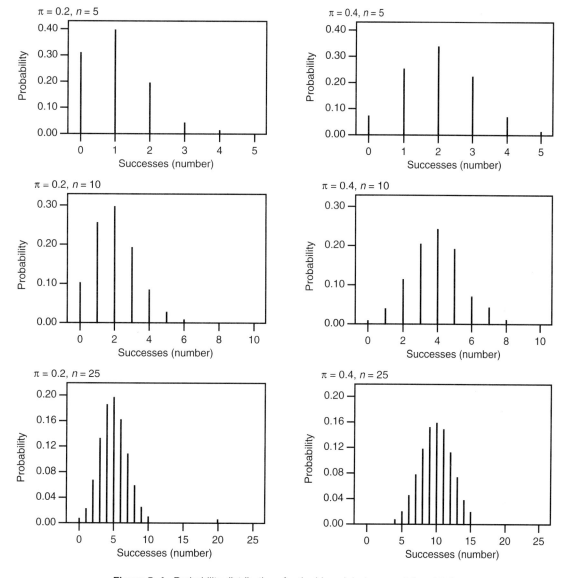

Figure 5–4. Probability distributions for the binomial when $\pi = 0.2$ and 0.4.

95% of the area under the standard normal, or z, distribution from the 2½% in each tail. The only prerequisite to using the z distribution is that the product of the proportion and the sample size (pn) be greater than 5 [and that $(1 - p)n$ be greater than 5 as well].

Using the preceding formula, the 95% confidence interval for the true proportion of patients who develop DVT after hip replacement surgery is

$$p \pm 1.96 \sqrt{\frac{p(1 - p)}{n}}$$
$$= 0.10 \pm 1.96 \sqrt{\frac{0.10(1 - 0.10)}{217}}$$
$$= 0.10 \pm 0.04$$

or 0.06–0.14. The investigators may therefore be 95% confident that the interval 0.06–0.14 (or 6–14%) contains the true proportion of hip replacement procedures in which patients develop DVT with the use of IPC. Just for practice, determine the values of the z distribution used for the 90% and 99% confidence intervals.

Various graphs and pictorial aids have been developed to help researchers test hypotheses about proportions. Figure A–1 in Appendix A is a graph that can be used to obtain estimates of 95% confidence intervals for the proportion. To use the graph, we locate the observed proportion on the horizontal axis and determine the points at which a vertical line extended upward from the observed proportion intersects the sample size lines. These intersection points are then projected on the vertical axis to determine the 95% confidence limits.

For our example, the observed proportion is 0.10, and the sample size is 217. Because no sample size of 217 occurs on the graph, we will use the next smallest sample size, 200, which results in a more **conservative** estimate. A vertical line drawn at $p = 0.10$ in Figure A–1 intersects the lines for a sample size of 200, and lines are projected onto the vertical axis. The projections indicate a confidence interval from approximately 0.06 to 0.15, similar in width to the one found in the preceding calculation.

5.4.2 The z Distribution to Test a Hypothesis about a Proportion

Recall that we can draw conclusions from samples using two methods: finding confidence intervals or testing hypotheses. Although we have already stated our preference for confidence intervals, suppose Woolson and Watt (1991) wanted to perform a statistical test to learn whether the observed proportion of procedures in which proximal DVT develops with the use of IPC therapy was less than the proportion observed when this therapy was not used. The best way to test this research hypothesis is with a clinical trial in which patients are randomized to treatment with IPC and compared with patients randomized to a placebo treatment or the usual standard of care. Their study did not have a concurrent control group, however, so the investigators compared their outcome with the 20–50% of patients given prophylactic therapy other than IPC and in whom DVT occurred, based on reported studies. Again we use the six-step procedure for testing hypotheses.

Step 1: State the research question in terms of statistical hypotheses. Suppose that Woolson and Watt (1991) wanted to know whether the observed proportion of 0.10 was significantly less than 0.20 (using the most conservative value reported in other studies). The z distribution can be used to test the hypothesis for this research question. Here we use the Greek letter π to stand for the hypothesized population proportion because the null hypothesis refers to the population:

H$_0$: The proportion of patients in the population who develop DVT is 0.20 or more, or $\pi \geq 0.20$.

H$_1$: The proportion of patients in the population who develop DVT is less than 0.20, or $\pi < 0.20$.

In this example, we are interested in concluding that IPC therapy is preferred only if the proportion of patients with DVT is less than the previously reported 20%; therefore, a one-tailed test to detect only a negative difference is appropriate. We would use a two-tailed test if we want to know whether the therapy results in either a reduced or an elevated rate of DVT.

Step 2: Decide on the appropriate test statistic. In this example, the sample size (217) times the proportion (0.10) is 22, and the sample size (217) times 1 minus the proportion (0.90) is 195. Because both are greater than 5, we can use the z test. The z test, just like the t test, takes the common form of the observed value of the statistic minus its hypothesized value divided by its standard error.

$$z = \frac{p - \pi}{\sqrt{\pi(1 - \pi)/n}}$$

Step 3: Select the level of significance for the statistical test. For this one-tailed test, we use $\alpha = 0.025$ so our conclusion will be consistent with the 95% confidence interval found earlier. (For a two-tailed test, we would use $\alpha = 0.05$ to be consistent with the 95% confidence interval.)

Step 4: Determine the value the test statistic must attain to be declared significant. A one-tailed test with the alternative hypothesis in the negative direction (less than the null hypothesis) places the entire rejection area in the lower part of the probability distribution. The value of z that divides the normal distribution into the lower 2½% and upper 97½% is −1.96 (Table A–2). The null hypothesis that the true population proportion is greater than or equal to 0.20 is therefore rejected if the observed value of z is less than −1.96 (see Figure 5–5). Recall that researchers sometimes skip this step and, instead, look at the P value from the computer program for the statistical test.

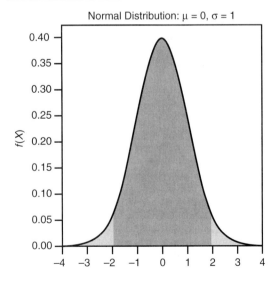

Figure 5–5. Defining areas of acceptance and rejection in the standard normal distribution (z) using $\alpha = 0.05$. (Graph produced using the Visualizing Continuous Distributions module in Visual Statistics, a program published by McGraw-Hill Companies; used with permission.)

Step 5: Perform the calculations. The null hypothesis says the proportion equals 0.20, so this is the value we use for the true proportion, not the proportion we observed among the 217 patients in the sample, 0.10. Substituting these values in the z test (and using four decimal places for greater accuracy) gives

$$z = \frac{0.1014 - 0.20}{\sqrt{0.20(1 - 0.20)/217}} = \frac{-0.0986}{0.0272} = -3.63$$

Step 6: Draw and state the conclusion. Because the observed value of z, −3.63, is less than the critical value, −1.96, the decision is to reject the null hypothesis that the proportion of patients with DVT is ≥0.20. The probability of observing a proportion as small as 0.10 if the true DVT rate is ≥0.20 is less than 2.5 in 100, or 1 in 40. The conclusion is that IPC during and after total hip replacement appears to result in a proximal DVT less often than would occur without this therapy, with $P < 0.025$.

The actual P value associated with this hypothesis test is found by determining how likely z is to be −3.63 or less. Using Table A–2, the area in one tail of the z distribution is 0.001 when $z = \pm 3.00$; because −3.63 is less than −3.00, the P value is reported as $P < 0.001$. Even when computer programs report a very low probability, the lowest P value researchers typically present is 0.001.

Does this mean that intermittent pneumatic compression during hip replacement surgery causes patients to be less likely to have a DVT? Or is it possible that the patients in this study would have had a low proportion of DVTs whether or not the physicians used IPC? We really do not know the answer to this question because the study was not randomized and no control group of patients was included that did not receive IPC. The results are persuasive, compared with other reported studies, but we cannot conclude causation from historical controls.

5.4.3 Continuity Correction

The z distribution is continuous and the binomial distribution is discrete, and many statisticians recommend making a small correction to the test statistic to create a more accurate approximation. This **continuity correction** involves subtracting $\frac{1}{2}n$ from the **absolute value** of the numerator of the z statistic. (Recall that the absolute value of a number is positive, regardless of whether the number itself is positive or negative.) The test statistic is

$$z = \frac{|P - \pi| - (1/2n)}{\sqrt{\pi(1 - \pi)/n}}$$

In our example, the equation becomes

$$z = \frac{|0.1014 - 0.20| - [1/(2 \times 217)]}{\sqrt{0.20(1 - 0.20)/217}}$$

$$= \frac{|-0.0986| - 0.0023}{0.0272}$$

$$= \frac{-0.0964}{0.0272} = -3.54$$

The continuity correction has minimal effect because of the large sample size, so we reach the same conclusion as before.

Not using the continuity correction makes the value of z a little too liberal, allowing us to reject the null hypothesis a little more often than we should. Using the continuity correction makes the value of z a little too conservative, allowing us to retain the null hypothesis more often than we should. Which is better? To be honest, even statisticians do not agree on the answer to this. In the past, we suggested not using the continuity correction, but because more and more articles in the medical literature include the continuity correction, we are more likely to recommend it today.

5.5 MEANS WHEN THE SAME GROUP IS MEASURED TWICE

Earlier in this chapter, we found confidence intervals for means and proportions. We also illustrated research questions that investigators ask when they want to compare one group of subjects to a known or assumed population mean or proportion. In actuality, these latter situations do not occur very often in medicine (or, indeed, in most other fields). We discussed these methods because they are relatively simple statistics, and minor modifications of these tests can be used for research questions that do occur with great frequency.

In this section and the next, we concentrate on studies in which the same group of subjects is observed twice using **paired designs** or **repeated-measures designs.** Typically in these studies, subjects are measured to establish a baseline (sometimes called the *before* measurement); then, after some intervention or at a later time, the same subjects are measured again (called the *after* measurement). The research question asks whether the intervention makes a difference. In this design, each subject serves as his or her own control. The observations in these studies are called *paired* observations because the before and after measurements made on the same people (or on matched pairs) are paired in the analysis. We sometimes call these *dependent* observations as well, because, if we know the first measurement, we have some idea of what the second measurement will be (as we will see later in this chapter).

Sometimes the second measurement is made shortly after the first. In other studies a considerable time passes before the second measurement. In the study by Gelkopf and colleagues (1994), 3 months elapsed between measurements because the intervention itself lasted 3 months. Henderson and colleagues (1997), however, interviewed elderly people in 1990–1991 and then interviewed them again 3–4 years later. The goal of paired designs is to control for extraneous factors that might influence the result; then, any differences caused by the intervention will not be masked by the differences among the subjects themselves.

5.5.1 Why Researchers Use Repeated-Measures Studies

Because paired designs can be very powerful in detecting significant differences, they are used very frequently, as illustrated by the following example.

Suppose a researcher wants to evaluate the effect of a new diet on weight loss. Furthermore, suppose the population consists of only six people who have used the diet for 2 months; their weights before and after the diet are given in Table 5–5. To estimate the amount of weight loss, the researcher selects a random sample of three patients to determine their mean weight before the diet and then selects an independent random sample of three patients to determine their mean weight after the diet. Just by chance, the random sample of patients in the before-diet sample includes patients 2, 3, and 6; their mean weight is (89 + 83 + 95)/3 = 89 kg. Also just by chance, the random sample of patients in the after-diet sample consists of patients 1, 4, and 5; their mean weight after the diet is (95 + 93 + 103)/3 = 97 kg. (Of course, we contrived the makeup of the random samples in this example to make a point, but they really could occur by chance.) The researcher would conclude that the patients gained an average of 8 kg on the diet. What is the problem here?

The means for the two independent random samples indicate that the patients gained weight, but, in fact, they each lost 5 kg on the diet. We know the conclusion based on these random samples is incorrect because we can examine the entire population and determine the actual differences; but in real life, we can rarely observe the population. The problem is that the characteristic being studied (weight) is quite *variable* from one patient to another; in this small population of six patients, weight varied from 83 to 108 kg before the diet program began. Furthermore, the amount of change, 5 kg, is relatively small compared with the variability among patients and is overwhelmed (or overshadowed) by this variability. The researcher needs a way to control for variability among patients.

Table 5–5. Illustration of observations in a paired design (before and after measurements).

Patient	Weight Before (kg)	Weight After (kg)
1	100	95
2	89	84
3	83	78
4	98	93
5	108	103
6	95	90

The solution, as you may have guessed, is to select a single random sample of patients and measure their weights both before and after the diet. Because the measurements are taken on the same patients, the true change is more likely to be observed. The paired design allows researchers to detect change more easily by controlling for extraneous variation among the observations. Many biologic measurements exhibit wide variation among individuals, and the use of the paired design is thus especially appropriate in the health field.

The statistical test that researchers use when the same subjects are measured on a numerical (interval) variable before and after an intervention is called the **paired t test,** because the observations on the same subject are paired with one another to find the difference. This test is also called the **matched groups t test** and, sometimes, the dependent groups t test.

The good news is that paired, or before-and-after, designs are easy to analyze. Instead of having to find the mean and standard deviation of both the before and the after measurements, we need find only the mean and standard deviation of the *differences* between the before-and-after measurements. Then, the t distribution we used for a single mean (described in Sections 5.2 and 5.3) can be used to analyze the differences themselves.

To illustrate, examine the mean weights of the six subjects in the weight-loss example. Before the diet, the mean weight was 95.5 kg; after the diet, the mean was 90.5 kg. The difference between the means, 95.5 − 90.5 = 5 kg, is exactly the same as the mean weight loss, 5 kg, for each subject. The standard deviation of the differences, however, is not equal to the difference between the standard deviations in the before-and-after measurements. The differences between each before-and-after measurement must be analyzed to obtain the standard deviation of the differences. Actually, the standard deviation of the differences is almost always smaller than the standard deviation in the before measurements and in the after measurements. This is because the two sets of measurements are generally correlated, meaning that the lower values in the before measurements are associated with the lower values in the after measurements and similarly for the higher values. For example, in this illustration, the standard deviations of the weights both before and after the diet program are 8.74, whereas the standard deviation of the differences is 0. Why is this the case? Because we made the before-and-after measurements perfectly correlated. Of course, as with the t distribution used with one mean, we must assume that the differences are normally distributed.

5.5.2 Confidence Intervals for the Mean Difference in Paired Designs

One way to evaluate the effect of an intervention in a before-and-after study is to form a confidence interval (CI) for the mean difference. To illustrate, we

Table 5–6. Information on two groups of schizophrenic patients.

	Neutral-Film Group	Humorous-Film Group
Number of patients		
Males	14	14
Females	3	3
Age		
Mean (standard deviation)	43.8 (13.6)	47.1 (13.8)
Number of years hospitalized		
Mean (standard deviation)	13.0 (11.0)	16.1 (11.9)
Social support variables		
Mean (standard deviation)		
Sum of family and staff		
Before	3.2 (2.8)	4.4 (2.7)
After	3.1 (3.1)	5.6 (3.5)
Family		
Before	1.8 (2.0)	2.3 (1.9)
After	1.4 (1.7)	2.1 (2.0)
Staff		
Before	0.7 (1.2)	1.2 (1.3)
After	0.9 (1.4)	2.5 (2.6)

Source: Adapted and reproduced from Table 1, with permission of the author and publisher, from Gelkopf M, Sigal M, Kramer R: Therapeutic use of humor to improve social support in an institutionalized schizophrenic inpatient community. *J Socl Psychol* 1994;**134**(2):175–182.

use data from the study in which researchers designed an experiment to learn whether or not watching comedies had an effect on the therapeutic relationship between staff and patients with chronic schizophrenia (Gelkopf et al, 1994). Patients listed the staff members who gave them emotional or instrumental support both before and after the experiment. Some descriptive information on the two groups is given in Table 5–6.

The number of staff listed can be considered a numerical variable, so we use means and standard deviations. If we focus on the group shown humorous films, we see that the mean number of staff the patients listed as supportive before they saw the films was 1.2 (stan-

dard deviation 1.3) After the 3-month study period, the number had increased to 2.5 (standard deviation 2.6). We want to know whether this increase could happen by chance. To examine the mean difference in a paired study, we need the raw data so we can find the mean and standard deviation of the differences between the before-and-after scores. The before, after, and difference scores are given in Table 5–7.

For patients in this study, the mean of the 17 differences is 1.35 (indicating that, on average, the number of staff rated as supportive increased after patients watched the comedies), and the standard deviation of the differences is 2.09. The calculations for the mean and the standard deviation of the differences use the

Table 5–7. Differences between after and before measures of staff support by two groups of schizophrenic patients.

Patient	Neutral-Film Group			Humorous-Film Group		
	Before	After	Difference	Before	After	Difference
1	1	0	−1	2	2	0
2	0	0	0	0	0	0
3	4	4	0	0	3	3
4	1	1	0	0	1	1
5	0	0	0	2	5	3
6	1	1	0	3	2	−1
7	0	0	0	3	2	−1
8	0	0	0	3	10	7
9	0	0	0	0	0	0
10	0	0	0	2	4	2
11	1	2	1	1	1	0
12	0	0	0	1	4	3
13	3	3	0	0	0	0
14	1	1	0	0	0	0
15	0	0	0	3	4	1
16	0	0	0	0	1	1
17	0	4	4	0	4	4

Source: Data, reproduced with permission of the author and publisher, from Gelkopf M, Sigal M, Kramer R: Therapeutic use of humor to improve social support in an institutionalized schizophrenic inpatient community. *J Soc Psychol* 1994;**134**(2):175–182.

same formulas as in Chapter 3 except that we replace the symbol X (used for an observation on a single subject) with the symbol d to stand for the difference in the measurements for a single subject. Then, the mean difference $\bar{d}$ is the sum of the differences divided by the number of subjects, or $\bar{d} = \Sigma d/n$. Using the differences d's instead of X's and the mean difference $\bar{d}$ instead of $\bar{X}$, we can find the standard deviation of the differences by the following formula:

$$SD_d = \sqrt{\frac{\Sigma(d - \bar{d})^2}{n - 1}}, \text{ or } 2.09$$

We suggest you confirm these calculations using the Gelkopf.xls data set on the CD-ROM. You can compute the differences, the mean, and the standard deviation of the differences.

Just as when we have one group of observations and find the standard error of the mean by dividing the standard deviation SD by the square root of the sample size, we find the standard error of the mean differences by dividing the standard deviation of the differences SD_d by the square root of n, $(SD_d/\sqrt{n} = 2.09/\sqrt{17} = 0.507)$. Finding a 95% confidence interval for the mean difference is just like finding a 95% confidence interval for the mean of one group, except again we use the mean difference and the standard error of the mean differences instead of the mean and standard error of the mean. We also use the t distribution with $n - 1$ degrees of freedom to evaluate research hypotheses about mean differences, just as we did about the mean in one group. To illustrate, if we want to calculate a 95% confidence interval for the mean difference in number of supportive staff, we use the value of t for $n - 1 = 17 - 1 = 16$ degrees of freedom, which is 2.12 from Appendix A–3. Using these values in the formula for a 95% confidence interval for the true population difference gives

Difference ± Confidence factor × Standard error of the difference

or

$$\bar{d} \pm t_{(n-1)} \times \frac{SD_d}{\sqrt{n}} = 1.35 \pm 2.12 \times \frac{2.09}{\sqrt{17}}$$
$$= 1.35 \pm 2.12 \times 0.507$$
$$= 1.35 \pm 1.075 = 0.275 \text{ to } 2.425$$

This confidence interval can be interpreted as follows. We are 95% sure that the *true mean difference* in number of staff rated as supportive after watching humorous movies for 3 months (compared with evaluations before watching the movies) is between 0.275 and 2.425. Logically, because the entire interval is greater than zero, we can be 95% sure that the mean difference is greater than zero. In plain words, it appears that humorous movies helped to increase the patients' opinions of the supportiveness of their staff.

Can you tell from the calculations for the 95% CI in this example how small a difference could be observed and still be statistically significant? Because we subtracted 1.075 from the observed mean difference to calculate the lower limit of the confidence interval, if the mean difference is less than 1.075, the 95% confidence interval will include zero (1.074 − 1.075 = −0.001). In this situation we would conclude the films had no effect. Of course, the same reasoning would apply if the difference was negative; for example, if the mean difference was −1.074, the confidence interval would also contain zero (the upper limit would be −1.074 + 1.075 = +0.001).

5.5.3 The Paired t Test for the Mean Difference

As with means, we can use the same distribution (the t distribution) for both confidence intervals and hypothesis tests about mean differences. Again, we use data from Presenting Problem 3, in which researchers designed an experiment to test whether watching comedies has an effect on the therapeutic relationship between staff and patients with chronic schizophrenia (Gelkopf, Sigal, and Kramer, 1994).

Step 1: State the research question in terms of statistical hypotheses. The statistical hypothesis for a paired design is usually stated as follows, where the Greek letter delta (δ) stands for the difference in the population:

H_0: The true difference in the number of supportive staff is zero, or the films do not affect scores, or, in symbols, $\delta = 0$.

H_1: The true difference in the number of supportive staff is not zero, or the films do affect scores, or, in symbols, $\delta \neq 0$.

We are interested in rejecting the null hypothesis of no difference in two situations: when the program significantly increases patient perception of support levels, and when the program significantly decreases perception of support levels; it is a two-tailed test.

Step 2: Decide on the appropriate test statistic. When the purpose is to see if a difference exists between before and after measurements in a paired design, and the observations are measured on a numerical (either interval or ratio) scale, the test statistic is the t statistic for comparing the means between two paired groups, assuming the differences are normally distributed. We almost always want to know if a change occurs, or, in other words, if the difference is zero. If we wanted to test the hypothesis that the mean difference is equal to some value other than zero, we would need to subtract that value (instead of zero) from the mean difference in the numerator of the following formula:

$$t = \frac{\bar{d} - 0}{SD_d / \sqrt{n}}$$

with $n - 1$ degrees of freedom, where $\bar{d}$ stands for the mean difference and $SD_d / \sqrt{n}$ for the standard error of the mean differences as explained earlier.

Step 3: Select the level of significance for the statistical test. Let us use $\alpha = 0.01$.

Step 4: Determine the value the test statistic must attain to be declared significant. The value of t that divides the distribution into the central 99% is 2.921, with 0.5% of the area in each tail with $n - 1 = 16$ degrees of freedom. We therefore reject the null hypothesis that the program does not make a difference if the value of the t statistic is less than -2.921 or greater than $+2.921$.

Step 5: Perform the calculations. Substituting our numbers (mean difference of 1.35, hypothesized difference of 0, standard deviation of 2.09, and a sample size of 17), the observed value of the t statistic is

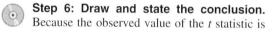

$$t = \frac{\bar{d} - \delta}{SD_d / \sqrt{n}} = \frac{1.35 - 0}{2.09 / \sqrt{17}} = \frac{1.35}{0.507} = 2.67$$

Step 6: Draw and state the conclusion. Because the observed value of the t statistic is 2.67, less than the critical value 2.921, we cannot reject the null hypothesis that mean scores given support staff by patients before and after seeing humorous films are unchanged. In other words, watching the humorous films is interpreted as having no effect on patient perceptions of staff support ($P > 0.01$). This conclusion is different from the one we concluded with the 95% confidence interval. Why? Use the CD-ROM and the Gelkopf and colleagues (1994) data set to calculate a t test of the mean difference using $\alpha = 0.05$. Now is the conclusion the same? As you will see, we came to a different conclusion because we used a lower or more stringent P value. If we used $\alpha = 0.05$, the critical value would be 2.12, and we would reject the null hypothesis.

5.6 PROPORTIONS WHEN THE SAME GROUP IS MEASURED TWICE

Researchers might want to ask two types of questions when a measurement has been repeated on the same group of subjects. Sometimes they are interested in knowing how much the first and second measurements agree with each other; other times they want to know only whether a change has occurred following an intervention or the passage of time. We discuss the first situation in detail in this section and then cover the second situation briefly.

5.6.1 Measuring Agreement between Two People

Frequently in the health field, a practitioner must interpret a procedure as indicating the presence or the absence of a disease or abnormality; that is, the observation is a yes-or-no outcome, a nominal measure. A common strategy to show that measurements are reliable is to repeat the measurements and see how much they agree with each other. As will be discussed more fully in Chapter 13, when one person observes the same subject twice and the observations are compared, the degree of agreement is called **intrarater reliability** (*intra-* meaning within). When two or more people observe the same subject, their agreement is called **interrater reliability** (*inter-* meaning between). A common way to measure interrater reliability when the measurements are nominal is to use the kappa statistic (see definition in following section). If the measurements are on a numerical scale, the correlation between the measurements is found. We will discuss the correlation coefficient in Chapter 8.

In Presenting Problem 4, Garneau and his colleagues (1991) interpreted magnetic resonance images (MRI) of the shoulders of 15 symptomatic patients. Two radiologists made independent evaluations; in other words, one radiologist did not know the results of the other radiologist's determination. Their initial evaluations of positive or negative for labral tear from Table 5–8 (ignoring whether there really was a tear) have been rearranged in Table 5–9. Radiologist A diagnosed six of the images as positive; radiologist B diagnosed nine as positive; they agreed on three of these images.

We can describe the degree of agreement between the two radiologists as follows. Three of fifteen (20%) is an underestimate because they also agreed that three of the images were negative. The total observed agreement [(3 + 3)/15 = 40%] is an overestimate, because it ignores the fact that, with only two categories (positive and negative), they would agree by chance part of the time. We must therefore adjust their observed agreement for chance agreement and see how much they agree beyond the level of chance.

To find the percentage of images they would agree on by chance we use a straightforward application of one of the probability rules we discussed in Chapter 4. If the radiologists make independent assessments of each image, we can use the multiplication rule for two independent events to see how likely it is that they agree merely by chance.

The statistic most often used to measure agreement between two observers on a binary variable is **kappa** (κ), defined as the agreement beyond chance divided by the amount of possible agreement beyond chance. Reviewing the data in Table 5–9, radiologist A said six, or 40%, of the images were positive, and radiologist B said nine, or 60%, were positive. Using the multiplication rule, they would therefore agree that by chance 40% × 60%, or 24%, of the images were positive. Similarly, by chance alone the radiologists would agree that 60% × 40%, or another 24%, were negative. Any two radiologists would therefore agree by chance in their assessments on 24% + 24%, or

Table 5–8. Subject-specific evaluations of labral tears in symptomatic patients.

Patient	Standard of Reference[a]	Radiologist A		Radiologist B	
		First Evaluation[b,c]	Second Evaluation	First Evaluation	Second Evaluation
1	+, II	TP*	TP*	TP*	TP*
2	+, II	TP	FN	TP*	TP
3	+, II	FN	TP	TP*	TP
4	+, II	FN	TP*	TP*	TP*
5	+, I	TP*	TP*	TP	TP*
6	+, I	TP*	TP*	FN	TP*
7	+, I	FN	TP*	TP	TP
8	+, I	FN	FN	TP	FN
9	+, I	FN	FN	FN	FN
10	–	TN	FP	TN	TN
11	–	TN	FP	TN	TN
12	–	TN	FP	FP	FP
13	–	TN	FP	FP	FP
14	–	FP	FP	TN	FP
15	–	FP	FP	TN	FP

[a]+ indicates positive at surgery or arthroscopy for labral tear; – indicates negative at surgery or arthroscopy for labral tear or presumed normal. I indicates grade I labral tear (labrum separated from articular surface); II indicates grade II labral tear (labrum absent).
[b]TP indicates true-positive findings; FN false-negative findings; FP false-positive findings; and TN true-negative findings.
[c]* indicates a correct determination of grade, based on arthroscopy or surgery.
Source: Adapted and reproduced, with permission from the author and publisher, from Garneau RA et al: Glenoid labrum: Evaluation with MR imaging. *Radiology* 1991;**179:**519–522.

48%, of the images. In actuality, the radiologists agreed on (3 + 3)/15, or 40%, of the 40 images, so their level of agreement beyond chance was 0.40 – 0.48, or –0.08, the numerator of κ. In this example, agreement beyond chance is negative because, in fact, these radiologists agreed less often than would occur by chance.

The potential agreement beyond chance is simply 100% minus the chance agreement of 48%, or, using proportions, 1 – 0.48 = 0.52. κ in this example is therefore –0.08/0.52 = –0.154. The formula for kappa and our calculations are as follows:

$$\kappa = \left(\frac{\text{Observed} - \text{Expected agreement}}{1 - \text{Expected agreement}} \right)$$

$$= \left(\frac{O - E}{1 - E} \right)$$

$$= \frac{0.40 - 0.48}{1 - 0.48} = \frac{-0.08}{0.52}$$

$$= -0.154$$

Sackett and associates (1991) point out that the level of agreement varies considerably depending on the clinical task, ranging from 57% agreement with a κ of 0.30 for two cardiologists examining the same electrocardiograms from different patients, to 97% agreement with a κ of 0.67 for two radiologists examining the same set of mammograms. Byrt (1996) has proposed the following guidelines for interpreting kappa:

0.93–1.00	Excellent agreement
0.81–0.92	Very good agreement
0.61–0.80	Good agreement
0.41–0.60	Fair agreement
0.21–0.40	Slight agreement
0.01–0.20	Poor agreement
≤0.00	No agreement

When κ is zero, agreement is only at the level expected by chance. When κ is negative, as in the previous example, the observed level of agreement is less than we would expect by chance alone. This example illustrates the need for studies on interobserver agreement to be carefully designed so that precise criteria and adequate numbers of images are included in the study (Freedman et al, 1993).

Table 5–9. Observed agreement on magnetic resonance imaging.

		Radiologist B		Radiologist A Totals
		Positive	Negative	
Radiologist A	**Positive**	3	3	6
	Negative	6	3	9
Radiologist B	**Totals**	9	6	15

Source: Adapted and reproduced, with permission of the author and publisher, from Garneau RA et al: Glenoid labrum: Evaluation with MR imaging. *Radiology* 1991;**179:**519–522.

The 2×2 table in Table 5–9 is reproduced by NCSS in Table 5–10, along with the calculation of kappa. Most of the time, we are interested in the kappa statistic as a descriptive measure and not whether it is statistically significant. The NCSS statistical program reports the value of t for the kappa statistic; we can use the tables in Appendix A if we want to know the probability. Alternatively, we can use the probability calculator in NCSS.

5.6.2 Proportions in Studies with Repeated Measurements and the McNemar Test

In studies in which the outcome is a binary (yes/no) variable, researchers may want to know whether the proportion of subjects with (or without) the characteristic of interest changes after an intervention or the passage of time. In these types of studies, we need a statistical test that is not only similar to the paired t test, but also appropriate with nominal data. The McNemar test can be used for comparing paired proportions.

The researchers in Presenting Problem 5 (Henderson et al, 1997) wanted to know whether changes occurred in the status of elderly people who were interviewed twice, the second time happening 3–4 years after the first interview. We will cover this study in more detail when we discuss regression in Chapters 8 and 10, but we focus on it here because it also illustrates the McNemar test. One of the variables in the interview was marital status, and it is reasonable to ask whether the proportion of elderly who were married changed over the study period. Here we have a binary variable: people are either married or not.

Data on marital status (for the subjects for whom the investigators had the information at both interviews) is displayed in a 2×2 table in Table 5–11. The authors refer to the baseline data as wave 1 and the follow-up as wave 2. At wave 1, 336, or 56.6%,

Table 5–10. Comparison of radiographic readings by two radiologists.

Cross Tabulation Report

Radiologist B	Radiologist A		
	Negative	Positive	Total
Negative	3	6	9
Positive	3	3	6
Total	6	9	15

The number of rows with at least one missing value is 0.

Chi-Square Statistics Section

Kappa reliability test	−0.153846
Kappa's standard error	0.238337
Kappa's t value	−0.645497

Source: Data, used with the permission of the author and publisher, from Garneau RA et al: Glenoid labrum: Evaluation with MR imaging. *Radiology* 1991;**179**:519–522. Table produced with NCSS 97, a registered trademark of the Number Cruncher Statistical System; used with permission.

Table 5–11. Number of elderly depressed at the first interview (wave 1) and the second interview (wave 2) 3–4 years later.

Married at Wave 1 × Married at Wave 2 Crosstabulation

Count

		Married at Wave 2		
		No	Yes	Total
Married at Wave 1	No	257	1	258
	Yes	45	291	336
	Total	302	292	594

Source: Data, reproduced with permission of the author and publisher, from Henderson AS et al: The course of depression in the elderly: A longitudinal community-based study in Australia. *Psychol Med* 1997;**27**:119–129. Table produced with SPSS, a registered trademark of SPSS, Inc; used with permission.

of the people interviewed were married, but at wave 2 the number had decreased to 292, or 49.2%. Forty-five people who were married at the time of wave 1 were no longer married at wave 2 (lower left cell of the table), and 1 person who was not married at wave 1 married in the intervening time (upper right cell).

The null hypothesis is that the proportions of married elderly people are the same at the two different time periods. The alternative hypothesis is that the paired proportions are not equal. The McNemar test for paired proportions is very easy to calculate; it uses only the numbers in the cells where before-and-after scores change; that is, the upper right and lower left cells. For the numerator we find the absolute value of the difference between the top right and the bottom left cells in the 2×2 table and square the number. In our example this is the absolute value of $|1 - 45| = 44^2 = 1936$. For the denominator we take the sum of the top right and bottom left cells: $1 + 45 = 46$. Dividing 1936 by 46 gives 42.01; in symbols the equation is

$$\text{McNemar} = \frac{(|b - c|)^2}{b + c} = \frac{(|1 - 45|)^2}{1 + 45} = \frac{(44)^2}{46} = 42.09$$

If we want to use $\alpha = 0.05$, we compare the value of the McNemar test to the critical value of 3.84 to decide if we can reject the null hypothesis that the paired proportions are equal. (We explain more about how we determined this value when we discuss chi-square in the next chapter.) Because 42.09 is larger than 3.84, we can reject the null hypothesis and conclude that there is a difference in the proportion of elderly people who were married at the two interview times.

Results from the NCSS program for the McNemar test are given in Table 5–12. Note that NCSS reports the P value as zero. Does this mean there is zero probability the marital status did not change? Not really; it is just that statistical programs report P values to only a given number of decimal places.

Table 5–12. Analysis using the McNemar statistic for the number of elderly depressed subjects at the first interview (wave 1) and the second interview (wave 2) 3–4 years later.

Cross Tabulation Report

	Married at Wave 2		
Married at Wave 2	No	Yes	Total
No	257	1	258
Yes	45	291	336
Total	302	292	594

The number of rows with at least one missing value is 0.

Chi-Square Statistics Section

McNemar's test statistic	42.086957
McNemar's degrees of freedom	1.000000
McNemar's probability level	0.000000

Warning: At least one cell had a value less than 5.

Source: Data, used with the permission of the author and publisher, from Henderson AS et al: The prevalence of depressive disorders and the distribution of depression symptoms in later life: A survey using Draft ICD-10 and DSM-III-R. *Psychol Med* 1997;**27**:119–129. Table produced with NCSS 97, a registered trademark of the Number Cruncher Statistical System; used with permission.

As with the chi-square statistic, it is possible to use a continuity correction with the McNemar test. The correction involves subtracting 1 from the absolute value in the numerator before squaring it. In our example this is the absolute value of $|1 - 45| - 1 = 44 - 1 = 43$, and $43^2 = 1849$. For the denominator we take the sum of the top right and bottom left cells: $1 + 45 = 46$. Dividing 1849 by 46 gives 40.20; the calculations are

$$\text{McNemar} = \frac{(|1 - 45| - 1)^2}{1 + 45}$$
$$= \frac{(43)^2}{46} = 40.20$$

5.7 A SINGLE GROUP WHEN THE OBSERVATIONS ARE NOT NORMALLY DISTRIBUTED

If observations are quite skewed, the t distribution should not be used, because the values that are supposed to separate the upper and lower 2½% of the area of the distribution do not really do so. In this situation, either we can **transform** or **rescale** the observations, or we can use nonparametric methods.

5.7.1 Transforming or Rescaling Observations

Transforming observations expresses their values on another scale. To take a simple example, if weight is measured in pounds, we can multiply by 2.2 to get weight in kilograms. The main reason for knowing about **transformations** is that they sometimes make it possible to use statistical tests that otherwise would be inappropriate. You already know about several transformations. For example, we introduced the standard normal, or z, distribution in Chapter 4, which we obtain by subtracting the mean from each observation and then dividing by the standard deviation. The z transformation is a linear transformation; it rescales a distribution with a given mean and standard deviation to a distribution in which the mean is 0 and the standard deviation is 1. The basic bell shape of the distribution itself is not changed by this transformation.

Nonlinear transformations change the shape of the distribution. We also talked about rank ordering observations when we discussed ordinal scales in Chapter 3. This transformation ranks observations from lowest to highest (or vice versa). The rank transformation can be very useful in analyzing observations that are skewed, and many of the **nonparametric** methods we discuss in this book use ranks as their basis.

Other nonlinear transformations can be used to straighten out the relationship between two variables

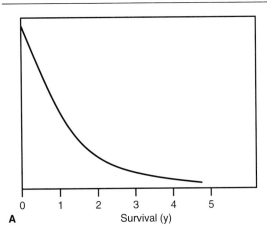

A   Survival (y)

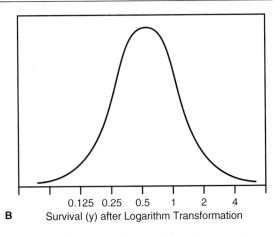

B   Survival (y) after Logarithm Transformation

Figure 5–6. Example of logarithm transformation for survival of patients with cancer of the prostate metastatic to bone.

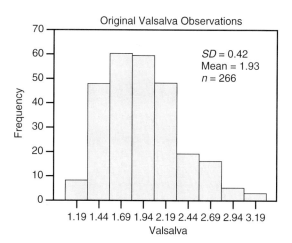
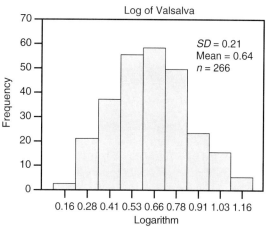

Figure 5–7. Distributions of Valsalva ratio before and after a logarithm transformation has been applied. (Data, used with permission, from Gelber et al: Cardiovascular autonomic nervous system tests: Determination of normative values and effect of confounding variables. *J Auton Nerv Syst* 1997;**67**:40–44. Analysis produced with SPSS; used with permission.)

by changing the shape of the skewed distribution to one that more closely resembles the normal distribution. Consider the survival time of patients who are diagnosed with cancer of the prostate. A graph of possible values of survival time (in years) for a group of patients with prostate cancer metastatic to the bone is given in Figure 5–6A. The distribution has a substantial positive skew, so methods that assume a normal distribution would not be appropriate. Figure 5–6B illustrates the distribution if the logarithm[2] of survival time is used instead, that is, $Y = \log(X)$, where Y is the transformed value (or exponent) related to a given value of X. This is the log to base 10.

Another log transformation uses the transcendental number e as the base and is called the **natural log,** abbreviated ln. Log transformations are frequently used with laboratory values that have a skewed distribution. Gelber and colleagues (1997), featured in Presenting Problem 1 in Chapter 3, studied the Valsalva ratio (ratio of heart rate to deep breathing rate). They employed a log transformation to make Valsalva ratios more normally distributed. Figure 5–7 contains the distribution of Valsalva ratios as well as the transformed natural log values.

Another transformation that has much the same effect is the square root transformation, $Y = \sqrt{X}$. Although this transformation is perhaps not used as frequently in medicine as the log transformation, it can

be very useful when a log transformation overcorrects. In a study of women who were administered a paracervical block to diminish pain and cramping with cryosurgery (Harper, 1997, Presenting Problem 2 in Chapter 6), one of the variables used to measure pain was very skewed. The authors used a square root transformation and improved results.

We calculated the natural log and the square root of the pain score. A histogram of each is given in Figure 5–8. You can see that neither transformation is very close to a normal distribution. In this situation, the investigators might well choose a **nonparametric** procedure that does not make any assumptions about the shape of the distribution.

Transformations have other uses as well. If you are interested in learning more about transformations, see the discussion by Murphy (1982).

5.7.2 The Sign Test for Hypotheses about the Median in One Group

An alternative to transforming data is to use statistical procedures called nonparametric methods. Nonparametric methods are based on weaker assumptions; they do not require the observations to follow any particular distribution nor do they require us to estimate any population values (parameters). They are therefore appropriately called **nonparametric** (ie, no parameters), or **distribution-free,** methods.

Recall the study by Dennison and coworkers (1997) from Presenting Problem 1 about energy consumption levels by 2-year-old children. Can we assume they are normally distributed? Figure 5–9 is a histogram of energy consumption. How would you describe the distribution? It is somewhat positively skewed, or skewed to the right. Should we have used

---

[2]Remember from your high school or college math courses that the log of a number is the power of 10 that gives the number. For example, the log of 100 is 2 because 10 raised to the second power (10^2) is 100, the log of 1000 is 3 because 10 is raised to the third power (10^3) to obtain 1000, and so on. We can also think about logs as being exponents of 10 that must be used to get the number.

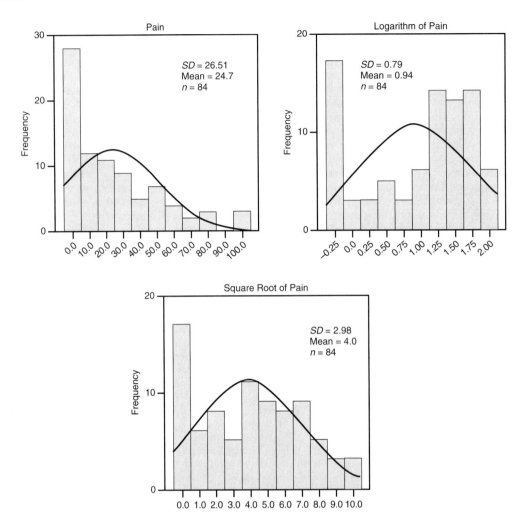

Figure 5–8. Original observations and two transformations of the pain score. (Data, used with permission, from Harper D: Paracervical block diminishes cramping associated with cryosurgery. *J Fam Pract* 1997;**44**:75–79. Analysis produced with SPSS; used with permission.)

the *t* test to compare the mean energy intake with that reported in the NHANES III study? Let us see the outcome if we use a method that requires no assumptions about the distribution.

The **sign test** is a nonparametric test that can be used with a single group using the median rather than the mean. For example, it might be more appropriate to ask: Did children in the study by Dennison and colleagues have the same median level of energy intake as the 1286 kcal reported in the NHANES III study? (Because we do not know the median in the NHANES data, we assume for this illustration that the mean and median values are the same.)

The logic behind the sign test is as follows: If the median energy intake in the population of 2-year-old children is 1286, the probability is 0.50 that any observation is less than 1286. (The probability is also

0.50 that any observation is greater than 1286.) We count the number of observations less than 1286 and can use the binomial distribution (introduced in Chapter 4) with $\pi = 0.50$. Table 5–13 contains the data on the energy level in 2-year-olds ranked from lowest to highest. From Table 5–13, there are 57 two-year-olds in the Dennison and coworkers study with energy levels lower than 1286 and 37 whose energy level was higher. The probability of observing $X = 57$ out of $n = 94$ values less than 1286 using the binomial distribution is

$$P(x) = \frac{n!}{x!(n-x)!}(\pi)^x(1-\pi)^{n-x}$$

$$P(57) = \frac{94!}{57!(94-57)!}(0.5)^{57}(1-0.5)^{94-57}$$

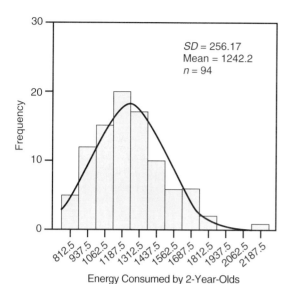

Figure 5–9. A histogram with a normal curve of energy consumption among 2-year-old children. (Data, used with permission, from Dennison BA, Rockwell HL, Baker SL: Excess fruit juice consumption by preschool-aged children is associated with short stature and obesity. *Pediatrics* 1997;**99**:15–22. Analysis produced with SPSS; used with permission.)

Rather than trying to calculate this probability, we use this example as an opportunity to use the z approximation to the binomial distribution to illustrate the sign test. We use the same level of α and use a two-tailed test so we can directly compare the results to the t test in Section 5.3.1.

Step 1: The null and alternative hypotheses are

H_0: The population median energy intake level in 2-year-old children is 1286 kcal, or MD = 1286.

H_1: The population median energy intake level in 2-year-old children is not 1286 kcal, or MD ≠ 1286.

Step 2: Assuming energy intake is not normally distributed, the appropriate test is the sign test; and because the sample size is large, we can use the z distribution. In the sign test we deal with frequencies instead of proportions, so the z test is rewritten in terms of frequencies.

$$z = \frac{|X - n\pi| - (1/2)}{\sqrt{n\pi(1 - \pi)}}$$

where X is the number of children with energy levels less than 1286 (57 in our example), or we could use the number with energy levels greater than 1286; it does not matter. The total number of children n is 94, and the probability π is 0.5, to reflect the 50% chance that any

observation is less than (or greater than) the median. Note that ½ is subtracted from the absolute value in the numerator; this is the continuity correction. We use ½ because this formula is for frequencies (compared with ½n in the formula using proportions).

Step 3: We use $\alpha = 0.05$ so we can compare the results with those found with the t test.

Step 4: The critical value of the z distribution for $\alpha = 0.05$ is ±1.96. So, if the z test statistic is less than −1.96 or greater than +1.96, we will reject the null hypothesis of no difference in median levels of energy intake.

Step 5: The calculations are

$$z = \frac{|57 - 94(0.5)| - 0.5}{\sqrt{94(0.5)(1 - 0.5)}}$$
$$= \frac{|57 - 47| - 0.5}{4.85}$$
$$= \frac{9.5}{4.85}$$
$$= 1.96$$

Step 6: The value of the sign test is 1.96 and is right on the line with +1.96. It is traditional that statisticians do not reject the null hypothesis unless the value of the test statistic exceeds the critical value, so we do not reject the null hypothesis that the median energy intake level in 2-year-olds in the Dennison and coworkers study is different from that in the NHANES III study.

Note the following two points. First, the value of the test statistic using the t test was −1.37. Looking at the formula tells us that the critical value of the sign test is positive because we use the absolute value in the numerator. Second, we drew the same conclusion when we used the t test. If we had not used the continuity correction, however, the value of z would be 10/4.85, or 2.06, and we would have rejected the null hypothesis. Here the continuity correction makes a difference in our conclusion.

⊙ Use the CD-ROM to rank the energy intake of the 5-year-old children and then compare the median with 1573 in the NHANES III study. Are the results the same as you obtained with the t test in Section 5.3.1?

A useful discussion of nonparametric methods is given in the article by Moses and associates (1984) and in the comprehensive text by Hollander and Wolfe (1998).

5.8 MEAN DIFFERENCES WHEN THE OBSERVATIONS ARE NOT NORMALLY DISTRIBUTED

Using the t test requires that we assume the differences are normally distributed, and this is especially important with small sample sizes, ($n < 30$). If there

Table 5–13. Rank ordering of 2-year-old children according to energy consumption.

Row	ID	Energy (ranked)	Row	ID	Energy (ranked)	Row	ID	Energy (ranked)
2	3	754.38	36	196	1133.09	79	65	1348.54
3	111	784.07	37	71	1138.43	80	161	1353.41
4	14	804.94	38	90	1140.86	82	12	1360.29
5	171	846.47	39	155	1142.86	83	1	1361.23
6	110	871.25	40	127	1156.89	84	75	1366.55
7	166	880.52	41	89	1173.30	86	61	1376.19
8	192	906.89	42	93	1175.76	87	27	1379.75
9	208	907.95	43	176	1177.24	89	98	1395.66
10	237	909.58	44	5	1184.59	90	197	1401.53
11	11	923.18	45	87	1191.05	95	135	1415.58
12	209	930.37	46	51	1192.12	98	58	1433.81
13	33	930.92	47	67	1192.35	100	129	1437.98
14	23	944.83	48	108	1192.69	105	70	1448.06
15	66	947.55	49	231	1194.34	107	8	1458.32
17	6	984.12	51	132	1213.32	112	73	1494.85
18	94	990.46	52	163	1229.13	115	179	1500.29
19	88	992.09	53	230	1235.56	116	105	1502.42
20	72	1009.83	54	199	1241.20	117	44	1510.70
21	76	1029.15	55	229	1248.31	120	35	1530.82
22	13	1035.34	56	36	1249.01	123	125	1553.70
23	112	1037.19	57	148	1253.14	129	28	1595.82
24	233	1054.41	58	183	1258.85	133	41	1627.34
25	207	1060.85	59	206	1259.94	135	21	1636.00
26	18	1074.43	63	138	1271.83	138	162	1653.48
27	82	1087.06	64	174	1285.44	141	10	1676.85
29	216	1096.98	65	39	1287.97	148	69	1727.23
30	106	1098.76	67	178	1290.07	150	109	1741.91
31	85	1108.74	68	19	1293.83	154	15	1785.38
32	146	1110.32	72	142	1308.86	155	101	1788.58
33	134	1110.85	75	37	1317.63	165	168	2154.31
34	7	1115.39	76	143	1321.53			
35	57	1122.28	78	92	1337.60			

Variables	Count	Mean	Median	Standard Deviation
Energy	94	1242.197	1221.225	256.1682

Source: Data, reproduced with permission of author and publisher, from Dennison BA, Rockwell HL, Baker SL: Excess fruit juice consumption by preschool-aged children is associated with short stature and obesity. *Pediatrics* 1997;**99**:15–22. Table produced using NCSS; used with permission.

is any reason to suspect that the distribution of the differences is quite skewed and therefore not normal in the population, several other methods are more appropriate. First, one of the transformations we discussed earlier can be used. More often, however, researchers in the health sciences use a nonparametric statistical test that does not require the normal distribution. For paired designs, we can use the sign test that we used with a single group, applying it to the differences. In addition, we can also use a nonparametric procedure called the **Wilcoxon signed rank test** (also called the Mann–Whitney U test). In fact, there is absolutely no disadvantage in using the Wilcoxon signed rank test in any situation with a small sample size, even when observations are normally distributed. The Wilcoxon test is almost as powerful (correctly rejecting the null hypothesis when it is false and thus concluding there is a difference when there really is one) as the *t* test. For paired comparisons, we recommend the Wilcoxon test over the sign test because it is more powerful.

5.8.1 The Wilcoxon Signed Rank Test for the Mean Difference

Using the Wilcoxon signed rank test requires either exhaustive calculations (comparing each observation to all the other observations and counting the number it exceeds) or employing extensive statistical tables. This may be one reason that many introductory statistics texts do not discuss the method. To overcome this disadvantage, two statisticians (Iman, 1974; Conover and Iman, 1981) developed a much simpler method that gives results very close to the Wilcoxon statistic. Their method requires us first to rank the differences and then to calculate the paired *t* statistic by using the ranks instead of the original differences. Because we much prefer to use computers and expect that you do as well, we present the following example simply to give you an idea of the logic behind the procedure.

Using the study by Gelkopf and colleagues (1994), we can compare our conclusion with that found with the paired *t* test. Suppose we believe that the differences in perceived staff support by patients who

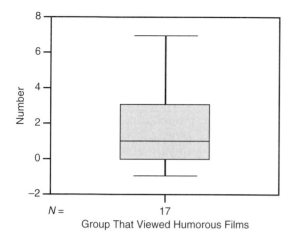

Figure 5–10. Box-and-whisker (boxplot) of changes in the number of staff listed as supportive before and after the intervention. (Data, used with permission, from Gelkopf M, Sigal M, Kramer R: Therapeutic use of humor to improve social support in an institutionalized schizophrenic inpatient community. *J Soc Psychol* 1994; **134**(2):175–182. Table produced with SPSS; used with permission.)

watched comedies are not normally distributed in the population. The differences in the sample certainly do not follow a normal distribution (see the box-and-whisker plot in Figure 5–10). In these situations, we need to use a nonparametric test to determine if significant change occurred in the perceptions of patients who watched comedies.

To use the Iman and Conover approximation, we find the absolute value of each difference. Table 5–14 gives the differences and absolute values of the differences for patients who saw the humorous films. Only two of the patients in this study listed fewer staff as supportive after seeing comedies (patients 6 and 7), so most of the absolute values in this example are the same as the original differences. Next, we treat all the differences as if they are positive and rank their values from lowest to highest (see the last column in Table 5–14). If there is no difference, such as with the first two patients in Table 5–14, we ignore the observations. When there are ties, we average the ranks for those subjects and use the average for each. For example, there are 11 subjects who had nonzero before-and-after differences, so there are 11 ranks we need to analyze. Five subjects (4, 6, 7, 15, and 16) had a difference of 1 in the scores they assigned staff. Because these values rank 1, 2, 3, 4, and 5, we give each of them a value of 3, the mean of these ranks. Finally, we go back and give each rank the same plus or minus sign as the original difference (thus the name, signed rank test).

In the Wilcoxon signed rank test positive and negative ranks tend to cancel one another out. In other words, if about the same number of patients decreased their opinion of staff support as increased it, the mean would be about zero.

Step 1: The null and alternative hypotheses, stated in terms of ranks, are

H_0: The difference in number of supportive staff is equal to zero.
H_1: The difference in number of supportive staff is not equal to zero.

Table 5–14. Differences between after and before measures of staff support patients who watched humorous films: Illustration of approximation of Wilcoxon signed rank test.

Patient Number	Before	After	Difference	Absolute Value	Rank Order[a]	Rank Order[b]
1	2	2	0	0	3.5	
2	0	0	0	0	3.5	
3	0	3	3	3	14	8
4	0	1	1	1	9	3
5	2	5	3	3	14	8
6	3	2	−1	1	−9	3
7	3	2	−1	1	−9	3
8	3	10	7	7	17	11
9	0	0	0	0	3.5	
10	2	4	2	2	12	6
11	1	1	1	0	3.5	
12	1	4	3	3	14	8
13	0	0	0	0	3.5	
14	0	0	0	0	3.5	
15	3	4	1	1	9	3
16	0	1	1	1	9	3
17	0	4	4	4	16	10

[a]Rank order including zero changes.
[b]Rank order omitting zero changes.
Source: Data reproduced, with permission of author and publisher, from Gelkopf M, Sigal M, Kramer R: Therapeutic use of humor to improve social support in an institutionalized schizophrenic inpatient community. *J Soc Psychol* 1994;**134**(2):175–182.

Step 2: To calculate the approximate Wilcoxon signed rank test, we use the signed ranks R instead of the differences d. Then we find the mean rank, the standard deviation of the ranks, and the standard error of the ranks (the standard deviation divided by the square root of the sample size). We substitute these values in the formula for the t test and proceed as usual.

$$t = \frac{\text{Mean rank} - 0}{\text{SD of ranks}/\sqrt{n}}$$

Step 3: We use $\alpha = 0.05$ so we can compare the results with those found with the paired t test.

Step 4: The critical value of the t distribution with $n - 1 = 10$ degrees of freedom is 2.228. So, if the t statistic is less than −2.228 or greater than +2.228, we will reject the null hypothesis of no difference in median number of supportive staff.

Step 5: In this example, the mean of the 11 signed ranks is 4.91, and the standard deviation is 4.78. Using these values in the t statistic formula gives

$$\begin{aligned} t &= \frac{\text{Mean rank} - 0}{\text{SD of ranks}/\sqrt{n}} \\ &= \frac{4.91 - 0}{4.78/\sqrt{11}} \\ &= \frac{4.91}{1.44} \\ &= 3.40 \end{aligned}$$

Step 6: Because 3.40 is greater than 2.228, the value from the t distribution with 10 degrees of freedom and $\alpha = 0.05$, the test is statistically significant. As it turns out, we come to the same conclusion we did with the paired t test on the original unranked observations, that viewing the humorous films had a positive effect on schizophrenic patients' perception of how supportive their staff is.

5.8.2 The Sign Test for Paired Samples

Recall that the sign test for one group involves testing whether the proportion of observations greater than the median observation is different from 0.50. The sign test can also be used with paired designs but on differences instead of single observations. We recommend the Wilcoxon signed rank test, but the following brief overview of the sign test for paired differences may be helpful.

For the sign test with before-and-after studies we use the differences between the number of staff listed as supportive before and after watching comedies. If we assume the films have no influence, then, on average, about half the patients will think that more staff are supportive after watching the comedies, and about half will think fewer staff are supportive.

Nine of the patients listed staff as more supportive after seeing the humorous films, two patients said they were less supportive, and six did not change their opinion (see Table 5–14). We ignore subjects who have no difference in before-and-after scores because they do not influence the conclusion one way or the other. Among the 11 patients who changed their opinions, we can say that the probability that any one patient lists more staff as supportive after the experiment is 0.5, assuming the films made no difference in their attitude toward the staff. In other words, we expect 50% of 11, or 5.5 patients, to change simply by chance. We want to know if 9 of 11 patients is different from 5.5 or whether we could observe 9 by chance. Because the sample size is relatively small, we illustrate the sign test using the binomial distribution.

$$\begin{aligned} P(X) &= \frac{n!}{n!(n-X)!}(0.5)^X(1-0.5)^{n-X} \\ &= \frac{11!}{9!(11-9)!}(0.5)^9(1-0.5)^{11-9} \\ &= \frac{11 \times 10 \times 9!}{9! \times 2 \times 1}(0.00195)(0.25) \\ &= 0.027 \end{aligned}$$

Because we calculated only whether 9 of 11 could occur by chance, the probability, 0.027, is for a one-tailed test. Doubling the probability gives 0.054. Based on the sign test, we conclude there is not enough evidence to say that humorous films had a positive effect on the patients who saw them. This conclusion is not consistent with our conclusion from both the paired t test and the Wilcoxon signed rank test.

We reproduced the output from NCSS illustrating both the Wilcoxon signed rank test and the sign test in Box 5–2 (page 103). Note that NCSS also performs tests to see if the assumption of normality is warranted. As we can see in this example, it is not. A histogram illustrating the distribution of the change in scores for staff is given in Box 5–2.

The P value for the sign test (called the Quantile test by NCSS) is 0.057, close to the value we observed. The actual numbers used in the Wilcoxon signed rank test are different from those we calculated because NCSS uses the exact formula and we used an approximation based on ranks. The conclusion is the same, however.

5.9 FINDING THE APPROPRIATE SAMPLE SIZE FOR RESEARCH

Researchers must learn how large a sample is needed before beginning their research because they may not otherwise be able to determine significance when it occurs. Earlier in this chapter, we talked about type I (α) errors and type II (β) errors, and we defined power $(1 - \beta)$ as the probability of finding significance when there really is a difference. We noted that low power can occur because the sample size is too small.

Readers of research reports also need to know what sample size was needed in a study. This is especially true when the results of a study are not statistically significant (a **negative** study), because the results would possibly have been significant if the sample size had been larger. Increasingly, editors of journals require authors to provide sample size information in the method section of the article. Institutional review boards (IRB) examine proposals before giving approval for research involving human and animal subjects. These review boards also require sample size estimates before they approve a study. Granting agencies require this information as well.

A variety of formulas can determine what size sample is needed, and several computer programs can estimate sample sizes for a wide range of study designs and statistical methods. A somewhat advanced discussion of the logic of sample size estimation in clinical research was reported by Lerman (1996).

Many people prefer to use a computer program to calculate sample sizes. The manuals that come with these programs are very helpful. We present typical computer output from some of these programs in the next two sections and in following chapters.

We also give formulas that protect against both type I and type II errors for two common situations: a study that involves one mean or one proportion, and a study that measures a group twice and compares the difference before and after an intervention. Although we recommend using computer programs instead of calculating numbers by hand, we suggest you work the following examples to better understand how to use the statistical programs.

5.9.1 Finding the Sample Size for Studies with One Mean

This section details the process for estimating the sample size for a study comparing the mean in one group to a standard value or norm.

To estimate sample size for a research study involving a single mean, answer the following four questions:

1. What level of significance (α level or P value) related to the null hypothesis is wanted?
2. What is the desired level of power (equal to $1 - \beta$)?
3. How large should the difference be between the mean and the standard value or norm ($\mu_1 - \mu_0$) for the difference to have clinical importance?
4. What is a good estimate of the standard deviation σ in the population?

Specifications of α for a null hypothesis and β for an alternative hypothesis permit us to solve for the sample size. These specifications lead to the follow-

ing two critical ratios, where z_α is the two-tailed value of z related to α, generally 0.05, and z_β is the one-tailed value of z related to β, generally 0.20.

$$z_\alpha = \frac{\bar{X} - \mu_0}{\sigma/\sqrt{n}} \quad \text{and} \quad z_\beta = \frac{\bar{X} - \mu_1}{\sigma/\sqrt{n}}$$

Solving these two critical ratios for the sample size n gives

$$n = \left[\frac{(z_\alpha - z_\beta)\sigma}{\mu_1 - \mu_0} \right]^2$$

We illustrate the calculations using data from the Dennison and coworkers (1997) study (Presenting Problem 1). Suppose that prior to beginning their study the investigators wanted to know whether observed mean juice consumption in 2-year-olds is different from 5 oz/day—either more or less. They might choose a type I error (concluding that a difference in mean juice consumption occurs when there is none) to be 0.05, and power of 0.80, the probability of detecting a true difference. They assume the standard deviation is about 3 oz. From the given information, what is the sample size needed to detect a difference of 1 or more ounces?

The two-tailed z value for α of 0.05 is ± 1.96 (from Table A–2); this is the critical value that divides the central 95% of the z distribution from 2½% in each tail (refer to Figure 5–5). The lower one-tailed z value related to β is approximately -0.84 (the critical value that separates the lower 20% of the z distribution from the upper 80%). With a standard deviation of 3 and the 1-oz difference the investigators want to be able to detect (consumption of ≤ 4 oz or ≥ 6 oz), the sample size is

$$
\begin{aligned}
n &= \left[\frac{[1.96 - (-0.84)]3}{6 - 5} \right]^2 \\
&= \left[\frac{(1.96 + 0.84)3}{1} \right]^2 \\
&= \left[\frac{8.40}{1} \right]^2 \\
&= 70.56, \text{ or } 71
\end{aligned}
$$

To say that a mean juice consumption of ≤ 4 oz/day or ≥ 6 oz/day is a significant departure from an assumed 5 oz/day (with standard deviation of 3), investigators will need a sample of 71.

The sample size must be 71 instead of 70 because statistical convention dictates that we always round up from a fractional result. Because the investigators were interested in detecting a rather small difference of 1 oz between juice intake in 2-year-old children and an assumed mean in the population, they need a moderately large sample. In Exercise 3 you are asked to calculate how large a sample would be needed if they wanted to detect a difference of 2 or more oz.

5.9.2 The Sample Size for Studies with One Proportion

This section presents the formula for estimating the approximate sample size needed to compare a proportion in a single sample with a standard value. Just as in estimating the sample size for a mean, the researcher must answer the same four questions to estimate the sample size needed for a single proportion.

1. What is the desired level of significance (the α level) related to the null hypothesis, π_0?

2. What level of power $(1 - \beta)$ is desired associated with the alternative hypothesis, π_1?

3. How large should the difference between the proportions $(\pi_1 - \pi_0)$ be for it to be clinically significant?

4. What is a good estimate of the standard deviation in the population? For a proportion, it is easy: the proportion itself, π, determines the estimated standard deviation. It is $\pi(1 - \pi)$.

The formula to determine the sample size is

$$ n = \left[\frac{z_\alpha \sqrt{\pi_0(1 - \pi_0)} - z_\beta \sqrt{\pi_1(1 - \pi_1)}}{\pi_0 - \pi_1} \right]^2 $$

where z_α is the *two-tailed* z value related to the null hypothesis and z_β is the lower *one-tailed* z value related to the alternative hypothesis.

To illustrate, we consider again Presenting Problem 2, Woolson and Watt's (1991) study of the use of IPC to prevent DVT following total hip replacement. In the methods section of their article, the investigators provide a statement about power: 70 patients in each group gives a probability of 0.80 of detecting a 20% difference (from an estimated frequency of 10%) between the three therapy groups with $P < 0.05$. We replicate their analysis to estimate the sample size needed to achieve an 80% power of detecting a decrease in rate of DVT from 30% to 10%, again with $P < 0.05$.

The two-tailed z value related to $\alpha = 0.05$ is ±1.96 (from Table A–2, the critical value dividing the central 95% of the z distribution from the 2½% in each tail; see Figure 5–5). The lower one-tailed z value related to β is approximately −0.84 (the critical value separating the lower 20% of the z distribution from the upper 80%). Then, the estimated sample size is

$$ n = \left[\frac{1.96 \sqrt{0.30 \times 0.70} - (-0.84) \sqrt{0.10 \times 0.90}}{0.30 - 0.10} \right]^2 $$

$$ = \left(\frac{1.15}{0.20} \right)^2 $$

$$ = 5.75^2 $$

from which, by squaring and rounding up, we get 34. Thus, we calculate that these physicians need use only 34 patients (or hip replacement procedures) to

determine whether IPC will decrease to 10% the percentage who develop postoperative DVT. Assuming there is no difference in the three therapies used in the study, the sample of 217 is more than adequate. Exercise 4 calculates the sample size needed if we use 20% instead of 30% as the previous rate.

5.9.3 Sample Sizes for Before-and-After Studies

When studies involve the mean in a group measured twice, generally the research question focuses on whether there has been a change, or stated another way, whether the mean difference varies from zero. As we saw in Section 5.5, we can use the same approach to finding confidence intervals and doing hypothesis tests for a mean in one group as for determining a change in the mean in one group measured twice. So, we can use the same formulas to find the desired sample size. The only difference from the previous illustration is that we test the change (or difference between the means) against a population value of zero. If you have access to one of the power computer programs, you can compare the result from the procedure to calculate the sample size for one mean with the result from the procedure to calculate the sample size for a mean difference, generally referred to as the paired *t* test. If you assume the standard deviations are the same in both situations, you will get the same number. Recall that the major advantage of the paired design is that, by using subjects as their own controls, the standard deviation of the differences is smaller than the standard deviation of the before-and-after measurements themselves. Thus, it is easier to find statistical significance.

Unfortunately, the situation is not as simple when the focus is on proportions. In this situation, we need to use different formulas to determine sample sizes for before-and-after studies. Because paired studies involving proportions occur less often than paired studies involving means, we refer you to the power programs for calculating sample sizes for paired proportions.

5.9.4 Computer Programs for Finding Sample Sizes

Using data from Dennison and coworkers (1997), we use the SamplePower program to calculate the sample size for a study involving one mean. Output from the program is given in Figure 5–11. (If you use this program, you can automatically get the sample size for 80% power by clicking on the binoculars icon in the tool bar.) SamplePower indicates we need *n* of 73, close to the value we calculated of 71. This program also generates a verbal statement (by pressing the icon that has lines on it and indicates it produces a report). Part of a power statement is also reproduced in Figure 5–11.

To find the sample size for a proportion, we use the nQuery program with data from Woolson and

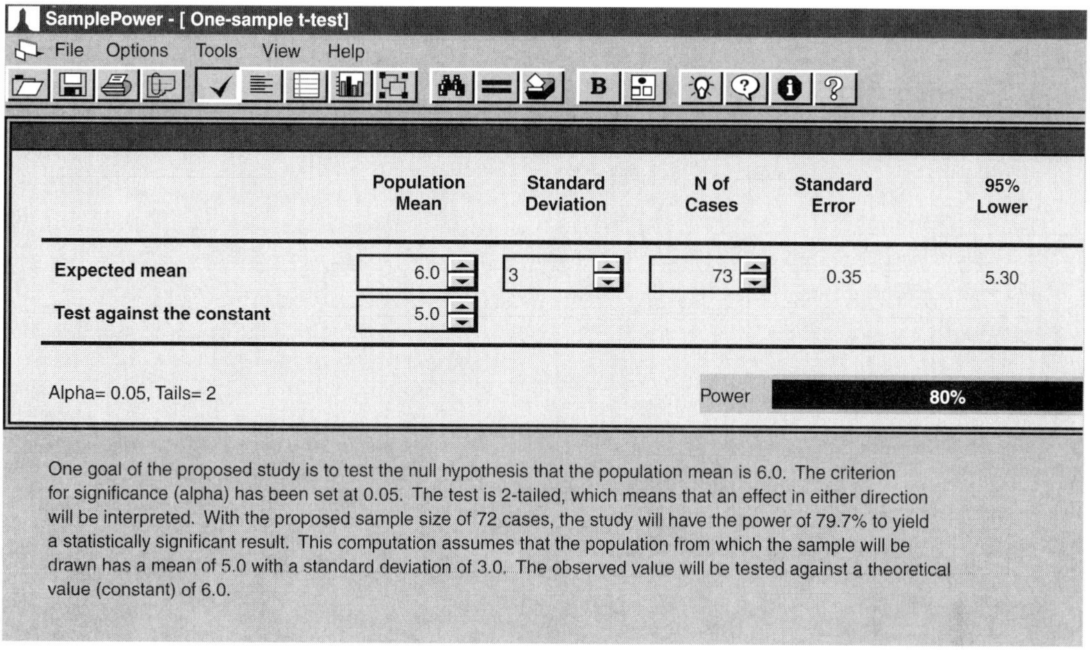

	Population Mean	Standard Deviation	N of Cases	Standard Error	95% Lower
Expected mean	6.0	3	73	0.35	5.30
Test against the constant	5.0				

Alpha= 0.05, Tails= 2   Power   80%

One goal of the proposed study is to test the null hypothesis that the population mean is 6.0. The criterion for significance (alpha) has been set at 0.05. The test is 2-tailed, which means that an effect in either direction will be interpreted. With the proposed sample size of 72 cases, the study will have the power of 79.7% to yield a statistically significant result. This computation assumes that the population from which the sample will be drawn has a mean of 5.0 with a standard deviation of 3.0. The observed value will be tested against a theoretical value (constant) of 6.0.

Figure 5–11. Computer output from the SamplePower program estimating a sample size for the mean juice consumption in 2-year-old children. (Data, used with permission, from Dennison BA, Rockwell HL, Baker SL: Excess fruit juice consumption by preschool-aged children is associated with short stature and obesity. *Pediatrics* 1997;**99**:15–22. Table produced with SamplePower 1.00, a registered trademark of SPSS, Inc.; used with permission.)

Watt (1991). Output from this procedure is given in Figure 5–12 and agrees with our findings that *n* needs to be 34 to give the power we want. nQuery also generates a statement, included in Figure 5–12.

Finally, we illustrate the output from the PASS program for finding the sample size for a mean. The program for one mean can be used for a paired design, and we show this with data from Gelkopf and colleagues (1994). Output from this procedure is given in Box 5–3. Recall that the change in the number of staff rated as supportive by patients is significant with a sample of 17 patients at $P < 0.05$ but not at $P < 0.01$. The output from PASS shows us that a sample size of 29 is needed to conclude that the observed findings are significant at $P < 0.01$. PASS also provides a graph of the relationship between power and sample size and generates a statement (not shown).

5.10 SUMMARY

This chapter illustrated a variety of methods for estimating and testing hypotheses about means and proportions. We also illustrated methods to use in paired or before-and-after designs in which the same subjects are measured twice. These studies are typically called repeated-measures designs. The next chapter

extends this discussion to research questions involving two independent groups of subjects.

We used observations on children whose juice consumption and overall energy intake was studied by Dennison and coworkers (1997). We formed a 95% confidence interval for the mean daily fruit juice consumed by 2-year-old children and found it to be 4.99–6.95 oz/day. We illustrated hypothesis testing about the mean in one group by asking whether the mean energy intake in 2-year-olds was different from the norm found in a national study. The equivalence of the conclusions drawn when using confidence intervals and when doing hypothesis tests was discussed.

In the study published by Woolson and Watt (1991), the investigators concluded that intermittent compression during and after surgery reduces the rate of proximal vein thrombosis after total hip replacement. This finding was consistent with the results of our comparing the observed proportion of patients who developed proximal vein thrombosis with the proportion observed in previous studies (ie, historical controls). The authors also noted that the number of patients in their study did not permit them to conclude that the effectiveness of intermittent compression could be augmented by oral administration of aspirin or heparin; that is, their study did not have sufficient power to detect the observed difference

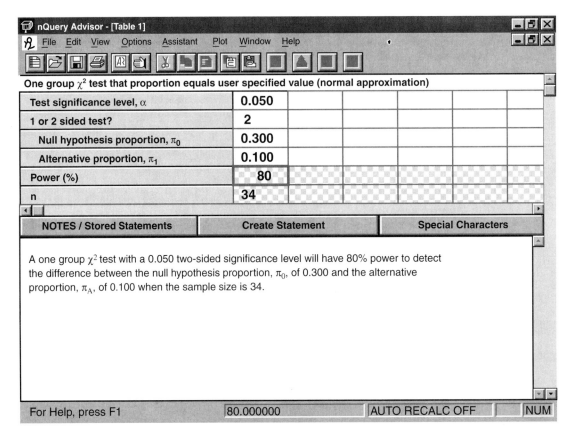

One group χ^2 test that proportion equals user specified value (normal approximation)

Test significance level, α	**0.050**						
1 or 2 sided test?	**2**						
Null hypothesis proportion, π_0	**0.300**						
Alternative proportion, π_1	**0.100**						
Power (%)	**80**						
n	**34**						

NOTES / Stored Statements	Create Statement	Special Characters

A one group χ^2 test with a 0.050 two-sided significance level will have 80% power to detect the difference between the null hypothesis proportion, π_0, of 0.300 and the alternative proportion, π_A, of 0.100 when the sample size is 34.

For Help, press F1   80.000000   AUTO RECALC OFF   NUM

Figure 5–12. Computer output from the nQuery program estimating a sample size for the number of patients needed in the study of deep venous thrombosis. (Data, used with permission, from Woolson ST, Watt JM: Intermittent pneumatic compression to prevent proximal deep venous thrombosis during and after total hip replacement. *J Bone Joint Surg* 1991;**73-A:**507–511.)

with aspirin or heparin. A related study by Schulman and associates (1997) compared the probability of recurrence of DVT in patients who were treated for 6 months versus those who received indefinite treatment. Long-term treatment reduced the incidence of recurrence from over 20% to less than 5%.

To illustrate the usefulness of paired or before-and-after studies, we used data from the study by Gelkopf and colleagues (1994) in which one group of chronic schizophrenic patients watched comedy films for 3 months. The investigators wanted to know whether or not using humor created a more positive relationship between staff and patients. We analyzed the number of staff patients listed as supportive before and after the 3-month period, and we looked at their research question in two ways. First, we used the *t* statistic to form a 95% confidence interval for the change in perceived support by patients who watched humorous films and concluded that there appears to be a beneficial effect in the group that watched comedies. Second, we performed a paired *t*

test for the difference in the before-and-after observations and found that the difference was not statistically significant at $P < 0.01$. We conclude, therefore, that the program makes a difference at $P < 0.05$ but not at $P < 0.01$.

Gelkopf and colleagues (1994) actually did a more complex analysis of the data in their study. They used a method called analysis of covariance to control for any differences between the two groups on their scores at the beginning of the study, and then they compared the groups. Analysis of covariance is a powerful method, which we discuss in Chapter 10. Their analysis showed that the experimental group (viewing comedy films exclusively) perceived an increase in support from the staff but not from other patients. No improvements occurred in family networks or friendships. The authors concluded that humor creates a positive atmosphere, improving the therapeutic alliance between patients and staff.

Two procedures are used when subjects are measured twice and the proportion with a given characteris-

Box 5–3. Computer output from the PASS program estimating a sample size for the number of patients needed in the study of humorous films.

One-Sample *t*-Test Power Analysis

Subject Sample size for Gelkopf and colleagues study
Numeric results for one-sample *t*-test
Null hypothesis: Mean 0 = Mean 1
Alternative hypothesis: Mean 0 < or > Mean 1
The standard deviation was assumed to be known.

Power	N	α	β	Mean 0	Mean 1	σ
0.618	20	0.010	0.382	0.00	1.35	2.10
0.670	22	0.010	0.330	0.00	1.35	2.10
0.717	24	0.010	0.283	0.00	1.35	2.10
0.759	26	0.010	0.241	0.00	1.35	2.10
0.796	28	0.010	0.204	0.00	1.35	2.10
0.828	30	0.010	0.172	0.00	1.35	2.10

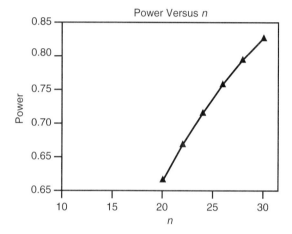

Data, used with permission, from Gelkopf M, Sigal M, Kramer R: Therapeutic use of humor to improve social support in an institutionalized schizophrenic inpatient community. *J Soc Psychol* 1994;**134**(2):175–182. Analyzed with PASS 6.0, a registered trademark of the Number Cruncher Statistical System; used with permission.

tic is of interest. The kappa statistic measures the amount of agreement between two observers and adjusts for agreement that occurs simply by chance. Kappa is frequently used to compare agreement among radiologists, as in the study by Garneau and coworkers (1991), and among people who interpret other diagnostic procedures. On other occasions, investigators want to know whether the proportion of subjects changes after an intervention. In this situation, the McNemar test is used, as with changes in the marital status in the study of elderly by Henderson and colleagues (1997).

We explained alternatives to use when observations are not normally distributed. Among these are several kinds of transformations, with the log (logarithmic transformation) being fairly common, especially for biologic variables. We also discussed nonparametric tests. These tests make no assumptions about the distribution of the data. We illustrated the sign test for

testing hypotheses about the median in one group and the Wilcoxon signed rank test for paired observations. The Wilcoxon signed rank test can also be used to analyze numerical outcomes that are normally distributed, and its power is almost as great as that of the *t* test. Finally, we illustrated the sign test for paired groups. Because it is not as sensitive to differences as the Wilcoxon test, it is used less frequently.

We concluded the chapter with a discussion of the important concept of power. We outlined the procedures for estimating the sample size for research questions involving one group and illustrated the use of three statistical programs that make the process much easier.

In the next chapter, we move on to research questions that involve two independent groups. The methods you learned in this chapter are not only important for their use with one group of subjects, but they also serve as the basis for the methods in the next chapter.

A summary of the statistical methods discussed in this chapter is given in Appendix C. These flowcharts can help both readers and researchers determine which statistical procedure is appropriate for comparing means.

EXERCISES

1. Using the study by Dennison and coworkers (1997), find the 99% confidence interval for the mean fruit juice consumption among 2-year-olds and compare the result with the 95% confidence interval we found (4.99–6.95).
   a. Is it wider or narrower than the confidence interval corresponding to 95% confidence?
   b. How could Dennison and coworkers increase the precision with which the mean level of juice consumption is measured?
   c. Recalculate the 99% confidence interval assuming the number of children is 200. Is it wider or narrower than the confidence interval corresponding to 95% confidence?

2. Using the study by Dennison and coworkers, test whether the mean consumption of soda in 2-year-olds differs from zero. What is the *P* value? Find the 95% confidence interval for the mean and compare the results to the hypothesis test.

3. Using the Dennison and coworkers study, determine the sample size needed if the researchers wanted 80% power to detect a difference of ≥2 oz in fruit juice consumption among 2-year-olds (assuming the standard deviation is 3 oz). Compare the results with the sample size needed for a difference of 1 oz.

4. What sample size is needed if Woolson and Watt (1991) wanted to know if the observed 10% of patients who develop postoperative DVT differed from an assumed norm of 20%? How does this number compare with the number we found assuming a norm of 30%?

5. Our calculations indicated that a sample size of 71 is needed to detect a difference of ≥1 oz from an assumed mean of 5 oz in the Dennison and coworkers study, assuming a standard deviation of 3 oz. Dennison and coworkers had 94 children in their study and found a mean juice consumption of 5.97 oz. Because 94 is larger than 71, we expect that a 95% CI for the mean would *not* contain 5. The CI we found was 4.99–6.95, however, and because this CI contains 5, we cannot reject a null hypothesis that the true mean is 5. What is the most likely explanation for this seeming contradiction?

6. Using the data from the Gelkopf and colleagues study (1994), how large would the mean difference need to be to be considered significant at the 0.05 level if only ten patients were included

in the group of patients who saw comedies? *Hint:* Use the formula for one mean and solve for the difference.

7. Two physicians evaluated a sample of 50 mammograms and classified them as negative (needing no follow-up) versus positive (needing follow-up). Physician 1 determined that 30 mammograms were negative and 20 were positive, and physician 2 found 35 negative and 15 positive. They agreed that 25 were negative. What is the agreement beyond chance?

8. Use the data from the Gelkopf and colleagues study to determine if a change occurs in the number of staff rated as supportive by the neutral-film group. This group watched a variety of films, not exclusively humorous ones.
   a. First, examine the distribution of the changes in scores. Is the distribution normal so we can use the paired *t* test, or is the Wilcoxon test more appropriate?
   b. Second, use the paired *t* test to compare the before-and-after measures of staff support; then, use the *t* test for one sample to compare the difference to zero. Compare the answers from the two procedures. You may use the data set on the CD-ROM or refer to Table 5–7 for the data.

9. Using the Canberra Interview for the Elderly (CIE), Henderson and colleagues (1997) collected data on depressive symptoms and cognitive performance for 545 people. The interview was given at baseline and again 3–4 years later. The CIE reports the depression measure on a scale from 1 to 17.
   a. Use the data set in the folder entitled "Henderson" on the CD-ROM to examine the distribution of the depression scores at baseline and later. What statistical method is preferred for determining if a change occurs in depression scores?
   b. We recoded the depression score as depressed versus not depressed. Use the McNemar statistic to see if the proportion of depressed people is different at the end of the study.
   c. Do the conclusions agree? Discuss why or why not.

10. Dennison and coworkers also studied 5-year-old children. Use the data set in the CD-ROM folder marked "Dennison" to evaluate fruit juice consumption in 5-year-olds.
   a. Are the observations normally distributed?
   b. Perform the *t* test and sign test for one group. Do these two tests lead to the same conclusion? If not, which is the more appropriate?
   c. Produce a box plot for 2-year-olds and for 5-year-olds and compare them visually. What do you think we will learn when we compare these two groups in the next chapter?

11. If you have access to the statistical program Visual Statistics, use the data set on the CD-ROM for Presenting Problem 2 to determine how the distribution changes as the proportion and the sample size change. What happens as the proportion gets closer to 0? to 0.5? to 1? And what happens as the sample size increases? Decreases? Try some situations in which the proportion times the sample size is quite small (eg, 0.2×10). What happens to the shape of the distribution then?

12. Following is a report that appeared in the April–June 1999 *Chance News* from the Chance Web site at http://www.dartmouth.edu/~chance/chance_news/recent_news/chance_news_8.05.html#polls

Read the information and answer the discussion questions.

"Election Had Too Many Polls and Not Enough Context"

We do not often see a newspaper article criticizing the way it reports the news but this is such an article. Schachter writes about the way newspapers confuse the public with their tracking of the polls. He starts by commenting that the polls are "crude instruments which are only modestly accurate". The truth is in the margin of error, which is "ritualistically repeated in the boilerplate paragraph that newspapers plunk about midway through poll stories (and the electronic media often ignore)."

He remarks that when the weather forecaster reports a 60% chance of rain tomorrow, few people believe the probability of rain is exactly 60%. But when a pollster says that 45% of the voters will vote for Joe Smith, people believe this and feel that the poll failed if Joe got only 42%. They also feel that something is wrong when the polls do not agree.

Schacter reviews how the polls did in the recent Ottawa election and finds that they did quite a good job taking the margin of error into account—"much better than the people reporting, actually."

In a more detailed analysis of the polls in this election, Schachter gives examples to show that, when newspapers try to explain each chance fluctuation in the polls, they often miss the real reason voters change their minds.

Schachter concludes by saying: "It's amusing to consider what might happen if during an election one media outlet reported all the poll results as a range. Instead of showing the Progressive Conservatives at 46%, for example, the result would be shown as 44–50%. That imprecision would silence many of the pollsters who like to pretend they understand public opinion down to a decimal point. And after the initial confusion, it might help the public to see polls for what they are: useful, but crude, bits of information."

(Harvey Schachter, *The Ottawa Citizen,* 5 June, 1999)

DISCUSSION QUESTIONS:

1. What do you think about the idea of giving polls as intervals rather than as specific percentages? Would this help also in weather predictions?

2. Do you agree that weather predictions of the temperature are understood better than poll estimates? For example, what confidence interval would you put on a weather predictor's 60% chance for rain?

Research Questions about Two Separate or Independent Groups

PRESENTING PROBLEMS

Presenting Problem 1. Severe uterovaginal prolapse may be surgically treated with a variety of operations designed to correct pelvic support defects. These surgical procedures may be performed using either a vaginal or an abdominal approach. A few studies have compared these two approaches. Benson and colleagues (1996) designed a randomized clinical trial to test the hypothesis that either a vaginal or an abdominal approach is equally effective.

Women were considered candidates for the study if they had cervical prolapse to or beyond the hymen or vaginal vault inversion greater than 50% of its length. Over a 2-year period, women were assigned on the basis of a random number table to have pelvic reconstruction surgery by either a vaginal or an abdominal approach. Surgical outcomes were noted as optimally effective, satisfactorily effective, or unsatisfactorily effective based on an assessment of prolapse symptoms and integrity of the vaginal support during a Valsalva strain maneuver. The patients were examined postoperatively at 6 months and then annually for up to 5 years. Other outcome measures included charges for hospital stay, length of stay, and time required in the operating room. Although a sample size necessary to show a clinically significant difference of 20% with power of 80% and an alpha level of 0.05 was 124 women, the study was aborted for ethical reasons when an interim analysis revealed a disparity in outcomes between the two groups after a total of 88 patients had been enrolled.

We use these data to form a confidence interval for the difference in time required in the operating room. We also use operating room times to compare the variability in two groups. Data on several variables are given in Section 6.2 and on the CD-ROM.

Presenting Problem 2. Cryosurgery is a commonly used therapy for treatment of cervical intraepithelial neoplasia (CIN). The procedure is associated with pain and uterine cramping. Symptoms are mediated by the release of prostaglandins and endoperoxides during the thermodestruction of the cervical tissue. The most effective cryosurgical procedure, the so-called 5-minute double freeze, produces signifi-

cantly more pain and cramping than other cryosurgical methods. It is important to make this procedure as tolerable as possible.

The purpose of Harper's (1997) study was to compare the perceptions of both pain and cramping in women undergoing the procedure with and without a paracervical block. All of the participants received naproxen sodium 550 mg prior to surgery. Those getting the paracervical block were injected with 1% lidocaine with epinephrine at 9 and 3 o'clock at the cervicovaginal junction to infiltrate the paracervical branches of the uterosacral nerve.

Within 10 min of completing the cryosurgical procedure, the intensity of pain and cramping were assessed on a 100-mm visual analog scale (VAS), in which 0 represented no pain or cramping and 100 represented the most severe pain and cramping. Patients were enrolled in a nonrandom fashion (the first 40 women were treated without anesthetic and the next 45 with a paracervical block), and there was no placebo treatment.

We use data on intensity of cramping and pain to illustrate the t test for comparing two groups and the nonparametric Wilcoxon rank sum test. The investigator also wanted to compare the proportion of women who had no pain or cramping at the first and second freezes. We use these observations to illustrate the chi-square test. Data from the study are given in Sections 6.2.4 (means and standard deviations of pain and cramping scores) and 6.3.6 (number of patients experiencing pain or cramping).

Presenting Problem 3. Sleep-disordered breathing (SDB), including obstructive sleep apnea and central sleep apnea, is a common problem in patients undergoing rehabilitation after a stroke. This group of breathing disorders is characterized by periodic reductions in the depth of breathing (hypopnea), periodic cessation of breathing (apnea), or a continuous reduction in ventilation.

Good and colleagues (1996) evaluated 48 patients admitted to a stroke rehabilitation ward to determine the prevalence of SDB and its effect on clinical outcomes. They documented the patients' sleep histories, as well as the presence of morning and excessive daytime sleepiness. Objective measures included arterial oxyhemoglobin desaturation (SaO_2) in all patients and polysomnography in 19 patients. The Barthel index, a standardized scale that measures mobility and activities of daily living, was recorded at admission, at discharge, and at 3 and 12 months after stroke onset. Another primary outcome measure was the ability to return home at discharge and to live at home 3 and 12 months after the stroke. The authors wanted to know if oxygen desaturation has an effect on the patient's ability to live at home after discharge from the hospital.

6.1 PURPOSE OF THE CHAPTER

In the previous chapter, we looked at statistical methods we can use when the research question involves:

1. A single group of subjects and the goal is to estimate the proportion or mean or we want to compare an observed value to a norm or standard.

2. A single group that is measured twice and the goal is to estimate how much the proportion or mean in the group changes between measurements.

In contrast, the procedures in this chapter are used to determine if a difference exists between two groups. We introduce methods for comparing proportions and means in two **independent** groups, that is, knowing the observations for one group does not provide any information about the observations in the second group. In all instances, we assume the groups represent random samples from the larger population to which researchers want to apply the conclusions.

When observations are numerical (either interval or ratio variables) and the research question asks whether the means of two groups are equal, we can use either the two-sample (independent-groups) *t* **test** or, when we are concerned about meeting assumptions for the *t* test, the **Wilcoxon rank sum test.** Benson and colleagues (1996) wanted to know if patients spent different amounts of time in the operating room depending on whether they underwent vaginal or abdominal reconstructive surgery for the treatment of pelvic support defects. As another example, Harper (1997) used the Wilcoxon test to investigate whether receiving a paracervical block resulted in differences in the amount of pain and cramping experienced by women undergoing cryotherapy. We will use data from these studies to illustrate confidence intervals, the *t* test, and the Wilcoxon method. In addition, we suggest an "eyeball" test for means and standard errors presented in graphs.

We can use several methods when observations are nominal or categorical and summarized as proportions and the research question asks whether the proportions in two independent groups are equal. Presenting Problem 3 illustrates this situation. Good and his colleagues (1996) wanted to know whether oxygen desaturation in patients who had a stroke was re-

lated to the patient's being able to be discharged home or to an extended care facility. They defined an index of desaturation (DI) as the number of desaturation events per hour and focused their attention on DI $\geq$ 10/h versus > 10/h. We can use the *z* distribution to form a confidence interval or test proportions. We can also merely count the number of observations and use the chi-square test instead.

Various uses of chi-square and Fisher's exact test, which are useful when sample sizes are small, are discussed. Finally, we reiterate the importance of estimating the sample size needed to help us draw the right conclusions (called determining the power of the statistical test) and illustrate methods for two independent groups.

6.2 DECISIONS ABOUT MEANS IN TWO INDEPENDENT GROUPS

When trying to answer research questions about the means in two separate groups, the appropriate statistic to use is the *t* test for two independent groups. Usually, the research question involves comparing two means to see if they are equal or if one mean is greater than the other mean. For example, Benson and colleagues (1996) in Presenting Problem 1 wanted to know if operating room time differed for patients undergoing vaginal versus abdominal reconstructive surgery to treat pelvic support defects. We noted in Chapter 5 that the *z* test can be used to analyze questions involving means if the *population standard deviation is known.* This, however, is rarely the case in applied research, and researchers typically use the *t* test to analyze research questions involving two independent means.

A survey of statistical methods used in original papers appearing in the *New England Journal of Medicine* (Emerson and Colditz, 1983) reported that 44% used *t* tests. A similar review of four surgical journals (Reznick et al, 1987) indicated that 22% of surgical articles also use *t* tests. Other surveys report that *t* tests are used in 5% of the articles in otolaryngology journals (Hokanson et al, 1987b); 7% of pathology articles (Hokanson et al, 1987a); and 10–15% of articles in psychiatry (Hokanson et al, 1986b), oncology (Hokanson et al, 1986a), family practice (Fromm and Snyder, 1986), obstetrics and gynecology (Welch and Gabbe, 1996), and circulatory physiology (Williams et al, 1997). The nonparametric procedures we introduce in this chapter are used in 3–18% of the articles in the same journals. Furthermore, Williams and coworkers (1997) noted a number of problems in using the *t* test, including no discussion of assumptions, in more than 85% of the articles. Welch and Gabbe (1996) noted errors in using the *t* test when a nonparametric procedure is called for and in using the chi-square test when Fisher's exact test should be employed. Thus, being able to evaluate the use of tests comparing means and proportions—whether they are used properly and how to interpret the results—is an important skill for medical practitioners.

6.2.1 Comparing Two Means Using Confidence Intervals

The means and standard deviations from selected variables are given in Table 6–1. In this chapter, we analyze the operating room time (in minutes) for patients who had the vaginal procedure to correct pelvic defects and those who had the abdominal procedure. We want to know what average difference in time is required in the operating room by these two groups of patients. The variable for time is numerical, and we know that means provide an appropriate way to describe the average with numerical variables. We can find the mean operating room time for each set of patients and form a confidence interval for the difference in the times.

The form for a confidence interval for the difference between two means is

Confidence interval = Mean difference ± Number related to confidence level desired (often 95%) × Standard error of the difference

If we use symbols to illustrate a confidence interval for the difference between two means and let $\overline{X}_1$ stand for the mean of the first group and $\overline{X}_2$ for the mean of the second group, then we can write the difference between the two means as $\overline{X}_1 - \overline{X}_2$.

As you know from the previous chapter, the number related to the level of confidence is the critical value from the t distribution. For two means, we use the t distribution with $(n_1 - 1)$ degrees of freedom

corresponding to the n_1 subjects in group 1 plus $(n_2 - 1)$ degrees of freedom corresponding to the n_2 subjects in group 2 for a total of $(n_1 + n_2 - 2)$ degrees of freedom.

With two groups, we also have two standard deviations. One assumption for the t test, however, is that the standard deviations in the two groups are equal (discussed in Section 6.2.3). We achieve a more stable estimate of the true standard deviation in the population if we average the two separate standard deviations to obtain a **pooled standard deviation** that is based on a larger sample size. The pooled standard deviation may be thought of as average standard deviation, but it is actually a weighted average of the two variances (squared standard deviations) with weights based on the sample sizes. Once we have the pooled standard deviation, we use it in the formula for the standard error of the difference between two means, the last term in the preceding equation for a confidence interval.

The standard error of the mean difference tells us how much we can expect the differences between two means to vary if a study is repeated many times. First we discuss the logic behind the standard error and then we illustrate its use with data from the study by Benson and colleagues.

The formula for the pooled standard deviation looks complicated, but it is simply a weighted average of the squared standard deviations (or variances) in each group. We first square the standard deviation in each group (SD_1 and SD_2) to obtain the variance, multiply each variance by the number in that group minus 1, and add to get $(n_1 - 1) SD_1^2 + (n_2 - 1) SD_2^2$. Of course, the standard deviations, SD_1 and SD_2, are based on the samples because we do not know the

Table 6–1. Means and standard deviations on variables from the study on reconstructive surgery for pelvic defects.

Variable	Group	N	Mean	Standard Deviation	Standard Error of Mean
Age	Vaginal	48	63.5625	9.3055	1.3431
	Abdominal	40	66.1500	9.6571	1.5269
Parity	Vaginal	48	2.5625	1.3977	0.2017
	Abdominal	40	3.3000	1.5055	0.2380
Hemoglobin change	Vaginal	48	2.5792	0.9496	0.1371
	Abdominal	40	2.9525	0.9766	0.1544
Discomfort rating	Vaginal	42	4.3810	1.8993	0.2931
	Abdominal	34	5.2941	2.0528	0.3520
Time to recurrence	Vaginal	30	11.5667	11.4762	2.0953
	Abdominal	15	17.8667	11.8072	3.0486
Operating room time	Vaginal	48	195.6250	38.3198	5.5310
	Abdominal	40	214.7750	46.8065	7.4008
Hospital charge	Vaginal	28	$6536.8929	$851.0053	$160.8249
	Abdominal	19	$8047.7895	$2623.3058	$601.8276
Hospital stay	Vaginal	48	5.1667	1.1547	0.1667
	Abdominal	40	5.3750	1.1252	0.1779

Source: Reproduced, with permission, from Benson JT et al: Vaginal versus abdominal reconstructive surgery for the treatment of pelvic support defects: A prospective randomized study with long-term outcome evaluation. *Am J Obstet Gynecol* 1996;**175**:1418–1422.

true population standard deviations, σ_1 and σ_2. Next we divide by the sum of the number of subjects in each group minus 2.

$$\frac{(n_1 - 1)SD_1^2 + (n_2 - 1)SD_2^2}{n_1 + n_2 - 2}$$

Finally, we take the square root to find the pooled standard deviation.

$$SD_p = \sqrt{\frac{(n_1 - 1)\ SD_1^2 + (n_2 - 1)\ SD_2^2}{n_1 + n_2 - 2}}$$

The pooled standard deviation is used to calculate the standard error of the difference. In words, the standard error of the difference between two means is the pooled standard deviation, SD_p, multiplied by the square root of the sum of the reciprocals of the sample sizes. In symbols, the standard error of the mean difference is

$$SE_{(\bar{x}_1 - \bar{x}_2)} = SD_p \sqrt{\left(\frac{1}{n_1} + \frac{1}{n_2}\right)}$$

Recall from Chapter 5 that the formula for the standard error of a single mean is

$$SE_{\bar{x}} = \frac{SD}{\sqrt{n}} = SD\sqrt{\frac{1}{n}}$$

Perhaps you noticed the correspondence between the formulas for the standard error of a mean and the standard error for the difference between two means. The standard deviation, SD, is replaced by the pooled standard deviation, SD_p; and the square root of the reciprocal of n, $\sqrt{1/n}$, is replaced by the square root of the reciprocal of n_1 plus the reciprocal of n_2.

We use the data on operating room times from Benson and colleagues to illustrate the calculation of the pooled standard deviation, although we always use a computer to do the actual computation. Forty-eight patients underwent the vaginal procedure, and 40 had the abdominal procedure (See Table 6–1). Substituting 48 and 40 for the two sample sizes and 38.32 and 46.81 for the two standard deviations in the formula for the pooled standard deviation, we have

Pooled $SD =$
$$SD_p = \sqrt{\frac{(48 - 1)38.32^2 + (40 - 1)46.81^2}{48 + 40 - 2}}$$
$$= 42.38$$

Does it make sense that the value of the pooled standard deviation is always between the two sample standard deviations? In fact, if the sample sizes are equal, it is the mean of the two standard deviations (see Exercise 4).

Finally, to find the standard error of the difference, we substitute 42.38 for the pooled standard deviation and 48 and 40 for the sample sizes and obtain

$$SE_{(\bar{x}_1 - \bar{x}_2)} = 42.38 \sqrt{\left(\frac{1}{48} + \frac{1}{40}\right)}$$
$$= 42.38 \times 0.214 = 9.07$$

The standard error of the difference in operating room times required for the two procedures is therefore 9.07. The standard error is really just the standard deviation of the differences in means if we repeated the study many times. It indicates that we can expect the mean differences in a large number of similar studies to have a standard deviation of about 9 min.

Now we have all the information needed to find a confidence interval for the mean difference in operating room times. From Table 6–1, the mean operating room times were 195.63 min for patients having the vaginal procedure and 214.78 min for patients having the abdominal procedure. To find the 95% confidence limits for the difference between these means (195.63 − 214.78 = −19.15), we use the two-tailed value from the t distribution for 48 + 40 − 2 = 86 degrees of freedom (Appendix A–3) that separates the central 95% of the t distribution from the 5% in the tails. The value we want is between 2.00 (corresponding to 60 degrees of freedom) and 1.98 (for 120 degrees of freedom). To find a more accurate value, we can interpolate between 2.00 and 1.98 and obtain approximately 1.99 for the value of t. Note that the value for t is very close to the value for z, 1.96, because the degrees of freedom, based on the sample sizes, is relatively large.

Using these numbers in the formula for 95% confidence limits, we have −19.15 ± (1.99) (9.07) = −19.15 ± 18.05 or −37.20 to −1.10. Interpreting this confidence interval, we can be 95% confident that the interval from −37.20 to −1.10 contains the true mean difference in operating room times.[1] Because the interval from −37.20 to −1.10 does not contain the value 0, it is not likely that the mean difference is 0. Table 6–2 illustrates the NCSS procedure for comparing two means and determining a confidence interval (see the shaded line). The confidence interval found by NCSS is −37.19 to −1.11, slightly different from ours due to rounding. Use the data set in the Benson folder and compare your results.

---

[1]To be precise, the confidence interval is interpreted as follows: 95% of such confidence intervals contain the true difference between the two means if repeated random samples of operating room times are selected and 95% confidence intervals are calculated for each sample.

Table 6–2. Confidence interval for operating room times.

Variable   OR TIME

Descriptive Statistics Section

Variable	Count	Mean	Standard Deviation	Standard Error	95% Lower Confidence Limit of Mean	95% Upper Confidence Limit of Mean
GROUP2=1	48	195.625	38.31983	5.530992	184.4981	206.7519
GROUP2=2	40	214.775	46.80647	7.400753	199.8056	229.7444

Confidence-Limits of Difference Section

Variance Assumption	df	Mean Difference	Standard Deviation	Standard Error	95% Lower Confidence Limit of Mean	95% Upper Confidence Level of Mean
Equal	86	−19.15	42.37955	9.072919	−37.18637	−1.11363
Unequal	75.25	−19.15	60.49178	9.23921	−37.55444	−0.7455618

Note: t alpha (equal) = 1.9879, t alpha (unequal) = 1.9920

Equal-Variance t-Test Section

Alternative Hypothesis	t Value	Probability Level	Decision (5%)	Power ($\alpha = 0.05$)	Power ($\alpha = 0.01$)
Difference <> 0	−2.1107	0.037704	Reject H_0	0.550598	0.306520
Difference < 0	−2.1107	0.018852	Reject H_0	0.673347	0.401740
Difference > 0	−2.1107	0.981148	Accept H_0	0.000092	0.000005

Difference: (GROUP2=1) − (GROUP2=2)

Tests of Assumption Section

Assumption	Value	Probability	Decision (5%)
Skewness normality (GROUP=A)	0.8513	0.394626	Cannot reject normality
Kurtosis normality (GROUP=A)	0.4929	0.622103	Cannot reject normality
Omnibus normality (GROUP=A)	0.9676	0.616448	Cannot reject normality
Skewness normality (GROUP=V)	0.9047	0.365649	Cannot reject normality
Kurtosis normality (GROUP=V)	0.7623	0.445874	Cannot reject normality
Omnibus normality (GROUP=V)	1.3995	0.496705	Cannot reject normality
Variance-ratio equal-variance test	*1.4920*	*0.195606*	*Cannot reject equal variances*
Modified-Levene equal-variance test	1.3932	0.241122	Cannot reject equal variances

Source: Reproduced, with permission, from Benson JT et al: Vaginal versus abdominal reconstructive surgery for the treatment of pelvic support defects: A prospective randomized study with long-term outcome evaluation. *Am J Obstet Gynecol* 1996;**175**:1418–1422. Table produced using NCSS 97, a registered trademark of the Number Cruncher Statistical System; used with permission.

6.2.2 An "Eyeball" Test Using Error Bar Graphs

Readers of the literature and those attending presentations of research findings find it helpful if information is presented in graphs and tables, and most researchers use them whenever possible. One easy graphic method to compare the means of two or more independent groups is fairly accurate when sample sizes are ten or greater (Browne, 1979).

We briefly introduced error bar plots in Chapter 3 when we talked about the different graphs that can be used to display data for two or more groups, and error bar plots are the basis for the graphic test. The 95% confidence interval for each group is found, and each confidence interval is placed on a graph. One of the following three results always occurs:

1. The top of one error bar does not overlap with the bottom of the other error bar, as illustrated in Fig-

ure 6–1A. When this occurs, we can be 95% sure that the means in two groups are significantly different.

2. The top of one 95% error bar overlaps the bottom of the other so much that the mean value for one group is contained within the limits for the other group (see Figure 6–1B). This indicates that no statistically significant difference occurs between the groups.

3. If 95% error bars overlap some but not as much as in situation 2, as in Figure 6–1C, we do not know if the difference is significant unless we form a confidence interval or do a statistical test for the difference between the two means.

To use the eyeball method for the mean operating room times, we find the 95% confidence interval for the mean in each individual group. Recall that the 95% confidence limit for a single mean is

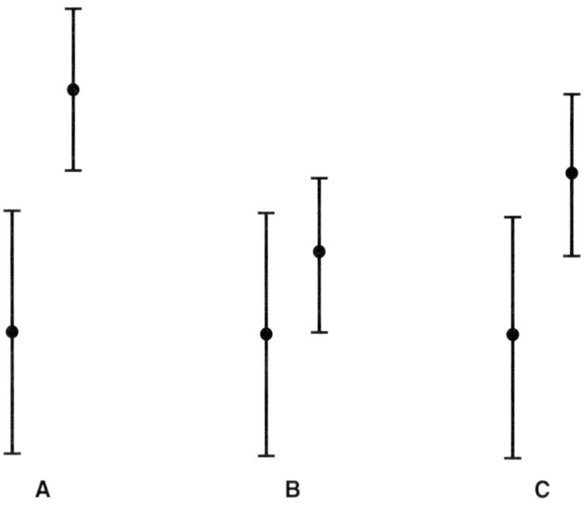

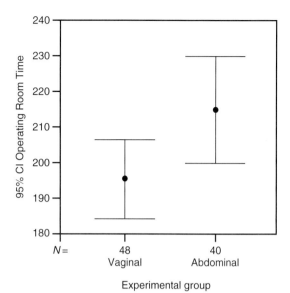

Figure 6–1. Visual assessment of differences between two independent groups, using 95% confidence limits.

Confidence interval = Mean ± Confidence factor
× Standard error of the mean

(Chapter 5 illustrates how to find a 95% confidence interval for a single mean.) We suggest you use the CD-ROM to find the 95% confidence interval for a single mean to check the following calculations. The 95% confidence interval for mean operating room time for patients having the vaginal procedure is

$$195.63 \pm (2.013)\left(\frac{38.32}{\sqrt{48}}\right) = 195.63 \pm 11.13$$
$$= 184.50 \text{ to } 206.76$$

For patients having the abdominal procedure, the 95% confidence interval for the mean operating room time is

$$214.78 \pm (2.021)\left(\frac{46.81}{\sqrt{40}}\right) = 214.78 \pm 14.96$$
$$= 199.82 \text{ to } 229.74$$

These two confidence intervals are shown in Figure 6–2. This example illustrates the situation in Figure 6–1C: The graphs overlap (ie, 206.76 and 199.82 overlap), but not enough to include the mean of either group (ie, neither 195.63 nor 214.78). In this situation, we have two choices: Find the confidence interval for the difference between the two means as in the previous section, or perform a statistical test of the difference between the two means, a procedure we will illustrate in the next section.

A word of caution is needed here. When the sample size in each group is greater than ten, the 95% confidence intervals are approximately equal to the

Figure 6–2. Illustration of error bars. (Data, used with permission, from Benson JT et al: Vaginal versus abdominal reconstructive surgery for the treatment of pelvic support defects: A prospective randomized study with long-term outcome evaluation. *Am J Obstet Gynecol* 1996;**175:**1418–1422. Plot produced with SPSS 97, a registered trademark of SPSS, Inc. Used with permission.)

---

mean ±2 standard errors (*SE*), so graphs of the mean ±2 standard errors can be used for the eyeball test. Some authors, however, instead of using the mean ±2 standard errors, present a graph of the mean ±1 standard error or the mean ±2 standard deviations (*SD*). Plus or minus one standard error gives only a 68% confidence interval for the mean. Plus or minus 2 standard deviations results in the 95% interval in which the *individual* measurements are found *if the observations are normally distributed.* Although nothing is inherently wrong with these graphs, they cannot be interpreted as just outlined. Readers have to check graph legends very carefully before using the eyeball test to interpret published graphs.

6.2.3 Assumptions for the *t* Distribution

Three assumptions are needed to use the *t* distribution for either determining confidence intervals or testing hypotheses. We very briefly mention them here and then we outline some options to use if the observations do not meet the assumptions.

1. As is true with one group, the *t* test assumes that the observations in *each group* follow a normal distribution. Violating the assumption of normality gives *P* values that are lower than they should be, making it easier to reject the null hypothesis and say there is a difference when none really exists. At the

same time, confidence intervals are narrower than they should be, so conclusions based on them may be wrong. What is the solution to the problem? Fortunately, this issue is of less concern if the sample sizes are at least 30 in each group. With smaller samples that are not normally distributed, a **nonparametric** procedure called the **Wilcoxon rank sum** test is a better choice. We discuss this method in Section 6.2.6.

2. Secondly, the standard deviations (or variances) in the two samples are assumed to be equal (statisticians call them homogeneous variances). This is true because the null hypothesis states that the two means are equal, which is actually another way of saying that the observations in the two groups are from the same population. In the population from which they are hypothesized to come, there is only one standard deviation; therefore, the standard deviations in the two groups must be equal if the null hypothesis is true. What is the solution when the standard deviations are not equal? Fortunately, this assumption can be ignored when the sample sizes are equal (Box, 1953). This is one of several reasons many researchers try to have fairly equal numbers in each group. (Statisticians say the t test is **robust** with equal sample sizes.) Some statistical methods test whether standard deviations are equal before doing a t test, and many computer programs automatically provide this information when they do a t test. These tests are discussed in Section 6.2.5.

3. The final assumption is one of independence, meaning that knowing the values of the observations in one group tells us nothing about the observations in the other group. In contrast, consider the paired group design discussed in Chapter 5, in which knowledge of the value of an observation at the time of the first measurement does tell us something about the value at the time of the second measurement. For example, we would expect a subject who has a relatively low value at the

first measurement to have a relatively low second measurement as well. For that reason, the paired t test is sometimes referred to as the dependent groups t test. No statistical test can determine whether independence has been violated, however, so the best way to ensure two groups are independent is to design and carry out the study properly.

6.2.4 Comparing Means in Two Groups with the t Test

In the study on uterine cryosurgery, Harper (1997) wanted to compare the severity of pain and cramping perceived by women undergoing the usual practice of cryosurgery with the perception of pain of women who received a paracervical block prior to the cryosurgery. She used a visual analog scale from 0 to 100 to represent the amount of pain or cramping, with higher scores indicating more pain or cramping. Means and standard deviations for various pain and cramping scores are reported in Table 6–3.

A reasonable research question is whether women who received a paracervical block prior to the cryosurgery had less severe total cramping with cryosurgery than women who did not have a paracervical block. Stating the research question in this way implies that the researcher is interested in a directional or one-tailed test, testing only whether the severity of cramping is less in the group with a paracervical block. From Table 6–3, the mean total cramping score is 35.60 on a scale from 0 to 100 for women who had the paracervical block versus 51.41 for women who did not have the block. This difference could occur by chance, however, and we need to know the probability that a difference this large would occur by chance before we can conclude that these results will generalize to similar populations of women.

The sample sizes are larger than 30 and are fairly similar, so the issues of normality and equal vari-

Table 6–3. Means and standard deviations on variables from the study on paracervical block prior to cryosurgery.

Variable	Group	N	Mean	Standard Deviation	Standard Error of Mean
First cramping score	No block	39	48.51	28.04	4.49
	Block	45	32.88	25.09	3.74
First pain score	No block	39	38.82	28.69	4.59
	Block	45	33.33	29.77	4.44
Second cramping score	No block	39	32.10	28.09	4.50
	Block	45	25.60	27.86	4.15
Second pain score	No block	39	23.77	26.14	4.19
	Block	45	25.33	27.27	4.07
Total cramping score	No block	39	51.41	28.11	4.50
	Block	45	35.60	28.45	4.24
Total pain score	No block	39	43.49	29.06	4.65
	Block	45	38.58	27.74	4.14

Source: Reproduced, with permission, from Harper DM: Paracervical block diminishes cramping associated with cryotherapy. *J Fam Pract* 1997;**44**:71–75.

ances are of less concern and the t test for two independent groups can be used to answer this question. Let us designate women with a paracervical block as group 1 and those without a paracervical block as group 2. The six steps in testing the hypothesis are as follows:

Step 1: H_0: Women who had a paracervical block prior to cryosurgery did not experience less total cramping on the average than women who had no block, as measured by cramping score. In symbols, we express it as

$$\overline{X}_1 \ge \overline{X}_2 \quad \text{or} \quad \overline{X}_1 - \overline{X}_2 \ge 0$$

H_1: Women who had a paracervical block prior to cryosurgery experienced less total cramping on the average than women who had no block, as measured by cramping score. In symbols, we express it as

$$\overline{X}_1 < \overline{X}_2 \quad \text{or} \quad \overline{X}_1 - \overline{X}_2 < 0$$

As an aside, see how awkwardly the null hypothesis is stated, especially with a one-tailed test. The null hypothesis is generally what the investigators want to disprove and the alternative hypothesis is what they really expect to occur.

Step 2: The t test can be used for this research question (assuming the observations follow a normal distribution, the standard deviations in the population are equal, and the observations are independent). The t statistic for testing the mean difference in two independent groups is the difference between the means in the numerator and the standard error of the mean difference in the denominator; in symbols it is

$$t_{(n_1 + n_2 - 2)} = \frac{(\overline{X}_1 - \overline{X}_2)}{SD_p \sqrt{[(1/n_1) + (1/n_2)]}}$$

where there are $(n_1 - 1) + (n_2 - 1) = (n_1 + n_2 - 2)$ degrees of freedom and SD_p is the pooled standard deviation. (See Section 6.2.1 for details on how to calculate SD_p.)

Step 3: Let us use an α of 0.01 so there will be only 1 chance in 100 that we will incorrectly conclude that a difference exists in the cramping score if there really is none.

Step 4: The degrees of freedom are $(n_1 + n_2 - 2)$ $= 45 + 39 - 2 = 82$. For a one-tailed test, the critical value separating the lower 1% of the t distribution from the upper 99% is approximately -2.39 (using the more conservative value for 60 degrees of freedom in Table A–3). So, the decision is to reject the null hypothesis if the observed value of t is less than -2.39. See Figure 6–3.

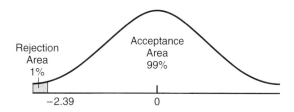

Figure 6–3. Areas of acceptance and rejection for testing hypothesis on mean total cramping in patients with and without paracervical block ($\alpha = 0.01$, one-tailed).

Step 5: The calculations for the t statistic follow. First, the pooled standard deviation is 28.27 (see Exercise 2). Then the observed value for t is

$$t_{(45 + 39 - 2)} = \frac{(35.60 - 51.41)}{28.27\sqrt{[(1/45) + (1/39)]}}$$
$$= \frac{-15.81}{(28.27)(0.219)} = -2.56$$

Please check our calculations using the CD-ROM and the data set in the Harper folder.

Step 6: The observed value of t, -2.56, is less (or more extreme) than the critical value of -2.39, so we can reject the null hypothesis. In plain words, there is enough evidence in this study to conclude that, on the average, women who had a paracervical block prior to cryosurgery experienced less total cramping than women who did not have the block. Note that our conclusion refers to women *on the average* and does not mean that every woman with a paracervical block would experience less cramping.

Remember that one of the required assumptions for using the t test for independent groups is that the standard deviations are equal. The next section discusses methods to test whether this assumption is warranted.

6.2.5 Comparing Variation in Independent Groups

The t test for independent groups assumes equal standard deviations or variances, called homogeneous variances, as do the analysis of variance procedures to compare more than two groups discussed in Chapter 7. We can ignore this assumption if the sample sizes are approximately equal. If not, many statisticians recommend testing to see if the standard deviations are equal. If they are not equal, the degrees of freedom for the t test can be adjusted downward, making it more difficult to reject the null hypothesis, or a nonparametric method, such as the Wilcoxon rank sum test (illustrated in the next section), can be used.

6.2.5.a The *F* Test for Equal Variances: One statistical test for the equality of two variances is called the *F* test. This test can be used to determine if two standard deviations are equal, because the standard deviation is the square root of the variance, and if the variances are equal, so are the standard deviations. Some computer programs calculate the *F* test. This test has some major shortcomings, as we discuss later on; however, an illustration is worthwhile because the *F* test is the statistic used to compare more than two groups (analysis of variance, the topic of Chapter 7).

To calculate the *F* test, the *larger* variance is divided by the *smaller* variance to obtain a ratio, and this ratio is then compared with the critical value from the *F* distribution (corresponding to the desired significance level). If two variances are about equal, their ratio will be about 1. If their ratio is significantly greater than 1, we conclude the variances are unequal. Note that we guaranteed the ratio is at least 1 by putting the larger variance in the numerator. How much greater than 1 does *F* need to be to conclude that the variances are unequal? As you might expect, the significance of *F* depends partly on the sample sizes, as is true with most statistical tests.

Sometimes common sense indicates no test of homogeneous variances is needed. For example, the standard deviations of the total cramping scores in the study by Harper are approximately 28.1 and 28.5, so the variances are 789.6 and 812.3. The practical significance of this difference is nil, so a statistical test for equal variances is unnecessary, and the *t* test is an appropriate choice. As another example, consider the standard deviations of charges for hospital stay from the study by Benson and colleagues (1996) given in Table 6–1: $851 for the group with the vaginal procedure and $2623 for the group with the abdominal procedures. This difference is so great (the *variance* in the abdominal group is almost ten times larger) that the *t* test should not be used, so again no statistical test is needed. The standard deviations of operating room times are 38.3 and 46.8, however, and this difference has practical significance, so a statistical test will be helpful in deciding the best approach to analysis. The null hypothesis for the test of equal variances is that the variances are equal. Using the operating room time variances to illustrate the *F* test, $38.3^2 = 1466.9$ and $46.8^2 = 2190.2$, and the *F* ratio is (putting the larger value in the numerator) $2190.2/1466.9 = 1.49$.

Although this ratio is greater than 1, you know by now that we must ask whether a value this large could happen by chance, assuming the variances are equal. The *F* distribution has two values for degrees of freedom: one corresponding to the numerator degrees of freedom and one corresponding to the denominator degrees of freedom, each equal to the sample size minus one. The *F* distribution for our example has $40 - 1 = 39$ degrees of freedom for the numerator and $48 - 1 = 47$ degrees of freedom for the denominator. Using $\alpha = 0.05$, the critical value of

the *F* distribution from Table A–4 is approximately 1.66. (We used 40 degrees of freedom for the numerator and interpolated between 40 and 60 degrees of freedom for the denominator.) Because the result of the *F* test is 1.49, smaller than 1.66, we do not reject the null hypothesis of equal variances. We can therefore proceed with the *t* test. Figure 6–4 shows a graph of the *F* distribution to illustrate this hypothesis test.

If the *F* test is significant and the hypothesis of equal variances is rejected, the standard deviations from the two samples cannot be pooled for the *t* test because pooling assumes they are equal. When this happens, one approach is to use separate variances and decrease the degrees of freedom for the *t* test (using a formula called the Satterthwaite correction). Reducing the degrees of freedom requires a larger observed value for *t* in order to reject the null hypothesis; in other words, a larger difference between the means is required. The Satterthwaite correction makes the *t* test more conservative; we can think of it as a penalty for violating the assumption of equal standard deviations when we have unequal sample sizes. Alternatively, a nonparametric procedure may be used. It also may be possible to transform the data to another scale (as described in Chapter 5) in which the variances are equal. NCSS gives the *F* test, called the variance ratio equal-variance test, in the Tests of Assumptions section in the *t* test analysis procedure; see the italicized line in Table 6–2.

6.2.5.b The Levene Test for Equal Variances:
The major problem with using the *F* test is that it is

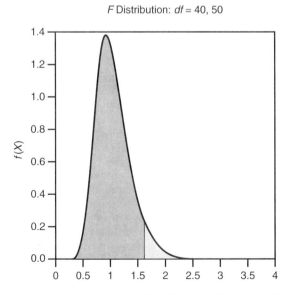

Figure 6–4. Illustration of *F* distribution with 40 and 50 degrees of freedom (with $\alpha = 0.05$ critical area, one-tailed). (Graph produced with Visual Statistics software; used with permission.)

Table 6–4. Computer listing from JMP on testing the equality of variances.

Level	Count	Standard Deviation	Mean Absolute Difference to Mean	Mean Absolute Difference to Median
Abdominal	40	46.80647	37.00250	36.62500
Vaginal	48	38.31983	29.98438	29.95833

Test	F Ratio	df Numerator	df Denominator	Probability > F
O'Brien [0.5]	1.5457	1	86	0.2171
Brown-Forsythe	1.3932	1	86	0.2411
Levene	1.6347	1	86	0.2045
Bartlett	1.6959	1	?	0.1928

Source: Data, used with permission, from Benson JT et al: Vaginal versus abdominal reconstructive surgery for the treatment of pelvic support defects: A prospective randomized study with long-term outcome evaluation. *Am J Obstet Gynecol* 1996;**175**:1418–1422. Plot produced using JMP Statistics and Graphics Guide, a registered trademark of the SAS Institute, Inc; used with permission.

very sensitive to data that are not normal. Statisticians say the F test is not **robust** to departures from normality. In other words, the F test may appear significant because the data are not normally distributed and not because the variances are unequal.

Several other procedures can be used to test the equality of standard deviations, and most computer programs provide options to the F statistic. A good alternative is the Levene test. For two groups, the Levene test is a t test of the absolute value of the distance each observation is from the mean in that group (not a t test of the original observations). So, in essence, it tests the hypothesis that the average deviations (of observations from the mean in each group) are the same in the two groups. If the value of the Levene test is significant, the conclusion is that, on average, the deviations from the mean in one group exceed those in the other.

For example, designating the group having the vaginal procedure as group 1, the absolute value of the difference between each observation and the mean OR time is

$$|X - \bar{X}_1| = |X - 195.625|$$

Similarly, the absolute value of the difference between each observation and the mean OR time in group 2, the group having the abdominal procedure, is

$$|X - \bar{X}_2| = |X - 214.775|$$

Applying the t test to these absolute values results in the Levene test. The Levene test is a good approach whether or not the data are normally distributed.

The Levene test can also be used for testing the equality of variances when more than two groups are being compared. Both the Statistical Package for the Social Sciences (SPSS) and the JMP statistical software from the SAS Institute report this statistic, and NCSS reports the modified Levene test in which the mean in each group in the preceding formula is replaced with the median in each group.

Table 6–4 is the computer output produced when

JMP is used to test the equality of variances. Note that JMP provides four tests and that the probability is similar for all of them. Because the P value of the Levene test is greater than 0.05, 0.2045 in this example, we do not reject the hypothesis of equal variances and proceed with the t test.

If the Levene test is significant, the hypothesis of equal average deviations is rejected and the t test is not appropriate. Some computer programs give another test, called the Welch test, for the means in two independent groups, which can be used instead of the t test. Alternatively, a nonparametric procedure may be used, as we illustrate in the following section.

Use the CD-ROM to test the equality of variances for hospital charges. This test is found in the t test procedure in SPSS and NCSS and in the model fitting procedure in JMP.

6.2.6 Comparing Means with the Wilcoxon Rank Sum Test

Sometimes a researcher wants to compare two independent groups, for which one or more of the assumptions for the t test is seriously violated. The following options are available. In Chapter 5 we discussed transforming the observations in a single group that are not normally distributed to another scale. Transforming observations can also be done when two groups are being analyzed. In particular, transformations can be effective when standard deviations are not equal. Researchers in the health field more often use a nonparametric test instead of transforming the values and then using the t test. The test goes by various names: Wilcoxon rank sum test, Mann–Whitney U Test, or Mann–Whitney–Wilcoxon rank sum test.[2] The text by Hollander and Wolfe (1998) provides information on many nonparametric tests, as does the text by Conover (1998).

---

[2]As an aside, the different names for this statistic occurred when a statistician, Wilcoxon, developed the test at about the same time as a pair of statisticians, Mann and Whitney. Unfortunately for readers of the medical literature, there is still no agreement on which name to use for this test.

In essence, this test tells us whether medians (as opposed to means) are different. The test is very time-consuming to calculate and, as with the Wilcoxon signed rank test for paired groups in Chapter 5, an approximate test that uses the ranks of the observations can be used instead (Conover and Iman, 1981). Because the Wilcoxon rank sum test is available in most statistical computer packages, we only wish to acquaint you with the procedure.

To illustrate the Wilcoxon rank sum test, we use the total cramping scores from Presenting Problem 2 (Harper, 1997). The first step is to rank *all* the scores from lowest to highest (or vice versa), ignoring the group they are in. Table 6–5 lists the scores and their rankings. In this example, the lowest score is 0, given by subjects 5, 21, 46, 52, 55, 77, and 81. Ordinarily, these seven subjects would be assigned ranks 1, 2, 3, 4, 5, 6, and 7. When subjects have the same or tied

Table 6–5. Rank of total cramping scores from the study on paracervical block prior to cryosurgery.

Women without a Block			Women with a Paracervical Block		
Subject	Score	Rank	Subject	Score	Rank
1	14	19	40	50	50
2	88	79	41	70	66
3	37	36	42	66	63
4	27	28	43	50	50
5	0	4	44	75	72
6	40	38	45	5	14
7	35	35	46	0	4
8	40	38	47	6	15
9	49	48	48	20	22
10	44	43	49	2	10
11	78	74	50	78	74
12	4	12	51	52	53
13	100	84	52	0	4
14	31	31	53	98	83
15	34	34	64	5	14
16	44	43	55	0	4
17	73	70	56	24	25
18	55	56	57	45	45
19	2	10	58	52	53
20	72	68	59	25	26
21	0	4	60	87	78
22	83	77	61	45	45
23	97	82	62	40	38
24	65	62	63	27	28
25	72	68	64	22	23
26	95	81	65	17	20
27	53	54	66	57	57
28	50	50	67	9	18
29	62	60	68	61	59
30	32	33	69	47	47
31	43	41	70	47	47
32	27	28	71	72	68
33	68	64	72	1	8
34	63	61	73	41	40
35	23	24	74	2	10
36	83	77	75	19	21
37	75	72	76	7	16
38	92	80	77	0	4
39	55	56	78	32	33
			79	79	75
			80	58	58
			81	0	4
			82	70	66
			83	9	18
			84	30	30
Mean rank	49.2	36.7			
Standard deviation	23.7	33.5			

Source: Reproduced, with permission, from Harper DM: Paracervical block diminishes cramping associated with cryotherapy. *J Fam Pract* 1997;**44**:71–75.

scores, however, the practice is to assign the average rank, so each of these seven women is given the rank of 4. This process continues until all scores have been ranked, with the highest score, 100 by subject 13, receiving the rank of 84 because there are 84 subjects.

After the observations are ranked, the ranks are analyzed just as though they were the original observations; that is, the mean and standard deviation of the ranks are calculated for each group of women and these are then used to calculate the pooled standard deviation of the ranks and the t test.

The Wilcoxon rank sum method tests the hypothesis that the means of the ranks are equal in the two groups. Conceptually, the test proceeds as follows: If there is no significant difference between the two groups, some low ranks and some high ranks will occur in each group, that is, the ranks will be distributed across the two groups more or less evenly. In this situation, the means ranks will be similar as well. On the other hand, if a large difference occurs between the two groups, one group will have more subjects with higher ranks than the other group, and the mean of the ranks will be higher in that group.

Use the CD-ROM to do the t test on the rank variable in the Harper data set. To be consistent with the t test on the original observations reported in Section 6.2.4, use $\alpha = 0.01$ and do a one-tailed test to see if the paracervical block results in lower cramping scores.

Using NCSS, the t test on the rank of cramping scores is -2.42, less than the critical value of -2.39, so again we reject the null hypothesis and conclude the paracervical block had a beneficial result. The output from NCSS on both the Wilcoxon rank sum test on the original observations and the t test using the ranked data is given in Table 6–6. Note from the highlighted lines in Table 6–6 that the P value for the differences is 0.009364 when the Wilcoxon rank sum test is used and 0.008897 when the t test on the ranks is done instead. As we can see, using the t test on ranks is a good alternative if a computer program for the Wilcoxon test is not available.

This conclusion from the Wilcoxon rank sum test is the same that we reached using the t test on the original observations. Recall that the three assumptions for the t test are (1) observations are independent, (2) observations are normally distributed, and

Table 6–6. Illustration of t test of cramping score to obtain Wilcoxon rank sum and t test of ranks of cramping score.

A. Wilcoxon rank sum test on cramping score

Variable	Count	Mean	Standard Deviation	Standard Error
No block	39	51.41026	28.11135	4.50142
Paracervical block	45	35.6	28.45123	4.24126

Mann–Whitney U or Wilcoxon Rank Sum Test for Difference in Medians

Variable	Mann–Whitney U	Wilcoxon Sum Ranks	Mean of Wilcoxon Rank Sum	Standard Deviation of Wilcoxon Rank Sum
No block	1139.5	1919.5	1657.5	111.447
Paracervical block	615.5	1650.5	1912.5	111.447
Number sets of ties = 18	Multiplicity factor = 528			

Exact Probability Approximation without Correction

Alternative Hypothesis Level	Probability (5%)	Decision	z Value	Probability Level	Decision (5%)
Difference <> 0			2.3509	0.018728	Reject H_0
Difference < 0			2.3509	0.990636	Accept H_0
Difference > 0			2.3509	0.009364	Reject H_0

B. t Test on rank of total cramping score

Variable	Count	Mean	Standard Deviation	Standard Error
No block	39	49.21795	23.32460	3.734925
Paracervical block	45	36.67778	24.01802	3.580395

Equal-Variance t Test Section

Alternative Hypothesis	t Value	Probability Level	Decision (5%)
Difference <> 0	2.4186	0.017794	Reject H_0
Difference < 0	2.4186	0.991103	Accept H_0
Difference > 0	2.4186	0.008897	Reject H_0

Source: Data, used with permission, from Harper DM: Paracervical block diminishes cramping associated with cryotherapy. *J Fam Pract* 1997;**44:**71–75. Table produced using NCSS 97, a registered trademark of the Number Cruncher Statistical System; used with permission.

(3) the standard deviations (or variances) are the same in each group. Unless there is some reason to suspect otherwise, we assume the observations are independent, and we already concluded in Section 6.2.5 that the standard deviations in the two groups were not different.

We used box-and-whisker plots to evaluate the distribution of the observations (Figure 6–5). What do you conclude about the distributions? The medians (denoted by tiny circles) fall midway in the boxes that enclose the 25th to 75th percentile of scores in both groups, indicating a normal distribution. The positive tail for the scores for the women receiving a block is a little longer than the negative tail, indicating a slightly positive skew, but overall, the distributions are fairly normal. So, it appears that the assumptions for the t test are adequately met in this example, and, as we would expect, the t test and the nonparametric Wilcoxon rank sum test lead to the same conclusion.

The Wilcoxon rank sum test illustrated earlier and the signed rank test discussed in Chapter 5 are excellent alternatives to the t test. When assumptions are met for the t test and the null hypothesis is not true, the Wilcoxon test is almost as likely to reject the null hypothesis. Statisticians say the Wilcoxon test is as powerful as the t test. Furthermore, when the assumptions are not met, the Wilcoxon tests are more powerful than the t test. So, researchers find the Wilcoxon tests very useful.

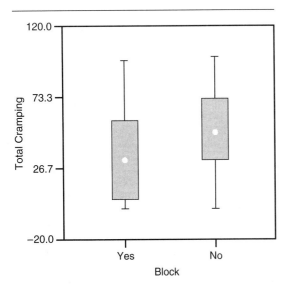

Figure 6–5. Illustration of box plots to compare distributions of cramping scores. (Data, used with permission, from Harper DM: Paracervical block diminishes cramping associated with cryotherapy. *J Fam Pract* 1997;**44:** 71–75. Table produced with NCSS 97, a registered trademark of the Number Cruncher Statistical System; used with permission.)

6.3 DECISIONS ABOUT PROPORTIONS IN TWO INDEPENDENT GROUPS

We now turn our attention to research questions in which the outcome is a counted or categorical variable. As discussed in Chapter 3, proportions are commonly used to summarize counted data. When the research question involves two independent groups, we can learn whether the proportions are different using any of three different methods:

1. Form a confidence interval for the difference in proportions using the z distribution.

2. Test the hypothesis of equal proportions by using the z test.

3. Test the hypothesis of expected frequencies by using a chi-square test.

The first two methods are extensions of the way we formed confidence intervals and used the z test for one proportion in Chapter 5. The chi-square method is new in this chapter, but we like this test because it is very versatile and easy to use. Although each approach gives a different numerical result, they all lead to the same conclusion about differences between two independent groups. The method that investigators decide to use depends primarily on how they think about and state their research question.

Articles in the medical literature often report use of the z and chi-square tests for proportions and frequencies. Literature reviews indicate their use ranges from 3% in pathology articles (Hokanson et al, 1987a) to 25% of the articles in family practice journals (Fromm and Snyder, 1986) and 30% in the *New England Journal of Medicine* (Altman, 1991b).

6.3.1 Confidence Interval for Comparing Two Independent Proportions

Table 6–7 gives information from the study by Good and colleagues (1996) on patients who had suffered a recent stroke. One of the primary outcome measures in this study was the patient's ability to be discharged home rather than to an extended care facility. Of special interest was the subset of patients who had an elevated desaturation index (DI >10/h). The investigators wanted to know if the proportion of patients discharged home was the same, regardless of the level of the desaturation index. To find a confidence interval for the difference in proportions, we first need to convert the numbers to proportions. In this example, the proportion of patients with a normal DI who were discharged home was 27/32 = 0.844, whereas the proportion of patients with an elevated DI who were discharged home was 8/15 = 0.533.

Recall that the general form for a confidence interval is

CI = Statistic ± Number related to the confidence level desired (often 95%) × Standard error of statistic

Table 6–7. Means and standard deviations on variables from the study of sleep-disordered breathing.

Variable	Group	N	Mean	Standard Deviation
Barthel index at admission	DI ≥ 10	15	30.3	16.5
	DI < 10	32	33.4	11.2
Barthel index at discharge	DI ≥ 10	15	50.7	24.0
	DI < 10	32	63.3	18.3
Barthel index at 3 months	DI ≥ 10	14	59.6	20.7
	DI < 10	30	77.8	19.0
Barthel index at 12 months	DI ≥ 10	13	64.2	21.3
	DI < 10	29	80.5	21.7
Able to be discharged home	DI ≥ 10	8		
	DI < 10	27		

Abbreviation: DI = desaturation index.
Source: Reproduced, with permission, from Good DC et al: Sleep-disordered breathing and poor functional outcome after stroke. *Stroke* 1996;**27**:252–259.

Normally, we think about using the binomial distribution when our research question involves proportions. Recall from Chapter 5 that the binomial distribution takes on a shape similar to the z distribution (the standard normal distribution) when the product of the proportion and the sample size gets large. If the product is 5 or more, the z test provides a good approximation to the binomial. We illustrated this method for research questions about one proportion in Chapter 5, and we can use a similar approach for research questions about two proportions, except that the product of the proportion and the sample size must be at least 5 in each group. To do this we let p_1 stand for the proportion of patients with a normal desaturation index (DI) in this study who were able to be discharged home and p_2 for the proportion of patients with an elevated DI who were able to be discharged home. These proportions are estimates of the proportions in the population, and the difference between the two proportions ($\pi_1 - \pi_2$ in the population) is estimated by $p_1 - p_2$ or $0.844 - 0.533 = 0.311$. The difference between two proportions is the statistic about which we want to form a confidence interval (the first term in the previous formula for a confidence interval).

As with all confidence intervals, the second term in the formula comes from the statistical tables and is determined by how confident we want to be. Generally, we form 95% confidence intervals, so referring to the z distribution in Table A–2 and locating the value that defines the central 95% of the z distribution, we find 1.96, a value that is probably becoming familiar by now.

The third term is the standard error of the difference between two proportions. Just as with the difference in two means, it is quite a chore to calculate the standard error of the difference in two proportions, so again we will illustrate the calculations to show the logic of the statistic but expect that you will always use a computer to calculate this value.

Recall from Chapter 5 that the standard error of one proportion is $\sqrt{p(1-p)/n}$. With two proportions, there are two standard errors and the standard error of the difference $p_1 - p_2$ is a combination of them.

$$SE(p_1 - p_2) = \sqrt{\left\{\left[\frac{p_1(1 - p_1)}{n_1}\right] + \left[\frac{p_2(1 - p_2)}{n_2}\right]\right\}}$$

Similar to the way two sample standard deviations are pooled when two means are compared, the two sample proportions are pooled to form a weighted average using the sample sizes as weights. The pooled proportion provides a better estimate to use in the standard error; it is designated simply as p without any subscripts and is calculated by adding the observed frequencies ($n_1p_1 + n_2p_2$) and dividing by the sum of the sample sizes, $n_1 + n_2$. When we substitute $p = (n_1p_1 + n_2p_2) \div (n_1 + n_2)$ for each of p_1 and p_2 in the preceding formula, we have the formula for the standard error of the difference: the square root of the product of three values: the pooled proportion p, 1 minus the pooled proportion $(1 - p)$, and the sum of the reciprocals of the sample sizes $(1/n_1) + (1/n_2)$. In symbols, the standard error for the difference in two proportions is

$$SE(p_1 - p_2) = \sqrt{p(1 - p)\left(\frac{1}{n_1} + \frac{1}{n_2}\right)}$$

The formula for the standard error of the difference between two proportions can be thought of as an average of the standard errors in each group. Putting all these pieces together, a 95% confidence interval for the difference in two proportions is $(p_1 - p_2) \pm 1.96 \times SE(p_1 - p_2)$. To illustrate, first find the standard error of the difference between the proportion of patients with a normal versus an elevated desaturation index who were discharged home. The two proportions are 0.844 and 0.533. The pooled, or average, proportion is therefore

$$p = \frac{n_1p_1 + n_2p_2}{n_1 + n_2}$$
$$= \frac{(32 \times 0.844) + (15 \times 0.533)}{32 + 15}$$
$$= 0.745$$

As you might expect, the value of the pooled proportion, like the pooled standard deviation, always lies between the two proportions.

Next, we substitute 0.745 for the pooled proportion, p, and use the sample sizes from this study to find the standard error of the difference between the two proportions.

$$SE(p_1 - p_2) = \sqrt{p(1-p)\left(\frac{1}{n_1} + \frac{1}{n_2}\right)}$$
$$= \sqrt{0.745(1-0.745)\left(\frac{1}{32} + \frac{1}{15}\right)}$$
$$= \sqrt{(0.745)\,(0.255)\,(0.098)} = 0.136$$

So, the 95% confidence interval for the difference in the two proportions is

$$95\%\ CI = (p_1 - p_2) \pm 1.96 \times SE(p_1 - p_2)$$
$$= (0.844 - 0.533) \pm 1.96 \times 0.136$$
$$= 0.311 \pm 0.267,\ \text{or}\ 0.044\ \text{to}\ 0.578$$

The interpretation of this confidence interval is similar to that for other confidence intervals: Although we observed a difference of 0.311, we have 95% confidence that the interval from 0.044 to 0.578 contains the true difference in the proportion of patients who were able to be discharged to their homes.

Because the entire confidence interval is greater than zero (ie, zero is *not* within the interval), we can conclude that the proportions are significantly different from each other at $P < 0.05$ (ie, because it is a 95% confidence interval). If, however, a confidence interval contains zero, there is not sufficient evidence to conclude a difference exists between the proportions. Please confirm these calculations using the CD-ROM, and obtain a 99% confidence interval as well. Are the two proportions significantly different at $P < 0.01$ as well?

6.3.2 The z Test and Two Independent Proportions

Recall that confidence intervals and hypothesis tests lead to the same conclusion. We use the same data on patients with normal and elevated levels of the desaturation index (DI) from the study by Good and colleagues (1996) to illustrate the z test[3] for the difference between two independent proportions. The six-step process for testing a statistical hypothesis

follows. The symbols π_1 and π_2 stand for the proportion in the population of patients.

Step 1: H_0: The proportion of patients with a normal DI discharged home is the same as the proportion of patients with an elevated DI discharged home, or $\pi_1 = \pi_2$.

H_1: The proportion of patients with a normal DI discharged home is not the same as the proportion of patients with an elevated DI discharged home, or $\pi_1 \neq \pi_2$.

Here, a two-tailed or nondirectional test is used because the researcher is interested in knowing whether a difference exists in either direction; that is, whether a larger or smaller proportion of patients with a normal DI was discharged home than was the proportion of patients with an elevated DI.

Step 2: The z test for one proportion, introduced in Chapter 5, can be modified to compare two independent proportions. Remember that it can be used whenever the observed frequencies are 5 or greater in each group. The test statistic, in words, is the difference between the observed proportions divided by the standard error of the difference. In terms of sample values,

$$z = \frac{p_1 - p_2}{\sqrt{p(1-p)[(1/n_1) + (1/n_2)]}}$$

where p_1 is the proportion in one group, p_2 is the proportion in the second group, and p (with no subscript) stands for the pooled, or average, proportion (defined in Section 6.3.1)

Step 3: Choose the level for a type I error (concluding there is a difference in the proportion discharged home when there really is no difference). We use $\alpha = 0.05$ so the findings will be consistent with those based on the 95% confidence interval in the previous section.

Step 4: Determining the critical value for a two-tailed test at $\alpha = 0.05$, the value of the z distribution that separates the upper and lower $2\frac{1}{2}\%$ of the area under the curve from the central 95% is ± 1.96 (from Table A–2). We therefore reject the null hypothesis of equal proportions if the observed value of the z statistic is less than the critical value of -1.96 or greater than $+1.96$. (Before continuing, based on the confidence interval in the previous section, do you expect the value of z to be greater or less than either of these critical values?)

Step 5: Calculations are

---

[3] The z test for the difference between two independent proportions is actually an approximate test. That is why we must assume the proportion times the sample size is greater than 5 in each group. If not, we must use the binomial distribution or, if np is really small, we might use the Poisson distribution (both introduced in Chapter 4).

$$z = \frac{p_1 - p_2}{\sqrt{p(1-p)[(1/n_1) + (1/n_2)]}}$$
$$= \frac{0.844 - 0.533}{\sqrt{0.745(1-0.745)[(1/32) + (1/15)]}}$$
$$= \frac{0.311}{0.136} = 2.287$$

Step 6: The observed value of z, 2.287, is greater than 1.96, so the null hypothesis—that the proportion of patients discharged home is the same regardless of whether their DI was normal or elevated—is rejected. And we can conclude that different proportions of patients were discharged home. In this situation, patients who had an elevated desaturation index were less likely to be able to be discharged home than those with a normal index. Note the consistency of this conclusion with the 95% confidence interval in the previous section.

To report results in terms of the P value, we find the area of the z distribution closest to 2.287 in Table A–2. The area between ±2.287 (first column in Table A–2) is between 0.976 and 0.979 (second column of Table A–2), so the P value is between 0.021 and 0.024; we recommend reporting either $0.01 < P < 0.05$, or $P < 0.03$. Few computer programs give procedures for the z test for two proportions. Instead, they produce an alternative method to compare two proportions: the chi-square test, the subject of the next section. NCSS has a procedure to test two proportions as one of the choices under "Other," and we suggest you confirm the preceding calculations using it.

6.3.3 Using Chi-Square to Compare Frequencies or Proportions in Two Groups

We can use the chi-square test to compare frequencies or proportions in two or more groups and in many other applications as well. Used in this manner, the test is referred to as the chi-square test for independence. This versatility is one of the reasons researchers so commonly use chi-square. In addition, the calculations are relatively easy to apply to data presented in tables. Like the z approximation, the chi-square test is an approximate test, and using it should be guided by some general principles we will mention shortly. After giving some background, we apply the chi-square test to a research question comparing two independent proportions, using data from the study by Good and colleagues (1996). Subsequently, we will show how to use the chi-square test with more than two groups.

Good and colleagues (1996) wanted to know whether the proportion of patients with a normal DI who were discharged home is the same as the proportion of patients with an elevated DI who were discharged home (see Table 6–7). Actually, we can state this research question two different ways:

1. Is there a difference in the proportion of patients who are discharged home with a normal DI versus an elevated DI? Stated this way, the chi-square test (just as the z test) can be used to test the equality of two proportions.

2. Is there an association (or relationship or dependency) between a patient's DI (normal or elevated) and whether the patient is capable of being discharged home? Stated this way, the chi-square test can be used to test whether one of the variables is associated with the other. When we state the research hypothesis in terms of independence, the chi-square test is generally (and appropriately) called the chi-square test for independence.

In fact, we use the same chi-square test regardless of how we state the research question—an illustration of the test's versatility.

6.3.3.a An Overview of the Chi-Square Test: Before using the chi-square test with the data from Good and colleagues, it is useful to examine an intuitive description of the test to understand the logic behind it. Table 6–8A contains data from a hypothetical study in which 100 patients are given an experimental treatment and 100 patients receive a control treatment. Fifty patients, or 25%, respond positively; the remaining 150 patients respond negatively. The numbers in the four cells are the observed frequencies in this hypothetical study.

Now, if no relationship exists between treatment and outcome, meaning that treatment and outcome are **independent,** we would expect approximately 25% of the patients in the treatment group and 25% of the patients in the control group to respond positively. Similarly, we would expect approximately 75% of the patients in the treatment group and approximately 75% in the control group to respond negatively. Thus, if no relationship exists between treatment and outcome, the frequencies should be as listed in Table 6–8B. The numbers in the cells of Table 6–8B are called **expected frequencies.**

The logic of the chi-square test follows:

1. The total number of observations in each column (treatment or control) and the total number of observations in each row (positive or negative) are considered to be given or fixed. (These column and row totals are also called **marginal frequencies.**)

2. If we assume that columns and rows are independent, we can calculate the number of observations expected to occur by chance—the **expected frequencies.** We find the expected frequencies by multiplying the column total by the row total and dividing by the grand total. For instance, in Table 6–8B the num-

Table 6–8. Hypothetical data for chi-square.

A. Observed Frequencies			
	Treatment	Control	Total
Positive	40	10	50
Negative	60	90	150
Total	100	100	200

B. Expected Frequencies			
	Treatment	Control	Total
Positive	25	25	50
Negative	75	75	150
Total	100	100	200

ber of treated patients expected to be positive by chance is $(100 \times 50)/200 = 25$. We put this expected value in cell (1, 1) where the first 1 refers to the first row and the second 1 refers to the first column.

3. The chi-square test compares the observed frequency in each cell with the expected frequency. If no relationship exists between the column and row variables (ie, treatment and response), the observed frequencies will be very close to the expected frequencies; they will differ only by small amounts.[4] In this instance, the value of the chi-square statistic will be small. On the other hand, if a relationship (or dependency) does occur, the observed frequencies will vary quite a bit from the expected frequencies, and the value of the chi-square statistic will be large.

Putting these ideas into symbols, O stands for the observed frequency in a cell and E for the expected frequency in a cell. In each cell, we find the difference and square it (just as we did to find the standard deviation—so, when we add them, the differences do not cancel each other—see Chapter 3). Next, we divide the squared difference by the expected value. At this point we have the following term corresponding to each cell:

$$\frac{(O - E)^2}{E}$$

Finally, we add the terms from each cell to get the chi-square statistic:

$$\chi^2_{(df)} = \sum \frac{(\text{Observed frequency} - \text{Expected frequency})^2}{\text{Expected frequency}}$$

$$= \sum \frac{(O - E)^2}{E}$$

where χ^2 stands for the chi-square statistic, and (df) stands for the degrees of freedom.

6.3.3.b The Chi-Square Distribution: The chi-square distribution, χ^2 (lower case Greek letter chi, pronounced like the "ki" in *kite*), like the t distribution, has degrees of freedom. In the chi-square test for independence, the number of degrees of freedom is equal to the number of rows minus 1 times the number of columns minus 1, or $df = (r - 1)(c - 1)$, where r is the number of rows and c the number of columns. (See Section 6.3.5.f for an illustration of degrees of freedom.) Figure 6–6 shows the chi-square distribution for 1 degree of freedom. As you can see, the chi-square distribution has no negative values. The mean of the chi-square distribution is equal to the degrees of freedom; therefore, as the degrees of freedom increase, the mean moves more to the right.

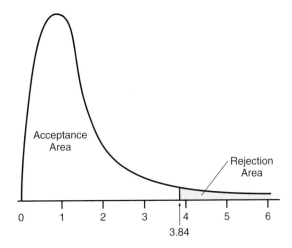

Figure 6–6. χ^2 distribution (with 1 df and $\alpha = 0.05$ critical value).

In addition, the standard deviation increases as degrees of freedom increase, so the chi-square curve spreads out more as the degrees of freedom increase. In fact, as the degrees of freedom become very large, the shape of the chi-square distribution becomes more like the normal distribution.

To use the chi-square distribution for hypothesis testing, we find the critical value in Table A–5 that separates the area defined by α from that defined by $1 - \alpha$. Table A–5 contains only upper-tailed values for χ^2 because they are the values generally used in hypothesis testing. Because the chi-square distribution is different for each value of the degrees of freedom, different critical values correspond to degrees of freedom. For example, the critical value for $\chi^2_{(1)}$ with $\alpha = 0.05$ is 3.841. If you have access to a computer program that produces statistical distributions, find the chi-square distribution and change the degrees of freedom. Note how the curve changes as the degrees of freedom change.

6.3.4 The Chi-Square Test for Independence

Now we apply the chi-square test to the observations in Table 6–7.

Step 1: H_0:   Level of DI and discharge home or elsewhere (ie, columns and rows) are independent.

        H_1:   Level of DI and discharge home or elsewhere (ie, columns and rows) are not independent.

Step 2: The chi-square test is appropriate for this research question because the observations are nominal data (frequencies).

Step 3: We use the traditional α of 0.05.

Step 4: The contingency table has two rows and two columns, so $df = (2 - 1)(2 - 1) = 1$. The critical

---

[4]We say small amounts because of what is called *sampling variability*—variation among different samples of patients who could be randomly selected for the study.

value in Table A–5 that separates the upper 5% of the χ^2 distribution from the remaining 95% is 3.841. The chi-square test for independence is almost always a one-tailed test to see whether the observed frequencies vary from the expected frequencies by more than the amount expected by chance. We therefore decide to reject the null hypothesis of independence if the observed value of χ^2 is greater than 3.841.

Step 5: The first step in calculating the chi-square statistic is to find the expected frequencies for each cell. The illustration using hypothetical data (see Table 6–8) showed that expected frequencies are found by multiplying the column total by the row total and dividing by the grand total:

$$\text{Expected frequency} = \frac{\text{Row total} \times \text{Column total}}{\text{Grand total}}$$

See Exercise 7 to learn why expected values are found this way.

As an illustration, multiplying the number of patients with a normal DI, 32, by the number of patients not discharged home, 12, and then dividing by the total number of patients, 47, gives $(32 \times 12)/(47) = 8.17$, the expected frequency for cell (1, 1), abbreviated $E(1, 1)$. The expected frequencies for the remaining cells in Table 6–7 follow and are listed in Table 6–9:

$$E(1, 2) = (15 \times 12)/47 = 3.83$$
$$E(2, 1) = (32 \times 35)/47 = 23.83$$
$$E(2, 2) = (15 \times 35)/47 = 11.17$$

One of the expected frequencies is less than 5, so we should proceed with caution with the chi-square test. (We explain why expected frequencies should not be too small in Section 6.3.5.)

Then, squaring the difference between the observed and expected frequencies in each cell, dividing by the expected frequency, and then adding them all to find χ^2 gives the following:

$$\chi^2 = \frac{(5 - 8.17)^2}{8.17} + \frac{(7 - 3.83)^2}{3.83}$$
$$+ \frac{(27 - 23.83)^2}{23.83} + \frac{(8 - 11.17)^2}{11.17}$$
$$= 1.23 + 2.62 + 0.42 + 0.90 = 5.17$$

Step 6: The observed value of $\chi^2_{(1)}$, 5.17, is greater than 3.841, so we can reject the null hypothesis of independence and conclude that a dependency or relationship exists between DI and ability to be discharged home. Because this study is not an experimental study, it is not possible to conclude that an abnormal DI *causes* the patient to be discharged someplace other than home. We can only say that DI and discharge location are associated. It is possible that another event, such as the patient's general physical condition, is the precipitating factor for both.

Use the CD-ROM to confirm these calculations. We reproduced output from the chi-square program in NCSS in Table 6–10.

6.3.5 Using Chi-Square Tests

Because of the widespread use of chi-square tests in the literature, it is worthwhile to discuss several aspects of these tests.

6.3.5.a Shortcut Chi-Square Formula for 2 × 2 Tables: A shortcut formula simplifies the calculation of χ^2 for 2 × 2 tables, because expected frequencies do not need to be computed. Table 6–11 gives the setup of the table for the shortcut formula.

The shortcut formula for calculating χ^2 from a 2 × 2 contingency table is

$$\chi^2 = \frac{n(ad - bc)^2}{(a + c)(b + d)(a + b)(c + d)}$$

Using this formula with data gives

$$\chi^2 = \frac{47[(5 \times 8) - (7 \times 27)]^2}{(5 + 27)(7 + 8)(5 + 7)(27 + 8)} = 5.18$$

This value for χ^2 agrees (within rounding error) with the value obtained in Section 6.3.4. In fact, the two approaches are equivalent for 2 × 2 tables.

6.3.5.b Small Expected Frequencies & Fisher's Exact Test: The chi-square procedure, like the test based on the z approximation, is an approximate method. Just as the z test should not be used unless np in both groups is greater than 5, the chi-square test should not be used when the *expected frequencies* are small. Look at the formula for chi-square:

$$\chi^2 = \sum \frac{(O - E)^2}{E}$$

Table 6–9. 2 × 2 Table for study on sleep disturbances.

	A. Observed Frequencies		
Discharged Home	Desaturation Index		
	Normal	High	Total
No	5	7	12
Yes	27	8	35
Total	32	15	47
	B. Expected Frequencies		
Discharged Home	Desaturation Index		
	Normal	High	Total
No	8.2	3.8	12.0
Yes	23.8	11.2	35.0
Total	32.0	15.0	47.0

Source: Adapted and reproduced, with permission, from Good DC et al: Sleep-disordered breathing and poor functional outcome after stroke. *Stroke* 1996;**27**:252–259.

Table 6–10. Illustration of output from χ^2 analysis.

A. Counts Section

	Desaturation Index		
Discharged Home	**Normal**	**High**	**Total**
No	5	7	12
Yes	27	8	35
Total	32	15	47

B. Expected Counts Assuming Independence Section

	Desaturation Index		
Discharged Home	**Normal**	**High**	**Total**
No	8.2	3.8	12.0
Yes	23.8	11.2	35.0
Total	32.0	15.0	47.0

C. Chi-Square Statistics Section

Chi-square	5.176	
Degrees of freedom	1.000	
Probability level	0.023	Reject H_0

WARNING: At less one cell had an expected value less than 5.

D. Fisher's Exact Test Section

	P_1	P_2
Proportions	0.156250	0.466667
Difference ($D_0 = P_1 - P_2$)		−0.310417
Correlation coefficient		−0.331849

E.

Hypothesis	Probability Level	Test Type	Calculation Method
H_0: $P_1 = P_2$			$D = P_1 - P_2$ for a table
H_a: $P_1 < P_2$	0.029733	One-tailed	Sum of probabilities of tables where $D <= D_0$
H_a: $P_1 > P_2$	0.995067	One-tailed	Sum of probabilities of tables where $D >= D_0$
H_a: $P_1 <> P_2$	0.034055	Two-tailed	Sum of probabilities of tables where $|D| >= D_0$

Source: Data, used with permission, from Good DC et al: Sleep-disordered breathing and poor functional outcome after a stroke. *Stroke* 1996;**27**:252–259. Table produced using NCSS 97, a registered trademark of the Number Cruncher Statistical System; used with permission.

It is easy to see that a small expected frequency in the denominator of one of the terms in the equation causes that term to be large, which, in turn, inflates the value of chi-square.

How small can expected frequencies be before we must worry about them? Although there is no ab-solute rule, most statisticians agree that an expected frequency of 2 or less means that the chi-square test should not be used; and many argue that chi-square should not be used if an expected frequency is less than 5. We suggest that if any expected frequency is less than 2 or if more than 20% of the expected frequencies are less than 5, then an alternative procedure called **Fisher's exact test** should be performed. (We emphasize that the *expected* values are of concern here, not the *observed* values. This point is often misunderstood, and researchers sometimes mistakenly think that the chi-square test cannot be performed if a zero or a very small observed value occurs in one of the cells.) If the contingency table of observations is larger than 2 × 2, categories should be combined to eliminate most of the expected values less than 5; this procedure is discussed further in Section 6.3.6.

For Fisher's exact test, the exact probability of the occurrence of the observed frequencies, given the assumption of independence and the size of the marginal frequencies (row and column totals), is computed for the 2 × 2 table. For example, using the

Table 6–11. Standard notation for chi-square 2 × 2 table.

	Treatment	Control	Total
Positive	a	b	$a + b$
Negative	c	d	$c + d$
Total	$a + c$	$b + d$	$a + b + c + d = n$

Shortcut formula for chi-square

$$\chi^2_{(1)} = \frac{n(ad - bc)^2}{(a + c)(b + d)(a + b)(c + d)}$$

Fisher's exact test

$$P = \frac{(a + b)!\,(c + d)!\,(a + c)!\,(b + d)!}{a!\,b!\,c!\,d!\,n!}$$

notation in Table 6–11, the probability P of obtaining the observed frequencies in the table is

$$P = \frac{(a+b)!\,(c+d)!\,(a+c)!\,(b+d)!}{a!\,b!\,c!\,d!\,n!}$$

Recall that ! is the symbol for factorial (introduced in Chapter 4); that is, $n! = n(n-1)(n-2)\cdots(3)(2)(1)$. Calculating the probability of the observed frequencies for the Good study in Table 6–10A gives

$$P = \frac{(12)!\,(35)!\,(32)!\,(15)!}{5!\,7!\,27!\,8!\,47!} = 0.025$$

In other words, the probability of observing the precise distribution in Table 6–10A is 0.025, given the row and column totals. The null hypothesis, however, tested with both the chi-square test and Fisher's exact test is that the observed frequencies or *frequencies more extreme* could occur by chance, given the fixed values of the row and column totals. For Fisher's exact test, the probability for each distribution of frequencies more extreme than those observed must therefore also be calculated, and the probabilities of all the more extreme sets are added to the probability of the observed set. For our example, then, we need to compute P for five additional situations: for frequencies more extreme than the 5 in row 1, column 1 of Table 6–10A, that is, for tables that have frequencies of 4, 3, 2, 1, and 0 in cell 1, 1.

Calculating Fisher's exact test is very tedious, and fortunately, computer programs typically give the value of this statistic for 2×2 tables. NCSS gives the P values for Fisher's exact test, and the output is reproduced in Table 6–10E; the value for a two-tailed test is 0.034. The approximate chi-square statistic calculated for this example in Section 6.3.4 was 5.17; the critical value for $P = 0.05$ is 3.84 and for $P = 0.01$ is 6.64; so we know the probability is between 0.01 and 0.05. Here, we see the exact probability given by Fisher's exact test is 0.034. Readers of medical journals need a basic understanding of the purpose of this statistic and not how to calculate it, that is, you need only remember that Fisher's exact test is used as an alternative to the chi-square test to examine association in 2×2 tables when expected frequencies are small.

6.3.5.c Continuity Correction: Some investigators report corrected chi-square values, called chi-square with **continuity correction** or chi-square with **Yates' correction.** This correction is similar to the one for the z test for one proportion discussed in Chapter 5; it involves subtracting ½ from the difference between observed and expected frequencies in the numerator of χ^2 before squaring; it has the effect of making the value for χ^2 smaller. (In the shortcut formula, $n/2$ is subtracted from the absolute value of $ad - bc$ prior to squaring.)

A smaller value for χ^2 means that the null hypothesis will not be rejected as often as it is with the larger, uncorrected chi-square; that is, it is more conservative. Thus, the risk of a type I error (rejecting the null hypothesis when it is true) is smaller; however, the risk of a type II error (not rejecting the null hypothesis when it is false and should be rejected) then increases. Some statisticians recommend the use of the continuity correction for all 2×2 tables (Yates, 1984); others caution against its use (Grizzle, 1967). Both corrected and uncorrected chi-square statistics are commonly encountered in the medical literature.

6.3.5.d Risk Ratios versus Chi-Square: Both the chi-square test and the z approximation test allow investigators to test a hypothesis about equal proportions or about a relationship between two nominal measures, depending on how the research hypothesis is articulated. It may have occurred to you that the risk ratios (**relative risk** or **odds ratio**) introduced in Chapter 3 (Section 3.7.4) could also be used with 2×2 tables when the question is about an association. The statistic selected depends on the purpose of the analysis. If the objective is to estimate the relationship between two nominal measures, then the relative risk or the odds ratio is appropriate. Furthermore, confidence intervals can be found for relative risks and odds ratios (illustrated in Chapter 8), which, for all practical purposes, accomplish the same end as a significance test. Confidence intervals for risk ratios are being used with increasing frequency in medical journals.

6.3.5.e Overuse of Chi-Square: Because the chi-square test is so easy to understand and calculate, it is sometimes used when another method is more appropriate. A common misuse of chi-square tests occurs when two groups are being analyzed and the characteristic of interest is measured on a numerical scale. Instead of correctly using the t test, researchers convert the numerical scale to an ordinal or even binary scale and then use chi-square. As an example, investigators brought the following problem to one of us.

Some patients who undergo a surgical procedure are more likely to have complications than other patients. The investigators had collected data on one group of patients who had complications following surgery and on another group of patients who did not have complications, and they wanted to know whether a relationship existed between the patient's age and the patient's likelihood of having a complication. The investigators had formed a 2×2 contingency table, with the columns being complication versus no complication, and the rows being patient age ≥45 years versus age <45 years. The investigators had performed a chi-square test for independence. The results, much to their surprise, indicated no relationship between age and complication.

The problem was the arbitrary selection of 45 years as a cutoff point for age. When a t test was performed, the mean age of patients who had complications was significantly greater than the mean age of patients who did not. Forty-five years of age, although meaningful perhaps from a clinical perspective related to other factors, was not the age sensitive to the occurrence of complications.

When numerical variables are analyzed with methods designed for ordinal or categorical variables, the greater specificity or detail of the numerical measurement is wasted. Investigators may opt to categorize a numerical variable, such as age, for graphic or tabular presentation; however, the analysis should be done on the correct scale.

6.3.5.f Illustration of Degrees of Freedom: The chi-square test provides a nice illustration of the concept of degrees of freedom. Suppose we have a contingency table with three rows and four columns and marginal frequencies, such as Table 6–12. How many cells in the table are "free to vary" (within the constraints imposed by the marginal frequencies)?

In column 1, the frequencies for rows 1 and 2 can be any value at all, as long as neither is greater than their row total and their sum does not exceed 100, the column 1 total. The frequency for row 3, however, is determined once the frequencies for rows 1 and 2 are known; that is, it is 100 minus the values in rows 1 and 2. The same reasoning applies for columns 2 and 3. At this point, however, the frequencies in row 3 as well as all the frequencies in column 4 are determined. Thus, there are $(3 - 1) \times (4 - 1) = 2 \times 3 = 6$ degrees of freedom. In general, the degrees of freedom for a contingency table are equal to the number of rows minus 1 times the number of columns minus 1, or, symbolically, $df = (r - 1) \times (c - 1)$.

6.3.6 Using Chi-Square to Compare Frequencies or Proportions in More Than Two Groups

Remember that we can use either the z test or the chi-square test when only two groups are being analyzed. When frequency tables have more than two rows and two columns, the z test is no longer applicable. We can still use chi-square, however, regardless of the number of levels or categories within each variable.

For example, in Presenting Problem 2, Harper (1997) wanted to examine the relationship between the severity of cramping or pain after having a paracervical block versus having no block prior to the cryosurgery. Table 6–13 gives the results in a 2×4 contingency table with the cramping or pain combinations as columns and whether or not a paracervical block was used as the rows.

We use the chi-square statistic regardless of whether we state the research question in terms of proportions or frequencies. For example, Harper could ask whether the proportion of women who reported the different combinations of pain and cramping is the same regardless of whether they had a paracervical block. Alternatively, Harper could ask whether cramping or pain is associated with paracervical block.

The chi-square statistic for the Harper data in Table 6–13 is exactly the same formula as used earlier:

$$\chi^2_{(df)} = \sum \frac{(O - E)^2}{E}$$

except that the degrees of freedom are different. There are eight terms in the formula for χ^2 in this example, one for each of the eight cells of the 2×4 table, so the degrees of freedom are $(r - 1)(c - 1) = (2 - 1)(4 - 1) = 3$.

The following are abbreviated steps for the chi-square hypothesis test. Refer to Table 6–13 for the contingency table, and be sure and confirm these calculations using the CD-ROM.

Step 1: H₀: The occurrence of pain or cramping is independent of whether a paracervical block was used prior to cryosurgery.

H₁: The occurrence of pain or cramping is not independent of whether a paracervical block was used prior to cryosurgery.

Step 2: The chi-square test is appropriate for this research question because the observations are nominal data (frequencies).

Step 3: For this test, let us use an α of 0.01.

Step 4: The contingency table has two rows and four columns, so $df = (2 - 1)(4 - 1) = 3$. The critical value separating the upper 1% of the χ^2 distribution from the remaining 99% with $3df$ is 11.345 (Table A–5). So, χ^2 must be greater than 11.345 in order to reject the null hypothesis of independence.

Step 5: After calculating the expected frequencies for the cells in Table 6–13, we calculate χ^2:

$$\chi^2 = \frac{(1 - 1.86)^2}{1.86} + \frac{(3 - 2.14)^2}{2.14} + \frac{(1 - 1.86)^2}{1.86}$$
$$+ \frac{(3 - 2.14)^2}{2.14} + \frac{(4 - 3.71)^2}{3.71} + \frac{(4 - 4.29)^2}{4.29}$$
$$+ \frac{(33 - 31.57)^2}{31.57} + \frac{(35 - 36.43)^2}{36.43}$$
$$= 0.40 + 0.34 + 0.40 + 0.34 + 0.02$$
$$+ 0.02 + 0.07 + 0.06 = 1.65$$

Table 6–12. Illustration of degrees of freedom in chi-square.

Rows	Columns 1	Columns 2	Columns 3	Columns 4	Total
1	*	*	*		75
2	*	*	*		100
3					225
Total	100	100	100	100	

Table 6–13. Tables of observed and expected frequencies from the study on paracervical block prior to cryosurgery.

	Occurrence of Pain or Cramping: Observed Values				
Block	No Pain/No Cramping	Pain/ No Cramping	No Pain/Cramping	Pain/Cramping	Total
No	1	1	4	33	39
Yes	3	3	4	35	45
Total	4	4	8	68	84

	Occurrence of Pain or Cramping: Expected Values				
Block	No Pain/No Cramping	Pain/ No Cramping	No Pain/Cramping	Pain/Cramping	Total
Yes	1.86	1.86	3.71	31.57	39.00
No	2.14	2.14	4.29	36.43	45.00
Total	4.00	4.00	8.00	68.00	84.00

Source: Reproduced, with permission, from Harper DM: Paracervical block diminishes cramping associated with cryotherapy. *J Fam Pract* 1997;**44:**71–75.

Step 6: The observed value of χ^2 with $3df$, 1.65, is far less than the critical value of 11.345, so we do not reject the null hypothesis. We can conclude that this study does not provide sufficient evidence of a dependency or relationship between simply the occurrence of pain and cramping after the first freeze and whether the woman had a paracervical block.

The output from NCSS is given in Table 6–14. Use the chi-square program on the CD-ROM, and compare the outcome you obtain to the results in Table 6–14.

The astute reader has probably wondered about the number of small expected values in Table 6–13: Six of the eight cells have an expected value less than 5, and two of the cells have an expected value less

than 2. Chi-square is therefore not appropriate because the small expected values make the value of chi-square too large. In this example, even with an inflated value, the chi-square statistic is much smaller than the critical value. The appropriate strategy, however, is to collapse the cells of the table so no cells will have expected values less than 2. In this example, we suggest combining the first three conditions (no pain or cramping, cramping only, pain only) and compare that with both pain and cramping.

The previous illustration of chi-square had only two rows and four columns, but contingency tables can have any number of rows and columns. Of course, the sample size needs to increase as the number of categories increases to keep the expected values of an acceptable size.

6.3.7 The Chi-Square Goodness-of-Fit Test

We described several situations in which chi-square is appropriate, but another application of the chi-square statistic is worth briefly noting: the goodness-of-fit test. The goodness-of-fit test is used to describe how closely observations fit an expected distribution (which might be based on theory or previous observations). For example, chi-square can be used to test whether observations follow a binomial or a normal distribution. The procedure involves dividing the theoretical distribution into intervals and finding the expected frequency in each interval. Then the observed frequencies within each interval are compared with the expected ones.

Sometimes the comparison is with an external set of observations, and in this situation, the external observations are used as the expected frequencies. For example, suppose a group of psychiatrists want to know if the frequency of problems, such as depression, learning disabilities, or family conflict, in their patients are similar to the national norms. The actual numbers of patients seen with each type of problem, the observed frequencies, are compared with the numbers of patients reported by psychiatrists nation-

Table 6–14. Occurrence of pain and cramping after cryosurgery.

Chi-Square Statistics Section

Chi-square	1.638612	
Degrees of freedom	3.000000	
Probability level	0.650667	Accept H_0
Phi	0.139669	
Cramer's V	0.139669	
Pearson's contingency coefficient	0.138326	
Tschuprow's T	0.106125	
Lambda A . . Rows dependent	0.000000	
Lambda B . . Columns dependent	0.000000	
Symmetric lambda	0.000000	
Kendall's tau-B	–0.039013	
Kendall's tau-B (with correction for ties)	–0.094990	
Kendall's tau-C	–0.051398	
Gamma	–0.235294	

WARNING: At least one cell had an expected value less than 5.

Source: Data, used with permission, from Harper DM: Paracervical block diminishes cramping associated with cyrotherapy. *J Fam Pract* 1997;**44:**71–75. Table produced using NCSS 97, a registered trademark of the Number Cruncher Statistical System; used with permission.

ally. The chi-square statistic itself is calculated as shown earlier.

6.4 FINDING SAMPLE SIZES FOR PROPORTIONS IN TWO GROUPS

In Chapter 5 we discussed the importance of having enough subjects in a study to find significance if a difference really occurs. We saw that a relationship exists between sample size and being able to conclude that a difference exists; that is, as the sample size increases, the power to detect an actual difference also increases. The process of estimating the number of subjects for a study is called finding the **power** of the study. Knowing the sample sizes needed is helpful in determining whether a negative study is negative because the sample size was too small. More and more journal editors now require authors to provide this key information.

Just as with studies involving only one group, a variety of formulas can be used to estimate how large a sample is needed, and several computer programs are available for this purpose as well. The formulas given in the following section protect against both type I and type II errors for two common situations: when a study involves two means or two proportions.

6.4.1 Finding the Sample Size for Studies about Means in Two Groups

This section presents the process to estimate the approximate sample size for a study comparing the means in two independent groups of subjects. The researcher needs to answer four questions, the first two of which are the same as those presented in Chapter 5 for one group:

1. What level of significance (α level or P value) related to the null hypothesis is wanted?

2. How great should the chances be of detecting an actual difference; that is, what is the desired level of power (equal to $1 - \beta$)?

3. How large should the difference between the mean in one group and the mean in the other group be for the difference to have clinical importance; that is, $(\pi_1 - \pi_2)$?

4. What is a good estimate of the standard deviations, σ_1 and σ_2, in the two populations? To simplify this process, we assume that the standard deviations in the two populations are equal.

To summarize, if $\mu_1 - \mu_2$ is the magnitude of the difference to be detected between the two groups, σ is the estimate of the standard deviation in each group, z_α is the two-tailed value of z related to α, and z_β is the lower one-tailed value of z related to β, then the sample size needed in *each* group is

$$n = 2\left[\frac{(z_\alpha - z_\beta)\,\sigma}{\mu_1 - \mu_2}\right]^2$$

To illustrate this formula, recall that Benson and his colleagues (1996) in Presenting Problem 1 compared the operating room times for 48 women who had an abdominal procedure with the times for 40 who had a vaginal procedure to correct uterovaginal prolapse. We found the 95% confidence interval for the difference in mean operating times (19.15 min) in Section 6.2.1. The 95% CI, −37.20 to −1.10, does not contain 0, so we conclude that a difference exists between the mean operating room times in the two groups. Suppose the investigators determined, prior to beginning their study, that they wished to have a large enough sample of patients to be able to detect a mean difference of 20 min or more. Assume they were willing to accept a type I error (incorrectly concluding that a difference in operating room times existed) of 0.05 and wanted to be able to detect a true difference with 0.80 probability ($\beta = 0.20$). Based on their clinical experience, they estimated the standard deviation of operating room times as 45 min. Using these values, what sample size is needed?

The two-tailed z value for α of 0.05 is ±1.96 and the lower one-tailed z value for β of 0.20 is −0.84 (the critical value separating the lower 20% of the z distribution from the upper 80%). From the given estimates, the sample size for each group is

$$n = 2\left[\frac{(z_\alpha - z_\beta)\,\sigma}{\mu_1 - \mu_2}\right]^2$$
$$= 2\left\{\frac{[1.96 - (-0.84)]45}{20}\right\}^2$$
$$= 2\left(\frac{126}{20}\right)^2 = 2 \times 39.69, \text{ or rounding up, } 2 \times 40 = 80$$

Thus, 80 women are needed in each group if the investigators want to have an 80% chance (or 80% power) of detecting a difference of ≥ 20 min in operating room times. The output from the PASS program for two means is given in Box 6–1. The plot makes it easy to see the relationship between the sample size (N_1) and power.

Harper (1997) performed a power analysis. She calculated the number of patients needed to have a power of 80% to detect a difference of 20 mm on the visual analog scale (VAS) at the 0.05 level of significance. The estimate was 35 women in each group, but this was based on an estimated standard deviation of 30 mm. After 35 patients were enrolled, the investigator calculated the standard deviation and found it to be larger than anticipated; therefore, she increased the study size to 40 women to maintain the same 80% power.

6.4.1.a Shortcut Estimate of Sample Size: We developed a rule of thumb for quickly estimating the sample sizes needed to compare the means of two groups. First, determine the ratio of the standard devi-

---

Box 6–1. Two-sample *t* test power analysis using PASS: Estimates of *N*s for operating room times.

Numeric results for two-sample *t* test
Null hypothesis: Mean$_1$=Mean$_2$
Alternative hypothesis: Mean$_1$<>Mean$_2$
The sigmas were assumed to be known and equal.
The *N*s were forced to be equal.

Power	N_1	N_2	Alpha	Beta	Mean$_1$	Mean$_2$	Sigma$_1$	Sigma$_2$
0.74838	70	70	0.05000	0.25162	215.00	195.00	45.00	45.00
0.80260	80	80	0.05000	0.19740	215.00	195.00	45.00	45.00
0.84648	90	90	0.05000	0.15352	215.00	195.00	45.00	45.00
0.88154	100	100	0.05000	0.11846	215.00	195.00	45.00	45.00
0.90925	110	110	0.05000	0.09075	215.00	195.00	45.00	45.00
0.93092	120	120	0.05000	0.06908	215.00	195.00	45.00	45.00

Power Versus *N*1

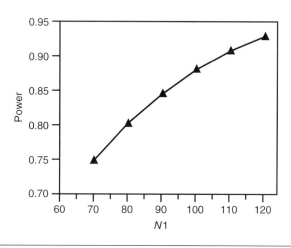

---

ation to the difference to be detected between the means $[\sigma/(\mu_1 - \mu_2)]$; then, square this ratio. For a study with a *P* value of 0.05, an experiment will have a 90% chance of detecting an actual difference between the two groups if the sample size in each group is approximately 20 times the squared ratio. For a study with the same *P* value but only an 80% chance of detecting an actual difference, a sample size of approximately 15 times the squared ratio is required. In the previous example, we would have $15 \times (45/20)^2$, or 76 subjects, a slight underestimate. Exercise 8 allows you to learn how this rule of thumb was obtained.

Note that these estimates assume that the sample sizes are equal in the two groups. It is possible to use unequal sample sizes, but the formulas are more complicated. Many computer programs, including PASS and nQuery, provide estimates for unequal sample sizes.

6.4.2 Finding the Sample Size for Studies about Proportions in Two Groups

This section presents the formula for estimating the approximate sample size needed in a study with two groups when the outcome is expressed in terms of proportions. Just as with studies involving two means, the researcher must answer four questions.

1. What is the desired level of significance (the α level) related to the null hypothesis, π_0?

2. What should be the chance of detecting an actual difference, that is, what power $(1 - \beta)$ is desired should be associated with the alternative hypothesis, π_1?

3. How large should the difference be between the proportion in one group and the proportion in the other group $(\pi_1 - \pi_2)$ for it to be clinically significant?

4. What is a good estimate of the standard deviation in the population? For a proportion, it is easy: The null hypothesis assumes the proportions are equal, and the proportion itself determines the estimated standard deviation: $\pi (1 - \pi)$.

To simplify matters, we again assume that the sample sizes are the same in the two groups. The symbol π_1 denotes the proportion in one group, and π_2 the proportion in the other group. Then, the formula for *n* is

$$n = \left[\frac{z_\alpha \sqrt{2\pi_1(1-\pi_1)} - z_\beta \sqrt{\pi_1(1-\pi_1) + \pi_2(1-\pi_2)}}{\pi_1 - \pi_2} \right]^2$$

where z_α is the two-tailed z value related to the null hypothesis and z_β is the lower one-tailed z value related to the alternative hypothesis.

To illustrate, use the study by Good and colleagues (1996) of patients who suffered a recent stroke. Among patients with a normal desaturation index, 27 of 32 were discharged to their own home (0.844) compared with 8 of 15 patients with an elevated index (0.533). We found that the 95% confidence interval for the difference in proportions was 0.044 to 0.578, and because the interval does not contain 0, we concluded a difference existed in the proportion that was discharged to their own home. We suppose that the investigators, prior to doing the study, wanted to estimate the sample size needed to detect a significant difference if the proportions discharged home were 0.85 and 0.55. They are willing to accept a type I error (or falsely concluding that a difference exists when none really occurred) of 0.05, and they wanted a 0.90 probability of detecting a true difference.

The two-tailed z value related to α is +1.96, and the lower one-tailed z value related to β is −1.645, the value that separates the lower 10% of the z distribution from the upper 90%. Then, the estimated sample size is

$$n = \left[\frac{1.96\sqrt{(2 \times 0.85 \times 0.15)} - (-1.645)\sqrt{(0.85 \times 0.15) + (0.55 \times 0.45)}}{0.85 - 0.55} \right]^2$$

$$= \left(\frac{1.997}{0.3} \right)^2 = 6.657^2$$

$$= 44.316, \text{ or } 45 \text{ in each group}$$

This sample size is fairly large, and chances are that the investigators will compromise and recalculate the sample size with less power or a larger difference (see Exercise 9).

We use the nQuery program with data from Good and colleagues to illustrate finding the sample size for the difference in two proportions. The table and plot produced by nQuery are given in Figure 6–7 and that n needs to be slightly larger than our estimate to give the power we want.

6.5 SUMMARY

This chapter has focused on statistical methods that are useful in determining whether two independent groups differ on some important measure. In the next chapter, we extend the discussion to studies that involve more than two groups.

The t test is used when the outcome is measured on a numerical scale. If the distribution of the obser-

vations is skewed or if the standard deviations in the two groups are different, the Wilcoxon rank sum test is the procedure of choice. In fact, it is such a good substitute for the t test that some statisticians recommend it for almost all situations.

The chi-square test is used with counts or frequencies when two groups are being analyzed, but the chi-square is very versatile and can be used with more than two groups. We also discussed what to do when sample sizes are small, commonly referred to as small expected frequencies. We recommend Fisher's exact test with a 2 × 2 table and collapsing rows or columns with a larger table. We briefly touched on a number of other issues related to the use of chi-square in medical studies.

In Presenting Problem 1, Benson and his colleagues (1996) wanted to know if a difference occurred in several outcomes, including discomfort rating, operating room time, and length of hospital stay. The researchers found an unexpected difference in surgical effectiveness between the two groups. In the vaginal treatment group, the surgical outcome was classified as optimal in 12 (29%), satisfactory in 16 (38%), and unsatisfactory in 14 (33%). In the abdominal treatment group, these respective outcomes were 22 (58%), 10 (26%), and 6 (16%). The length of time to determine unsatisfactory surgical outcome was significantly shorter for the vaginal group (11.2 months) than for the abdominal group (22.1 months). Reoperation was performed in 20 women, 14 from the vaginal treatment group and 6 from the abdominal group.

Nonclinical outcome measures included a mean charge for hospital stay of $6537 for the vaginal group and $8048 for the abdominal group. The abdominal procedure required an average of 19 min longer than the vaginal approach in this study (215 min vs 196 min). We illustrated the logic of the pooled standard deviation, needed to form a confidence interval for the difference in operating room times. The 95% confidence interval for the difference did not contain zero, indicating that this difference was statistically significant at $P < 0.05$.

Presenting Problem 2 used the study by Harper (1997) to illustrate the t test for two independent groups. Harper wanted to know whether women undergoing cryosurgery who had a paracervical block before the surgery experienced less pain and cramping than women who did not have the block. We compared the scores that women assigned to the degree of cramping they experienced with the procedure. Women who had the paracervical block had significantly lower scores, indicating they experienced less severe cramping. We used the same data to illustrate the Wilcoxon rank sum test and came to the same conclusion. The Wilcoxon test is recommended when assumptions for the t test (normal distribution, equal variances) are not met. The investigator reported that women receiving paracervical block perceived less cramping than those that did not re-

nQuery Advisor - [Table 2]

File Edit View Options Assistant Plot Window Help

Two group χ^2 test of equal proportions (odds ratio = 1) (equal n's)

Test significance level, α	0.050		
1 or 2 sided test?	2		
Group 1 proportion, π_1	0.850		
Group 2 proportion, π_2	0.550		
Odds ratio, $\psi = \pi_2(1-\pi_1)/[\pi_1(1-\pi_s)]$	0.216		
Power (%)	90		
n per group	47		

NOTES / Stored Statements	Create Statement	Special Characters

For Help, press F1   90.000000   AUTO RECALC OFF   NUM

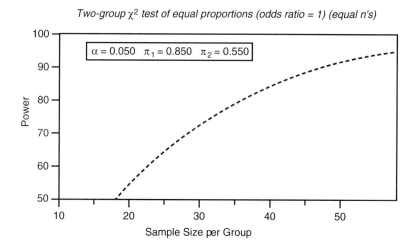

Two-group χ^2 test of equal proportions (odds ratio = 1) (equal n's)

$\alpha = 0.050 \quad \pi_1 = 0.850 \quad \pi_2 = 0.550$

Power

Sample Size per Group

Figure 6–7. Two-sample test for proportions power analysis using nQuery Advisor; used with permission.

ceive it, a result that is consistent with our analysis. The paracervical block did not decrease the perception of pain, however.

Turning to research questions involving nominal or categorical outcomes, we introduced the z statistic for comparing two proportions and the chi-square test. Sleep-disordered breathing (SDB) is common in patients undergoing rehabilitation after stroke. In Good and colleagues' (1996) study of sleep-disordered breathing and clinical outcomes, investigators were interested in learning whether an elevated desaturation index was a factor in whether patients were deemed capable of being discharged to their own home. They observed that 84% of patients with a desaturation index ≤ 10 could go to their own home, compared with 53% of those with a desaturation index > 10. A 95% confidence interval for the difference between 84% and 53% did not contain zero, indicating a significant difference in this clinical outcome. We used the same data to illustrate the z test for two proportions and came to the same conclusion, illustrating once more the equivalence between the conclusions reached using confidence intervals and statistical tests.

The chi-square test uses observed frequencies and compares them to the frequencies that would be expected if no differences existed in proportions. We again used the data from Good and colleagues (1996) to illustrate the chi-square test for two groups, that is, for observations that can be displayed in a 2×2 table. Once more, the results of the statistical test indicated that a difference existed in proportions of patients discharged to their own home, depending on their desaturation index.

Data from the Harper study (1997) on cryosurgery were used to illustrate the chi-square test for more than two groups. Harper wanted to know if having a paracervical block was associated with different combinations of cramping and pain. She divided the women into four groups: those that had both pain and cramping, pain only, cramping only, or neither. The chi-square statistic indicated no statistically significant association between the occurrence of pain or cramping and paracervical block. Thus, although the block may affect the degree of cramping, it was not associated with the simple occurrence of combinations of cramping and pain.

The importance of sample size calculations was again stressed. We illustrated formulas and computer programs that estimate the sample sizes needed when two independent groups of subjects are being compared.

A summary of the statistical methods discussed in this chapter is given in Appendix C.

EXERCISES

1. How does a decrease in sample size affect the confidence interval? Recalculate the confidence interval for operating room times in Section 6.2, assuming that the means and standard deviations were the same but only 25 patients were in each group. Is the conclusion the same?

2. Calculate the pooled standard deviation for the total cramping score from Table 6–3.

3. Good and colleagues (1996) used the Barthel index (BI) to measure mobility and activities of daily living.

   a. Did patients with a desaturation index (DI) < 10 have the same mean BI at discharge as patients with a DI $\geq$ 10? Answer this question using a 95% confidence interval.

   b. Did a significant increase occur in BI from the time of admission until discharge for all the patients in the study (ie, ignoring the desaturation index)? Answer this question using a 95% confidence interval.

4. Show that the pooled standard deviation for two means is the average of the two standard deviations when the sample sizes are equal.

5. Use the data from Benson and colleagues (1996) to compare the operating room times for women having an abdominal versus a vaginal procedure. Compare the conclusion with the confidence interval in Section 6.2.

6. Collapse data from Harper in Table 6–13 into a 2×2 table by combining the three categories no pain/no cramping, pain/no cramping, and no pain/cramping. Does an association exist between the occurrence of both pain and cramping and whether the woman had a paracervical block prior to cryosurgery? Put the cramping variable as columns and the paracervical block variable as the rows.

   a. What conclusion is drawn if a chi-square test is performed using $\alpha = 0.05$?

   b. What conclusion is drawn about the relative risk of the occurrence of both pain and cramping with and without a paracervical block?

7. Use the rules for finding the probability of independent events to show why the expected frequency in the chi-square statistic is found by the following formula:

$$\text{Expected frequency} = \frac{\text{Row total} \times \text{Column total}}{\text{Grand total}}$$

8. How was the rule of thumb for calculating the sample size for two independent groups found?

9. Refer to the study by Good and colleagues (1996) on patients with stroke (Presenting Problem 3). How large a sample is needed to detect a difference of 0.85 versus 0.55 in the proportions discharged home with 80% power?

10. Compute the 90% and 99% confidence intervals for the difference in operating room times for the patients in the study by Ben-

son (1996). Compare these intervals with the 95% interval obtained in Section 6.2.1. What is the effect of lower confidence on the width of the interval? Of higher confidence?

11. Suppose investigators compared the number of cardiac procedures performed by 60 cardiologists in large health centers during one year to the number of procedures done by 25 cardiologists in midsized health centers. They found no significant difference between the number of procedures performed by the average cardiologist in large centers and those performed in midsized centers using the *t* test. When they reanalyzed the data using the Wilcoxon rank sum test, however, the investigators noted a difference. What is the most likely explanation for these two conflicting findings?

12. Leveno and coworkers (1986) studied the effects of electronic fetal monitoring during labor by comparing a group of women who universally had fetal monitoring with another group of women who had monitoring only when a risk to the fetus was apparent. An alternate-month study design was used in which monitoring was provided in all pregnancies during one month (universal monitoring) and then provided only for high-risk pregnancies during the next month (selective monitoring); the study was performed over a 36-month period. The investigators were interested in determining whether universal electronic monitoring would improve perinatal results. Data from this study are given in Table 6–15. Perform an appropriate statistical procedure to answer the following questions:
    a. Do the groups show a difference in the cesarean rate?
    b. Among low-risk pregnancies, does a difference exist in the proportion with abnormal fetal heart rate?

    c. Among low-risk pregnancies, is any difference apparent in neonatal deaths?
    d. The researchers concluded that low-risk pregnancies do not need continuous electronic fetal monitoring during labor. Do you agree?

13. Table 6–16 presents some of the findings from a randomized, double-blind, placebo-controlled study of the use of parenteral penicillin in patients with Lyme arthritis (Steere et al, 1985). Identify the appropriate statistical method for determining whether a difference exists between responders and nonresponders for the following conditions:
    a. History of erythema chronicum migrans (ECM)
    b. Previous use of antibiotic for ECM
    c. Months from ECM to treatment of arthritis
    d. Erythrocyte sedimentation rate (ESR) after treatment

14. Recall that in Chapter 5 exercises we examined box plots for daily juice consumption by 2- and 5-year-olds. We asked you to say whether you thought the two groups drank different amounts of juice. Now, use the *t* test to learn if the means are different.

15. **Group Exercise.** Refer to the study by Moore and coworkers (1991) to answer the following questions:
    a. What type of statistical method was used for comparing young and old men? For comparing each group to the baseline or placebo values? Was this an appropriate method?
    b. What was the major conclusion from the study? Was this conclusion justified? What additional information could the investigators have provided that would be useful in

Table 6–15. Observations on electronic fetal monitoring.

Observation	Selective Monitoring ($n = 17,409$)	Universal Monitoring ($n = 17,586$)
Number of cesarean sections	1777	1933
Number of low-risk pregnancies[a]	7330	7288
Number of neonatal deaths in low-risk pregnancies	5	4
Abnormal fetal heart rate in low-risk pregnancies	196	551

[a]Defined as a single fetus in a cephalic presentation; spontaneous, uncomplicated labor; and a birth weight greater than 2500 g.
Source: Adapted and reproduced, with permission, from Tables 2 and 6 in Leveno KJ et al: A prospective comparison of selective and universal electronic fetal monitoring in 34,995 pregnancies. *N Engl J Med* 1986;**315**:615–619.

Table 6–16. Information on patients with Lyme arthritis.

Patient Characteristics	Responders	Non-responders
Number of patients	$n = 18$	$n = 22$
History of ECM	16	11
Antibiotic therapy for ECM	8	1
Antibiotic therapy for arthritis	4	2
Mean ± standard deviation Months from ECM to treatment of arthritis	32 ± 15	34 ± 19
Months of active arthritis	12 ± 10	11 ± 7
ESR (mm/h) after treatment	13 ± 9	18 ± 10

Source: Adapted and reproduced, with permission, from Table 3 in Steere AC et al: Successful parenteral penicillin therapy of established Lyme arthritis. *N Engl J Med* 1985; **312**:869–874.

helping readers decide whether the conclusion was appropriate?

16. **Group Exercise.** Physicians and dentists may be at risk for exposure to blood-borne diseases during invasive surgical procedures. Some investigators undertook to determine the incidence of glove perforation during obstetric procedures and identify risk factors (Serrano et al, 1991). The latex gloves of all members of the surgical teams performing cesarean deliveries, postpartum tubal ligations, and vaginal deliveries were collected for study; 100 unused gloves served as controls. Each glove was tested by inflating it with a pressurized air hose to 1.5 to 2 times the normal volume and submerging it in water. Perforations were detected by the presence of air bubbles when gentle pressure was applied to the palmar surface. Among the 754 study gloves, 100 had holes; none of the 100 unused control gloves had holes. In analyzing the data, the investigators found that 19 of the gloves with holes were among the 64 gloves worn by scrub technicians. Obtain a copy of this paper from your medical library and use it to help answer the following questions:

a. What is your explanation for the high perforation rate in gloves worn by scrub technicians? What should be done about these gloves in the analysis?

b. Are there other possible sources of bias in the way this study was designed?

c. An analysis reported by the investigators was based on 462 gloves used by house staff. The levels of training, number of gloves used, and number of gloves with holes were as follows: Interns used 262 gloves, 30 with holes; year 2 residents used 71 gloves, 9 with holes; year 3 residents used 58 gloves, 4 with holes; and year 4 residents used 71 gloves, 17 with holes. Confirm that a relationship exists between training level and proportion of perforation, and explain the differences in proportions of perforations.

d. What conclusions do you draw from this study? Do your conclusions agree with those of the investigators?

Research Questions about Means in Three or More Groups

7

PRESENTING PROBLEMS

Presenting Problem 1. In recent years researchers have become increasingly interested in the neuromodulation of immune function. In 1987, Irwin and colleagues published the results of a cross-sectional study of the relationship between major life events and immune function. Subjects in the study included women whose husbands were undergoing treatment for metastatic lung cancer, women whose husbands had died of lung cancer in the preceding 1–6 months, and women whose husbands were in good health. Scores on the Social Readjustment Rating Scale and the Hamilton Rating Scale for Depression were recorded for each of the women; in addition, two measures of immune system function, natural killer (NK) cell activity and T-cell subpopulation numbers (T helper cells and T suppressor cells), were determined.

According to their scores on the Social Readjustment Rating Scale, the women were divided into three groups: those with low scores (≤54), those with moderate scores (55–99), and those with high scores (≥100). The relationships between scores on the Social Readjustment Scale and alterations in immune function were analyzed. We use the data from this study to determine whether natural killer (NK) cell activity and T-cell numbers are the same for women with low, moderate, and high scores. Data are given in Section 7.2.1. and on the CD-ROM.

Presenting Problem 2. Previous studies of hyperthyroid patients have demonstrated impaired glucose tolerance and hypersecretion of insulin, supporting the concept of insulin resistance or diminished insulin sensitivity in hyperthyroidism. Published data on insulin sensitivity in hyperthyroidism conflict, however: Both diminished and normal insulin-stimulated glucose use are reported. Although most patients with hyperthyroidism lose weight, some women with this disease are slightly overweight. The association between obesity and decreased insulin sensitivity is well known. Gonzalo and colleagues (1996) studied the effect of excess body weight on glucose tolerance, insulin secretion, and insulin sensitivity in hyperthyroid patients. Intravenous glucose tolerance tests were performed on 14 hyperthyroid women, 6 of whom were overweight, and in 19 volunteers with normal thyroid levels matched for age and weight.[1]

The investigators wanted to know if differences existed in various outcomes depending on thyroid level and body mass index. We use the measurement on insulin sensitivity to illustrate the use of two-way analysis of variance. Data are given in Section 7.5.1 and are in a folder entitled "Gonzalo" on the CD-ROM.

Presenting Problem 3. The study by Good and colleagues (1996), Presenting Problem 3 in Chapter 6, examined sleep-disordered breathing in patients undergoing rehabilitation after a stroke. We used data from this study to learn if there was a difference in the proportion of patients discharged home with a normal desaturation index (DI) versus those with an elevated DI. These investigators studied other variables as well, including the Barthel index, a standardized scale that measures mobility and activities of daily living. This index was recorded at admission, at discharge, and at 3 and 12 months after stroke onset.

We use these data to illustrate a study design in which measurements are made repeatedly over time.

7.1 PURPOSE OF THE CHAPTER

Many research projects in medicine employ more than two groups, and the chi-square tests for three or more groups discussed in Chapter 6 are appropriate when the outcome is a categorical (or counted) measure. When the outcome is numerical, however, means are used, and the t tests discussed in Chapters 5 and 6 are applicable only for the comparison of two groups. For example, in the study by Irwin and colleagues (1987), the mean NK cell activity (measured

---

[1]The term *matching* generally means that one patient is matched with the control subject to ensure the groups are similar on the matching variable. Sometimes, two control subjects are selected for each patient. Fourteen patients and 19 controls were included in this study, and we expect the authors meant that the controls were selected so that the overall age and BMI distributions were similar to those in the patients.

in lytic units) is examined for three groups of women: those with low, moderate, and high scores on the Social Readjustment Rating Scale. Other studies, such as that by Gonzalo and colleagues (1996), examine the influence of more than one factor. These researchers were interested in differences in insulin sensitivity and the dependence of those differences on normal or elevated thyroid levels and on obesity. These situations call for a global, or omnibus, test to see whether any differences exist in the data prior to testing various combinations of means to determine individual group differences.

If a global test is not performed, multiple tests between different pairs of means will alter the α level for the experiment as a whole rather than for each comparison. For example, Marwick and colleagues (1999) studied the relationship between myocardial profusion imaging and cardiac mortality in men and women. Their goal was to compare the relationship with other variables they thought might influence the prognosis. Important factors included the number of involved coronary vessels (zero to three) and whether the profusion defect was fixed or could be reversed. These investigators properly chose to use multivariate methods to analyze the data, methods we will discuss in Chapter 10. Had they not done so, simply comparing men and women on the 2×4 different combinations of these factors (zero vessels fixed, zero vessels reversible, one vessel fixed, one vessel reversible, etc) would produce eight P values. If each comparison is made by using $\alpha = 0.05$, the chance that each comparison will falsely be called significant is 5%; that is, a type I error may occur eight different times. Overall, therefore, the chance ($8 \times 5\%$) of declaring one of the comparisons incorrectly significant is 40%.[2]

One approach for analyzing data that include multiple observations is called the **analysis of variance,** abbreviated **ANOVA** or **anova.** This method protects the researcher against error "inflation" by first asking if any differences exist at all among means of the groups. If the result of the ANOVA is significant, the answer is yes, and the investigator is then free to make comparisons between pairs or combinations of groups.

The topic of analysis of variance is complex, and many textbooks are devoted to the subject. Its use in the medical literature is somewhat limited, however, ranging from a low of about 2% of the articles in oncology (Hokanson et al, 1986a) and pathology (Hokanson et al, 1987a) journals, to about 3–4% in various surgery journals (Reznick et al, 1987), to a high of almost 10% in the psychiatric literature (Hokanson et al, 1986b) and 14% in the *New England Journal of Medicine* (Altman, 1991b). We introduce ANOVA in this text to familiarize you with the terms used and to give you an idea of how these

analyses are performed. As with other procedures, our goal is to provide enough discussion so that you can identify situations in which ANOVA is appropriate and interpret the results. If you are interested in learning more about analysis of variance, consult Armitage (1987) and Dunn and Clark (1987). Except for very simple study designs, our best advice to researchers conducting a study that involves more than two groups or two or more variables is to consult a statistician to determine how best to analyze the data.

We approach the topic as follows: In Section 7.2, we give an overview of the logic involved in ANOVA; the results from Presenting Problem 1 are then used to illustrate the computations intuitively. Section 7.3 presents the traditional approach and the formulas used in ANOVA; they are illustrated for Presenting Problem 1. Section 7.4 discusses some of the more commonly used methods for comparing means using ANOVA; these methods are called **multiple-comparison procedures.** Other ANOVA designs are discussed and illustrated in Section 7.5. As in the previous chapters, we use output from statistical computer programs as appropriate.

7.2 INTUITIVE OVERVIEW OF ANOVA

7.2.1 The Logic of ANOVA

In Presenting Problem 1, NK cell activity was measured for three groups of subjects: those who had low, medium, and high scores on the Social Readjustment Rating Scale. The original observations, sample sizes, means, and standard deviations provided by Irwin and his colleagues (1987) are given in Table 7–1.

Table 7–1. Natural killer cell activity (lytic units).[a]

	Low Score[b] (n = 13)	Moderate Score[b] (n = 12)	High Score[b] (n = 12)
	22.2	15.1	10.2
	97.8	23.2	11.3
	29.1	10.5	11.4
	37.0	13.9	5.3
	35.8	9.7	14.5
	44.2	19.0	11.0
	82.0	19.8	13.6
	56.0	9.1	33.4
	9.3	30.1	25.0
	19.9	15.5	27.0
	39.5	10.3	36.3
	12.8	11.0	17.7
	37.4		
Mean	40.23	15.60	18.06
Standard deviation	25.71	6.42	9.97

[a]One lytic unit is defined as the number of effector cells killing 20% of the target cells.
[b]The grouping is based on scores from the Social Readjustment Rating Scale.
Source: Observations, used with permission, from Irwin M et al: Life events, depressive symptoms, and immune function. *Am J Psychiatry* 1987;**144:**437–441.

---

[2]Actually, 40% is only approximately correct; it does not reflect the fact that some of the comparisons are not independent.

ANOVA provides a way to divide the total variation in NK cell activity for each subject into two parts. For example, let us denote a given subject's NK cell activity as X and consider how much X differs from the mean NK cell activity for all the subjects in the study, abbreviated $\overline{\overline{X}}$, where the double overbar denotes the grand (overall) mean of all subjects, regardless of which group they are in. This difference (symbolized $X - \overline{\overline{X}}$) can be divided into two parts: the difference between X and the mean of the group this subject is in, $\overline{X}_j$, and the difference between the group mean and the grand mean. In symbols, we write

$$(X - \overline{\overline{X}}) = (X - \overline{X}_j) + (\overline{X}_j - \overline{\overline{X}})$$

For example, subject 1 in the low-score group has an NK cell activity of 22.2 lytic units. The grand mean for all patients is 25.05, so subject 1 differs from the grand mean by $22.2 - 25.05$, or -2.85. This difference can be divided into two parts: the difference between 22.2 and the mean for the low group, 40.23; and the difference between the mean for the low group and the grand mean. Thus,

$$(22.2 - 40.23) + (40.23 - 25.05) = -18.03 + 15.18$$
$$= -2.85$$

Subject 1 appears to be "more different" from the mean of the low group than the mean of the low group is from the grand mean.

Although our example does not show exactly how ANOVA works, it is helpful for understanding the concept of dividing the variation into different parts. Here, we have been looking at simple differences related to just one observation; ANOVA considers the variation in all observations and divides it into (1) the variation between each subject and the subject's group mean and (2) the variation between each group mean and the grand mean. If the group means are quite different from one another, considerable variation will occur between them and the grand mean, compared with the variation within each group. If the group means are not very different, however, the variation between them and the grand mean will not be much more than the variation among the subjects within each group. The **F test** for two variances (discussed in Chapter 6) can therefore be used to test the ratio of the variance among means to the variance among subjects within each group.

The null hypothesis for the F test is that the two variances are equal; if they are, the variation among means is not much greater than the variation among individual observations within any given group. In this situation, we cannot conclude that the means are different from one another. Thus, we think of ANOVA as a test of the equality of means, even though the variances are being tested in the process. If the null hypothesis is rejected, we conclude that

not all the means are equal; however, we do not know which ones are not equal, which is why post hoc comparison procedures are necessary.

7.2.2 Illustration of Intuitive Calculations for ANOVA

Recall that the formula for the variance of the observations (or squared standard deviation; see Chapter 3) involves the sum of the squared deviations of each X from the mean $\overline{X}$:

$$SD^2 = \frac{\sum(X - \overline{X})^2}{n - 1}$$

A similar formula can be used to find the variance of means from the grand mean:

$$\text{Estimate of variance of means} = \frac{\sum n_j(\overline{X}_j - \overline{\overline{X}})^2}{j - 1}$$

where n is the number of observations in each group and j is the number of groups. This estimate is called the **mean square among groups,** abbreviated MS_A, and it has $j - 1$ degrees of freedom.

To obtain the variance within groups, we use a pooled variance like the one for the t test for two independent groups:

$$\text{Estimate of variance within groups} = \frac{\sum(n_j - 1)SD_j^2}{\sum(n_j - 1)}$$

This estimate is called the **error mean square** (or mean square within), abbreviated MS_E. It has $\sum(n_j - 1)$ degrees of freedom, or, if the sum of the number of observations is denoted by N, $N - j$ degrees of freedom. The F ratio is formed by dividing the estimate of the variance of means (mean square among groups) by the estimate of the variance within groups (error mean square), and it has $j - 1$ and $N - j$ degrees of freedom.

We will use the data on the NK cell activity to illustrate the calculations. In this example, the variable of interest (NK cell activity) is the **dependent variable,** and the grouping variable (score on Social Readjustment Rating Scale) is the **independent variable.** The data in Table 7–1 indicate that the mean NK cell activity for the low-score group is higher than the means for the moderate and high groups. If these three groups of women are viewed as coming from a larger population, then the question is whether mean NK cell activity levels differ in the population. Although differences exist in the means in Table 7–1, some differences in the samples would occur simply by chance, even when no variation existed in the population. The question is therefore reduced to whether the observed differences are large enough to convince us that they did not occur merely by chance but reflect real distinctions in the population.

The statistical hypothesis being tested, the null hypothesis, is that the mean NK cell activity is equal among women with low, moderate, and high scores. The alternative hypothesis is that a difference does exist; that is, not all the means are equal. The steps in testing the null hypothesis follow.

Step 1: H_0: The mean NK cell activity is equal in the three groups, or, in symbols, $\mu_1 = \mu_2 = \mu_3$

H_1: The means are not equal, or, in symbols, $\mu_1 \neq \mu_2$ or $\mu_2 \neq \mu_3$ or $\mu_1 \neq \mu_3$

Step 2: The test statistic in the test of equality of means in ANOVA is the F ratio, $F = MS_A/MS_E$, with $j - 1$ and $\Sigma(n_j - 1)$ degrees of freedom.

Step 3: We use $\alpha = 0.01$ for this statistical test.

Step 4: The value of the F distribution from Table A–4 with $j - 1 = 2$ degrees of freedom in the numerator and $\Sigma(n_j - 1) = 34$ degrees of freedom in the denominator, for $\alpha = 0.01$, is between 5.39 and 5.18; interpolation gives 5.31. The decision is therefore to reject the null hypothesis of equal means if the observed value of F is greater than 5.31 and falls in the rejection area (Figure 7–1).

Step 5: First we calculate the grand mean. Because we already know the means for the three groups, we can form a weighted average of these means to find the grand mean:

$$\overline{\overline{X}} = \frac{(13 \times 40.23) + (12 \times 15.6) + (12 \times 18.06)}{13 + 12 + 12}$$
$$= 25.05$$

The numerator of the MS_A is therefore

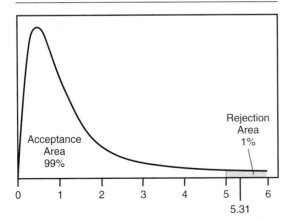

$$13(40.23 - 25.05)^2 + 12(15.60 - 25.05)^2$$
$$+ 12(18.06 - 25.05)^2 = (13 \times 230.43)$$
$$+ (12 \times 89.30) + (12 \times 48.86)$$
$$= 4653.57$$

The term MS_A is found by dividing the numerator by the number of groups minus 1, $(j - 1)$, which is 2 in this example; therefore,

$$MS_A = \frac{4653.57}{2} = 2326.79$$

The individual group variances are used to calculate the pooled estimate of the MS_E:

$$MS_E = \frac{\Sigma(n_j - 1)SD_j^2}{\Sigma(n_j - 1)}$$
$$= \frac{(12 \times 25.71^2) + (11 \times 6.42^2) + (11 \times 9.97^2)}{12 + 11 + 11}$$
$$= \frac{9478.84}{34} = 278.79$$

Finally, the F ratio is found by dividing the mean square among groups by the error mean square:

$$F = \frac{MS_A}{MS_E}$$
$$= \frac{2326.79}{278.79} = 8.35$$

Step 6: The observed value of the F ratio is 8.35, which is larger than 5.31 (the critical value from Table A–4). The null hypothesis of equal means is therefore rejected. We conclude that a difference does exist in mean NK cell activity among patients with low, moderate, and high scores on the Social Readjustment Rating Scale. Note that rejecting the null hypothesis does not tell us *which* group means differ, only that a difference exists; in Section 7.4, we illustrate different methods that can be used to learn which specific groups differ.

The results of ANOVA traditionally are presented in an ANOVA table similar to Table 7–2. The terms "sums of squares" and "mean squares" are discussed in the next section. When the results are given at this level of detail, we can easily determine exactly how the data were analyzed. Not all the authors, however, present this amount of detail; some simply list means and standard deviations along with F values or P values.

7.3 TRADITIONAL APPROACH TO ANOVA

In the preceding section, we presented a simple illustration of ANOVA by using formulas to estimate the variance among individual group means and the

Figure 7–1. Illustration of critical values in F distribution.

Table 7–2. ANOVA table for natural killer cell activity.[a]

Source of Variation	Sums of Squares	Degrees of Freedom	Mean Squares	F Ratio
Among groups	4,653.57	2	2326.79	8.35
Error	9,478.84	34	278.79	
Total	14,132.41	36		

[a]Figures are based on calculations from the intuitive overview. *Source:* Observations, used with permission, from Irwin M et al: Life events, depressive symptoms, and immune function. *Am J Psychiatry* 1987;**144**:437–441.

grand mean, called the mean square *among groups* (MS_A), and the variance *within* groups, called the mean square error or mean square *within groups* (MS_E). Traditionally in ANOVA, formulas are given for **sums of squares,** which are generally equivalent to the numerators of the formulas used in the preceding section; then, sums of squares are divided by appropriate degrees of freedom to obtain mean squares. Before illustrating the calculations for the data on NK cell activity (Presenting Problem 1), we define some terms and give the traditional formulas.

7.3.1 Terms & Formulas for ANOVA

In ANOVA, the term **factor** refers to the variable by which groups are formed, the **independent variable.** For example, in Presenting Problem 1, subjects were grouped using only one variable, the Social Readjustment Rating Scale; therefore, this study is an example of a one-factor ANOVA, called a one-way ANOVA. The number of groups defined by a given factor is referred to as the number of *levels* of the factor; the factor in Presenting Problem 1 has three levels: low, moderate, and high scores. In experimental studies in medicine, levels are frequently referred to as **treatments.**

Some textbooks approach analysis of variance from the perspective of models. The **model** for one-way ANOVA states that an individual observation can be divided into three components related to (1) the grand mean, (2) the group to which the individual belongs, and (3) the individual observation itself. To write this model in symbols, we let *i* stand for a given individual observation and *j* stand for the group to which this individual belongs. Then, X_{ij} denotes the observation of individual *i* in group *j*; for example, X_{11} is the first observation in the first group, and X_{53} is the fifth observation in the third group. The grand mean in the model is denoted by μ. The *effect* of being a member of group *j* may be thought of as the difference between the mean of group *j* and the grand mean; the effect associated with being in group *j* is written α_j. Finally, the difference between the individual observation and the mean of the group to which the observation belongs is written e_{ij} and is called the **error,** or

residual. Putting these symbols together, we can write the model for one-way ANOVA as

$$X_{ij} = \mu + \alpha_j + e_{ij}$$

which states that the *i*th observation in the *j*th group, X_{ij}, is the sum of three components: the grand mean μ; the effect associated with group *j*, α_j; and an error (residual), e_{ij}.

The size of an effect is, of course, related to the size of the difference between a given group mean and the grand mean. When inferences involve only specific levels of the factor included in the study, the model is called a **fixed-effects model.** The fixed-effects model assumes we are interested in making inferences only to the populations represented in the study, such as occurs, for example, if investigators wish to draw conclusions about three dosage levels of a drug. If, in contrast, the dosage levels included in the study are viewed as being randomly selected from all different possible dosage levels of the drug, the model is called a **random-effects model,** and inferences can be made to other levels of the factor not represented in the study.[3] Both models are used to test hypotheses about the equality of group means. The random-effects model, however, can also be used to test hypotheses and form confidence intervals about group variances, and it is also referred to as the components-of-variance model for this reason.

7.3.1.a Definitional Formulas: In Section 7.2.1, we showed that the variation of 22.2 lytic units from the grand mean of 25.05 (subject 1 in the low-score group) can be expressed as a sum of two differences: (1) the difference between the observation and the mean of the group it is in, plus (2) the difference between its group mean and the grand mean. This result is also true when the differences are squared and the squared deviations are added to form the sum of squares.

To illustrate, for one factor with *j* groups, we use the following definitions:

X_{ij} is the *i*th observation in the *j*th group.

$\overline{X}_j$ is the mean of all observations in the *j*th group.

$\overline{\overline{X}}$ is the grand mean of the observations.

Then, $\Sigma(X_{ij} - \overline{\overline{X}})^2$, the total sum of squares, or SS_T, can be expressed as the sum of $\Sigma(X_{ij} - \overline{X}_j)^2$, the error sum of squares (SS_E) and $\Sigma(\overline{X}_j - \overline{\overline{X}})^2$, the sum of squares among groups (SS_A).

[3]The calculations of sums of squares and mean squares are the same in both models, but the type of model determines the way the *F* ratio is formed when two or more factors are included in a study.

That is,

$$\Sigma(X_{ij} - \bar{\bar{X}})^2 = \Sigma(X_{ij} - \bar{X}_j)^2 + \Sigma(\bar{X}_j - \bar{\bar{X}})^2$$
$$\text{or} \quad SS_T = SS_E + SS_A$$

We do not provide the proof of this equality here, but interested readers can consult any standard statistical reference for more details (eg, Armitage, 1987; Daniel, 1998; Hays, 1997).

7.3.1.b Computational Formulas: Computational formulas are more convenient than definitional formulas when sums of squares are calculated manually or when using calculators, as was the situation before computers were so readily available. Additionally, computational formulas are preferred because they reduce round-off errors. Computational formulas can be derived from definitional ones, but because the algebra is complex we do not explain it here. If you are interested in the details, consult the previously mentioned texts for derivations.

The symbols in ANOVA vary somewhat from one text to another; the following formulas are similar to those used in many books and are the ones we will use to illustrate calculations for ANOVA. Let N be the total number of observations in all the groups, that is, $N = \Sigma n_j$. Then, the computational formulas for the sums of squares are

$$SS_T = \sum(X_{ij} - \bar{\bar{X}})^2 = \sum X_{ij}^2 - \frac{\left(\sum X_{ij}\right)^2}{N}$$

$$SS_A = \sum(\bar{X}_j - \bar{\bar{X}})^2 = \sum n_j\bar{X}_j^2 - \frac{\left(\sum X_{ij}\right)^2}{N}$$

and SS_E is found by subtraction: $SS_E = SS_T - SS_A$.

The sums of squares are divided by the degrees of freedom to obtain the mean squares:

$$MS_A = \frac{SS_A}{j - 1}$$

where j is the number of groups or levels of the factor, and

$$MS_E = \frac{SS_E}{N - j}$$

where j is the number of groups or levels of the factor, and N is the total sample size.

7.3.2 One-Way ANOVA

Presenting Problem 1 is an example of a one-way ANOVA model in which only one independent variable occurs: the score on the Social Readjustment Rating Scale. Three levels of scores occur: low, mod-

erate, and high; and the mean number of lytic units is examined for women at each level. (See Table 7–1.)

7.3.2.a Illustration of Traditional Calculations: To calculate sums of squares by using traditional ANOVA formulas, we must obtain three terms:

1. We square each observation (X_{ij}) and add, to obtain ΣX_{ij}^2.
2. We add the observations, square the sum, and divide by N, to obtain $(\Sigma X_{ij})^2/N$.
3. We square each mean ($\bar{X}_j$), multiply by the number of subjects in that group (n_j), and add, to obtain $\Sigma n_j\bar{X}_j^2$.

These three terms using the data in Table 7–1 are

$$\sum X_{ij}^2 = 22.2^2 + 97.8^2 + \cdots + 36.3^2 + 17.7^2$$
$$= 37,353.65$$

$$\frac{\left(\sum X_{ij}\right)^2}{N} = \frac{(22.2 + 97.8 + \cdots + 36.3 + 17.7)^2}{13 + 12 + 12}$$
$$= \frac{926.9^2}{37}$$
$$= 23,220.10$$

and

$$\sum n_j\bar{X}_j^2 = (13 \times 40.23^2) + (12 \times 15.60^2) + (12 \times 18.06^2)$$
$$= 27,874.17$$

Then, the sums of squares are

$$SS_T = \sum X_{ij}^2 - \frac{\left(\sum X_{ij}\right)^2}{N}$$
$$= 37,353.65 - 23,220.10$$
$$= 14,133.55$$

$$SS_A = \sum n_j\bar{X}_j^2 - \frac{\left(\sum X_{ij}\right)^2}{N}$$
$$= 27,874.25 - 23,220.10$$
$$= 4654.15$$

$$SS_E = SS_T - SS_A$$
$$= 14,133.55 - 4654.15$$
$$= 9479.40$$

Next, the mean squares are calculated.

$$MS_A = \frac{SS_A}{j - 1} = \frac{4654.15}{2} = 2327.08$$

$$MS_E = \frac{SS_E}{N - j} = \frac{9479.40}{34} = 278.81$$

Slight differences between these results and the results for the mean squares calculated in Section 7.2.2

are due to round-off error. Otherwise, the results are the same regardless of which formulas are used.

Finally, the F ratio is determined.

$$F = \frac{MS_A}{MS_E} = \frac{2327.08}{278.81} = 8.35$$

The calculated F ratio is compared with the value from the F distribution with 2 and 34 degrees of freedom at the desired level of significance. As we found in Section 7.2.2, for $\alpha = 0.01$, the value of F (2, 34) is 5.31. Because 8.35 is greater than 5.31, the null hypothesis is rejected; and we conclude that mean NK activity is not the same for patients who score low, moderate, and high on the Social Readjustment Rating Scale.

The formulas for one-way ANOVA are summarized in Table 7–3.

7.3.2.b Assumptions in ANOVA: Analysis of variance uses information about the means and standard deviations in each group. Like the t test, ANOVA is therefore a parametric method, and some important assumptions are made.

1. The values of the dependent or outcome variable are assumed to be normally distributed within each group, that is, at each level of the factor or independent variable. In our example, this assumption requires that mean NK activity be normally distributed in each of the three patient groups.

2. The population variance is the same in each group, that is, $\sigma_1^2 = \sigma_2^2 = \sigma_3^2$. In our example, this means that the variance (or squared standard deviation) of mean NK activity should be the same in each of the three patient groups.

3. The observations are a random sample, and they are independent; that is, the value of one observation is not related in any way to the value of another observation. In our example, the value of one patient's mean NK activity level must have no influence on that of any other patient.

Not all these assumptions are equally important. For example, the results of the F test are not affected by moderate departures from normality, especially for a large number of observations in each group or sample, that is, the F test is **robust** with respect to violations of the assumption of normality. If the observations are extremely skewed, however, especially for small samples, the Kruskal–Wallis nonparametric procedure, discussed later in this chapter, should be used.

The F test is more sensitive to the second assumption of equal variances, also called **homogeneity** of variances. Concern about this assumption is eliminated, however, if sample sizes are equal (or close to equal) in each group (Box, 1953; 1954). For this reason, investigators try to design studies with equal sample sizes. If they cannot, as is sometimes the situation in observational studies, two other solutions are possible. The first is to transform data within each group to obtain equal variances, using one of the transformations discussed in Chapter 5. The second solution is to select samples of equal sizes randomly from each group, although many investigators do not like this solution because perfectly good observations are thrown away. Investigators should consult a statistician for studies with greatly unequal variances and unequal sample sizes.

The last assumption is particularly important. In general, investigators should be certain that they have **independent observations.** Independence is a problem primarily with studies involving repeated measurements of the same subjects, and they must be handled in a special way, as we discuss later in this chapter.

As a final comment, recall that the fixed-effects model assumes that each observation is really a sum, consisting of the grand mean, the effect of being a member of the particular group, and the error (residual) representing any unexplained variation. Some studies involve observations that are proportions, rates, or ratios; and for these data, the assumption about sums does not hold.

7.3.3 Interpretation of Presenting Problem 1

The analysis of variance table for the NK cell activity using NCSS is shown in Table 7–4. The among-group factor is designated by A (group) in the first row of the table. We see that the value for the sum of squares for the among factor, 4654.16, is very close to the value we obtained in Section 7.3.2 (4654.15). Similarly, the mean squares and the F ratio correspond to those we calculated. NCSS also provides the power of the sample size to detect a difference of this magnitude among the groups.

The findings for Presenting Problem 1 as published by Irwin and colleagues (1987) are reproduced in Table 7–5. The table provides much useful infor-

Table 7–3. Formulas for one-way ANOVA.

Source of Variation	Sums of Squares	Degrees of Freedom	Mean Squares	F Ratio
Among groups	$SS_A = \Sigma n_j \bar{X}_j^2 - \dfrac{(\Sigma X_{ij})^2}{N}$	$j - 1$	$MS_A = \dfrac{SS_A}{j-1}$	$F = \dfrac{MS_A}{MS_E}$
Error	$SS_E = SS_T - SS_A$	$N - j$	$MS_E = \dfrac{SS_E}{N-j}$	
Total	$SS_T = \Sigma X_{ij}^2 - \dfrac{(\Sigma X_{ij})^2}{N}$	$N - 1$		

Table 7–4. Analysis of variance table for natural killer cell activity.

Source Term	df	Sums of Squares	Mean Squares	F Ratio	Probability Level	Power
A (group)	2	4654.16	2327.08	8.35	0.001	0.95
S (A)	34	9479.40	278.81			
Total (adjusted)	36	14133.55				
Total	37					

Source: Data, used with permission, from Irwin M et al: Life events, depressive symptoms, and immune function. *Am J Psychiatry* 1987;**144**:437–441. Table produced with NCSS 97, a registered trademark of the Number Cruncher Statistical System; used with permission.

mation, including sample sizes, means, and standard deviations (SD) for each group on each dependent measure, and results from the ANOVA.

The first measure in the table, Social Readjustment Rating Scale score, was actually the independent variable used to form the groups for ANOVA. These results are given to assure the reader that the division of the subjects into three groups did, in fact, result in groups that were significantly different, both clinically and statistically.

Why was ANOVA performed on the next three measures: age, race, and blood samples? Generally, this type of information is presented to demonstrate that groups are similar with respect to baseline measures that could have a possible confounding effect. The designation n.s. in the column headed by *P* stands for not significant.

The authors chose not to present *F* ratios for measures that were not significant. In fact, when *F* ratios are given, they help the reader determine the chances that a type II error (not rejecting a false hypothesis)

occurred. That is, we can be more confident that the measures do not differ if the *F* ratios that are not significant have a value closer to 1 than if the *F* ratios are larger than 1.

The two measures that are significant in the analysis of Presenting Problem 1 are the Hamilton depression score and the NK cell activity, the first with $P < 0.003$ and the second with $P < 0.001$. Thus, the probability of observing a difference this large merely by chance (ie, if no difference exists between the low, moderate, and high groups) is less than 3 in 1000 and less than 1 in 1000, respectively. NK cell activity was used to illustrate computations in this chapter, and the value of the *F* ratio (8.35) agrees with the results from our analysis. The authors used the Newman–Keuls comparison procedure and reported that the low group differed significantly from the high and moderate groups on mean NK cell activity and mean Hamilton depression score, but the moderate and high groups did not differ from each other. No differences existed between the groups on the other

Table 7–5. Age, race, depression score, and immune variables of women with low, moderate, and high Social Readjustment Rating Scale scores.

	Group						ANOVA	
	Low (n = 13)[a]		Moderate (n = 12)[a]		High (n = 12)[a]		F	
Measure	Mean	SD	Mean	SD	Mean	SD	(df = 2, 34)	P
Social Readjustment Rating Scale score	31.9	16.4	81.7	11.1	126.6	24.7	84.4	< 0.001
Age (years)	54.8	9.5	55.3	6.3	57.8	9.4	—	n.s.
Race[b]	0.7	0.2	0.8	0.2	0.8	0.2	—	n.s.
Number of blood samples	3.6	0.6	3.8	0.9	3.8	0.9	—	n.s.
Hamilton depression score	5.3	5.2	14.7	7.5	12.0	6.8	6.8	< 0.003
Natural killer cell activity (lytic units)	40.2	25.7	15.6	6.4	18.1	10.0	8.3	< 0.001
Absolute number of lymphocytes (cells/mL × 10)	1.8	0.5	2.2	0.5	2.5	0.8	—	n.s.
Percent Th cells[c]	34.0	6.5	38.0	9.8	37.0	8.4	—	n.s.
Percent Ts cells[c]	27.0	8.7	23.0	8.4	26.0	8.5	—	n.s.
Th-to-Ts ratio[c]	1.6	0.6	2.0	0.6	1.6	0.4	—	n.s.

[a]Low = 54 or less; moderate = 55–99; high = 100 or more.
[b]0 = black; 1 = white.
[c]n = 9 in low-score group; n = 9 in moderate-score group; n = 10 in high-score group.
Abbreviations: n.s. = not significant; Th = T helper; Ts = T suppressor/cytotoxic.
Source: Reproduced, with permission, from Table 1 in Irwin M et al: Life events, depressive symptoms, and immune function. *Am J Psychiatry* 1987;**144**:437–441.

immune function variables analyzed, total lympho-cyte count and T-cell subpopulations. We discuss the Newman–Keuls statistic in the next section.

The investigators controlled for possible **confounding variables** by excluding women who had a history of any chronic medical disorder associated with altered immune function or the abuse of alcohol or other substances. They concluded that women who were undergoing major life changes, such as bereavement, had lower NK cell activity than women who were not experiencing such events. Additional analyses indicated that the severity of depressive symptoms, as measured by the Hamilton Rating Scale for Depression, was associated with impaired NK cell activity, a decrease in T suppressor cells, and an increase in the ratio of T helper to T suppressor cells.

Graphs help readers appreciate the magnitude of results from a study. To illustrate this point, we used NCSS to produce a box plot of the values for NK cell activity in Figure 7–2. The analysis of variance indicates that at least one difference exists among the groups. Based on the box plot, what is your best guess as to which groups differ? In the next section we examine statistical tests that help answer this question.

7.4 MULTIPLE-COMPARISON PROCEDURES

The discussion thus far has ignored studies in which the investigator has a limited number of specific comparisons, called planned, or **a priori,** comparisons, in mind prior to designing the study. In this special situa-

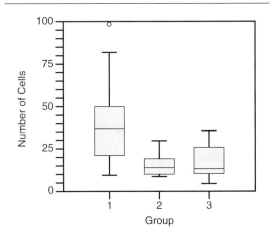

Figure 7–2. Box plot of NK cell activity. (Data, used with permission, from Irwin M et al: Life events, depressive symptoms, and immune function. *Am J Psychiatry* 1987; **144**:437–441. Table produced using NCSS 97, a registered trademark of the Number Cruncher Statistical System; used with permission.)

tion, comparisons can be made without performing an ANOVA first, although in actual practice, most investigators prefer to perform an ANOVA anyway. Typically, investigators want the freedom and flexibility of making comparisons afforded by the **posteriori,** or **post hoc,** methods. Before discussing these types of comparisons, however, we need two definitions.

A **comparison** or **contrast** between two means is the difference between the means, such as $\mu_1 - \mu_2$. Comparisons or contrasts can also involve more than two means. For example, suppose a study undertaken to compare a new drug with a placebo uses two dosage levels. The investigators may wish to compare the mean response for dosage 1 with the mean response for placebo, $\mu_1 - \mu_P$, as well as the mean response for dosage 2 with the mean response for placebo, $\mu_2 - \mu_P$. In addition, they may wish to compare the overall effect of the drug with the effect of placebo $[(\mu_1 + \mu_2)/2] - \mu_P$. Note that in all examples, the *coefficients* of the means add to 0; that is, rewriting the first comparison slightly gives $(1)\mu_1 + (-1)\mu_2$ and $(1) + (-1) = 0$; rewriting the last comparison gives $(\frac{1}{2})\mu_1 + (\frac{1}{2})\mu_2 + (-1)\mu_P$ and $(\frac{1}{2}) + (\frac{1}{2}) + (-1)$ again is 0.

The second definition involves the distinction between two different kinds of comparisons or contrasts. Two comparisons or contrasts are **orthogonal** if they do not use the same information. For example, suppose a study involves four different therapies: 1, 2, 3, and 4. Then, comparisons between $\mu_1 - \mu_2$ and between $\mu_3 - \mu_4$ are orthogonal because the information used to compare groups 1 and 2 is not the same information used to compare groups 3 and 4. In a sense, the questions asked by two orthogonal comparisons may be considered independent from each other. Conversely, comparisons of $\mu_1 - \mu_2$ and $\mu_1 - \mu_3$ are not orthogonal because they use redundant information; that is, observations in group 1 are used in both comparisons.

7.4.1 A Priori, or Planned, Comparisons

When comparisons are planned, they may be undertaken without first performing ANOVA. When the comparisons are all orthogonal, the *t* test for independent groups (see Chapter 6) may be used to compare two groups with the following modification: Instead of using the pooled standard deviation SD_p in the denominator of the *t* ratio, we use the error mean square MS_E. When sample sizes are equal, denoted by *n*, the *t* ratio becomes

$$t = \frac{(\bar{X}_i - \bar{X}_j)}{\sqrt{2MS_E/n}}$$

with $N - j$ degrees of freedom, where N is the total number of observations, $n_1 + n_2$, in the two groups.

7.4.1.a Adjusting the α Level Downward: When several planned comparisons are made, the probability of obtaining significance by chance is increased; that is, the probability of a type I error increases. For example, for four independent comparisons, all at $\alpha = 0.05$, the probability of one or more significant results is $4 \times 0.05 = 0.20$. One way to compensate for multiple comparisons is to decrease the α level, and one way to decrease the α level is to divide α by the number of comparisons made. For example, if four independent comparisons are made and the investigator wants to maintain the overall probability of a type I error at 0.05, this value is divided by 4 to obtain a comparison-wise α of $0.05/4 = 0.0125$. Using this method, each orthogonal comparison must be significant at the 0.0125 level to be declared statistically significant.

7.4.1.b The Bonferroni t Procedure: Another approach for planned comparisons is the **Bonferroni t method,** also called Dunn's multiple-comparison procedure. This approach is more versatile because it is applicable for both orthogonal and nonorthogonal comparisons. The Bonferroni t method increases the critical F value needed for the comparison to be declared significant. The amount of increase depends on the number of comparisons and the sample size.

To illustrate, consider the three groups of patients defined by scores on the Social Readjustment Rating Scale (Presenting Problem 1). The pairwise differences for mean NK cell activity for these three groups are listed in Table 7–6. These data will be used to illustrate all multiple comparisons in this section so that results of the different procedures can be compared. To simplify the comparisons, we will assume that 12 subjects are in the group with low scores, although 13 actually were in that group.

In the Bonferroni t procedure, $\sqrt{2MS_E/n}$ is multiplied by a factor related to the number of comparisons made and the degrees of freedom for the error mean square. In this example, three pairwise comparisons are possible, and there are 34 degrees of freedom. For $\alpha = 0.01$, the multiplier is 3.17. (If you are interested in more detail, consult Kirk, 1995.) Therefore,

$$3.17 \times \sqrt{\frac{2MS_E}{n}} = 3.17 \times \sqrt{\frac{2 \times 278.81}{12}}$$
$$= 3.17 \times 6.82$$
$$= 21.62$$

where the value for MS_E comes from our calculations in Section 7.3. All differences between pairs are compared with 21.62, and if they exceed this value, the differences are significantly different from 0 with $\alpha = 0.01$. Two of the pairwise differences in Table 7–6 are greater than 21.62, those between $\bar{X}_{low}$ and $\bar{X}_{high}$ and between $\bar{X}_{low}$ and $\bar{X}_{mod}$. We therefore conclude that persons with low scores on the Social Readjustment Rating Scale have a higher mean NK cell activity than persons with high or moderate scores on the scale; no differences exist, however, between the high and moderate groups. Is this conclusion consistent with your best guess after looking at the box plots in Figure 7–2?

7.4.2 Posteriori, or Post Hoc, Comparisons

Post hoc comparisons (the Latin term means "after this") are made after an ANOVA has resulted in a significant F test. The t test introduced in Chapter 5 should *not* be used for these comparisons. The problem with using t tests for post hoc comparisons is that they do not take into consideration the number of comparisons being made, the possible lack of independence (nonorthogonality) of the comparisons, and the post hoc (unplanned) nature of the comparisons.

Several procedures are available for making post hoc comparisons. Four of them are recommended by statisticians, depending on the particular research design, and two others are not recommended but are commonly used nonetheless. The data from Presenting Problem 1, as summarized in Table 7–6, are again used to illustrate these six procedures. As with the Bonferroni t method, special tables are needed to find appropriate multipliers for these tests when computer programs are not used for the analysis; excerpts from the tables are reproduced in Table 7–7 corresponding to $\alpha = 0.01$.

7.4.2.a Tukey's HSD Procedure: The first procedure we discuss was developed by the same statistician who gave us stem-and-leaf plots and box-and-whisker plots, and he obviously has a sense of humor. The procedure is called the Tukey test, or **Tukey's HSD** (honestly significant difference) test, so named because some post hoc procedures make significance too easy to obtain. It is applicable only for pairwise

Table 7–6. Differences between means of natural killer cell activity for groups based on Social Readjustment Rating Scale.

	$\bar{X}_{low}$	$\bar{X}_{high}$	$\bar{X}_{mod}$
$\bar{X}_{low}$	—	22.17	24.63
$\bar{X}_{high}$		—	2.46
$\bar{X}_{mod}$			—

Table 7–7. Excerpts from tables for use with multiple-comparison procedures for $\alpha = 0.01$.

Error df	Number of Means or Steps for Studentized Range		Number of Means for Dunnett's Test	
	2	3	2	3
30	3.89	4.45	2.46	2.72
34[a]	3.87	4.42	2.45	2.71
40	3.82	4.37	2.42	2.68

[a]Found by interpolation.

comparisons, but it permits the researcher to compare all pairs of means. A study by Stoline (1981) found it to be the most accurate and powerful procedure to use in this situation. Recall that power is the ability to detect a difference if one actually exists, so high power means that the null hypothesis is correctly rejected more often.

The HSD statistic, like the Bonferroni t, has a multiplier that is based on the number of treatment levels and the degrees of freedom for error mean square (in our example, 3 and 34, respectively). In Table 7–7, under the column for 3 and studentized range,[4] we find the multiplier 4.42. The HSD statistic is

$$HSD = \text{Multiplier} \times \sqrt{\frac{MS_E}{n}}$$

where n is the sample size in each group. Thus,

$$HSD = 4.42 \times \sqrt{\frac{278.81}{12}}$$
$$= 21.31$$

The differences in Table 7–6 are now compared with 21.31 and declared to be significantly different if they exceed this value. From the table, we see that the differences between the low and high groups and between the low and moderate groups are greater than 21.31. The conclusion is therefore the same as for the Bonferroni t—that persons with low scores on the Social Readjustment Rating Scale have a higher mean NK cell activity than persons with high or moderate scores on the scale; no differences exist, however, between the high and moderate groups. Tukey's procedure can also be used to form confidence intervals about the mean difference (as can the Bonferroni t method). For instance, the 99% confidence interval for the mean difference in NK cell activity between low and moderate groups is

$$(\bar{X}_{low} - \bar{X}_{mod}) \pm 21.31, \text{ or } 3.32 \text{ to } 45.94$$

7.4.2.b Scheffé's Procedure: **Scheffé's procedure** is the most versatile of all the post hoc methods because it permits the researcher to make all types of comparisons, not simply pairwise ones. For example, Scheffé's procedure allows us to compare the overall mean of two or more dosage levels with a placebo. A price is extracted for this flexibility, however: A higher critical value is used to determine significance. Thus, Scheffé's procedure is also the most conservative of the multiple-comparison procedures.

[4]The studentized range distribution was developed for a test of the largest observed difference in a set of means, essentially a test of significance of the range of the means. It is used as the basis for several post hoc comparisons.

The formula, which looks somewhat complicated, is

$$S = \sqrt{(j-1)\,F_{\alpha,df}}\,\sqrt{MS_E \sum \frac{C_j^2}{n_j}}$$

where j is the number of groups, $F_{\alpha,df}$ is the critical value of F used in ANOVA, MS_E is the error mean square, and $\sum (C_j^2/n_j)$ is the sum of squared coefficients divided by sample sizes in the contrast of interest. For example, in the contrast defined by $X_{low} - X_{high}$, $\sum C_j^2/n_j = (1)^2/12 + (-1)^2/12 = 0.167$; this value is the same for all pairwise comparisons listed in Table 7–6.[5]

The critical value for F at $\alpha = 0.01$ with 2 and 34 degrees of freedom was found to be 5.31 in Section 7.2. Substituting values in S yields

$$S = \sqrt{(j-1)\,F_{\alpha,df}}\,\sqrt{MS_E \sum \frac{C_j^2}{n_j}}$$
$$= \sqrt{2 \times 5.31}\,\sqrt{278.81 \times 0.167}$$
$$= 3.259 \times 6.824$$
$$= 22.24$$

Any contrast greater than 22.24 is therefore significant. As we see from Table 7–6, the difference in means between low and high groups is 22.17 and just barely misses being significant by the Scheffé test. Because the Scheffé test is the most conservative of all post hoc tests, 22.24 is the largest critical value required by any of the multiple-comparison procedures. Confidence intervals can also be formed by using the Scheffé procedure.

7.4.2.c The Newman–Keuls Procedure: Next, we examine the **Newman–Keuls procedure.** It was the one used by Irwin and colleagues (1987) in their analysis in Presenting Problem 1 and is commonly used in basic science research. Newman–Keuls uses a stepwise approach to testing differences between means and can be used only to make pairwise comparisons. The procedure ranks means from lowest to highest, and the number of steps that separate pairs of means is noted. For our example, the rank orders and the number of steps are given in Figure 7–3. In this procedure, the mean differences are compared with a critical value that depends on the number of steps between the two means, the sample size, and the number of groups being compared. In addition, the testing must be done in a prescribed sequence.

[5]This term is changed, however, if, say, the mean of the low group is compared with the mean of the moderate and high groups combined, that is, $\bar{X}_{low} - [(\bar{X}_{mod} + \bar{X}_{high})/2]$. In this situation,

$$\sum \frac{C_j^2}{n_j} = \frac{(1)^2}{12} + \frac{(-\frac{1}{2})^2}{12} + \frac{(-\frac{1}{2})^2}{12}$$
$$= 0.125$$

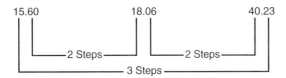

Figure 7–3. Ranking of means and steps for Newman–Keuls test.

The critical value also uses the studentized range, but the value corresponds to the number of steps between the means (instead of the number of means, as in the Tukey test); this value is multiplied by $\sqrt{MS_E/n}$ as in the Tukey test. The value from Table 7–7 corresponding to two steps with 34 degrees of freedom is 3.87; the value for three steps is 4.42. The critical values for this example are therefore

$$\text{Newman-Keuls} = \text{Multiplier} \times \sqrt{\frac{MS_E}{n}}$$

$$\text{Newman-Keuls} = 3.87 \times \sqrt{\frac{MS_E}{n}}$$

$$= 3.87 \times 4.82$$

$$= 18.65$$

$$\text{Newman-Keuls} = 4.42 \times \sqrt{\frac{MS_E}{n}}$$

$$= 4.42 \times 4.82$$

$$= 21.31$$

The critical value for three steps is the same as the critical value for Tukey's HSD test, but the critical value for two steps is less. As with the other procedures, the conclusion is that persons with low scores on the Social Readjustment Rating Scale have a higher mean NK cell activity than persons with high or moderate scores, but no differences exist between the high and moderate groups. Although the conclusions are the same as in Tukey's test, we can see that using the Newman–Keuls procedure with several groups may permit the investigator to declare a difference between two means to be significant when the difference would not be significant in Tukey's HSD test. The primary disadvantage of the Newman–Keuls procedure is that it is not possible to form confidence intervals for mean differences.

7.4.2.d Dunnett's Procedure: The fourth procedure recommended by statisticians is called **Dunnett's procedure,** and it is applicable *only* in situations in which the investigator wants to compare several treatment means with a single control mean. No comparisons are permitted between the treatment means themselves, so this test has a very specialized application. In this special situation, however, Dunnett's test is convenient because it has a relatively low critical value. The size of the multiplier depends on the number of groups, including the control group, and the degrees of freedom for error mean square. The formula is

$$\text{Dunnett's test} = \text{Multiplier} \times \sqrt{\frac{2MS_E}{n}}$$

Even though Dunnett's test is not applicable to our example, we will determine the critical value for the sake of comparison. From Table 7–7, under the column for Dunnett's test and three groups, we find the multiplier 2.71. Multiplying it by $\sqrt{2MS_E/n}$ gives 2.71 × 6.82, or 18.48, a value almost 2 units lower than Tukey's value and almost 4 units lower than Scheffé value.

7.4.2.e Other Tests: Two procedures that appear in the medical literature but that are *not* recommended by statisticians are Duncan's new multiple-range test and the least significant difference test. Duncan's new multiple-range test uses the same principle as the Newman–Keuls test; however, the multipliers in the formula are smaller, so statistically significant differences are found with smaller mean differences. Duncan argued that the likelihood of finding differences is greater when a larger number of groups is used, and he increased the power of the test by using smaller multipliers. But his test, as a result, is too liberal and rejects the null hypothesis too often. Thus, it is not recommended by statisticians.

The least significant difference (LSD) test is one of the oldest multiple-comparison procedures. As with the other post hoc procedures, it requires a significant F ratio from the ANOVA to make pairwise comparisons. Instead of using an adjustment to make the critical value larger, however, as the other tests have done, the LSD test uses the t distribution corresponding to the number of degrees of freedom for error mean square. Statisticians do not recommend this test because, with a large number of comparisons, the α levels of each comparison are inflated and differences that are too small may be incorrectly declared significant.

As you can see, the multiple-comparison procedures are tedious to calculate; fortunately, they are available in most statistical software programs. Output from the recommended multiple-comparison procedures using the NCSS program is reproduced in Table 7–8. NCSS takes a slightly different approach to calculating the critical values by adjusting the critical value of the t statistic itself. The approach we used adjusts the value that includes the standard error term. We suggest you replicate the analysis using the CD-ROM. Do the conclusions agree with our findings?

7.5 ADDITIONAL ILLUSTRATIONS OF THE USE OF ANOVA

In this section, we extend the use of analysis of variance to several other important designs used in the

Table 7–8. Multiple comparisons for natural killer cell activity using NCSS.

Bonferroni (All-Pairwise) Multiple-Comparison Test

Response: Cell
Term A: Group
$\alpha = 0.050$ Error Term = S (A) $df = 34$ $MS_E = 278.8058$ Critical Value = 2.518259

Group	Count	Mean	Different from Groups
2	12	15.6	1
3	12	18.05833	1
1	13	40.23077	2, 3

Newman–Keuls Multiple-Comparison Test

Response: Cell
Term A: Group
$\alpha = 0.050$ Error Term = S (A) $df = 34$ $MS_E = 278.8058$

Group	Count	Mean	Different from Groups
2	12	15.6	1
3	12	18.05833	1
1	13	40.23077	2, 3

Sheffé's Multiple-Comparison Test

Response: Cell
Term A: Group
$\alpha = 0.050$ Error Term = S (A) $df = 34$ $MS_E = 278.8058$ Critical Value = 2.559648

Group	Count	Mean	Different from Groups
2	12	15.6	1
3	12	18.05833	1
1	13	40.23077	2, 3

Tukey–Kramer Multiple-Comparison Test

Response: Cell
Term A: Group
$\alpha = 0.050$ Error Term = S (A) $df = 34$ $MS_E = 278.8058$ Critical Value = 3.465454

Group	Count	Mean	Different from Groups
2	12	15.6	1
3	12	18.05833	1
1	13	40.23077	2, 3

Source: Data, used with permission, from Irwin M et al: Life events, depressive symptoms, and immune function. *Am J Psychiatry* 1987;**144**:437–441. Table produced with NCSS 97, a registered trademark of the Number Cruncher Statistical System; used with permission.

health field. Many experimental designs for ANOVA are possible. Most designs, however, are combinations of a relatively small number of designs: randomized factorial designs, randomized block designs, and Latin square designs. The principle of randomized assignment resulted from the work of two statisticians in the early 20th century, Ronald Fisher and Karl Pearson, who had considerable influence on the development and the direction of modern statistical methods. For this reason, the term "randomized" occurs in the names of many designs; and, of course, one of the assumptions is that a random sample has been assigned to the different treatment levels. In this section, we will describe several designs sometimes used for an ANOVA.

7.5.1 Two-Way ANOVA: Factorial Design

Two-way ANOVA is similar to one-way ANOVA except that two factors (or two independent vari-

ables) are analyzed. For example, in the study described in Presenting Problem 2, Gonzalo and colleagues (1996) wanted to know if a difference existed in insulin sensitivity depending on thyroid level or body mass index (BMI). They defined hyperthyroidism as an increase in serum thyroxine, free thyroxine index, and suppressed serum thyroid-stimulating hormone levels; overweight was defined as BMI > 25 (body mass index is calculated as weight in kilograms divided by height in meters squared, kg/m^2). Raw data are given in Table 7–9. In this example, both factors are measured at two levels on all subjects and are said to be *crossed.*

Because two factors are analyzed in this study (thyroid level and BMI), each measured at two levels (hyperthyroid vs controls and overweight vs normal weight), $2 \times 2 = 4$ treatment combinations are possible: overweight hyperthyroid subjects, overweight controls, normal weight hyperthyroid subjects, and normal

Table 7–9. Insulin sensitivity for women in different groups

| | Normal Thyroid | | Hyperthyroid | |
	Normal Weight	Overweight	Normal Weight	Overweight
	0.97	0.76	0.56	0.19
	0.88	0.44	0.89	0.11
	0.66	0.48	0.55	0.13
	0.52	0.39	0.66	0.21
	0.38	1.10	0.11	0.32
	0.71	0.19	0.27	0.01
	0.46	0.19	0.56	
	0.29	0.19	0.80	
	0.68			
	0.96			
	0.97			
N	11.00	8	8	6
Mean	0.68	0.47	0.55	0.16
SD	0.25	0.32	0.26	0.10
	All Control Women		**All Hyperthyroid Women**	
N	19		14	
Mean	0.59		0.38	
SD	0.29		0.28	
	All Overweight Women		**All Normal Weight Women**	
N	14		19	
Mean	0.34		0.63	
SD	0.29		0.25	

Source: Data, used with permission, from Gonzalo MA et al: Glucose tolerance, insulin secretion, insulin sensitivity and glucose effectiveness in normal and overweight hyperthyroid women. *Clin Endocrinol* 1996;**45:**689–697.

weight controls. Three questions may be asked in this two-way ANOVA:

1. Do differences exist between hyperthyroid subjects and controls? If so, the means for each treatment combination might resemble the hypothetical values given in Table 7–10A, and we say a difference exists in the *main effect* for thyroid status. The null hypothesis for this question is that insulin sensitivity is the same in hyperthyroid subjects and in controls ($\mu_H = \mu_C$).

2. Do differences exist between overweight and normal weight subjects? If so, the means for each treatment combination might be similar to those in Table 7–10B, and we say a difference occurs in the *main effect* for weight. The null hypothesis for this question is that insulin sensitivity is the same in overweight subjects and in normal weight subjects ($\mu_O = \mu_N$).

3. Do differences exist owing to neither thyroid status nor weight alone but to the combination of factors? If so, the means for each treatment combination might resemble those in Table 7–10C, and we say an **interaction** effect occurs between the two factors. The null hypothesis for this question is that any difference in insulin sensitivity between overweight hyperthyroid subjects and overweight controls is the same as the difference between normal weight hyperthyroid subjects and normal weight controls ($\mu_{OH} - \mu_{OC} = \mu_{NH} - \mu_{NC}$).

This study can be viewed as two separate experiments on the same set of subjects for each of the first two questions. The third question can be answered, however, only in a single experiment in which both factors are measured and more than one observation is made at each treatment combination of the factors (ie, in each cell).

The topic of interactions is important and worth pursuing a bit further. Figure 7–4A is a graph of *hypothet-*

Table 7–10. Possible results for hypothetical data in two-way ANOVA: Means for each treatment combination.

A. Difference between Patients and Controls

Subjects	Weight	
	Over	Normal
Patients	1.00	1.00
Controls	0.50	0.50

B. Difference between Over and Normal Weight Subjects

Subjects	Weight	
	Over	Normal
Patients	0.50	1.00
Controls	0.50	1.00

C. Differences owing Only to Combination of Factors

Subjects	Weight	
	Over	Normal
Patients	0.50	1.00
Controls	1.00	0.50

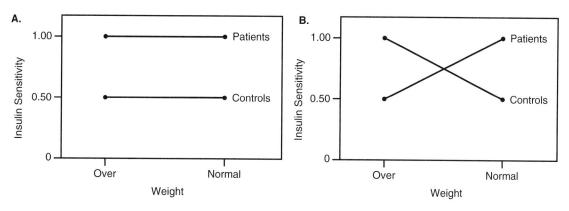

Figure 7–4. Graphs of interaction. **A:** No interaction; effects are additive. **B:** Significant interaction; effects are multiplicative.

ical mean insulin sensitivity levels from Table 7–10A for hyperthyroid and control, overweight and normal weight women. When lines connecting means are parallel, no interaction exists between the factors of thyroid status and weight status, and the effects are said to be *additive*. If the interaction is significant, however, as in Table 7–10C, the lines intersect and the effects are called *multiplicative*. Figure 7–4B illustrates this situation and shows that main effects, such as thyroid status and overweight status, are difficult to interpret when significant interactions occur. For example, if the interaction is significant, any conclusions regarding increased insulin sensitivity depend on both thyroid status and weight; any comparison between women with hyperthyroidism and controls depends on the weight of the subject. Although this example illustrates an extreme interaction, many statisticians recommend that the interaction be tested first and, if it is significant, main effects *not* be tested.

The calculations in two-way ANOVA are tedious and will not be illustrated in this book. They are conceptually similar to the calculations in the simpler one-way situation, however: The total variation in observations is divided, and sums of squares are determined for the first factor, the second factor, the interaction of the factors, and the error (residual), which is analogous to the within-group sums of squares in one-way ANOVA.

7.5.1.a Summary of Presenting Problem 2: The results from the study by Gonzalo and colleagues (1996) are given in Table 7–11. The table gives the findings for several variables, including the one in which we are interested, the sensitivity to insulin, abbreviated SI. The means and standard errors are given for each of the four individual groups as well as for the total group with hyperthyroidism and the total control group (without hyperthyroidism). Note that the table contains the standard errors of the mean, not the standard deviations. In other words, the mean insulin sensitivity is 0.55 L/min pmol $\times 10^4$ for the eight women who are of normal weight with hyperthyroidism, but we do not know the value of the standard deviation until we multiply the standard error, 0.09, by the square root of the sample size.

Refer again to Table 7–9 for the means and standard deviations for each of the four individual groups

Table 7–11. β-Cell function and intravenous glucose tolerance test.

Subjects	Glucose AUC (min mmol/L)	Δ Insulin AUC 0–10 min (min pmol/L)	Δ Insulin AUC 10–20 min (min pmol/L)	SG (10^2/min)	SI (L/min pmol 10^4)
NW-HT ($n = 8$)	1050 ± 57	3943 ± 704	2188 ± 217	2.2 ± 0.3	0.55 ± 0.09
OW-HT ($n = 6$)	1121 ± 22[a,b]	9036 ± 3375	4895 ± 1405[c]	3.8 ± 1.1	0.16 ± 0.04[a,b]
Total-HT ($n = 14$)	1080 ± 34[d]	6126 ± 1587	3348 ± 691	2.8 ± 0.5	0.38 ± 0.07[d]
NW-C ($n = 11$)	981 ± 25	4035 ± 396	1906 ± 219	3.3 ± 0.6	0.68 ± 0.07
OW-C ($n = 8$)	1026 ± 32	5309 ± 1657	3399 ± 663	4.3 ± 0.7	0.47 ± 0.11
Total-C: ($n = 19$)	1000 ± 20	4571 ± 723	2535 ± 343	3.7 ± 0.4	0.59 ± 0.07

Abbreviations: NW = normal weight; OW = overweight; HT = hyperthyroid patients; C = control subjects; AUC = area under the curve. Data presented as mean ± SEM.
[a]$P < 0.05$ OW-HT versus NW-HT.
[b]$P < 0.05$ OW-HT versus OW-C.
[c]$P < 0.05$ OW-C versus NW-C.
[d]$P < 0.05$ total-HT versus total-C.

of women and for the two thyroid groups and two weight groups as well. The mean insulin sensitivity is 0.59 for control women and 0.38 for hyperthyroid women. For overweight women, mean insulin sensitivity is 0.34, compared with 0.63 for normal weight women. When the means are examined for each individual group, normal weight control women have the highest sensitivity, and overweight women with hyperthyroidism have the lowest sensitivity. Two-way analysis of variance can help us make sense of all these means and see which are significantly different. The results are given in Table 7–12.

The computer output produced by SPSS lists a great deal of information, but we focus on the rows labeled as *main effects* and *two-way interactions*. We first examine the interaction effect, listed as Hyperthyroid * overweight in the table; the mean square is 0.06 (6.091E-02 in scientific notation), the F statistic is 0.958, and the P value is 0.336 (in the column labeled Significance). Because the P value is greater than 0.05, the null hypothesis of no interaction is not rejected, so we conclude there is no evidence of significant interaction between hyperthyroidism and weight status. A graph of the interaction is given in Figure 7–5. If the interaction were significant, we would stop at this point and not proceed to interpret the main effects of thyroid and weight status. The lines in Figure 7–5 do not cross, however, so we are able to consider the main effects. Note that the graph in Figure 7–5 is simply the mean values given in Table 7–9 for the four individual groups.

The hyperthyroid main effect has 1 degree of freedom (because two thyroid groups are being analyzed), so the mean square is the same as the sum of squares, 0.374 in Table 7–12. The F statistic for this effect is 5.883, and the P value is 0.022. We therefore reject the null hypothesis of equal mean insulin sensitivity for the two groups defined by thyroid status and conclude that women who are hyperthyroid have a lower sensitivity than those with normal thyroid levels. Similarly, the overweight main effect is significant, with a P value of 0.002, so we conclude that being overweight has an effect on insulin sensitivity as well.

7.5.2 Randomized Factorial Designs

The studies discussed in this chapter thus far are examples of randomized **factorial designs** with one or two factors. Randomized factorial designs with three or more factors are possible as well, and the ideas introduced in Section 7.5.1 generalize in a logical way. For example, a study examining thyroid level, weight, and gender (with more than one observation per treatment combination) has sums of squares and mean squares for thyroid level, weight, and gender; for the interactions between thyroid level and weight, between weight and gender, and between thyroid level and gender; and, finally, for the interaction among all three factors. Studies that employ more than three or four factors are rare in medicine because of the large number of subjects needed. For example, a study with three factors, each with two levels as we just described, has $2 \times 2 \times 2 = 8$ treatment combinations; if one factor has two levels, another has three levels, and the third has four levels, then $2 \times 3 \times 4 = 24$ different treatment combinations are possible. Finding an equal number of subjects for each treatment combination can be difficult.

7.5.3 Randomized Block Designs

A factor is said to be **confounded** with another factor if it is impossible to determine which factor is responsible for the observed effect. Age is frequently a confounding factor in medical studies, so investigators often age-match control subjects with treatment subjects. Randomized **block designs** are useful when a confounding factor contributes to variation.

In the **randomized block design,** subjects are first subdivided into homogeneous blocks; subjects from each block are then randomly assigned to each level of the experimental factor. This type of study is espe-

Table 7–12. Analysis of variance for study of insulin activity.[a,b]

			Unique Method				
			Sum of Squares	df	Mean Squares	F	Significance
Insulin sensitivity	Main effects	(Combined)	1.070	2	0.535	8.412	0.001
		Hyperthyroid	0.374	1	0.374	5.883	0.022
		Overweight	0.711	1	0.711	11.180	0.002
	2-way interactions	Hyperthyroid * overweight	6.091E-02	1	6.091E-02	0.958	0.336
	Model		1.071	3	0.357	5.614	0.004
	Residual		1.845	29	6.361E-02		
	Total		2.916	32	9.113E-02		

[a]Insulin sensitivity by hyperthyroid, overweight.
[b]All effects entered simultaneously.
Source: Data, used with permission, from Gonzalo MA et al: Glucose tolerance, insulin secretion, insulin sensitivity and glucose effectiveness in normal and overweight hyperthyroid women. *Clin Endocrinol* 1996;**45:**689–697. Output produced with SPSS, a registered trademark of SPSS, Inc.; used with permission.

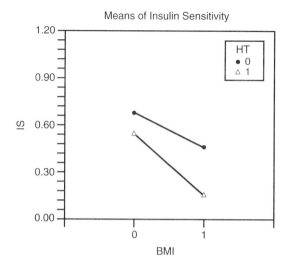

Figure 7–5. Graph of interaction for study of insulin sensitivity. (Data, used with permission, from Gonzalo MA et al: Glucose tolerance, insulin secretion, insulin sensitivity and glucose effectiveness in normal and overweight hyperthyroid women. *Clin Endocrinol* 1996;**45**:689–697. Output produced using NCSS 97, a registered trademark of the Number Cruncher Statistical System; used with permission.)

cially useful in laboratory experiments in which investigators are concerned about genetic variation and its effect on the outcome being studied. Litters of animals are defined as the blocks, and littermates are then randomly assigned to the different levels of treatment. In this experiment, blocking is said to control for genetic differences. In studies involving humans, blocking on age or severity of a condition is often useful. Investigators may also want to have more than one subject from each block assigned to each treatment level.

Sometimes, investigators cannot control for possible confounding factors in the design of a study. The procedure called **analysis of covariance** allows investigators to control statistically for such factors in the analysis; this procedure is discussed in Chapter 10.

7.5.4 Latin Square Designs

Latin square designs employ the blocking principle for two confounding (or nuisance) factors. The levels of the confounding factors are assigned to the rows and the columns of a square; then, the cells of the square identify treatment levels. For example, suppose that both age and body weight are important blocking factors in an experiment that has three dosage levels of a drug as the treatment. Then, three blocks of age and three blocks of body weight form a Latin square with nine cells, and each dosage level appears one or more times for each age–weight com-

bination. Table 7–13 illustrates this design. The Latin square design can be powerful, because only nine subjects are needed and yet two possible confounding factors have been controlled.

7.5.5 Nested Designs

In the factorial designs described previously, the factors are **crossed,** meaning that all levels of one factor occur within all levels of the other factors. Thus, all possible combinations are included in the experiment, as in the study described in Presenting Problem 2.

In some situations, however, crossed factors cannot be employed; so **hierarchical,** or *nested,* designs are used instead. In hierarchical designs, one or more of the treatments is nested within levels of another factor. Nesting is needed when entire sets of subjects must be given the same treatment, often because of administrative concerns. For example, educational experimentation is difficult to perform in medical schools because classes are often small, and medical students communicate with one another about their educational experiences. Thus, an investigator who wants to compare two methods of teaching physical examination skills, say, may opt for designing a cooperative study among six medical schools. Medical schools are randomly assigned to one of the two teaching methods, three schools for each method. Medical schools are then said to be nested within teaching conditions, and it is impossible to determine interaction effects between medical school and teaching condition.

7.5.6 Repeated-Measures Designs

Recall from Chapter 5 that the paired t test should be used when the same sample of subjects is observed on two occasions. This design is powerful because it controls for individual variation; and for both biologic and psychologic measurements, individual variation can be large. The counterpart to the paired t test in ANOVA is the **repeated-measures** (or split-plot) **design.** In this design, subjects serve as their own controls, so that the variability owing to individual differences is eliminated from the error (residual) term, increasing the chances of observing significant differences between levels of treatment. In this sense, repeated-measures designs have the same goal as designs using blocks. The repeated measurements may

Table 7–13. Latin square design with three dosage levels (D1, D2, D3).

Body Weight (kg)	Age level (years)		
	< 50	50–70	> 70
< 60	D1	D2	D3
60–90	D2	D3	D1
> 90	D3	D1	D2

be the same treatment level measured more than once, or they may involve the same subjects measured more than once under different levels of a treatment.

Unlike the randomized-block design, the treatments in a repeated-measures design are always applied in the same order rather than in random order. The analysis is the same as for the randomized-block design, however, even though the randomization method is different. The individuals become the blocks and the repeated-measures variable (the variable representing time) becomes the treatment.

The study of stroke patients by Good and colleagues (1996) had repeated measures of mobility and daily living using the Barthel index. Measurements were collected at four periods: at admission to the hospital, at discharge, and at 3 and 12 months after stroke. It would be useful to know if a difference exists in the pattern of changes over time for the 21 patients who were hypertensive, compared with the 21 who had normal blood pressure. (Five of the 47 patients did not have all measures of the Barthel index, so they have been omitted from the analysis.) The means and standard deviations of the Barthel index at each time are given in Table 7–14.

The results of a repeated-measures analysis of Barthel index are given in Table 7–15. The measure that is repeated, the Barthel index in this example, is called the *within-subjects measure;* and the variable that defines different groups is called the *between-subjects measure.* The SPSS procedure used, called the general linear model, is very versatile because it can use any analysis of variance design, but it is also very complicated. For our discussion, we ignore much of the printout and concentrate only on that portion reproduced in Table 7–15.

Certain assumptions made in repeated-measures ANOVA involve the relationship among the measures that are repeated, the Barthel index in our example. SPSS performs a test of this assumption, called a test of sphericity; it is analogous to testing whether the variances are equal when comparing two groups with the *t* test. Recall that we briefly discussed this assumption in Chapter 6 and mentioned that, if the variances are not equal, a formula called the Satterthwaite correction is used to reduce the degrees of freedom for the *t* test. If the sphericity test indicates the assumption is violated, then an analogous adjustment is made to the degrees of freedom in repeated-measures ANOVA, using one of several formulas. The top section of Table 7–15 gives the results of the analysis so we can see if the within-subjects factor is significant. If the assumption of sphericity is rejected (as it actually was in our example), SPSS gives the Greenhouse–Geisser and the Huynh–Feldt corrections. A lower bound correction is also available, which is the most conservative conclusion possible. In our example, all three indicate that a significant difference exists in the Barthel index measures over time. Although a *P* value of 0.000 is shown, statisticians recommend that it be stated as <0.001, because it is always remotely possible that our conclusion is incorrect.

The set of numbers in Table 7–15 associated with the block entitled BARTHEL*HYPERTE2 shows the results of the test of the interaction between the Barthel index and hypertension. Because this interaction is significant, we conclude that the pattern of changes in the Barthel index over the four time periods is not the same for patients with hypertension as for those without hypertension. Looking at the means in Table 7–14, we see that the values for patients with hypertension increase more rapidly over time and continue to increase after the 3-month measurement.

The second section of Table 7–15, entitled Test of Between-Subjects Effects, gives the results of the ANOVA for the between-subjects factor of hypertension; that is, it compares patients with and without hypertension. The results are not significant at the traditional 0.05 level (*P* value = 0.085), indicating that the Barthel index *collapsed over the time periods* was not different for patients with and without hypertension. Because a significant interaction occurred, however, we do not draw any conclusions

Table 7–14. Means and standard deviations at the three times the Barthel index was measured.

Hypertension		Admission BI	Discharge BI	3-Month BI	12-Month BI
No	Mean	33.3333	57.1429	67.8571	67.8571
	N	21	21	21	21
	Standard deviation	13.4474	18.1364	18.4778	22.8348
Yes	Mean	32.8571	64.7619	78.8095	83.0952
	N	21	21	21	21
	Standard deviation	13.1882	20.3394	20.4270	20.2161
Total	Mean	33.0952	60.9524	73.3333	75.4762
	N	42	42	42	42
	Standard deviation	13.1572	19.4196	20.0203	22.6535

Abbreviation: BI = Barthel index.
Source: Data, used with permission, from Good DC et al: Sleep-disordered breathing and poor functional outcome after stroke. *Stroke* 1996;**27**:252–259. Output produced with SPSS, a registered trademark of SPSS, Inc.; used with permission.

Table 7–15.   Illustration of repeated-measures analysis of Barthel index.

Tests of Within-Subjects Effects

Measure: MEASURE_1

Source		Type III Sum of Squares	df	Mean Square	F	Significance
BARTHEL	Sphericity assumed	47880.952	3	15960.317	173.306	0.000
	Greenhouse–Geisser	47880.952	1.873	25562.723	173.306	0.000
	Huynh–Feldt	47880.952	2.011	23810.767	173.306	0.000
	Lower-bound	47880.952	1.000	47880.952	173.306	0.000
BARTHEL*HYPERTE2	Sphericity assumed	1392.857	3	464.286	5.041	0.003
	Greenhouse–Geisser	1392.857	1.873	743.620	5.041	0.010
	Huynh-Feldt	1392.857	2.011	692.655	5.041	0.009
	Lower-bound	1392.857	1.000	1392.857	5.041	0.030
Error(BARTHEL)	Sphericity assumed	11051.190	120	92.093		
	Greenhouse–Geisser	11051.190	74.923	147.500		
	Huynh–Feldt	11051.190	80.436	137.391		
	Lower-bound	11051.190	40.000	276.280		

Tests of Between-Subjects Effects

Measure: MEASURE_1
Transformed variable: Average

Source	Type III Sum of Squares	df	Mean Square	F	Significance
Intercept	619285.714	1	619285.714	554.510	0.000
HYPERTE2	2916.667	1	2916.667	2.612	0.114
Error	44672.619	40	1116.815		

Source: Data, used with permission, from Good DC et al: Sleep-disordered breathing and poor functional outcome after stroke. *Stroke* 1996;**27**:252–259. Output produced with SPSS, a registered trademark of SPSS, Inc.; used with permission.

about this factor. We suggest that you use the CD-ROM to replicate this analysis.

Recall that another assumption in ANOVA is that the observations be independent of one another. This assumption is frequently not met in repeated-measures ANOVA; therefore, certain other assumptions concerning the dependent nature of the observations must be made and tested. We will not discuss these assumptions here. From an interpretation perspective, readers of the medical literature merely need to know that repeated-measures ANOVA should be used in studies that repeat measurements on the same subjects.

7.6 NONPARAMETRIC ANOVA

Nonparametric ANOVA is not a different design but a different method of analysis. Recall from Chapters 5 and 6 that if the assumptions for the *t* tests are seriously violated, then nonparametric methods such as the Wilcoxon rank sum test for two independent groups or the signed rank test for paired designs should be used instead. A similar situation holds in ANOVA. Even though the *F* test is robust with respect to violating the assumption of normality and, if the sample sizes are equal, the assumption of equal variances, in some situations transforming observations to a logarithm scale or using nonparametric pro-

cedures is advisable. For example, when observations from small samples greatly depart from the normal distribution or when markedly unequal variances occur along with different sample sizes, nonparametric ANOVA should be considered.

Like the nonparametric procedures discussed in Chapters 5 and 6, the nonparametric methods in ANOVA are based on the analysis of ranks of observations rather than on original observations. For one-way ANOVA, the nonparametric procedure is the Kruskal–Wallis one-way ANOVA by ranks. Post hoc comparisons between pairs of means may be made by using the Wilcoxon rank sum test, with a downward adjustment of the α level to compensate for multiple comparisons, as described in Section 7.4.1. When more than two related samples are of interest, as in repeated measures, the nonparametric procedure of choice is the Friedman two-way ANOVA by ranks. The term "two" in Friedman two-way ANOVA refers to (1) levels of the factor (or treatment) and (2) the repeated occasions on which the subjects were observed. In the Good and colleagues (1996) example, the levels of the factor are hypertension versus no hypertension, and the repeated occasions are the Barthel index measured four times during the study. As a follow-up procedure to make pairwise comparisons, the Wilcoxon signed rank test with adjusted degrees of freedom can be used.

7.7 SAMPLE SIZES FOR ANOVA

It is just as important to look at the sample size needed for ANOVA as it is when studying only one or two groups. Unfortunately, the procedures in the power analysis programs are not as simple to use as the ones for means and proportions. As noted several times in this chapter, if you are planning a study in which an ANOVA is appropriate, it is a good idea to see a statistician prior to beginning.

We used the nQuery Advisor program to find the estimated sample size for the study by Irwin and coworkers (1987). We used the results they observed to determine the number in each group required for 80% power. Using this program required us to calculate the variance of the means and the pooled standard deviation.

The formula used by nQuery to find the variance (V) of the means is $V = \Sigma (\overline{X}_j - \overline{\overline{X}})^2 / G$, where $\overline{X}_j$ is the mean of the jth group, $\overline{\overline{X}}$ is the overall mean, and G is the number of groups. Without showing the calculations, this estimate is 122.87, using the means from the Irwin and coworkers study in Table 7–1. The pooled standard deviation is calculated in the same manner as for two groups, illustrated in Chapter 6; for this example, it is 16.7. The result of the power analysis is that a sample size of nine in each group was adequate to achieve 80% power of finding a difference in NK cell activity, if one truly exists. nQuery produces the following statement:

> When the sample size in each of the three groups is nine, a one-way analysis of variance will have 80% power to detect at the 0.050 level a difference in means characterized by a variance of means, $V = \Sigma (\overline{X}_j - \overline{\overline{X}})^2 / G$ of 122.870, assuming that the common standard deviation is 16.700.

Table 7–16. Hamilton depression scores for groupings based on Social Readjustment Rating Scale score.

Subject	Low	Moderate	High
1	1.2	20.0	15.2
2	11.3	19.0	15.0
3	12.3	0	19.2
4	13.3	17.0	3.8
5	8.7	13.6	0.7
6	0.8	20.7	19.3
7	2.3	19.5	21.0
8	0.5	15.4	7.0
9	3.0	3.0	9.0
10	2.7	7.3	18.0
11	12.0	24.5	7.5
12	0.3	16.5	8.0
13	1.0		
Mean	5.3	14.7	12.0
Standard deviation	5.2	7.5	6.8

Source: Observations, used with permission, from Irwin M et al: Life events, depressive symptoms, and immune function. *Am J Psychiatry* 1987;**144**:437–441.

7.8 SUMMARY

In the study described in Presenting Problem 1, the investigators were interested in the relationship between major life events and immune function. Women were divided into three groups according to their scores on the Social Readjustment Rating Scale. We used the data on natural killer (NK) cell activity to illustrate concepts and calculations involved in one-way analysis of variance. We found that indeed differences existed among groups in NK cell activity; post hoc procedures further indicated that the major difference occurs between women with low scores on the Social Readjustment Rating Scale; that is, they differ from women with moderate and high scores. The authors also found significant differences on the Hamilton depression score; no differences were found, however, for women of different ages or races or for other immune function variables analyzed.

Gonzalo and colleagues (1996) found no significant differences in glucose tolerance and insulin sensitivity in the nonoverweight hyperthyroid patients compared with the matched controls. We confirmed the findings for insulin sensitivity using two-way analysis of variance. The investigators also reported that, in those hyperthyroid patients with excessive weight, glucose tolerance and insulin sensitivity were significantly lower than in their matched controls.

Data from the study by Good and colleagues (1996) were used to illustrate repeated-measures analysis of variance. We found that the pattern of changes in the Barthel index over time is different for patients with hypertension versus for those without hypertension. Ignoring the time factor, the ANOVA indicated that the Barthel index was not different for patients with and without hypertension.

Determining which ANOVA study design or method is most appropriate for a given investigation is often difficult. Making this decision requires knowledge of the area being investigated and of experimental design methods. Considerations must include the kind of data to be collected (nominal, ordinal, interval), the number of treatments to be included and whether obtaining estimates of interaction effects is important, the number of treatment levels to be included and whether they should be fixed or random, the possibility of blocking on confounding factors, the number of subjects needed and whether that number is adequate for the proposed designs, and the ramifications of violating assumptions in ANOVA. Although Flowchart C–2 in Appendix C gives some guidelines for elementary designs, selecting the best design requires communication between investigators and statisticians, and the best design may be impossible because of one or more of the considerations just listed.

Although all the post hoc procedures described in

Section 7.4 are used in health research, some methods are better than others for specific study designs. For pairwise comparisons (between pairs of means), Tukey's test is the first choice and the Newman–Keuls procedure is second. When several treatment means are to be compared with a single control but no comparisons among treatments are desired, Dunnett's test is best. For nonpairwise comparisons, such as $[(\mu_1 + \mu_2)/2] - \mu_3$, Scheffé's procedure is best. Duncan's new multiple-range test and the least significant difference test are not recommended.

Readers of the medical literature may have difficulty judging whether the best design was used in a study. Authors of journal articles do not always provide sufficient detail on experimental design, and it may not be possible to know the constraints present when the study was designed. In these situations, the reader can only judge the reputation of the authors and their affiliations and evaluate the scholarly practices of the journal in which the study is published. Some journal editors are increasingly requiring authors to specify their study designs and methods of analysis, and we hope they will continue their efforts.

EXERCISES

1. Use the data on the Hamilton depression score in Table 7–16 to perform a one-way ANOVA, using $\alpha = 0.01$. Interpret the results of your analysis.

2. Use the data in Table 7–16 and the values in Table 7–7 to perform Tukey's HSD test and Scheffé's post hoc test for comparing three means, or use the data in the file folder called "Irwin" in the CD-ROM. Compare the conclusions drawn with these two procedures.

3. A study was undertaken comparing drug use by physicians, pharmacists, medical students, and pharmacy students. Are the following sets of comparisons independent or dependent?
   a. Physicians with pharmacists and medical students with pharmacy students
   b. Medical students with physicians and physicians with pharmacists
   c. Medical students with physicians and pharmacists with pharmacy students
   d. Medical students with physicians, medical students with pharmacists, and medical students with pharmacy students

4. Characteristics of sleep apnea in hypertensive men and control patients were studied by Fletcher and associates (1985). The men with hypertension were subdivided into those with and without apnea. The mean and the standard deviation of total number of minutes of disordered breathing are given in Table 7–17. Use the shortcut formulas given in Section 7.2.2 to per-

Table 7–17. Total number of minutes of disordered breathing.

Group	Total Number of Minutes		
	n	Mean	Standard Deviation
Controls	34	3.9	4.7
Nonapneic hyptertensives	32	4.7	3.9
Apneic hypertensives	14	16.4	10.1

Source: Adapted and reproduced, with permission, from Fletcher EC et al: Undiagnosed sleep apnea in patients with essential hypertension. *Ann Intern Med* 1985;**103**:190–195.

form an ANOVA on these data. What are your conclusions? What assumption is violated in using ANOVA in this example?

5. Medical researchers are interested in the relationship between alcohol use along with other life-style characteristics and the development of diseases, such as cancer and hypertension. The hypothetical data in Table 7–18 could result from an ANOVA in a study comparing the mean blood pressures of patients who consume different amounts of alcohol.
   a. What type of ANOVA is represented in Table 7–18?
   b. What is the total variation?
   c. How many groups of patients were in the study? How many patients were in the study?
   d. What is the value of the *F* ratio?
   e. What is the critical value at 0.01?
   f. What conclusion is appropriate?

6. Francis and colleagues (1985) studied the relationship between acetylcholine synthesis in brain biopsy specimens in patients with Alzheimer's disease and a rating of their cognitive impairment. They also compared the differences in neurochemical markers of various neurotransmitters in brain tissue taken during autopsy from 48 patients with either early onset (age < 80 years) or late onset (age ≥ 80 years) of Alzheimer's disease and 34 controls of similar ages. Their data from brain tissue samples obtained at autopsy are shown in Table 7–19. The authors appropriately used a logarithmic trans-

Table 7–18. ANOVA on mean blood pressures.

Source of Variation	Sums of Squares	*df*	Mean Squares	*F*
Among groups	800	3	—	—
Within groups	1200	36	33.3	
Total	—			

Table 7–19. Neurochemical changes of temporal cortex in Alzheimer and matched control patients.

	Means and Standard Deviations			
	Early Onset (<80 years)		Late Onset (≥80 years)	
	Controls	Patients	Controls	Patients
n	14	19	20	29
Choline acetyltransferase[a]	99.7 ± 18.7	39.3 ± 33.1[b]	101.9 ± 41.6	42.1 ± 25.8[b]
Serotonin	1392 ± 868	504 ± 397[b]	915 ± 474	625 ± 420[b]
Norepinephrine	646 ± 385	230 ± 214[b]	549 ± 264	340 ± 280[b]
3-Methoxy-4-hydroxyphenylglycol	1451 ± 935	2187 ± 1268[b]	2126 ± 962	1768 ± 953
5-Hydroxyindoleacetic acid	6714 ± 3079	5423 ± 3308	8673 ± 4244	7094 ± 5649

[a]Choline acetyltransferase values are expressed as picomoles per hour per milligram (pmol/h/mg) of protein; all other values are expressed as femtomoles per milligram (fmol/mg) of protein.
[b]$P < 0.05$ between patients and controls in at least significant difference test.
Source: Adapted and reproduced, with permission, from Table 1 in Francis PT et al: Neurochemical studies of early-onset Alzheimer's disease: Possible influence on treatment. *N Engl J Med* 1985;**313**:7–11.

formation on the data for serotonin and 5-hydroxyindoleacetic acid in order to obtain observations that were normally distributed before they performed the ANOVA.

a. What are the main effects in this study?

b. Which of the five dependent variables have a potential interaction among the main factors?

c. What post hoc comparison method was used in this study?

d. What other information in the table is impor-

tant to define the type of analysis that is appropriate?

7. Use the data from the study by Gonzalo and colleagues (1996) to perform a two-way analysis of variance for the outcome of glucose level.

a. What is the P value for the interaction between thyroid status and weight to be significant?

b. What is the P value for the main effects?

c. State the conclusion in words.

Research Questions about Relationships among Variables

8

PRESENTING PROBLEMS

Presenting Problem 1. Presenting Problem 2 in Chapter 3 described a study by Hébert and colleagues (1997) that measured disability and functional changes in 655 residents of a community in Quebec, Canada. Subjects were age 75 years and older, and data were collected at baseline and again after 1 and 2 years. The Functional Autonomy Measurement System (SMAF), a 29-item rating scale measuring functional disability in five areas, was administered along with a questionnaire measuring health, cognitive function, and depression.

We used observations on mental ability for women 85 years or older at baseline and 2 years later to illustrate the correlation coefficient in Chapter 3 and found it to be 0.58. In this chapter we illustrate the statistical methods used to determine whether this value is significantly different from zero. The data for this research question were given in Chapter 3, Table 3–19.

Presenting Problem 2. Hypertension, defined as systolic pressure greater than 140 mm Hg or diastolic pressure greater than 90 mm Hg, is present in 20–30% of the U. S. population. Recognition and treatment of hypertension has significantly reduced the morbidity and mortality associated with the complications of hypertension. A number of finger blood pressure devices are marketed for home use by patients as an easy and convenient way for them to monitor their own blood pressure.

How correct are these finger blood pressure machines? Nesselroad and colleagues (1996) studied these devices to determine their accuracy. They measured blood pressure in 100 consecutive patients presenting to a family practice office who consented to participate. After being seated for 5 min, blood pressure was measured in each patient using a standard blood pressure cuff of appropriate size and with each of three automated finger blood pressure devices. The data were analyzed by calculating the correlation coefficient between the value obtained with the blood pressure cuff and the three finger devices and by calculating the percentage of measurements with each automated device that fell within the ±4 mm Hg margin of error of the blood pressure cuff.

We use the data to illustrate correlation and scatterplots. We also illustrate a test of hypothesis about two dependent or related correlation coefficients. Data are given in Section 8.4.1.

Presenting Problem 3. Symptoms of forgetfulness and loss of concentration can be a result of natural aging and are often aggravated by fatigue, illness, depression, visual or hearing loss, or certain medications. A phenomenon called anticipatory dementia is characterized as the fear that normal, age-associated memory change is the harbinger of Alzheimer's disease. Studies suggest a link between loss of memory and various measures of well-being.

Hodgson and Cutler (1997) wished to examine the consequences of anticipatory dementia. They stated their research question as follows: Does an association exist between anticipatory dementia and well-being? They studied 25 men and women with a living parent with a probable diagnosis of Alzheimer's disease, a condition in which genetic factors are known to be important. A control group of 25 men and women who did not have a parent with dementia was selected for comparison. A directed interview and questionnaire were used to measure concern about developing Alzheimer's disease and to assess subjective memory functioning. Four measures of each individual's sense of well-being were used in the areas of depression, psychiatric symptomatology, life satisfaction, and subjective health status. We use this study to illustrate biserial correlation and show its concordance with the t test. Observations from the study are given in Section 8.5.3.d, and the data are in a folder on the CD-ROM entitled "Hodgson."

Presenting Problem 4. The study of hyperthyroid women by Gonzalo and coinvestigators (1996) was a presenting problem in Chapter 7. Recall that the study reported the effect of excess body weight in hyperthyroid patients on glucose tolerance, insulin secretion, and insulin sensitivity. The study included 14 hyperthyroid women, 6 of whom were overweight, and 19 volunteers with normal thyroid levels of similar ages and weight. The investigators in this study also examined the relationship between insulin sensitivity and body mass index for hyperthyroid and control women. (See Figure 3 in Gonzalo and coinvestigators' article.) We revisit this study to calculate and compare two regression lines. Original observations are given in Chapter 7, Table 7–9.

8.1 AN OVERVIEW OF CORRELATION & REGRESSION

In Chapter 3 we introduced methods to describe the association or relationship between two variables. In this chapter we review these concepts and extend the idea to predicting the value of one characteristic from the other. We also present the statistical procedures used to determine whether a relationship between two characteristics is significant. Some typical applications in the health field are used to illustrate the concepts of correlation and regression. These methods were reported as being used in 6–7% of articles in surgery journals (Reznick et al, 1987) and 20% of articles in the *New England Journal of Medicine* (Emerson and Colditz, 1983), although their use subsequently increased to 35% (Altman, 1991b) and is probably higher by the time you read this chapter. Two probability distributions introduced previously—namely, the *t* distribution and the chi-square distribution—can be used for statistical tests in correlation and regression. As a result, much of the material in this chapter will be familiar to you.

In Presenting Problem 1, investigators wanted to know the relationship between mental ability in elderly women over a 2-year period. In Presenting Problem 2, practicing physicians were interested in whether the finger devices currently on the market provide accurate estimates of blood pressure, and in Presenting Problem 3, the focus was on the relationship between satisfaction with life and the fear of developing Alzheimer's disease. Gonzalo and colleagues (1996) in Presenting Problem 4, in addition to analyzing their data on insulin activity using analysis of variance (illustrated in Chapter 7), were interested in the relationship between body mass index (BMI) and insulin sensitivity. When the goal is merely to establish a relationship (or association) between two measures, as in these studies, the correlation coefficient (Pearson product moment correlation coefficient, introduced in Chapter 3) is the statistic most often used. Recall that the correlation coefficient is a measure of the linear relationship between two variables measured on a numerical scale.

In addition to establishing a relationship, investigators often want to predict an outcome. For instance, it would make sense to use the finger device blood pressure reading to predict a person's blood pressure as measured by the traditional cuff method (Presenting Problem 2). Similarly, researchers in Presenting Problem 4 wanted to predict a woman's insulin sensitivity, given her BMI. In each of these situations, one of the variables, such as finger device blood pressure or BMI, is considered to be the **independent,** or **explanatory, variable,** and cuff blood pressure or in-

sulin sensitivity is the **dependent, response,** or **outcome variable.**

Generally, the explanatory characteristic is the one that occurs first or is easier or less costly to measure. The statistical method of **linear regression** is used; this technique involves determining an equation for predicting the value of the outcome variable from values of the explanatory variable. One of the major differences between correlation and regression therefore is the purpose of the analysis—whether it is merely to describe a relationship or to predict a value. Several important similarities also occur, however. As we will see in this chapter, if the means and the standard deviations of both characteristics are known, we can calculate the correlation coefficient from the regression equation and vice versa. In addition, if the correlation coefficient is statistically significant, the regression equation will also be statistically significant. Many of the same assumptions are required for correlation and regression, and both measure the extent of a linear relationship between the two characteristics.

8.2 CORRELATION

Figure 8–1 illustrates several hypothetical **scatterplots** of data to demonstrate the relationship between the size of the correlation coefficient *r* and the shape of the scatterplot. When the correlation is near zero, as in Figure 8–1E, the pattern of plotted points is somewhat circular. When the degree of relationship is small, the pattern is more like an oval, as in Figures 8–1D and 8–1B. As the value of the correlation gets closer to either +1 or −1, as in Figure 8–1C, the plot has a long, narrow shape; at +1 and −1, the observations fall directly on a line, as for $r = +1.0$ in Figure 8–1A.

The scatterplot in Figure 8–1F illustrates a situation in which a strong but nonlinear relationship exists. For example, with temperatures less than 10–15°C, a cold nerve fiber discharges few impulses; as the temperature increases, so do numbers of impulses per second until the temperature reaches about 25°C. As the temperature increases beyond 25°C, the numbers of impulses per second decrease once again, until they cease at 40–45°C. The correlation coefficient, however, measures only a linear relationship, and it has a value close to zero in this situation.

One of the reasons for producing scatterplots of data as part of the initial analysis is to identify nonlinear relationships when they occur. Otherwise, if researchers calculate the correlation coefficient without examining the data, they can miss a strong, but nonlinear, relationship, such as the one between temperature and number of cold nerve fiber impulses.

8.2.1 Calculating the Correlation Coefficient

We use the study by Hébert and colleagues (1997) to extend our knowledge about correlation; for spe-

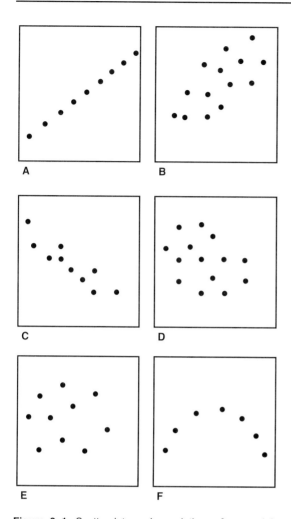

Figure 8–1. Scatterplots and correlations. **A:** $r = +1.0$; **B:** $r = 0.7$; **C:** $r = -0.9$; **D:** $r = -0.4$; **E:** $r = 0.0$; **F:** $r = 0.0$.

cific details on calculating the **correlation coefficient,** refer to Chapter 3, Section 3.7. Also, refer to Chapter 3, Table 3–19 for observations on the mental ability scores of 51 women who were 85 years or older at the beginning of the study.

Recall that the formula for the Pearson product moment correlation coefficient, symbolized by r, is

$$r = \frac{\Sigma(X - \overline{X})(Y - \overline{Y})}{\sqrt{\Sigma(X - \overline{X})^2 \Sigma(Y - \overline{Y})^2}}$$

where X stands for the independent variable and Y for the outcome variable.

As we discussed earlier, a valuable first step in looking at the relationship between two numerical characteristics is to examine the relationship graphically. Figure 8–2 is a scatterplot of the data, with

mental ability score at time 1 on the X-axis and mental ability score at time 3 on the Y-axis. We see from Figure 8–2 that a positive relationship exists between these two characteristics: Small values for mental ability at time 1 are associated with small values for mental ability at time 3. The same relationship exists for large values at the two times. The question of interest is whether the observed relationship is statistically significant. (A large number of duplicate or overlapping data points occur, especially for women who scored 0 at both times. We used the option in SYSTAT to add a small amount of randomness in the placement of the data points, called slight random jitter by SYSTAT, with the result that the points do not overlap completely.)

The extent of the relationship can be found by calculating the correlation coefficient. Using the data from Table 3–19 in Chapter 3, the correlation between mental ability at times 1 and 3 is

$$r = \frac{\Sigma(X - \overline{X})(Y - \overline{Y})}{\sqrt{\Sigma(X - \overline{X})^2 \Sigma(Y - \overline{Y})^2}}$$

$$= \frac{179.0588}{\sqrt{(220.3529)(428.5098)}}$$

$$= 0.5827$$

The correlation is 0.58, indicating a moderate to good relationship between scores on mental

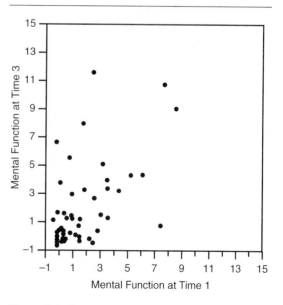

Figure 8–2. Scatterplot of mental ability scores. (Data, used with permission, from Hébert R, Brayne C, Spiegelhalter D: Incidence of functional decline and improvement in a community-dwelling very elderly population. *Am J Epidemiol* 1997;**145:**935–944. Plot produced with SYSTAT; used by permission.)

ability. Use the CD-ROM to confirm our calculations. Also, see Chapter 3, Section 3.7, for a review of the properties of the correlation coefficient.

8.2.2 Interpreting the Size of *r*

The size of the correlation required for statistical significance is, of course, related to the sample size. With a very large sample of subjects, such as 2000, even small correlations, such as 0.06, are significant. A better way to interpret the size of the correlation is to consider what it tells us about the strength of the relationship.

8.2.2.a The Coefficient of Determination: The correlation coefficient can be squared to form the statistic called the **coefficient of determination.** For the elderly women, the coefficient of determination is $(0.58)^2$, or 0.34. This result means that 34% of the variation in the values for one of the measures, such as mental ability at time 3, may be accounted for by knowing the mental ability of the women at time 1. This concept is demonstrated by the Venn diagrams in Figure 8–3. For the left diagram, $r^2 = 0.25$; so 25% of the variation in A is accounted for by knowing B (or vice versa). The middle diagram illustrates $r^2 = 0.50$, and the diagram on the right represents $r^2 = 0.34$ for our example.

The coefficient of determination tells us how strong the relationship really is. In the health literature, however, confidence limits or results of a statistical test for significance of the correlation coefficient are also commonly presented.

8.2.2.b The *t* Test for Correlation: The symbol for the correlation coefficient in the population (the population parameter) is ρ (lower case Greek letter rho). In a random sample, ρ is estimated by r. If several random samples of the same size are selected from a given population and the correlation coefficient r is calculated for each, we expect the r's to vary from one another but to follow some sort of distribution about the population value ρ, and, in fact, they do. Unfortunately, the sampling distribution of the correlation does not behave as nicely as the sampling distribution of the mean, which is normally distributed for large samples.

Part of the problem is what we might describe as a ceiling effect when the correlation approaches either –1 or +1. If the value of the population parameter is, say, 0.8, the sample values can exceed 0.8 only up to 1.0, but they can be less than 0.8 all the way to –1.0. The maximum value of 1.0 acts as a ceiling in keeping the sample values from varying considerably above 0.8 and results in a **skewed distribution.** When the population parameter is zero, however, the ceiling effects are equal, and the sample values are approximately distributed according to the *t* distribution.

The *t* distribution can therefore be used to test the hypothesis that the true value of the population parameter ρ is equal to zero. The following mathematical expression involving the correlation coefficient, often called the *t* ratio, has been found to have a *t* **distribution** with $n - 2$ degrees of freedom:

$$t = \frac{r\sqrt{n - 2}}{\sqrt{1 - r^2}}$$

Let us use this *t* ratio to test whether the observed value of $r = 0.58$ is sufficient evidence with 51 observations to conclude that the true population value of the correlation ρ is different from zero.

Step 1: H_0: No relationship exists between mental ability at time 1 and time 3 in elderly women; that is, the true correlation is zero: $\rho = 0$.

H_1: A relationship does exist between mental ability at time 1 and time 3 in elderly women; that is, the true correlation is not zero: $\rho \neq 0$.

Step 2: Because the null hypothesis is a test of whether ρ is zero, the *t* ratio may be used when the assumptions for correlation (discussed later on) are met.

Step 3: Suppose the investigators chose $\alpha = 0.01$ for this example.

Step 4: The degrees of freedom are $n - 2 = 51 - 2 = 49$. The value of a *t* distribution with 49 degrees of freedom that divides the area into the central 99% and the upper and lower 1% is approximately 2.68 (found by interpolation in Table A–3). We therefore reject the null hypothesis of zero correlation if (the absolute value of) the observed value of *t* is greater than 2.68.

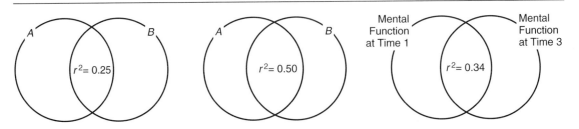

Figure 8–3. Illustration of r^2, proportion of explained variance.

Step 5: The calculation is

$$t = \frac{0.58 \sqrt{49}}{\sqrt{1 - 0.58^2}}$$
$$= 4.98$$

Step 6: The observed value of the t ratio with 49 degrees of freedom is 4.98, which is greater than 2.68. The null hypothesis of zero correlation is therefore rejected; that is, the relationship between mental ability at the beginning of the study as measured by the SMAF and mental ability 2 years later is large enough to conclude that these two variables are associated in the population of elderly women.

8.2.2.c Fisher's z Transformation to Test the Correlation: Investigators frequently use a significance test to determine whether $\rho = 0$, and this test is typically done by computer programs. Often, however, interest actually lies in whether the correlation is equal to another value. For example, consider a diagnostic test that gives accurate numerical values but is invasive and somewhat risky for the patient. Suppose that researchers develop an alternative testing procedure, and they want to demonstrate that the new procedure is as accurate as the test in current use. To do so, they must select a sample of patients and perform both the current test and the new procedure on each patient. An appropriate statistic for demonstrating the relationship between the current test and the new procedure is the correlation coefficient, so the next step is to calculate this statistic. Finally, the researchers want to show that the correlation measures more than a chance relationship.

Is it reasonable in this illustration to determine whether the observed correlation was significantly greater than zero, or is it more appropriate to establish that the correlation exceeded some minimum value acceptable to physicians who use the diagnostic test? If the latter approach is preferable, either a test of hypothesis can be performed to show that the correlation is greater than some value, such as 0.90, or a confidence interval about the observed correlation can be calculated. In either case, we can use a procedure called **Fisher's z transformation,** which allows us to test any null hypothesis—not just $\rho = 0$ as with the t test—and also to form confidence intervals.

To test the statistical significance of the correlation coefficient when the population parameter is not equal to zero, we must transform the correlation and then use the standard normal (z) distribution. We need a transformation because, as we mentioned earlier, the distribution of sample values of the correlation is skewed when $\rho \neq 0$. Although this method is a bit complicated, it is actually more flexible than the t test. Fisher's z transformation was proposed by the same statistician (Ronald Fisher) who developed Fisher's exact test for 2×2 contingency tables (discussed in Chapter 6).

Fisher's z transformation is

$$z(r) = \frac{1}{2} \ln \left(\frac{1 + r}{1 - r} \right)$$

where ln represents the natural logarithm. Table A–6 gives the z transformation for different values of r, so we do not actually need to use the formula. With moderate-sized samples, this transformation follows a normal distribution, and the following expression for the z test can be used:

$$z = \frac{z(r) - z(\rho)}{\sqrt{1/(n - 3)}}$$

To illustrate Fisher's z transformation for testing the significance of ρ, we evaluate the relationship between mental ability scores from Presenting Problem 1. For women 85 years or older, the correlation between these two measures was 0.58. The investigators may have expected a moderate-sized correlation between these two measures; let us suppose they want to know whether the correlation in the women 85 or older is significantly larger than 0.50. A one-tailed test of the null hypothesis that $\rho \leq 0.50$, which they hope to reject, may be carried out as follows.

Step 1: H_0: The relationship between mental ability at time 1 and time 3 in elderly women is ≤ 0.50; that is, the true correlation $\rho \leq 0.50$.

H_1: The relationship between mental ability at time 1 and time 3 in elderly women is >0.50; that is, the true correlation $\rho > 0.50$.

Step 2: Fisher's z transformation may be used with the correlation coefficient to test any hypothesis.

Step 3: Let us again use $\alpha = 0.01$ for this example.

Step 4: The alternative hypothesis specifies a one-tailed test. The value of the z distribution that divides the area into the lower 99% and the upper 1% is approximately 2.326 (from Table A–2). We therefore reject the null hypothesis that the correlation is ≤ 0.50 if the observed value of z is >2.326.

Step 5: The first step is to find the transformed values for $r = 0.58$ and $\rho = 0.50$ from Table A–6; these values are 0.663 and 0.549, respectively. Then, the calculation for the z test is

$$z = \frac{z(0.58) - z(0.50)}{\sqrt{1/(51 - 3)}}$$
$$= \frac{0.663 - 0.549}{\sqrt{1/48}}$$
$$= 0.79$$

Step 6: The observed value of the z statistic, 0.79, is less than 2.326. The null hypothesis that the correlation is 0.50 or less is therefore retained. The conclusion is that the correlation between mental ability scores at time 1 and 2 years later is significantly different from zero, as we saw in the previous section, but the evidence is insufficient to conclude it is greater than 0.50.

8.2.2.d Confidence Interval for the Correlation: A major advantage of Fisher's z transformation is that **confidence intervals** can be formed. The transformed value of the correlation is used to calculate confidence intervals in a manner similar to the calculations presented in previous chapters; however, after the limits are determined, they must be transformed back to values corresponding to the correlation coefficient.

To illustrate, we calculate a 95% confidence interval, using the z distribution in Table A–2 to find the critical value, for the correlation coefficient 0.58 in Presenting Problem 1. The confidence interval is

z Transform of $r \pm$ Confidence coefficient $\times$ Standard error

$$z \text{ Transform of } r \pm 1.96 \times \sqrt{1/(n-3)}$$
$$= 0.663 \pm (1.96)(0.144)$$
$$= 0.663 \pm 0.283$$
$$= 0.380 \text{ to } 0.946$$

Transforming the values 0.380 and 0.946 back to correlations by using Table A–6 gives, approximately, $r = 0.36$ and $r = 0.74$. The 95% confidence interval for the observed correlation of 0.58 is therefore 0.36 to 0.74; that is, we are 95% confident that the true value of the correlation in the population is contained within this interval. Note that the confidence interval is not symmetric about the sample value of 0.58, because the distribution of the correlation coefficient is skewed (not symmetric). Also note that 0.50 is in this interval, so we know the observed correlation of 0.58 is not different from 0.50 at $P = 0.05$ (or at $P = 0.01$ as shown in the preceding hypothesis test).

8.2.3 Assumptions in Correlation

The assumptions needed to draw valid conclusions about the correlation coefficient are that the sample was randomly selected and the two variables, X and Y, vary together in a joint distribution that is normally distributed, called the bivariate normal distribution. Just because each variable is normally distributed when examined separately, however, does not guarantee that, jointly, they have a bivariate normal distribution. Some guidance is available: If either of the two variables is *not* normally distributed, Pearson's product moment correlation coefficient is *not* the most appropriate method. Instead, either one or both of the variables may be transformed so that they more closely follow a normal distribution, as discussed in Chapter 5, or the Spearman rank correlation may be calculated. This topic is discussed in Section 8.4.

8.3 COMPARING TWO CORRELATION COEFFICIENTS

On occasion, investigators want to know if a difference exists between two correlation coefficients. Here are two specific instances: (1) comparing the correlations between the same two variables that have been measured in two independent groups of subjects and (2) comparing two correlations that involve a variable in common in the same group of individuals. These situations are not extremely common; on the other hand, statistical programs do not generally include the procedures. We designed Microsoft Excel programs; see the folder "Calculations" on the CD-ROM.

8.3.1 Comparing Correlations in Two Independent Groups

Fisher's z transformation can be used to test hypotheses or form confidence intervals about the difference between the correlations between the same two variables in two independent groups. The results of such tests are also called **independent correlations.** For example, Gonzalo and colleagues (1996) in Presenting Problem 4 wanted to compare the correlation between BMI and insulin sensitivity in the 14 women with hyperthyroid levels ($r = -0.775$) with the correlation between BMI and insulin sensitivity in the 19 control women ($r = -0.456$). See Figure 8–4.

In this situation, the value for the second group replaces $z(\rho)$ in the numerator for the z test shown in the previous section, and $1/(n-3)$ is found for each

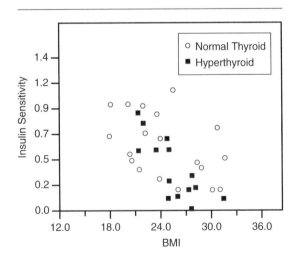

Figure 8–4. Scatterplot of BMI and insulin sensitivity. (Data, used with permission, from Gonzalo MA et al: Glucose tolerance, insulin secretion, insulin sensitivity and glucose effectiveness in normal and overweight hyperthyroid women. *Clin Endocrinol* 1996;**45:**689–697. Output produced using NCSS; used with permission.)

group and added before taking the square root in the denominator. The test statistic is

$$z = \frac{(z_{r_1} - z_{r_2})}{\sqrt{[1/(n_1 - 3)] + [1/(n_2 - 3)]}}$$

To illustrate, the values of z from Fisher's z transformation tables (A–6) for –0.775 and –0.456 are approximately 1.033 and 0.492 (with interpolation), respectively. Note that Fisher's z transformation is the same, regardless of whether the correlation is positive or negative. Using these values, we obtain

$$z = \frac{(1.033 - 0.492)}{\sqrt{[1/(14 - 3)] + [1/(19 - 3)]}}$$
$$= \frac{0.541}{\sqrt{0.091 + 0.063}}$$
$$= 1.38$$

Assuming we chose the traditional level of 0.05 for α, of the value of the test statistic, 1.38, is less than the critical value, 1.96, so we do not reject the null hypothesis of equal correlations. We decide that the evidence is insufficient to conclude that the relationship between BMI and insulin sensitivity is different for hyperthyroid women from that for controls. What is a possible explanation for the lack of statistical significance? It is possible that there is no difference in the relationships between these two variables in the population. When sample sizes are small, however, as they are in this study, it is always advisable to keep in mind that the study may have low power.

8.3.2 Comparing Correlations with Variables in Common in the Same Group

The second situation occurs when the research question involves correlations that contain the same variable (also called dependent correlations). For example, a very natural question for Nesselroad and colleagues (1996) was whether one of the finger devices was more highly correlated with the blood pressure cuff—considered to be the gold standard—than the other two. If so, this would be a product they might wish to recommend for patients to use at home. To illustrate, we compare the diastolic reading with device 1 and the cuff ($r_{XY} = 0.32$) to the diastolic reading with device 2 and the cuff ($r_{XZ} = 0.45$).

There are several formulas for testing the difference between two dependent correlations. We present the simplest one, developed by Hotelling (1940) and described by Glass and Stanley on pages 310–311 (1970). We will show the calculations for this example but, as always, suggest that you use a computer program. The formula follows the t distribution with $n - 3$ degrees of freedom; it looks rather forbidding and requires the calculation of several correlations:

$$t = (r_{XY} - r_{XZ})\sqrt{\frac{(n - 3)(1 + r_{YZ})}{2(1 - r_{XY}^2 - r_{XZ}^2 - r_{YZ}^2 + 2r_{XY}r_{XZ}r_{YZ})}}$$

We designate the cuff reading as X, device 1 as Y, and device 2 as Z. We therefore want to compare r_{XY} with r_{XZ}. Both correlations involve the X, or cuff, reading, so these correlations are dependent. To use the formula, we also need to calculate the correlation between device 1 and device 2, which is $r_{YZ} = 0.54$. Table 8–1 shows the correlations needed for this formula.

The calculations are

$$t = (0.32 - 0.45)\sqrt{\frac{(100 - 3)(1 + 0.54)}{2\left[\begin{array}{c}1 - (0.32)^2 - (0.45)^2 - (0.54)^2 \\ + 2(0.32)(0.45)(0.54)\end{array}\right]}}$$
$$= -0.13\sqrt{\frac{149.38}{2(0.40 + 0.56)}}$$
$$= -1.50$$

You know by now that the difference between these two correlations is not statistically significant because the observed value of t is –1.50, and |–1.50| = 1.50 is less than the critical value of t with 97 degrees of freedom, 1.99. This conclusion corresponds to that by Nesselroad and his colleagues in which they recommended that patients be cautioned that the finger blood pressure devices may not perform as marketed.

We designed a Microsoft Excel program for these calculations as well. It is included on the CD-ROM in a folder called "Calculations" and is entitled "z for 2 dept r's."

Table 8–1. Correlation matrix of diastolic blood pressures in all 100 subjects.

Pearson Correlations Section

	Cuff Diastolic	Device 1 Diastolic	Device 2 Diastolic	Device 3 Diastolic
Cuff	1.0000	**0.3209**	**0.4450**	0.3592
Diastolic	0.0000	0.0011	0.0000	0.0002
	100.0000	100.0000	100.0000	100.0000
Device 1	0.3210	1.0000	**0.5364**	0.5392
Diastolic	0.0011	0.0000	0.0000	0.0000
	100.0000	100.0000	100.0000	100.0000
Device 2	0.4450	0.5364	1.0000	0.5629
Diastolic	0.0000	0.0000	0.0000	0.0000
	100.0000	100.0000	100.0000	100.0000
Device 3	0.3592	0.5392	0.5629	1.0000
Diastolic	0.0002	0.0000	0.0000	0.0000
	100.0000	100.0000	100.0000	100.0000

Bolded values are needed for comparing two dependent correlations.
Source: Data, used with permission, from Nesselroad et al: Accuracy of automated finger blood pressure devices. *Fam Med* 1996;**28**:189–192. Output produced using NCSS; used with permission.

8.4 OTHER MEASURES OF CORRELATION

Several other measures of correlation are often found in the medical literature. Spearman's rho, the rank correlation introduced in Chapter 3, is used with ordinal data or in situations in which the numerical variables are not normally distributed. When a research question involves one numerical and one nominal variable, a correlation called the point–biserial correlation is used. With nominal data, the risk ratio, or kappa (κ), discussed in Chapter 5, can be used.

8.4.1 Spearman's Rho

Recall that the value of the correlation coefficient is markedly influenced by extreme values and thus does not provide a good description of the relationship between two variables when their distributions are skewed or contain outlying values. For example, consider the relationships among the various finger devices and the standard cuff device for measuring blood pressure from Presenting Problem 2. To illustrate, we use the first 25 subjects from this study, listed in Table 8–2 (see the file entitled "Nesselroad25").

It is difficult to tell if the observations are normally distributed without looking at graphs of the data. Some

statistical programs have routines to plot values against a normal distribution to help researchers decide whether a nonparametric procedure should be used. A normal probability plot for the cuff diastolic measurement is given in Figure 8–5. Use the CD-ROM to produce similar plots for the finger device measurements.

When the observations are plotted on a graph, as in Figure 8–5, it appears that the data are not unduly skewed. This conclusion is consistent with the tests given for the normality of a distribution by NCSS. Note the normal probability plot: If observations fall within the curved lines, the data can be assumed to be normally distributed.

As we indicated in Chapter 3, a simple method for dealing with the problem of extreme observations in correlation is to rank order the data and then recalculate the correlation on ranks to obtain the nonparametric correlation called **Spearman's rho,** or **rank correlation.** To illustrate this procedure, we continue to use data on the first 25 subjects in the study on blood pressure devices (Presenting Problem 2), even though the distribution of the values does not require this procedure. Let us focus on the correlation between the cuff and device 2, which we learned was 0.45 in Section 8.3.3.

Table 8–3 illustrates the ranks of the diastolic readings on the first 25 subjects. Note that each variable is ranked separately; when ties occur, the average of the ranks of the tied values is used.

The ranks of the variables are used in the equation for the correlation coefficient, and the resulting cal-

Table 8–2. Data on diastolic blood pressure for the first 25 subjects.

Subject	Cuff Diastolic	Device 1 Diastolic	Device 2 Diastolic	Device 3 Diastolic
1	80	58	51	38
2	65	79	61	47
3	70	66	61	50
4	80	93	75	53
5	60	75	76	54
6	82	71	75	56
7	70	58	60	58
8	70	73	74	58
9	60	72	67	59
10	70	88	70	60
11	48	70	88	60
12	100	114	82	62
13	70	74	56	64
14	70	75	79	67
15	70	89	62	69
16	60	95	75	70
17	80	87	89	72
18	80	57	74	73
19	90	69	90	73
20	80	60	85	75
21	70	72	75	77
22	85	85	61	79
23	100	102	99	89
24	70	113	83	94
25	90	127	108	99

Source: Data, used with permission, from Nesselroad et al: Accuracy of automated finger blood pressure devices. *Fam Med* 1996;**28**:189–192. Output produced using NCSS; used with permission.

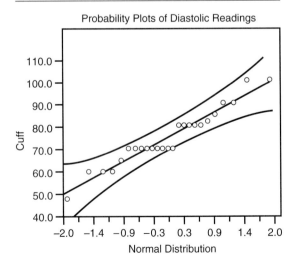

Figure 8–5. Diastolic blood pressure using cuff readings in 25 subjects. (Data, used with permission, from Nesselroad et al: Accuracy of automated finger blood pressure devices. *Fam Med* 1996;**28**:189–192. Output produced using NCSS; used with permission.)

Table 8–3. Rank order of the diastolic blood pressure for the first 25 subjects.

Row	Cuff Diastolic	Device 1 Diastolic	Device 2 Diastolic	Device 3 Diastolic
1	17.0	2.5	1.0	1.0
2	5.0	15.0	5.0	2.0
3	10.0	5.0	5.0	3.0
4	17.0	20.0	13.5	4.0
5	3.0	13.5	16.0	5.0
6	20.0	8.0	13.5	6.0
7	10.0	2.5	3.0	7.5
8	10.0	11.0	10.5	7.5
9	3.0	9.5	8.0	9.0
10	10.0	18.0	9.0	10.5
11	1.0	7.0	21.0	10.5
12	24.5	24.0	18.0	12.0
13	10.0	12.0	2.0	13.0
14	10.0	13.5	17.0	14.0
15	10.0	19.0	7.0	15.0
16	3.0	21.0	13.5	16.0
17	17.0	17.0	22.0	17.0
18	17.0	1.0	10.5	18.5
19	22.5	6.0	23.0	18.5
20	17.0	4.0	20.0	20.0
21	10.0	9.5	13.5	21.0
22	21.0	16.0	5.0	22.0
23	24.5	22.0	24.0	23.0
24	10.0	23.0	19.0	24.0
25	22.5	25.0	25.0	25.0

Source: Data, used with permission, from Nesselroad et al: Accuracy of automated finger blood pressure devices. *Fam Med* 1996;**28**:189–192. Output produced using NCSS; used with permission.

culation gives Spearman's rank correlation (r_S), also called Spearman's rho; that is,

$$r_S = \frac{\Sigma(R_X - \bar{R}_X)(R_Y - \bar{R}_Y)}{\sqrt{\Sigma(R_X - \bar{R}_X)^2}\ \sqrt{\Sigma(R_Y - \bar{R}_Y)^2}}$$

where R_X is the rank of the X variable, R_Y is the rank of the Y variable, and R_X and R_Y are the mean ranks for the X and Y variables, respectively. The rank correlation r_S may also be calculated by using other formulas, but this approximate procedure is quite good (Conover and Iman, 1981).

Calculating r_S for the ranked observations in Table 8–3 gives

$$r_S = \frac{416.5}{\sqrt{1227}\ \sqrt{1292.5}}$$
$$= 0.33$$

The value of r_S is smaller than the value of Pearson's correlation; this may occur when the bivariate distribution of the two variables is not normal. The t test, as illustrated for the Pearson correlation, can be used to determine whether the Spearman rank correlation is significantly different from zero. For example, the following procedure tests whether the value of Spear-

man's rho in the population, symbolized ρ_S (Greek letter rho with subscript S denoting Spearman) differs from zero.

Step 1: H_0:   The population value of Spearman's rho is zero; that is, $\rho_S = 0$.

     H_1:   The population value of Spearman's rho is not zero; that is, $\rho_S \neq 0$.

Step 2: Because the null hypothesis is a test of whether ρ_S is zero, the t ratio may be used.

Step 3: Let us use $\alpha = 0.05$ for this example.

Step 4: The degrees of freedom are $n - 2 = 25 - 2 = 23$. The value of the t distribution with 23 degrees of freedom that divides the area into the central 95% and the upper and lower 2½% is 2.069 (Table A–3). We therefore reject the null hypothesis of no correlation if (the absolute value of) the observed value of t is greater than 2.069.

Step 5: The calculation is

$$t = \frac{r\sqrt{n-2}}{\sqrt{1-r^2}}$$
$$= \frac{0.33\sqrt{23}}{\sqrt{1-0.33^2}}$$
$$= 1.677$$

Step 6: The observed value of the t ratio with 23 degrees of freedom is 1.677, less than 2.069. We therefore do not reject the null hypothesis. We conclude that a significant nonparametric correlation does not exist between the diastolic blood pressure measurements made by using the cuff and using the finger device 2.

Of course, if investigators want to test only whether Spearman's rho is greater than zero—that there is a significantly positive relationship—they can use a one-tailed test. For a one-tailed test with $\alpha = 0.05$ and 23 degrees of freedom, the critical value is 1.714, and the conclusion is the same.

It is easy to demonstrate that performing the above-mentioned test on the ranked data gives approximately the same results as the Spearman rho calculated the traditional way. We just used the Pearson formula on ranks and found that Spearman's rho for the sample of 25 subjects was 0.33 between the cuff measurement of diastolic pressure and finger device 2. Use the CD-ROM, and calculate Spearman's rho on the original data. You should also find that rho is 0.33 using the traditional methods of calculation.

To summarize, Spearman's rho is appropriate when investigators want to measure the relationship between: (1) two ordinal variables, or (2) two numerical variables when one or both are not normally distributed and investigators choose not to use a data transformation (such as taking the logarithm). Spearman's rank correlation is especially appropriate when outlying values occur among the observations.

8.4.2 Confidence Interval for the Odds Ratio & the Relative Risk

Chapter 3 introduced the **relative risk** (or risk ratio) and the **odds ratio** as measures of relationship between two nominal characteristics. Developed by epidemiologists, these statistics are used for studies examining risks that may result in disease. To discuss the odds ratio, recall the study discussed in Chapter 3 by Ballard and colleagues (1998) that examined the use of antenatal thyrotropin-releasing hormone (TRH). Data from this study were given in Chapter 3, Table 3–22. We calculated the odds ratio as 1.1 and said it means that an infant in the TRH group is 1.1 times more likely to develop respiratory distress syndrome than an infant in the placebo group. This finding is the opposite of what the investigators expected to find, and it is important to learn if the increased risk is statistically significant.

Significance can be determined in several ways. For instance, to test the significance of the relationship between treatment (TRH versus placebo) and the development of respiratory distress syndrome, investigators may use the chi-square test discussed in Chapter 6. In this situation, the degrees of freedom are equal to 1. The chi-square test for this example is left as an exercise (see Exercise 2). An alternative chi-square test, based on the natural logarithm of the odds ratio, is also available, and it results in values close to the chi-square test illustrated in Chapter 6 (Fleiss, 1999).

More often, articles in the medical literature use confidence intervals for risk ratios or odds ratios. Ballard and colleagues reported a 95% confidence interval for the odds ratio as (0.8 to 1.5). Let us see how they found this confidence interval.

The procedure for obtaining confidence intervals is a bit more complicated than usual because these ratios are not normally distributed, so calculating confidence intervals requires finding natural logarithms and antilogarithms. Many inexpensive calculators have these functions, however, so we briefly illustrate the procedure, first for the odds ratio and then for the relative risk. The formula for a 95% confidence interval for the odds ratio is

$$\exp\left[\ln(OR) \pm 1.96\sqrt{\frac{1}{a} + \frac{1}{b} + \frac{1}{c} + \frac{1}{d}}\right]$$

where exp denotes the exponential function, or antilogarithm, of the natural logarithm, ln, and a, b, c, d are the cells in a 2×2 table (see Table 6–11 in Chapter 6). The confidence interval for the odds ratio for risk of respiratory distress syndrome in infants who were given TRH from Table 3–22 is

$$\exp\left[\ln(1.074) \pm 1.96\right.$$
$$\left.\sqrt{\frac{1}{260} + \frac{1}{(392-260)} + \frac{1}{244} + \frac{1}{(377-244)}}\right]$$
$$= \exp(0.071 \pm 1.96\sqrt{0.023})$$
$$= \exp(-0.226, 0.368)$$
$$= 0.798 \text{ to } 1.445$$

This interval contains the value of the true odds ratio with 95% confidence. If the odds are the same in each group, the value of the odds ratio is approximately 1, indicating similar risks in each group. Because the interval contains 1, we may be 95% confident that the odds ratio risk may in fact be 1; that is, insufficient evidence exists to conclude that the risk of respiratory distress increases in infants who received TRH. By the same logic, this treatment has no protective effect. Of course, 90% or 99% confidence intervals can be formed by using 1.645 or 2.575 instead of 1.96 in the preceding equation.

To illustrate the confidence interval for the relative risk, we refer to the physicians' health study (Steering Committee of the Physicians' Health Study Research Group, 1989) summarized in Chapter 3 and Table 3–11. Recall that the relative risk for an MI in physicians taking aspirin was 0.581. The 95% confidence interval for the true value of the relative risk also involves logarithms:

$$\exp\left[\ln(RR)\right.$$
$$\left.\pm 1.96\sqrt{\frac{1-[a/(a+b)]}{a} + \frac{1-[c/(c+d)]}{c}}\right]$$

Again, the values for a, b, c, d are the cells in the 2×2 table illustrated in Table 6–11. Substituting values from Table 3–11, the 95% confidence interval for a relative risk of 0.581 is

$$\exp\left[\ln(0.581)\right.$$
$$\left.\pm 1.96\sqrt{\frac{1-(139/11,037)}{139} + \frac{1-(239/11,034)}{239}}\right]$$
$$= \exp[-0.543 \pm 1.96\sqrt{0.011}]$$
$$= \exp[-0.543 \pm 0.207]$$
$$= \exp[-0.750, -0.336]$$
$$= 0.472 \text{ to } 0.715$$

The 95% confidence interval does not contain 1, so the evidence indicates that the use of aspirin resulted in a reduced risk for MI. For a detailed and insightful discussion of the odds ratio and its advantages and disadvantages, see Feinstein (1985, Chapter 20) and Fleiss (1999, Chapter 5); for a discussion of both the odds ratio and the risk ratio, see Greenberg and coworkers (1996, Chapters 8 and 9).

The folder containing Microsoft Excel equations on the CD-ROM describes two routines for finding the 95% confidence limits for the OR and RR; they are called "CI for OR" and "CI for RR." You may find these routines helpful if you wish to find 95% confidence limits for odds ratios or relative risks for published studies that contain the summary data for these statistics.

8.4.3 Measuring Relationships in Other Situations

We have discussed how to measure and test the significance of relationships by using Pearson's product moment correlation coefficient, Spearman's nonparametric procedure based on ranks, and risk or odds ratios. Not all situations are covered by these procedures, however, such as when one variable is measured on a nominal scale and the other is numerical but has been classified into categories, when one variable is nominal and the other is ordinal, or when both are ordinal but only a few categories occur. In these cases, a contingency table is formed and the chi-square test is used, as illustrated in Chapter 6.

On other occasions, the numerical variable is not collapsed into categories. For example, Hodgson and Cutler (1997) studied 25 subjects who had a living parent with Alzheimer's disease and a matched group who had no family history of dementia. Subjects answered questions about their concern of developing Alzheimer's disease and the function of their memory. They also completed a questionnaire designed to evaluate their concerns about memory, the Memory Assessment Index (MAI). Data are given in Table 8–4.

These investigators were interested in the relationship between life satisfaction and performance on the MAI. Life satisfaction was measured as yes or no, and the MAI was measured on a scale from 0 = no memory problems to 12 = negative perceptions of memory and concern about developing dementia. When one variable is binary and the other is numerical, it is possible to evaluate the relationship using a special correlation, called the point–biserial correlation. If the binary variable is coded as 0 and 1, the Pearson correlation procedure can be used to find the point–biserial correlation. Box 8–1A gives the results of the correlation procedure using life satisfaction and MAI. The correlation is –0.37, and the *P* value is 0.008633.

Did you wonder why a *t* test was not used to see if a difference existed in mean MAI for those who were satisfied with their life versus those who were not satisfied? If so, you are right on target because a *t* test is another way to look at the research question. It simply depends on whether interest focuses on a relationship or a difference. What do you think the results of a *t* test would show? The output from the NCSS *t* test procedure is given in Box 8–1B. Of special interest is the *P* value (0.008633); it is the same as for the corre-

Table 8–4. Data on 50 subjects in the study on anticipatory dementia.

Sample[a]	Sex	Concerned[a]	MAI[b]	Life Satisf[a]	Health Status[a]
1	F	1	6	0	1
2	F	1	8	1	1
1	F	0	0	1	1
1	F	0	2	0	1
1	F	1	4	0	1
1	F	1	10	0	0
1	M	0	3	1	1
1	F	1	12	0	0
1	F	1	8	0	1
1	F	1	9	1	1
1	F	1	8	0	1
1	F	0	2	1	1
1	F	1	6	1	1
1	M	0	2	1	1
1	M	0	2	1	0
1	M	1	5	1	1
1	M	0	3	0	0
2	F	0	3	0	1
2	F	0	0	1	1
1	M	1	5	0	1
2	F	0	1	1	0
2	F	0	2	0	1
1	F	1	7	0	1
1	M	1	5	0	1
1	F	1	7	0	0
1	F	1	9	0	1
2	F	1	10	0	0
2	F	0	3	1	1
2	F	1	5	0	1
2	F	0	3	1	1
2	F	1	9	0	0
1	F	1	4	1	1
1	F	1	8	1	1
2	F	1	4	1	1
2	F	0	2	0	1
2	F	1	9	0	0
2	F	0	3	1	1
2	M	1	8	1	1
2	F	0	3	1	1
2	F	0	4	0	1
2	M	1	7	0	0
2	M	0	2	0	1
2	F	0	0	1	1
2	M	0	2	1	1
1	F	0	5	0	0
2	F	0	2	1	1
1	F	1	8	0	1
2	M	1	6	1	1
2	F	0	2	0	0
2	M	1	4	0	1

[a]Sample: 1=Alzheimer, 2=Control
Concerned: 0=No, 1=Yes
Life satisfaction: 0=Not satisfied, 1=Satisfied
Health status: 0=Excellent, 1=Not excellent
[b]MAI (Memory Assessment Index) on scale of 0=No memory problems to 12=Negative perceptions of memory and very concerned about developing dementia
Source: Data, used with permission, from Hodgson LG, Cutler SJ: Anticipatory dementia and well-being. *Am J Alzheimer's Dis* 1997;**12**:62–66. Output produced using NCSS; used with permission.

Box 8–1. Correlation and *t* test for life satisfaction and anticipatory dementia as measured by MAI.

A. Correlation Matrix

	Anticipatory Dementia	Life Satisfaction
Anticipatory Dementia	1.000000	–0.367601
	0.000000	0.008633
	50.000000	50.000000
Life Satisfaction	–0.367601	1.000000
	0.008633	0.000000
	50.000000	50.000000

B. *t* Test

	Count	Mean	Standard Deviation
LIFESAT=0	27	5.851852	2.931312
LIFESAT=1	23	3.652174	2.70704

Alternative Hypothesis	*t* Value	Probability Level	Decision (5%)	Power (α=0.05)
Difference <> 0	2.7386	0.008633	Reject H_0	0.765296

C. Box Plot

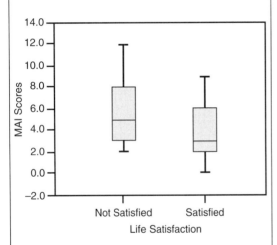

Source: Data, used with permission, From Hodgson LG, Cutler SJ: Anticipatory dementia and well-being. *Am J Alzheimer's Dis* 1997;**12**:62–66. Output produced using NCSS; used with permission.

lation. This illustrates an important principle: The point–biserial correlation between a binary variable and a numerical variable has the same level of significance as does a *t* test in which the groups are defined by the binary variable.

The point–biserial correlation is often used by test developers to help evaluate the questions on the test. For example, the National Board of Medical Examiners determines the point–biserial correlation between whether examinees get an item correct (a binary variable) and the examinee's score on the entire exam (a numerical variable). A positive point–biserial indicates that examinees who get the question correct tend to score high on the exam as a whole, whereas examinees who miss the question tend to score low generally. Similarly, a negative point–biserial correlation indicates that examinees who get the question correct tend to score low on the exam. The latter is clearly not a desirable situation; it is possible that the question is tricky or poorly worded because the better examinees are more likely to miss the question. You can see why this statistic is useful for test developers.

8.5 LINEAR REGRESSION

Remember that when the goal is to predict the value of one characteristic from knowledge of another, the statistical method used is **regression** analysis. This method is also called linear regression, simple linear regression, or least squares regression. Reviewing the history of these terms sheds some light on the nature of regression analysis.

The concepts of correlation and regression were developed by Sir Francis Galton, a cousin of Charles Darwin, who studied both mathematics and medicine in the mid-19th century (Walker, 1931). Galton was interested in heredity and wanted to understand why a population remains more or less the same over many generations with the "average" offspring resembling their parents; that is, why do successive generations not become more diverse. By growing sweet peas and observing the average size of seeds from parent plants of different sizes, he discovered regression, which he termed the "tendency of the ideal mean filial type to depart from the parental type, reverting to what may be roughly and perhaps fairly described as the average ancestral type." This phenomenon is more typically known as regression toward the mean. The term "correlation" was used by Galton in his work on inheritance in terms of the "co-relation" between such characteristics as heights of fathers and sons. The mathematician Karl Pearson went on to work out the theory of correlation and regression, and the correlation coefficient is named after him for this reason.

The term **linear regression** refers to the fact that correlation and regression measure only a straight-line, or linear, relationship between two variables. The term "simple regression" means that only one explanatory (independent) variable is used to predict an outcome. In **multiple regression,** more than one independent variable is included in the prediction equation.

Least squares regression describes the mathematical method for obtaining the statistical estimators in the regression equation. The important thing to remember is that when the term "regression" is used alone, it generally means linear regression based on the least squares method. The concept behind least squares regression is described in the next section. The application of regression is discussed in Section 8.5.2.

8.5.1 Least Squares Method

Several times previously in this text, we mentioned the linear nature of the pattern of points in a scatterplot. For example, in Figure 8–2, a straight line can be drawn through the points representing the values of mental function at time 1 and time 3 to indicate the direction of the relationship. The least squares method is a way to determine the equation of the line that provides a good fit to the points.

To illustrate the method, we consider the straight line in Figure 8–6. Elementary geometry can be used to determine the equation for any straight line. If the point where the line crosses, or *intercepts,* the Y-axis is denoted by a and the **slope** of the line by b, then the equation is

$$Y = a + bX$$

The slope of the line measures the amount of change in Y for each 1-unit change in X. If the slope is positive, Y increases as X increases; if the slope is negative, Y decreases as X increases; and vice versa. In the regression model, the slope in the population is generally symbolized by β_1, called the **regression coefficient;** and β_0 denotes the **intercept** of the regression line, that is, β_1 and β_0 are the population parameters in regression. In most applications, the points do not fall exactly along a straight line. For this reason, the regression model contains an *error term, e,* which is the distance the actual values of Y depart from the regression line. Putting all this together, the regression equation is given by

$$Y = \beta_0 + \beta_1 X + \varepsilon$$

When the regression equation is used to describe the relationship in the sample, it is often written as

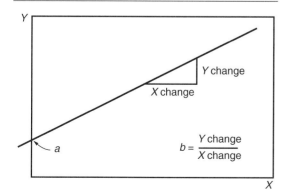

Figure 8–6. Geometric interpretation of a regression line.

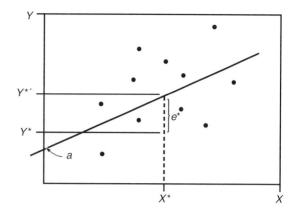

Figure 8–7. Least squares regression line.

$$Y' = b_0 + b_1 X \quad \text{or} \quad Y' = a + bX$$

We use the latter symbols in this chapter so we can avoid the need for subscripts.

For a given value of X, say X^*, the predicted value of Y^* is found by extending a horizontal line from the regression line to the Y-axis as in Figure 8–7. The difference between the actual value for Y^* and the predicted value, $e^* = Y^* - Y^{*'}$, provides a criterion for judging how well the line fits the data points. The least squares method determines the line that minimizes the sum of the squared vertical differences between the actual and predicted values of the Y variable; that is, β_0 and β_1 are determined so that $\Sigma (Y - Y')^2$ is minimized. The formulas for β_0 and β_1 are found,[1] and in terms of the sample estimates b and a, these formulas are

$$b = \frac{\Sigma(X - \overline{X})(Y - \overline{Y})}{\Sigma(X - \overline{X})^2}$$

$$a = \overline{Y} - b\overline{X}$$

8.5.2 Calculating the Regression Equation

Two approaches are possible for calculating the regression equation by hand. The first approach uses raw data and the formulas for a and b given in the preceding equations. This approach requires many calculations, regardless of whether these formulas or alternative computational formulas are used. The second method takes advantage of the relationship be-

---

[1] The procedure for finding β_0 and β_1 involves the use of differential calculus. The partial derivatives of the preceding equations are found with respect to β_0 and β_1; the two resulting equations are set equal to zero to locate the minimum values; these two equations in two unknowns, β_0 and β_1, are solved simultaneously to obtain the formulas for β_0 and β_1.

tween r and b. When the correlation has a positive value, the slope of the regression line drawn through the observations is also positive. Similarly, a negative correlation is associated with a negative slope. If the correlation is zero, the regression line is horizontal with a slope of zero. Thus, the formulas for the correlation coefficient and the regression coefficient are closely related. If r has already been calculated, it can be multiplied by the ratio of the standard deviation of Y to the standard deviation of X, SD_Y/SD_X to obtain b (see Exercise 9). Thus,

$$b = r \frac{SD_Y}{SD_X}$$

Similarly, if the regression coefficient is known, r can be found by

$$r = b \frac{SD_X}{SD_Y}$$

Of course, a far more practical way to obtain the regression equation is by using a computer, and except for illustration purposes, we assume anyone doing regression analysis uses a computer.

In the study described in Presenting Problem 4, the investigators wanted to predict insulin sensitivity from BMI in a group of women. Original observations were given in Chapter 7, Table 7–9. For now we ignore the different groups of women and examine the entire sample regardless of thyroid and weight levels.

Before calculating the regression equation for these data, let us create a scatterplot and practice "guesstimating" the value of the correlation coefficient from the plot (although it is difficult to estimate the size of r accurately when it is between -0.5 and $+0.5$ unless the sample size is quite large [Sokal and Rohlf, 1994]). Figure 8–8 is a scatterplot with BMI score as the explanatory X variable and insulin sensitivity as the response Y variable. How large do you think the correlation is?

If we knew the correlation between BMI and insulin sensitivity, we could use it to calculate the regression equation. Because we do not, we assume the needed terms have been calculated; they are

$$\Sigma(X - \overline{X})(Y - \overline{Y}) = -0.614$$
$$\Sigma(X - \overline{X})^2 = 14.182$$
$$\overline{X} = 24.921 \quad \text{and} \quad \overline{Y} = 0.503$$

Then,

$$b = \frac{\Sigma(X - \overline{X})(Y - \overline{Y})}{\Sigma(X - \overline{X})^2}$$
$$= \frac{-0.614}{14.182} = -0.0433$$

$$a = \overline{Y} - b\overline{X} = 0.503 - (-0.0433)(24.921)$$
$$= 0.503 + 1.079 = 1.5817$$

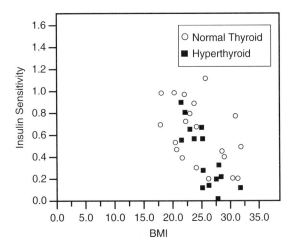

Figure 8–8. Scatterplot of observations on body mass index and insulin sensitivity. (Data, used with permission, from Gonzalo MA et al: Glucose tolerance, insulin secretion, insulin sensitivity and glucose effectiveness in normal and overweight hyperthyroid women. *Clin Endocrinol* 1996;**45**:689–697. Output produced using NCSS; used with permission.)

In this example, the insulin sensitivity scores are said to be regressed on BMI scores, and the regression equation is written as $Y' = 1.5817 - 0.0433X$, where Y' is the predicted insulin sensitivity score, and X is the BMI.

Figure 8–9 illustrates the regression line drawn through the observations. The regression equation has a positive intercept of $+1.58$, so that theoretically a patient with 0 BMI would have an insulin sensitivity of 1.58, even though, in the present example, a 0 BMI is not possible. The slope of -0.043 indicates that each time a woman's BMI increases by 1, her predicted insulin sensitivity decreases by approximately 0.043. For example, as the BMI increases from 20 to 30, insulin sensitivity decreases from about 0.73 to about 0.3. Whether the relationship between BMI and insulin sensitivity is significant is discussed in the next section.

8.5.3 Assumptions & Inferences in Regression

In the previous section, we worked with a sample of observations instead of the population of observations. Just as the sample mean $\overline{X}$ is an estimate of the population mean μ, the regression line determined from the formulas for a and b in the previous section is an estimate of the regression equation for the underlying population.

As in Chapters 6 and 7, in which we performed statistical tests to determine how likely it was that the observed differences between two means occurred by chance, in regression analysis, we must perform sta-

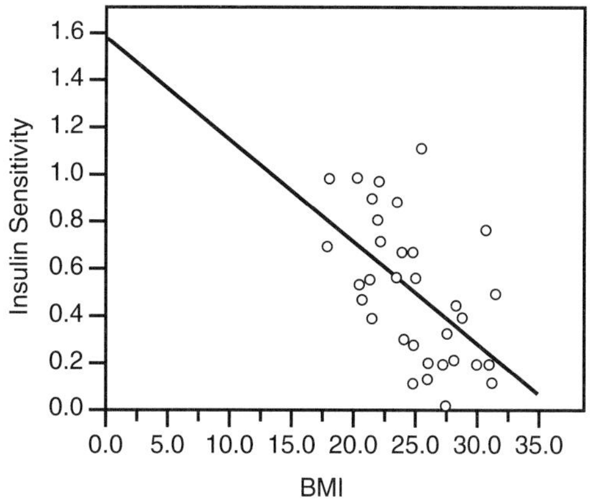

Figure 8–9. Regression of observations on body mass index and insulin sensitivity. (Data, used with permission, from Gonzalo MA et al: Glucose tolerance, insulin secretion, insulin sensitivity and glucose effectiveness in normal and overweight hyperthyroid women. *Clin Endocrinol* 1996;**45**:689–697. Output produced using NCSS; used with permission.)

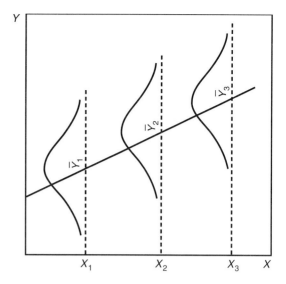

Figure 8–10. Assumption of equal variances of *Y*'s for all values of *X*.

tistical tests to determine the likelihood of any observed relationship between *X* and *Y* variables. Again, the question can be approached in two ways: using hypothesis tests or forming confidence intervals. Before discussing these approaches, however, we present the assumptions required in regression analysis.

If we are to use a regression equation, the observations must have certain properties. Thus, for each value of the *X* variable, the *Y* variable is assumed to have a normal distribution, and the mean of the distribution is assumed to be the predicted value, *Y'*. In addition, no matter the value of the *X* variable, the standard deviation of *Y* is assumed to be the same. These assumptions are rather like imagining a large number of individual normal distributions of the *Y* variable, all of the same size, one for each value of *X*. The assumption of this equal variation in the *Y*'s across the entire range of the *X*'s is called **homogeneity,** or **homoscedasticity.** It is analogous to the assumption of equal variances (homogeneous variances) in the *t* test for independent groups, as discussed in Chapter 6. If the variability of the *Y*'s differs by a large amount, transformations or other modifications must be made before regression can be performed. Figure 8–10 is a schematic drawing of these assumptions.

Another assumption of regression is the straight-line, or linear, assumption. It requires that the mean values of *Y* corresponding to various values of *X* fall on a straight line, as indicated in Figure 8–10. The values of *Y* are assumed to be independent of one another. This assumption is not met when repeated measurements are made on the same subjects; that is,

a subject's measure at one time is not independent from the measure of that same subject at another time. Finally, as with other statistical procedures, we assume the observations are a random sample from the population of interest.

Regression is a robust procedure and may be used in many situations in which the assumptions are not met, as long as the measurements are fairly reliable and the correct regression model is used. (Other regression models are discussed in Chapter 10.) Meeting the regression assumptions generally causes fewer problems in experiments or clinical trials than in observational studies because reliability of the measurements tends to be greater in experimental studies. Special procedures can be used when the assumptions are seriously violated, however; and as in ANOVA, researchers should seek a statistician's advice before using regression if questions arise about its applicability.

8.5.3.a The Standard Error of the Estimate: Regression lines, like other statistics, can vary. After all, the regression equation computed for any one sample of observations is only an estimate of the true population regression equation. If other samples are chosen from the population and a regression equation is calculated for each sample, these equations will vary from one sample to another with respect to both their slopes and their intercepts. An estimate of this variation is symbolized $S_{Y \cdot X}$ and is called the standard error of regression, or the **standard error of the estimate.** It is based on the squared deviations of the predicted *Y*'s from the actual *Y*'s and is found as follows:

$$S_{Y \cdot X} = \sqrt{\frac{\Sigma(Y - Y')^2}{n - 2}}$$

The computation of this formula is quite tedious; and although more user-friendly computational forms exist, we assume that you will use a computer program to calculate the standard error of the estimate. Because both the slope and the intercept can vary, it makes sense to perform a statistical test on each one. In each situation, a t test can be used, and the standard error of the estimate is part of the formula. It is also used in determining confidence limits. To present these formulas and the logic involved in testing the slope and the intercept, we illustrate the test of hypothesis for the intercept and the calculation of a confidence interval for the slope, using the BMI–insulin sensitivity regression equation determined earlier.

8.5.3.b Inference about the Intercept: To test the hypothesis that the intercept departs significantly from zero, we use the following procedure:

Step 1: H_0: $\beta_0 = 0$ (The intercept is zero)
H_1: $\beta_0 \neq 0$ (The intercept is not zero)

Step 2: Because the null hypothesis is a test of whether the intercept is zero, the t ratio may be used if the assumptions are met. The t ratio uses the standard error of the estimate, defined earlier, to calculate the standard error of the intercept (the denominator of the t ratio):

$$t = \frac{a - \beta_0}{\sqrt{S_{Y \cdot X}^2 \{(1/n) + [\overline{X}^2 / \Sigma(X - \overline{X})^2]\}}}$$

Step 3: Let us use α equal to the traditional value 0.05 for this example.

Step 4: The degrees of freedom are $n - 2 = 33 - 2 = 31$. The value of the t distribution with 31 degrees of freedom that divides the area into the central 95% and the combined upper and lower 5% is approximately 2.040 (from Table A–3). We therefore reject the null hypothesis of a zero intercept if (the absolute value of) the observed value of t is greater than 2.040.

Step 5: The calculation follows; we used a spreadsheet (Microsoft Excel) to calculate $S_{Y \cdot X} = 0.256$ and $\Sigma (X - \overline{X})^2 = 468.015$.

$$t = \frac{1.5817 - 0}{\sqrt{(0.256)^2 \{(1/33) + [(24.9212)^2 / 468.015]\}}}$$
$$= \frac{1.5817}{\sqrt{(0.0655)(1.3573)}}$$
$$= 5.30$$

Step 6: The absolute value of the observed t ratio is 5.30, which is greater than 2.040. The null hypothesis of a zero intercept is therefore rejected. We conclude that the evidence is sufficient to show that the intercept is significantly different from zero for the regression of insulin sensitivity on BMI.

As you know by now, it is also possible to form confidence limits for the intercept using the observed value and adding or subtracting the critical value from the t distribution multiplied by the standard error of the intercept.

8.5.3.c Inferences about the Regression Coefficient: Instead of illustrating the hypothesis test for the population regression coefficient, let us find a 95% confidence interval for β_1. The interval is given by

$$b \pm t_{(n-2)} \sqrt{S_{Y \cdot X}^2 \left[\frac{1}{\Sigma(X - \overline{X})^2}\right]}$$
$$= -0.0433 \pm 2.040 \sqrt{(0.256)^2 \left(\frac{1}{468.015}\right)}$$
$$= -0.0433 \pm 0.0241 = -0.0674 \text{ to } -0.0192$$

Because the interval excludes zero, we can be 95% confident that the regression coefficient is not zero but that it is between −0.0674 and −0.0192 or between about −0.07 and −0.02. Because the regression coefficient is significantly less than zero, can the correlation coefficient be equal to zero (see Exercise 3)? The relationship between b and r illustrated earlier and Exercise 3 should convince you of the equivalence of the results obtained with testing the significance of correlation and the regression coefficient. In fact, many authors in the medical literature perform a regression analysis and then report the P values to indicate a significant correlation coefficient.

The output from the SPSS regression program is given in Table 8–5. The program produces both the value of t and the associated P value, as well as 95% confidence limits. Do the results agree with those we found earlier? To become familiar with using regression, we suggest you replicate these results using the CD-ROM.

8.5.3.d Predicting with the Regression Equation: Individual and Mean Values: One of the important reasons for obtaining a regression equation is to predict future values for a group of subjects (or for individual subjects). For example, a clinician may want to predict insulin sensitivity from BMI for a group of women with newly diagnosed diabetes. Or the clinician may wish to predict the sensitivity for a particular woman. In either case, the variability associated with the regression line must be reflected in the prediction. The 95% confidence interval for a *predicted mean Y* in a group of subjects is

$$\text{Mean } Y' \pm t_{(n-2)} \sqrt{S_{Y \cdot X}^2 \left[\frac{1}{n} + \frac{(X - \overline{X})^2}{\Sigma(X - \overline{X})^2}\right]}$$

The 95% confidence interval for predicting a *single observation* is

Table 8–5. Computer output of regression of insulin sensitivity on body mass index.

Coefficients[a]

Mode 1		Unstandardized Coefficients		Standard Coefficients			95% Confidence Interval for B	
		B	Std. Error	Beta	t	Significance	Lower Bound	Upper Bound
1	(Constant)	1.582	0.299		5.294	0.000	0.972	2.191
	Body mass index	−0.043	0.012	−0.548	−3.652	0.001	−0.067	−0.019

[a]Dependent variable: insulin sensitivity.
Source: Data, used with permission, from Gonzalo MA et al: Glucose tolerance, insulin secretion, insulin sensitivity and glucose effectiveness in normal and overweight hyperthyroid women. *Clin Endocrinol* 1996;**45:**689–697. Output produced using SPSS, a registered trademark of SPSS, Inc; used with permission.

$$Y' \pm t_{(n-2)}\sqrt{S^2_{Y \cdot X}\left[1 + \frac{1}{n} + \frac{(X - \bar{X})^2}{\Sigma(X - \bar{X})^2}\right]}$$

Comparing these two formulas, we see that the confidence interval for predicting a single observation is wider than the interval for the mean of a group of individuals; 1 is added to the standard error term for the individual case. This result makes sense, because for a given value of X, the variation in the scores of individuals is greater than that in the mean scores of groups of individuals. Note also that the numerator of the third term in the standard error is the squared deviation of X from $\bar{X}$. The size of the standard error therefore depends on how close the observation is to the mean; the closer X is to its mean, the more accurate is the prediction of Y. For values of X quite far from $\bar{X}$, the variability in predicting the Y score is considerable. You can appreciate why it is difficult for economists and others who wish to predict future events to be very accurate!

Table 8–6 gives 95% confidence intervals associated with predicted mean insulin sensitivity levels and predicted insulin sensitivity levels for an individual corresponding to several different BMI values (and for the mean BMI in this sample of 33 women). Several insights about regression analysis can be gained by examining this table. First, note the differences in magnitude between the standard errors associated with the predicted mean insulin sensitivity and those associated with individual insulin sensitivity levels: The standard errors are much larger when we predict individual values than when we predict the mean value. In fact, the standard error for individuals is always larger than the standard error for means because of the additional 1 in the formula. Also note that the standard errors take on their smallest values when the observation of interest is the mean (BMI of 24.921 in our example). As the observation departs in either direction from the mean, the standard errors and confidence intervals become increasingly larger, reflecting the squared difference between the observation and the mean. If the confidence intervals are plotted as **confidence bands** about the regression line, they are closest to the line at the mean of X and curve away from it in both directions on each side of $\bar{X}$. Figure 8–11 shows the graph of the confidence bands.

Table 8–6 illustrates another interesting feature of the regression equation. When the mean of X is used in the regression equation, the predicted Y' is the mean of Y. The regression line therefore goes through the point (X, Y). Some elementary statistics texts give

Table 8–6. 95% Confidence intervals for predicted mean insulin sensitivity levels and predicted individual insulin sensitivity levels.

BMI	Insulin Sensitivity	Predicted	Predicting Means		Predicting Individuals	
			SE[a]	Confidence Interval	SE[b]	Confidence Interval
18.100	0.970	0.798	0.092	0.610 to 0.986	0.273	0.242 to 1.354
23.600	0.880	0.560	0.047	0.463 to 0.656	0.261	0.028 to 1.092
24.000	0.660	0.543	0.046	0.449 to 0.636	0.261	0.011 to 1.074
20.400	0.520	0.698	0.070	0.556 to 0.841	0.266	0.156 to 1.241
21.500	0.380	0.651	0.060	0.528 to 0.774	0.263	0.113 to 1.188
24.921	0.503	0.503	0.044	0.413 to 0.593	0.260	−0.027 to 1.033

Abbreviation: BMI = body mass index.
[a]Standard error for means.
[b]Standard error for individuals.

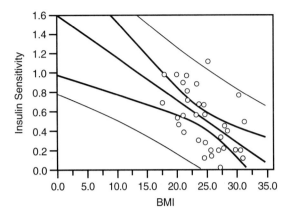

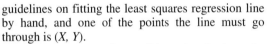

Figure 8–11. Regression of observations on body mass index and insulin sensitivity with confidence bands (heavy lines for means, light lines for individuals). (Data, used with permission, from Gonzalo MA et al: Glucose tolerance, insulin secretion, insulin sensitivity and glucose effectiveness in normal and overweight hyperthyroid women. *Clin Endocrinol* 1996;**45**:689–697. Output produced using NCSS; used with permission.)

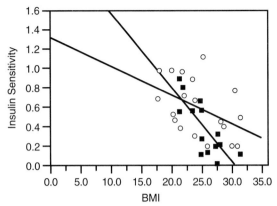

Figure 8–12. Separate regression lines for hyperthyroid (*squares*) and control (*circles*) women. (Data, used with permission, from Gonzalo MA et al: Glucose tolerance, insulin secretion, insulin sensitivity and glucose effectiveness in normal and overweight hyperthyroid women. *Clin Endocrinol* 1996; **45**:689–697. Output produced using NCSS; used with permission.)

guidelines on fitting the least squares regression line by hand, and one of the points the line must go through is (X, Y).

Now we can see why confidence bands about the regression line are curved. The error in the intercept means that the true regression line can be either above or below the line calculated for the sample observations, although it maintains the same orientation (slope). The error in measuring the slope therefore means that the true regression line can rotate about the point (X, Y) to a certain degree. The combination of these two errors results in the *concave* confidence bands illustrated in Figure 8–11. Sometimes journal articles have regression lines with confidence bands that are parallel rather than curved. These confidence bands are incorrect, although they may correspond to standard errors or to confidence intervals at their narrowest distance from the regression line.

8.5.4 Comparing Two Regression Lines

Sometimes investigators wish to compare two regression lines to see whether they are the same. For example, the investigators in Presenting Problem 4 were particularly interested in the relationship between BMI and insulin sensitivity in women who were hyperthyroid versus those whose thyroid levels were normal. The investigators determined separate regression lines for these two groups of women and reported them in Figure 3 of their article. We reproduced their regression lines in Figure 8–12.

As you might guess, researchers are often interested in comparing regression lines to learn whether the relationships are the same in different groups of

subjects. When we compare two regression lines, four situations can occur, as illustrated in Figure 8–13. In Figure 8–13A, the slopes of the regression lines are the same, but the intercepts differ. This situation occurs, for instance, in blood pressure measurements regressed on age in men and women; that is, the relationship between blood pressure and age is

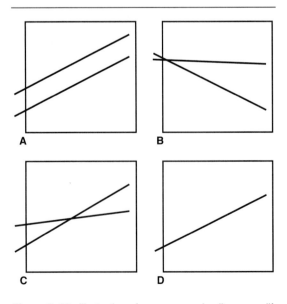

Figure 8–13. Illustration of ways regression lines can differ. **A:** Equal slopes and different intercepts. **B:** Equal intercepts and different slopes. **C:** Different slopes and different intercepts. **D:** Equal slopes and equal intercepts.

similar for men and women (equal slopes), but men tend to have higher blood pressure levels at all ages than women (higher intercept for men).

Figure 8–13B illustrates just the opposite situation: The intercepts are equal, but the slopes differ. This pattern may describe, say, the regression of platelet count on number of days following bone marrow transplantation in two groups of patients: those for whom adjuvant therapy results in remission of the underlying disease and those for whom the disease remains active. That is, prior to and immediately after transplantation, the platelet count is similar for both groups (equal intercepts), but at some time after transplantation, the platelet count remains steady for patients in remission and begins to decrease for patients not in remission (more negative slope for patients with active disease).

In Figure 8–13C, both the intercepts and the slopes of the regression lines differ. The investigators in Presenting Problem 4 reported a steeper decline in the slope of insulin sensitivity as the BMI increased in the hyperthyroid women than in the control group.[2] Although they did not specifically address any difference in intercepts, the relationship between BMI and insulin sensitivity resembles the situation in Figure 8–13C.

If no differences exist in the relationships between the predictor and outcome variables, the regression lines are similar to Figure 8–13D, in which the lines are coincident: Both intercepts and slopes are equal. This situation occurs in many situations in medicine and is considered to be the expected pattern (the null hypothesis) until it is shown not to apply by testing hypotheses or forming confidence limits for the intercept and slope.

From the four situations illustrated in Figure 8–13, we can see that three statistical questions need to be asked:

1. Are the slopes equal?
2. Are the intercepts equal?
3. Are both the slopes and the intercepts equal?

Statistical tests based on the t distribution can be used to answer the first two questions; these tests are illustrated in Kleinbaum and associates (1997). As these authors point out, however, the preferred approach is to use regression models for more than one independent variable—a procedure called multiple regression—to answer these questions. The procedure consists of pooling observations from both samples of subjects (eg, observations on both hyperthyroid and control women) and computing one regression line for the combined data. In addition, other regression coefficients are determined, coefficients that indicate whether it matters to which group

the observations belong. The simplest model—using the smallest possible number of explanatory variables to explain the observed phenomena adequately—is then selected. Because the regression lines were statistically different, the investigators in Presenting Problem 4 reported two separate regression equations.

8.6 USE OF CORRELATION & REGRESSION

Some of the characteristics of correlation and regression have been noted throughout the discussions in this chapter, and we recapitulate them here as well as mention other features. An important point to reemphasize is that correlation and regression describe *only* linear relationships. If correlation coefficients or regression equations are calculated blindly, without examining plots of the data, investigators can miss very strong, but nonlinear relationships.

8.6.1 Analysis of Residuals

A procedure useful in evaluating the fit of the regression equation is the analysis of residuals (Pedhazur, 1997). We calculated *residuals* when we found the difference between the actual value of Y and the predicted value of Y', or $Y - Y'$, although we did not use the term. A residual is the part of Y that is not predicted by X (the part left over, or the residual). The residual values, $Y - Y'$, are plotted on the Y-axis are plotted against the X values on the X-axis. The mean of the residuals is zero, and, because the slope has been subtracted in the process of calculating the residuals, the correlation between them and the X values should also be zero.

Stated another way, if the regression model provides a good fit to the data, as in Figure 8–14A, the values of the residuals are not related to the values of X. A plot of the residuals and the X values in this situation should resemble a patternless scatter of points corresponding to Figure 8–14B in which no correlation exists between the residuals and the values of X. If, in contrast, a curvilinear relationship occurs between Y and X, such as in Figure 8–14C, the residuals are negative for both small values and large values of X, because the corresponding values of Y fall below a regression line drawn through the data. They are positive, however, for midsized values of X because the corresponding values of Y fall above the regression line. In this case, instead of obtaining a random scatter, we get a plot like the curve in Figure 8–14D, with the values of the residuals being related to the values of X. Other patterns can be used by statisticians to help diagnose problems, such as a lack of homoscedasticity (equal variances) or various types of nonlinearity.

 Use the CD-ROM and the regression program to produce a graph of residuals for the data in

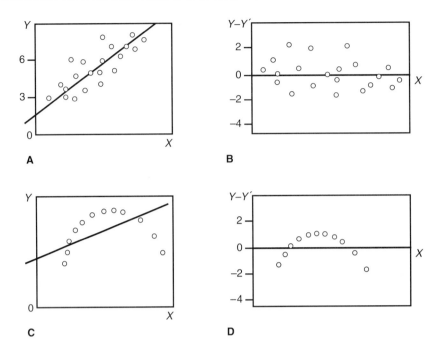

Figure 8–14. Illustration of analysis of residuals. **A:** Linear relationship between X and Y. **B:** Residuals versus values of X for relation in part **A. C:** Curvilinear relationship between X and Y. **D:** Residuals versus values of X for relation in part **C.**

Presenting Problem 4. Which of the four situations in Figure 8–14 is most likely? See Exercise 7.

8.6.2 Dealing with Nonlinear Observations

Several alternative actions can be taken if serious problems arise with nonlinearity of data. As we discussed previously, a *transformation* of the data may make the relationship linear, and regular regression methods can then be used on the transformed data. Another possibility, especially for a curve, is to fit a straight line to one part of the curve and a second straight line to another part of the curve, a procedure called *piecewise linear regression*. In this situation, one regression equation is used with all values of X less than a given value, and the second equation is used with all values of X greater than the given value. A third strategy, also useful for curves, is to perform polynomial regression; this technique is discussed in Chapter 10. Finally, more complex approaches called nonlinear regression may be used (Snedecor and Cochran, 1989).

8.6.3 Regression toward the Mean

The phenomenon called **regression toward the mean** often occurs in applied research and may go unrecognized. A good illustration of regression toward the mean occurred in the MRFIT study (Multi-

ple Risk Factor Intervention Trial Research Group, 1982), which was designed to evaluate the effect of diet and exercise on blood pressure in men with mild hypertension. To be eligible to participate in the study, men had to have a diastolic blood pressure of ≥90 mm Hg. The eligible subjects were then assigned to either the treatment arm of the study, consisting of programs to encourage appropriate diet and exercise, or the control arm, consisting of typical care. This study has been called a landmark trial and was reprinted in 1997 in the *Journal of the American Medical Association*. See Exercise 11.

To illustrate the concept of regression toward to the mean, we consider the hypothetical data in Table 8–7 for diastolic blood pressure in 12 men. If these men were being screened for the MRFIT study, only subjects 7 through 12 would be accepted; subjects 1 through 6 would not be eligible because their baseline diastolic pressure is <90 mm Hg. Suppose all subjects had another blood pressure measurement some time later. Because a person's blood pressure varies considerably from one reading to another, about half the men can be expected to have higher blood pressures and about half to have lower blood pressures, owing to random variation. Regression toward the mean tells us that those men who had lower pressures on the first reading are more likely to have higher pressures on the second reading. Similarly, men who had a diastolic blood pressure ≥90 on the

Table 8–7. Hypothetical data on diastolic blood pressure to illustrate regression toward the mean.

Subject	Baseline	Repeat
1	78	80
2	80	81
3	82	82
4	84	86
5	86	85
6	88	90
7	90	88
8	92	91
9	94	95
10	96	95
11	98	97
12	100	98

first reading are more likely to have lower pressures on the second reading. If the entire sample of men is remeasured, the increases and decreases tend to cancel each other. If, however, only a subset of the subjects is examined again, for example, the men with initial diastolic pressures >90, the blood pressures will appear to have dropped, when in fact they have not.

Regression toward the mean can result in a treatment or procedure appearing to be of value when it has had no actual effect; the use of a control group helps to guard against this effect. The investigators in the MRFIT study were aware of the problem of regression toward the mean and discussed precautions they took to reduce its effect.

8.6.4 Common Errors in Regression

A common error in regression analysis occurs when multiple observations on the same subject are treated as though they were independent. As a simple example, consider ten patients who have their weight and skinfold measurements recorded prior to beginning a low-calorie diet. We may reasonably expect a moderately positive relationship between weight and skinfold thickness. Suppose, however, that the same ten patients are weighed and measured again after 6 weeks on the diet. If all 20 observations are treated as though they were independent, several problems occur. First, the sample size will appear to be increased, which means that we are more likely to conclude significance. Second, because the relationship between weight and skinfold thickness in the same person is somewhat stable across minor shifts in weight, using both observations has the same effect as using duplicate measures, and this results in a correlation larger than it should be.

The magnitude of the correlation can also be erroneously increased by combining two different groups. For example, consider the relationship between height and weight. Suppose the heights and

weights of ten men and ten women are recorded, and the correlation between height and weight is calculated for the combined samples. Figure 8–15 illustrates how the scatterplot might look and indicates the problem that results from combining men and women in one sample. The relationship between height and weight appears to be more significant in the combined sample than it is when measured in men and women separately. Much of the apparent significance results because men tend both to weigh more and to be taller than women. Inappropriate conclusions may result from mixing two different populations—another common error to watch for in the medical literature.

8.6.5 Comparing Correlation & Regression

Correlation and regression have some similarities and some differences. First, correlation is scale-independent, but regression is not. That is, the correlation between two characteristics, such as height and weight, is the same whether height is measured in centimeters or inches and weight in kilograms or pounds. The regression equation resulting from regressing weight on height, however, depends on which scales are being used; that is, predicting weight measured in kilograms from height measured in centimeters gives different values for a and b from predicting weight in pounds from height in inches.

An important consequence of scale independence in correlation is that the correlation between X and Y is the same as the correlation between Y' and Y. They are equal because the regression equation itself, $Y' = a + bX$, is a simple rescaling of the X variable; that is, each value of X is multiplied by a constant value b

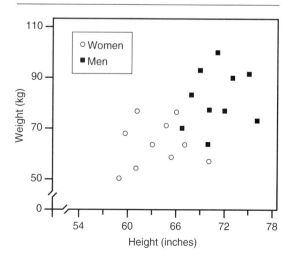

Figure 8–15. Hypothetical data illustrating spurious correlation.

and then a constant amount a is added. The fact that the correlation between the original variables X and Y is equal to the correlation between Y and the values of Y' obtained from the regression equation (ie, $r_{XY} = r_{Y'Y}$) provides a useful alternative method for testing the significance of the regression, as we will see in Chapter 10. Finally, the slope of the regression line has the same sign (+ or −) as the correlation coefficient (see Exercise 9).

8.6.6 Multiple Regression

Multiple regression analysis is a straightforward generalization of simple regression for applications in which two or more independent (explanatory) variables are used in the prediction equation. For example, in the study described in Presenting Problem 4, the investigators wanted to predict a woman's insulin sensitivity level based on her BMI. They also wanted to control for the age of the woman, however. The results from two analyses are given in Table 8–8. First, regression was done using the BMI to predict insulin sensitivity among hyperthyroid women; the resulting equation was

Predicted insulin sensitivity = 2.336 − 0.077 × BMI

Next, the regression was repeated using both BMI and age as independent variables. The results were

Predicted insulin sensitivity = 2.291 − 0.068 × BMI
− 0.004 × Age

As you can see, the addition of the age variable has relatively little effect; in fact, the P value for age is 0.30, indicating that age is not significantly associated with insulin sensitivity in this group of hyperthyroid women.

As an additional point, note that R^2 (called R-squared) is 0.601 for the first regression equation in Table 8–8. R^2 is interpreted in the same manner as the coefficient of determination, r^2, discussed in Section 8.2.2. This topic, along with multiple regression and other statistical methods based on regression, is discussed in detail in Chapter 10.

8.7 SAMPLE SIZES FOR CORRELATION & REGRESSION

As with other statistical procedures, it is important to have an adequate number of subjects in any study that involves correlation or regression. Complex formulas are required to estimate sample sizes for these procedures, but fortunately we can use statistical power programs to do the calculations.

Suppose that Hébert and colleagues (1997) wanted to know what sample size would be necessary to produce a confidence interval for the correlation of the mental ability scores at times 1 and 3 that would be within ±0.10 from the observed correlation coefficient. In other words, how many subjects are needed for a 95% confidence interval from 0.48 to 0.68 around the correlation of 0.58 found in their study? We used the nQuery Advisor program to illustrate the sample size needed in this situation; the output is given in Figure 8–16. A sample of 143 women would be necessary.

To illustrate the power analysis for regression, consider the regression equation to predict insulin sensitivity from BMI (Gonzalo et al, 1996). Recall that we found that a 95% confidence interval for the regression coefficient was between −0.0674 and −0.0192 in the entire sample of 33 women. Suppose

Table 8–8. Regression equations for hyperthyroid women using BMI versus BMI and age as predictor variables.

Regression Equation Section

Independent Variable	Regression Coefficient	Standard Error	t Value (H_0: B=0)	Probability Level	Decision (5%)
Intercept	2.336	0.462	5.054	0.0003	Reject H_0
BMI	−0.077	1.807E−02	−4.248	0.0011	Reject H_0
R^2	0.601				

Regression Equation Section

Independent Variable	Regression Coefficient	Standard Error	t Value (H_0: B=0)	Probability Level	Decision (5%)
Intercept	2.2905	0.461	4.973	0.0004	Reject H_0
Age	−4.463E−03	4.103E−03	−1.088	0.3000	Accept H_0
BMI	−6.782E−02	1.972E−02	−3.439	0.0055	Reject H_0
R^2	0.639				

Abbreviation: BMI = body mass index.
Source: Data, used with permission, from Gonzalo MA et al: Glucose tolerance, insulin secretion, insulin sensitivity and glucose effectiveness in normal and overweight hyperthyroid women. *Clin Endocrinol* 1996;**45**:689–697. Output produced using NCSS; used with permission.

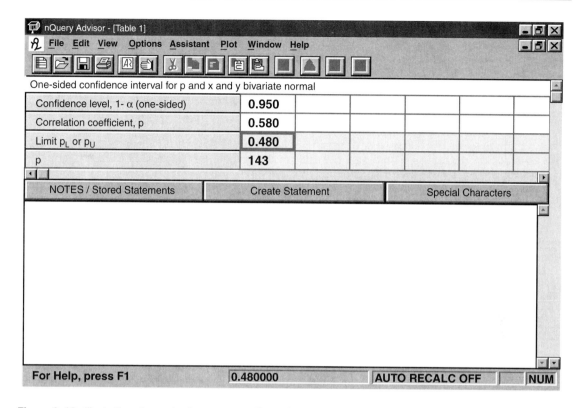

Figure 8–16. Illustration of sample size program nQuery Advisor. (Data, used with permission, from Hébert R, Brayne C, Spiegelhalter D: Incidence of functional decline and improvement in a community-dwelling very elderly population. *Am J Epidemiol* 1997;**145**:935–944. Figure produced using nQuery Advisor; used with permission.)

Gonzalo and colleagues wanted to know how many women would be needed for the regression. The power program PASS finds the sample size by estimating the number needed to obtain a given value for R^2 (or r^2 when only one independent variable is used). We assume they want the correlation between the actual insulin sensitivity and the predicted sensitivity to be at least 0.50, producing an r^2 of 0.25. The setup and output from the PASS program are given in Figures 8–17 and 8–18. From Figure 8-18, we see that a sample size of about 26 is needed in each group for which a regression equation is to be determined.

8.8 SUMMARY

Four presenting problems were used in this chapter to illustrate the application of correlation and regression in medical studies. The findings from the study described in Presenting Problem 1 demonstrate the relationship between measurements of mental ability in a group of elderly Canadian residents measured on two occasions (Hébert et al, 1997). We found that the correlation of 0.58 between these two measurements on women 85 years of age or older was statistically

significant. Thus, assuming no intervention, elderly women who exhibit decreased mental ability continue to do so over time.

In Presenting Problem 2, Nesselroad and colleagues (1996) evaluated three automated finger blood pressure devices marketed as being accurate devices for monitoring blood pressure. We examined the relationship among these devices and the standard method using a blood pressure cuff. The observed correlations were quite low, ranging from 0.32 to 0.45. We compared these two correlation coefficients and concluded that no statistical difference exists between them. Nesselroad also reported that the automated finger device measurements were outside of the ±4 mm Hg range obtained with the standard blood pressure cuff 75–81% of the time. These researchers appropriately concluded that people who want to monitor their blood pressure cannot trust these devices to be accurate.

Hodgson and Cutler (1997) reported results from their study of people's fears that normal age-associated memory change is a precursor of dementia. We examined the relationship between memory scores and whether people reported they were satisfied with their life. We demonstrated that the conclusions from com-

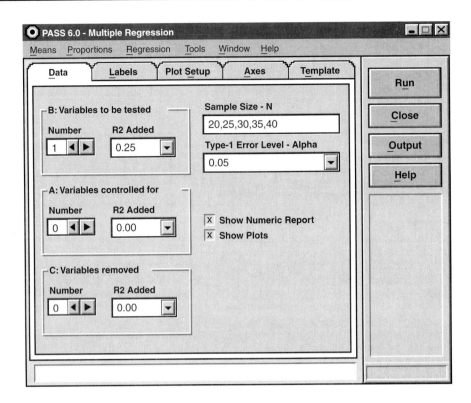

Figure 8–17. Illustration of setup for using the PASS sample size program for multiple regression using the data on insulin sensitivity. (Data, used with permission, from Gonzalo MA et al: Glucose tolerance, insulin secretion, insulin sensitivity and glucose effectiveness in normal and overweight hyperthyroid women. *Clin Endocrinol* 1996;**45:**689–697. Output produced using PASS; used with permission.)

puting the biserial correlation (the correlation between a numerical and a binary measure) and performing a *t* test are the same. Other results showed that the sense of well-being in these individuals is related to anticipatory dementia. Those with higher levels of anticipatory dementia are more depressed, have more psychiatric symptoms, have lower life satisfaction, and describe their health as being poorer than individuals not concerned about memory loss and Alzheimer's disease. Furthermore, women in the study demonstrated a relationship between anticipatory dementia and wellbeing that was not observed in men.

Data from Gonzalo and colleagues (1996) was used to illustrate regression, specifically the relationship between insulin sensitivity and BMI for hyperthyroid and control women. We found separate regression lines for hyperthyroid and for control women and observed that the relationships between insulin sensitivity and BMI are different in these two groups of women. The investigators also reported that overall glucose tolerance was not affected by hyperthyroidism in normal weight women.

The flowcharts for Appendix C summarize the methods for measuring an association between two

characteristics measured on the same subjects. Flowchart C–4 indicates how the methods depend on the scale of measurement for the variables, and flowchart C–5 shows applicable methods for testing differences in correlations and in regression lines.

EXERCISES

1. The extent to which stool energy losses are normalized in cystic fibrosis patients receiving pancreatic enzyme replacement therapy prompted a study by Murphy and colleagues (1991). They determined the amount of energy within the stools of 20 healthy children and 20 patients with cystic fibrosis who were comparatively asymptomatic while taking capsules of pancreatin, an enzyme replacement. Weighed food intake was recorded daily for 7 days for all study participants. Over the final 3 days of the study, all stools were collected. Measures of lipid content, total nitrogen content, bacterial content, and total energy content of the stools were recorded. Data for the cystic fibrosis chil-

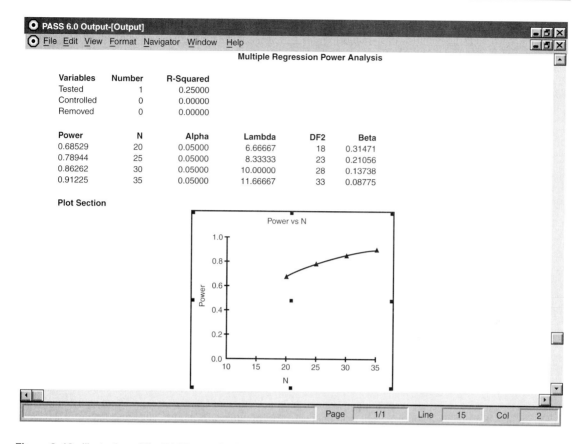

Figure 8–18. Illustration of the PASS sample size program for multiple regression using the data on insulin sensitivity. (Data, used with permission, from Gonzalo MA et al: Glucose tolerance, insulin secretion, insulin sensitivity and glucose effectiveness in normal and overweight hyperthyroid women. *Clin Endocrinol* 1996;**45**:689–697. Output produced using PASS; used with permission.)

dren are given in Table 8–9 and on the CD-ROM in a folder entitled "Murphy."

a. Find and interpret the correlation between stool lipid and stool energy.

b. Figure 8–19 is from the study by Murphy. What is the authors' purpose in displaying this graph? What can be interpreted about the relationship between fecal lipid and fecal energy for control patients? How does that relationship compare with the relationship in patients with cystic fibrosis?

2. a. Perform a chi-square test of the significance of the relationship between TRH and placebo and the subsequent development of respiratory distress syndrome using the data in Chapter 3, Table 3–22.

b. Determine 95% confidence limits for the odds ratio of 2.3 for the risk of death within 28 days of delivery among infants not at risk using the data in Table 3–21. What is your conclusion?

3. Calculate the correlation between BMI and insulin sensitivity for the entire sample of 33 women, using the results in Section 8.5.2 for *b*. The standard deviation of BMI is 3.82 and of insulin sensitivity is 0.030.

4. Goldsmith and colleagues (1985) examined 35 patients with hemophilia to determine whether a relationship exists between impaired cell-mediated immunity and the amount of factor concentrate used. In one of their studies, the ratio of OKT4 (helper T cells) to OKT8 (suppressor/cytotoxic T cells) was formed, and the logarithm of this ratio was regressed on the logarithm of lifetime concentrate use (Figure 8–20).

a. Why is the logarithm scale used for both variables?

b. Interpret the correlation.

c. What do the confidence bands mean?

5. Helmrich and coworkers (1987) conducted a study to assess the risk of deep vein thrombosis and pulmonary embolism in relation to the use

Table 8–9. Observations on stool lipid and stool energy losses in children with cystic fibrosis.

Subject	Fecal Lipid (g/day)	Fecal Energy (MJ/day)
1	10.0	2.1
2	11.0	1.1
3	9.9	1.1
4	9.8	0.9
5	15.5	0.7
6	5.0	0.4
7	10.7	1.0
8	13.0	1.5
9	13.8	1.2
10	16.7	1.4
11	3.2	1.0
12	4.0	0.5
13	6.0	0.9
14	8.9	0.8
15	9.1	0.6
16	4.1	0.5
17	17.0	1.2
18	22.2	1.1
19	2.9	0.9
20	5.0	1.0

Source: Modified and reproduced, with permission, from the table and Figure 3 in Murphy JL et al: Energy content of stools in normal healthy controls and patients with cystic fibrosis. *Arch Dis Child* 1991;**66**:495–500.

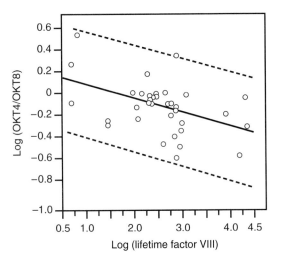

Figure 8–20. Regression of logarithm of OKT4:OKT8 on logarithm of factor concentrate use (Reproduced, with permission, from Goldsmith JM et al: Sequential clinical and immunologic abnormalities in hemophiliacs. *Arch Intern Med* 1985;**145**:431–434.)

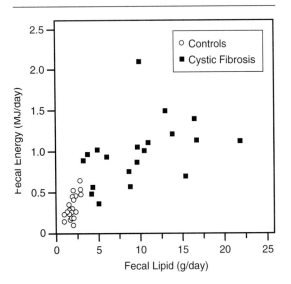

Figure 8–19. Stool lipid versus stool energy losses for the control subjects and cystic fibrosis patients. (Reproduced, with permission, from Figure 3 in Murphy JL et al: Energy content of stools in normal healthy controls and patients with cystic fibrosis. *Arch Dis Child* 1991;**66**: 495–500.)

of oral contraceptives. They were especially interested in the risk associated with low dosage (<50 µg estrogen) and confined their study to women under the age of 50 years. They administered standard questionnaires to women admitted to the hospital for deep vein thrombosis or pulmonary embolism as well as to a control set of women admitted for trauma and upper respiratory infections to determine their history and current use of oral contraceptives. Twenty of the 61 cases and 121 of the 1278 controls had used oral contraceptives in the previous month.

    a. What research design was used in this study?

    b. Find 95% confidence limits for the odds ratio for these data.

    c. The authors reported an age-adjusted odds ratio of 8.1 with 95% confidence limits of 3.7 and 18. Interpret these results.

6. The graphs in Figure 8–21 were published in the study by Einarsson and associates (1985).

    a. Which graph exhibits the strongest relationship with age?

    b. Which variable would be best predicted from a patient's age?

    c. Do the relationships between the variables and age appear to be the same for men and women; that is, is it appropriate to combine the observations for men and women in the same figure?

7. Use the CD-ROM regression program to produce a graph of residuals for the data in Presenting Problem 4. Which of the four situations in Figure 8–14 is most likely?

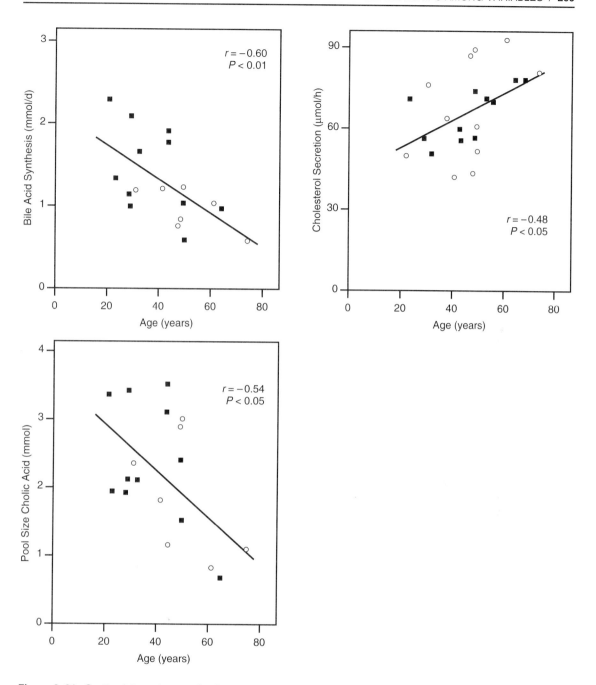

Figure 8–21. Scatterplots and regression lines for relation between age and hepatic secretion of cholesterol, total bile acid synthesis, and size of cholic acid pool for women (open circles) and men (filled circles). (Reproduced, with permission, from Einarsson K et al: Influence of age on secretion of cholesterol and synthesis of bile acids by the liver. *N Engl J Med* 1985;**313**:277–282.)

8. Explain why the mean of the predicted values, $\overline{Y'}$, is equal to $\overline{Y}$.

9. Develop an intuitive argument to explain why the sign of the correlation coefficient and the sign of the slope of the regression line are the same.

10. **Group Exercise.** The causes and pathogenesis of steroid-responsive nephrotic syndrome (also known as minimal-change disease) are unknown. Levinsky and colleagues (1978) postulated that this disease might have an immunologic basis because it may be associated with

atopy, recent immunizations, or a recent upper respiratory infection. It is also responsive to corticosteroid treatment. They analyzed the serum from children with steroid-responsive nephrotic syndrome for the presence of IgG-containing immune complexes and the complement-binding properties (C1q-binding) of these complexes. For purposes of comparison, they also studied these two variables in patients with systemic lupus erythematosus. You will need to consult the published article for details of the study; a graph from the study is reproduced in Figure 8–22.

a. What were the study's basic research questions?

b. What was the study design? Is it the best one for the study's purposes?

c. What was the rationale in defining the kinds of patients to be studied? How were subjects obtained?

d. Interpret the correlations for the two sets of patients in Figure 8–22. What conclusions do you draw about the relationships between C1q-binding and IgG complexes in patients with systemic lupus erythematosus? In patients with steroid-responsive nephrotic syndrome?

e. Discuss the use of the parallel lines surrounding the regression line; do they refer to means or individuals? (*Hint:* The standard error of regression is 11.95 and $(X - \overline{X})^2$ is 21,429.37).

f. Do you think the regression lines for the two sets of patients will differ?

g. Would the results from this study generalize? If so, to what patient populations, and what cautions should be taken? If not, what features of the study limit its generalizability?

11. **Group Exercise.** The MRFIT study (Multiple Risk Factor Intervention Trial Research Group, 1982), has been called a landmark trial; it was the first large-scale clinical trial, and it is rare to have a study that follows more than 300,000 men who were screened for the trial for a number of years. The *Journal of the American Medical Association* reprinted this article in 1997. In addition, the journal published a comment in the Landmark Perspective section by Gotto (1997). Obtain a copy of both articles.

a. What research design was used in the study?

b. Discuss the eligibility criteria. Are these criteria still relevant today?

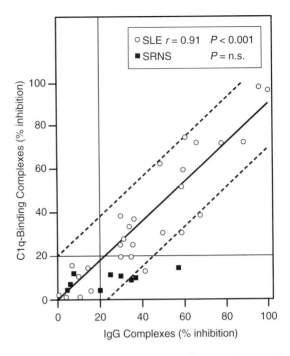

Figure 8–22. Scatterplot of C1q-binding complexes and IgG complexes in patients with systemic lupus erythematosus (SLE; open circles) and steroid-responsive nephrotic syndrome (SRNS; filled circles), illustrating the possibility of differences in regression lines for SLE and SRNS patients. (Reproduced, with permission, from Levinsky RJ et al: Circulating immune complexes in steroid-responsive nephrotic syndrome. *N Engl J Med* 1978;**298**:126–129.)

c. What were the treatment arms? Are these treatments still relevant today?

d. What statistical methods were used? Were they appropriate? One method, the Kaplan–Meier product-limit method, is discussed in Chapter 9.

e. Refer to Figure 1 in the original study. What do the lines in the figure indicate?

f. Examine the distribution of deaths given in Table 4. What statistical method is relevant to analyzing these results?

g. The perspective by Gotto discusses the issue of power in the MRFIT study. How was the power of the study affected by the initial assumptions made in the study design?

Analyzing Research Questions about Survival

9

PRESENTING PROBLEMS

Presenting Problem 1. To determine risk factors that predict which patients will decide to discontinue their life-saving dialysis, Bajwa and colleagues (1996) at the University of Alberta, Edmonton, performed a prospective study of patients undergoing chronic dialysis treatment. In Canada, discontinuation of dialysis is second only to cardiovascular disease as a cause of death in patients on long-term dialysis.

A prospective study of 235 chronic dialysis patients analyzed 300 sociodemographic, quality-of-life, medical, and dialysis variables over a period of 3½ years. Seventy-six patients (32%) died during the follow-up period. Thirteen (17%) died because of discontinuation of dialysis. We use data from this study to illustrate methods for analyzing survival data. A sample of 25 patients is used to show actual calculations, but results from the entire study are also given. Data from the study are available in a data set entitled "Bajwa" on the CD-ROM.

Presenting Problem 2. Between 1968 and 1975, a cardiac surgeon at Baylor College of Medicine performed coronary artery bypass surgery on 1698 patients (Lawrie et al, 1991). This carefully followed cohort is the subject of a study describing outcomes after 15–20 years. Follow-up activities included physician visits, questionnaires, and telephone interviews at regular intervals. Data were available on 92% of the patients 20 years after surgery. Multiple variables, including cholesterol and triglyceride levels, presence of hypertension or diabetes, and the number of diseased vessels, were analyzed with respect to survival. Diabetes mellitus and systolic blood pressure >160 mm Hg were associated with reduced survival rates, and 818 of the 1698 patients underwent a postoperative catheterization. The influence of the number of diseased vessels before surgery is shown in Section 9.7.

Presenting Problem 3. Prostate-specific antigen (PSA) is a serine protease glycoprotein secreted predominately by both normal and neoplastic prostate epithelia. It circulates in the bloodstream and can be measured by a variety of assays and consequently has become an important tool in the understanding of prostate cancer biology and growth. PSA value correlates with the stage of the prostate tumor at diagnosis and is an important prognostic variable. (See also Shipley et al, 1999, a presenting problem in Chapter 4.) An increasing PSA value after prostate cancer treatment is a sensitive indictor of relapse but does not discriminate between local recurrence and metastatic recurrence. Crook and coinvestigators (1997) studied the correlation between both the pretreatment PSA and posttreatment nadir PSA with the outcome in men with localized prostate cancer who were treated with external beam radiation therapy.

This was a prospective study of 207 men with localized adenocarcinoma of the prostate treated with radiation therapy. Pretreatment PSA values were obtained for all of the men, and posttreatment values were obtained at 3–6-month intervals for 5 years and yearly thereafter. Posttreatment prostate biopsies were done at 12 months. Patients with residual tumor had repeat biopsies about every 6 months, whereas those with negative biopsy results had repeat biopsies at 36 months or if a rising PSA value occurred.

The Gleason histologic scoring system was used to classify tumors on a scale of 2 to 10. A low score indicates a well-differentiated tumor, a medium score a moderately differentiated tumor, and a high score a poorly differentiated tumor. Tumors were also classified using the TNM (tumor, node, metastasis) staging system, called the T classification. A T1 tumor is a nonpalpable tumor identified by biopsy. A T2 tumor is palpable on digital rectal examination and limited to the prostate gland. T3 and T4 tumors have invaded adjacent prostate structures, such as the bladder neck or seminal vesicle. The median age of patients was 69 years, and the median duration of follow-up was 36 months. Sixty-eight of the 207 patients had a recurrence of prostate cancer: 20 had local recurrence, 24 had nodal or metastatic recurrence, 7 had both local and distant recurrence, and 17 had biochemical recurrence (elevated PSA with negative biopsy and metastatic workup). The prognostic importance of pretreatment PSA, posttreatment nadir PSA, the Gleason score, and the T classification were examined.

We summarize this study and present the results from the Kaplan–Meier survival analysis predicting recurrence. Data on the patients are given on the CD-ROM in the data set entitled "Crook."

9.1 PURPOSE OF THE CHAPTER

Many studies in medicine are designed to determine whether a new medication, a new treatment, or a new procedure will perform better than the one in current use. Although measures of short-term effects are of interest with efforts to provide more efficient health care, long-term outcomes, including mortality and major morbidity, are also important. For example, Presenting Problem 2 discusses 20-year survival rates among patients who had coronary bypass surgery. In Presenting Problem 1, the investigators with the data on dialysis patients want to examine survival in patients who discontinued versus those who continued dialysis. In both studies, the outcome was binary—survival or death of patients—and the desire is to estimate the length of time patients survive with specific types of treatment or under specific conditions. Often, studies focus on comparing survival times for two or more groups of patients, as is the case for the analysis by diseased vessel in the coronary bypass surgery article.

The methods of data analysis discussed in previous chapters are not appropriate for measuring length of survival for two reasons. First, investigators frequently must analyze data before all patients have died; otherwise, it may be many years before they know which treatment is better. When analysis of survival is done while some patients in the study are still living, the observations on these patients are called **censored observations,** because we do not know how long these patients will remain alive. Figure 9–1 illustrates a situation in which observations on patients B and E are censored.

The second reason special methods are needed to analyze survival data is that patients do not typically begin treatment or enter the study at the same time, as

they did for Figure 9–1. For example, in the dialysis study, patients entered the study at different times. When the entry time for patients is not simultaneous and when some patients are still in the study when the analysis is done, the data are said to be **progressively censored.** Figure 9–2 shows results for a study with progressively censored observations. The study began at time 0 months with patient A; then, patient B entered the study at time 7 months; patient C entered at time 8 months; and so on. Patients B and E were still alive at the time the data were analyzed at 40 months.

Analysis of survival times is sometimes called **actuarial,** or **life table, analysis.** Historically, astronomer Edmund Halley (of Halley's Comet fame) first used life tables in the 17th century to describe survival times of residents of a town. Since then, these methods have been used in various ways. For example, life insurance companies use life tables to determine the life expectancy of individuals, and this information is subsequently used to establish premium schedules. Insurers generally use cross-sectional data about how long people of different age groups are expected to live and use this information to develop a *current* life table. In medicine, however, most studies of survival use *cohort* life tables, in which the same group of subjects is followed for a given period. The data for life tables may come from cohort studies (either prospective or historical) or from clinical trials; the key feature is that the same group of subjects is followed for a prescribed time.

Analysis of survival data occurs to varying degrees in the medical literature, depending on the specialty of the journal. For example, these methods were used in only about 1% of articles published in psychiatry (Hokanson et al, 1986b) and pathology (Hokanson et al, 1987a); they were used in 12% of surgical articles (Reznick et al, 1987), 14% of oncology articles (Hokanson et al, 1986a), and 32% of original papers in the *New England Journal of Medicine* (Altman, 1991b).

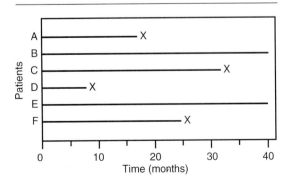

Figure 9–1. Example of censored observations (X means patient died).

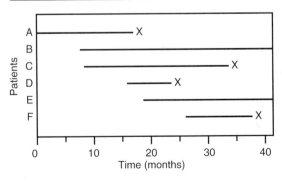

Figure 9–2. Example of progressively censored observations (X means patient died).

In this chapter, we examine two commonly used methods to determine survival curves—life (actuarial) tables and the Kaplan–Meier procedure—as well as a method to determine confidence limits about the curves. After discussing the concept of hazard rate, we examine ways survival curves may be compared. Then, survival analyses published by the authors of the studies described in Presenting Problems 2 and 3 are examined and interpreted. As with many statistical procedures, the computations involved in estimating survival curves and comparing them are tedious; we employ small samples to illustrate the logic of the method, assuming computer programs will always be used to perform these analyses.

9.2 WHY SPECIALIZED METHODS ARE NEEDED TO ANALYZE SURVIVAL DATA

Before illustrating the methods for analyzing survival data, let us consider briefly why some intuitive methods are not very useful or appropriate. To illustrate these points, we use the data on dialysis in Table 9–1. Two hundred and thirty-five patients were in the study, but for the purpose of illustration, we selected a sample of 25: 18 patients who remained on dialysis and 7 patients who discontinued dialysis.

Colton (1974, pp. 238–241) gives a creative presentation of some simple methods to analyze survival data; the arguments presented in this section are mod-eled on his discussion. Some methods appear at first glance to be appropriate for analyzing survival data, but closer inspection shows they are incorrect.

Suppose someone suggests calculating the mean length of time patients survive on dialysis. Using the data in Table 9–1, the mean survival time for all patients is 604.88, or 605 days. This value may be further broken down into mean survival time among patients who remained on dialysis (680 days) and mean survival time among patients who stopped dialysis (411 days), with the obvious but hardly enlightening conclusion that patients who remain on dialysis live longer than patients who stop dialysis.

The problem is that mean survival time depends on when the data are analyzed; it will change with each passing month until the point when all the subjects have died. Therefore, mean survival estimates calculated in this way are useful only when all the subjects have died or when the event being analyzed has occurred for all subjects. Almost always, however, investigators wish to analyze their data prior to that time.

An estimate of median length of survival time is also possible, and it can be calculated after only half of the subjects have died. Again, however, investigators often wish to evaluate the outcome prior to that time.

A concept sometimes used in epidemiology is the number of deaths per each 100 **person-years of observation.** To illustrate, we use the observations in Table 9–1 to determine the number of person-days of survival. Regardless of whether patients are alive or

Table 9–1. Survival of sample of 25 patients on dialysis.[a]

Patient	Days in Study	Stopped Hemodialysis	Outcome	Treatment
1	632	No	A	CAPD
2	619	No	A	CAPD
3	1016	No	A	HD
4	296	No	A	CAPD
5	1059	No	A	HD
6	828	No	A	HD
7	357	No	A	HD
8	1064	No	A	HD
9	695	No	A	CAPD
10	650	No	A	HD
11	1022	No	A	HD
12	166	No	D	HD
13	643	No	A	CAPD
14	1031	No	D	HD
15	1097	No	A	HD
16	228	No	D	HD
17	497	No	D	HD
18	346	No	A	CAPD
19	969	Yes	D	HD
20	576	Yes	D	CAPD
21	860	Yes	D	HD
22	158	Yes	D	HD
23	174	Yes	D	CAPD
24	76	Yes	D	CAPD
25	63	Yes	D	CAPD

Abbreviations: CAPD = continuous ambulatory peritoneal dialysis; HD = hemodialysis; A = alive; D = dead.
[a]Sample of 25 patients from the 235 patients.
Source: Data, used with permission, from Bajwa K, Szabo E, Kjellstrand CM: A prospective study of risk factors and decision making in discontinuation of dialysis. *Arch Intern Med* 1996;**156:**2571–2577. Table produced with NCSS; used with permission.

dead at the end of the study, they contribute to the calculation for however long they have been in the study. Patient 1 therefore contributes 632 days, patient 2 is in the study for 619 days, patient 3 for 1016 days, and so on. The total number of days patients have been observed is 15,122 days; converting to years by dividing by 365 days gives 41.4 person-years. The 11 patients who died during the period give 11/41.4 = 0.266, or 26.6 deaths per 100 person-years of observation. This number may be useful in comparing the results during this period with results during another period or results obtained by another investigator.

One problem with using person-years of observation, however, is that the same number is obtained by observing 1000 patients for 1 year or by observing 100 patients for 10 years. Although the number of subjects is involved in the calculation of person-years, it is not evident as an explicit part of the result; and no statistical methods are available to compare these numbers. Another problem is the inherent assumption that the risk of the event, for example, death or rejection, during any one unit of time is constant throughout the study, although several other survival methods also make this assumption.

Mortality rates (defined in Chapter 3) are a familiar way to deal with survival data, and they are used (especially in oncology) to estimate 3- and 5-year survival with various types of medical conditions. We cannot determine a mortality rate, however, using data on *all* patients until the specified length of time has passed. To illustrate, again using the data in Table 9–1, if we estimate the mortality rate as the number of patients who died divided by the number of patients in the study, we have 11/25 = 0.44, or 44%. We have the problem noted for mean length of survival, however; the mortality rate depends on when the data are analyzed. The mortality rate may be quite small if it is calculated early enough in a study; but it will be 100% if investigators wait long enough to analyze the data.

We can also calculate 1-year survival rates for the data on the dialysis patients. Among the 11 patients who died, 6 did so within 1 year of beginning dialysis. Among the 14 patients who were still alive at the time of analysis, only 11 patients were followed at least a year, and we do not know whether patients who were in the study less than 1 year will survive an entire year. One solution is to divide the number who died in the first 12 months, 6, by the total number in the study, 25, for an estimate of 0.24, or 24%. This estimate, however, is probably too low, because it assumes that all patients who were in the study less than 1 year will live at least 12 months.

An alternative solution is to subtract the number of patients who were not in the study for 12 months to obtain 6/(25 − 3) = 0.273, or 27.3%. This technique is similar to the approach used in cancer research in which 3- and 5-year mortality rates are based on only

those patients who were in the study at least 3 or 5 years. The shortcoming of this approach is that it ignores completely the contribution of those who were in the study less than 1 year. For example, patient 7 was in the study for 357 days, and this time is not counted at all. This approach is acceptable when a large number of patients is being followed; however, for small sample sizes—as often occurs early in the study of a new drug or procedure—we need to find a way to use information gained from all patients who entered the study. A reasonable approach should produce an estimate between 24% and 27.3%, which is exactly what actuarial life table analysis and Kaplan–Meier product limit methods do. They give credit for the amounts of time subjects survived up to the time when the data are analyzed.

9.3 ACTUARIAL, OR LIFE TABLE, ANALYSIS

Actuarial, or life table, analysis is also sometimes referred to in the medical literature as the Cutler–Ederer method (1958). The actuarial method is not computationally overwhelming and, at one time, was the predominant method used in medicine. The availability of computers makes it far less often used today, however, than the Kaplan–Meier product limit method discussed in the next section.

To illustrate the calculations involved in actuarial analysis, we arranged the length of time the 18 patients who remained on dialysis were in the study in a frequency table (Table 9–2). The time intervals used in the analysis are somewhat arbitrary but should be selected so that the number of censored observations in any interval is small; we group by 180-day intervals.

We use the observations in Table 9–2 to produce Table 9–3. The column headed n_i in Table 9–3 is the number of patients in the study at the beginning of the interval; all patients (18) began the study, so n_1 is 18. During the first time interval, from the time they entered the study up to 180 days later, 1 patient died (patient 12), referred to as "terminating," so $d_1 = 1$. The proportion terminating is 1/18 = 0.0556. The proportion surviving is 1 − 0.0556 = 0.9444, and, because we are still on the first period, the cumulative survival is also 0.9444.

Now we move to the second interval in Table 9–3, beginning at 180 days. Because 1 patient died during the first interval, the number of patients remaining at the beginning of the second interval is 17. During days 180–360, patient 16 died, so $d_2 = 1$, and 3 patients (patients 4, 18, and 7) began the interval and are still alive but have been in the study less than 360 days. These patients are treated as "withdrawals" (even though this term is not truly descriptive); therefore, $w_2 = 3$. The proportion terminating at the second interval is not 1/17 because, although 17 patients began the interval, 3 patients did not complete it. The actuarial method counts patients who were in the

Table 9–2. Survival of sample of 18 patients who remained on dialysis.

Patient	Days in Study	Stopped Hemodialysis	Outcome
12	166	No	D
16	228	No	D
4	296	No	A
18	346	No	A
7	357	No	A
17	497	No	D
2	619	No	A
1	632	No	A
13	643	No	A
10	650	No	A
9	695	No	A
6	828	No	A
3	1016	No	A
11	1022	No	A
14	1031	No	D
5	1059	No	A
8	1064	No	A
15	1097	No	A

Source: Data, used with permission, from Bajwa K, Szabo E, Kjellstrand CM: A prospective study of risk factors and decision making in discontinuation of dialysis. *Arch Intern Med* 1996;**156:**2571–2577. Table produced with NCSS; used with permission.

study at the beginning of the interval but not at the end of it, either because they were not in the study that long or because they were lost to follow-up. This method assumes that patients withdraw randomly throughout the interval; therefore, on the average, they withdraw halfway through the time represented by the interval. In a sense, this method gives patients who "withdraw" credit for being in the study for half of the period. Thus, the denominator of the proportion is reduced by half of the number of patients who withdraw during the period. In our example, the proportion terminating is $1/[17 - (3/2)] = 1/15.5$, or 0.0645. Again, the proportion surviving is $1 - 0.0645$, or 0.9355. The cumulative proportion surviving is 0.9444×0.9355, or 0.8835. This computation procedure continues until the table is completed.

Note that p_i is the probability of surviving interval i only; and to survive interval i, a patient must have survived all previous intervals as well. Thus, p_i is an example of a conditional probability; that is, the probability of surviving interval i is dependent, or conditional, on surviving until that point, or p_i equals probability (surviving interval i, given survival of previous intervals). This probability is sometimes called the **survival function.** Recall from Chapter 4 that if one event is conditional on a previous event, the probability of their joint occurrence is found by multiplying the probability of the conditional event by the probability of the previous event. The cumulative probability of surviving interval i plus all previous intervals is therefore found by multiplying p_i by $p_{i-1}, p_{i-2}, \cdots p_1$.

The results from an actuarial analysis can help answer questions that may help clinicians counsel patients or their families. For example, we might ask, If X is the length of time survived by a patient selected at random from the population represented by these

dialysis patients, what is the probability that X is 12 months or greater? From Table 9–3, the probability is 0.88, or almost 9 out of 10, that a patient will live for at least 12 months.

Journal articles do not present the results from life table analysis as we have in Table 9–3; rather, the results are usually presented in a survival curve. The solid line in Figure 9–3 is a survival curve for the sample of 18 dialysis patients who continued dialysis treatment. Typically, as the interval from entry into the study becomes longer, the number of patients who were in the study that long becomes increasingly smaller. This means that the standard deviation of the estimate of the proportion surviving gets increasingly larger. Sometimes the number of patients remaining in the study is printed under the time line. Some authors provide graphs with dashed lines on either side of the survival curve that represent 95% **confidence bands** for the curve. The confidence limits become wider as time progresses, reflecting decreased confidence in the estimate of the proportion as the sample size decreases. These practices are desirable, but not all computer programs provide them.

The formula for obtaining confidence bands assumes that under mild censoring and for sufficiently large sample sizes, the proportion surviving at any interval is approximately normally distributed. It uses *Greenwood's formula* for the **standard error** (Greenwood, 1926) and is as follows:

$$SE(S_i) = S_i \sqrt{\Sigma \frac{q_i}{n_i - d_i - (w_i/2)}}$$

The actuarial method involves two assumptions about the data. The first is that all withdrawals during

Life Table
Survival Variable TIME

Table 9–3. Life table for sample of 18 patients who remained on dialysis.

Interval Start Time	n_i Number Entering This Interval	w_i Number Withdrawing during Interval	d_i Number of Terminal Events	Number Exposed to Risk	$q_i = d_i / [n_i - (w_i/2)]$ Proportion Terminating	$p_i = 1 - q_i$ Proportion Surviving	$S_i = p_i p_{i-1} p_{i-2} \cdots p_i$ Cumulative Proportion Surviving at End
0	18	0	1	18	0.0556	0.9444	0.9444
180	17	3	1	15.5	0.0645	0.9355	0.8835
360	13	0	1	13	0.0769	0.9231	0.8156
540	12	5	0	9.5	0.0000	1.0000	0.8156
720	7	1	0	6.5	0.0000	1.0000	0.8156
900	6	4	1	4	0.2500	0.7500	0.6117
1080	1	1	0	0.5	0.0000	1.0000	0.6117

Source: Data, used with permission, from Bajwa K, Szabo E, Kjellstrand CM: A prospective study of risk factors and decision making in discontinuation of dialysis. *Arch Intern Med* 1996;**156**:2571–2577. Output produced with SPSS; used with permission.

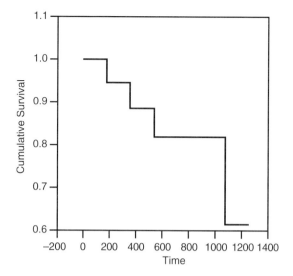

Figure 9–3. Survival curve for sample of 18 patients from the 235 patients. (Used, with permission, from Bajwa K, Szabo E, Kjellstrand CM: A prospective study of risk factors and decision making in discontinuation of dialysis. *Arch Intern Med* 1996;**156:**2571–2577. Figure produced with SPSS; used with permission.)

a given interval occur, on average, at the midpoint of the interval. This assumption is of less consequence when short time intervals are analyzed; however, considerable bias can occur if the intervals are large, if many withdrawals occur, and if withdrawals do not occur midway in the interval. The Kaplan–Meier method introduced in the next section overcomes this problem. The second assumption is that, although survival in a given period depends on survival in all previous periods, the probability of survival at one period is independent of the probability of survival at others. This condition, although probably violated somewhat in much medical research, does not appear to cause major concern to biostatisticians.

9.4 KAPLAN–MEIER PRODUCT LIMIT METHOD

The Kaplan–Meier method of estimating survival is similar to actuarial analysis except that time since entry in the study is not divided into intervals for analysis. For this reason, it is especially appropriate in studies involving a small number of patients. Depending on the number of patients who died, the **Kaplan–Meier product limit method** may involve fewer calculations than the actuarial method, primarily because survival is estimated each time a patient dies, so withdrawals are ignored. An illustration from Presenting Problem 1 on dialysis patients should clarify this statement.

The first step is to list the times when death occurred, as in the column "Day of Death" in Table 9–4. In the dialysis study, one patient died on day 166, one on day 228, one on day 497, and one on day 1031. Then, at the time of each death, the number of patients who are still alive and remain in the study is entered under the column "Number of Patients." For example, 18 patients were alive and in the study at least 166 days, so 18 is entered into this column. One patient died at day 166, so 1 is entered under the column "Number of Deaths. By the time the third patient died at 497 days, only 13 patients were still in the study, and so forth. Patients who are lost to follow-up and those who are still alive but not for the given length of time merely drop out of the calculations by no longer being considered, as patients 4, 18, and 7 do by 497 days. This process continues as illustrated in Table 9–4.

The probability of death is calculated each time a patient dies and is $q_i = d_i/n_i$. As in the actuarial method, the probability of survival at month i is $p_i = 1 - q_i$, and the cumulative survival is $S_i = p_i p_{i-1} p_{i-2} \cdots p_1$.

For example, at day 166, the probability of death is $1/18 = 0.0556$, and the probability of survival is $1 - 0.0556 = 0.9444$. At day 228, the probability of death is $1/17 = 0.0588$, and the probability of survival is 0.9412; however, the cumulative probability of survival is $0.9444 \times 0.9412 = 0.8889$. The complete calculations are given in Table 9–4. Note that the Kaplan–Meier procedure gives exact survival proportions because it uses exact survival times; the actuarial method gives approximations because it groups survival times into intervals. Prior to the widespread use of computers, the actuarial method was much easier to use for a very large number of observations.

The standard error of the cumulative survival estimate S_i is similar to the standard error for an actuarial curve. For the Kaplan–Meier product limit estimate, the standard error is

Table 9–4. Kaplan–Meier product limit estimates of survival for the sample of 18 patients who remained on dialysis.

Day of Death	Number of Patients	Number of Deaths	$q_i = d_i/n_i$	$p_i = 1 - q_i$	$S_i = p_i p_{i-1} p_{i-2} \cdots p_1$
166	18	1	0.0556	0.9444	0.9444
228	17	1	0.0588	0.9412	0.8889
497	13	1	0.0769	0.9231	0.8205
1031	4	1	0.2500	0.7500	0.6154

Source: Data, used with permission, from Bajwa K, Szabo E, Kjellstrand CM: A prospective study of risk factors and decision making in discontinuation of dialysis. *Arch Intern Med* 1996;**156:**2571–2577. Table produced with NCSS; used with permission.

Table 9–5. Calculations for confidence bands for Kaplan-Meier curve for the sample of 18 patients who remained on dialysis.

Day of Death	n_i	d_i	$\dfrac{d_i}{n_i(n_i - d_i)}$	$\sum\left[\dfrac{d_i}{n_i(n_i - d_i)}\right]$	S_i	$S_i\sqrt{\sum\dfrac{d_i}{n_i(n_i - d_i)}}$	1.96SE
166	18	1	0.00327	0.00327	0.9444	0.05399	0.10582
228	17	1	0.00368	0.00694	0.8889	0.07408	0.14519
497	13	1	0.00641	0.01335	0.8205	0.09482	0.18585
1031	4	1	0.08333	0.09669	0.6154	0.19136	0.37506

Source: Data, used with permission, from Bajwa K, Szabo E, Kjellstrand CM: A prospective study of risk factors and decision making in discontinuation of dialysis. *Arch Intern Med* 1996;**156**:2571–2577. Table produced with NCSS; used with permission.

$$SE(S_i) = S_i\sqrt{\sum \dfrac{d_i}{n_i(n_i - d_i)}}$$

For example, at day 166, 18 patients are still in the study and 1 death has occurred, so

$$\dfrac{d_i}{n_i(n_i - d_i)} = \dfrac{1}{18 \times 17}$$
$$= 0.00327$$

and the standard error is

$$SE(S_i) = S_i\sqrt{\sum \dfrac{d_i}{n_i(n_i - d_i)}}$$
$$= 0.9444 \sqrt{0.00327} = 0.05399$$

The remaining calculations are given in Table 9–5.

Figure 9–4 is a graph of the Kaplan–Meier product limit curve for the sample of 18 patients who continued dialysis. In this graph, the curve is step-like because the proportion of patients surviving changes precisely at the points when a subject dies.

Table 9–6 shows the analysis of these same 18 patients produced by the NCSS computer program. Note that the program lists the length of time each patient is in the study but calculates the survival function and its standard error only for the days corresponding to patient deaths. The figure also contains the analysis for the seven patients who discontinued dialysis. Because all of these patients died, the calculations are done for every patient.

Figure 9–5 is a graph of the Kaplan–Meier product limit curves for both groups of patients. This graph illustrates the vast difference in survival for those patients who remain on dialysis versus those who stop. Although this is just a sample, we will see that survival curves of the entire sample of 235 patients are not dissimilar.

Before continuing with the discussion, we present the analysis of the entire sample of 235 patients in the dialysis study by Bajwa and colleagues (1996). Two hundred twenty-two patients continued with dialysis, and 13 patients opted to discontinue. The Kaplan–Meier survival curves are given in Figure 9–6.

The difference in the survival curves for the two groups appears to be large, based on Figure 9–6. As with all similar statements, however, we know it is important to perform a statistical test to evaluate the degree of any differences. We illustrate this analysis in the next section.

 Use the CD-ROM and replicate our analysis to produce the survival curves.

9.5 COMPARING TWO SURVIVAL CURVES

Although some journal articles report survival statistics for only one group, more often investigators wish to compare survival between two or more samples of patients. To illustrate the computations involved in comparing two survival distributions, we compare survival times for patients who continued

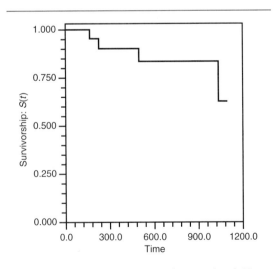

Figure 9–4. Kaplan–Meier curve for sample of 18 patients who continued dialysis. (Used, with permission, from Bajwa K, Szabo E, Kjellstrand CM: A prospective study of risk factors and decision making in discontinuation of dialysis. *Arch Intern Med* 1996;**156**:2571–2577. Figure produced with NCSS; used with permission.)

Table 9–6. Kaplan–Meier analysis for sample of 25 patients from the 235 patients.

Survival Analysis Report

Time variable	TIME
Censor variable	CENS
Group variable	STOP

Kaplan–Meier Product Limit Survival Distribution. STOP = 0

Rank	Sample Size	Time	Survivorship S(t)	Standard Error of S(t)	Hazard Fn H(t) = −log (S(t))	Standard Error of H(t)
1	18	166.0	0.944444	0.053990	0.057158	0.246026
2	17	228.0	0.888889	0.074074	0.117783	0.306186
3	16	296.0+				
4	15	346.0+				
5	14	357.0+				
6	13	497.0	0.820513	0.094821	0.197826	0.375289
7	12	619.0+				
8	11	632.0+				
9	10	643.0+				
10	9	650.0+				
11	8	695.0+				
12	7	828.0+				
13	6	1016.0+				
14	5	1022.0+				
15	4	1031.0	0.615385	0.191352	0.485508	0.710837
16	3	1059.0+				
17	2	1064.0+				
18	1	1097.0+				

Kaplan–Meier Product Limit Survival Distribution. STOP = 1

Rank	Sample Size	Time	Survivorship S(t)	Standard Error of S(t)	Hazard Fn H(t) = −log (S(t))	Standard Error of H(t)
1	7	63.0	0.857143	0.132260	0.154151	0.424288
2	6	76.0	0.714286	0.170747	0.336472	0.578502
3	5	158.0	0.571429	0.187044	0.559616	0.756850
4	4	174.0	0.428571	0.187044	0.847298	1.009133
5	3	576.0	0.285714	0.170747	1.252763	1.446254
6	2	860.0	0.142857	0.132260	1.945910	2.545730
7	1	969.0	0.000000	0.000000	0.000000	0.000000

Source: Data, used with permission, from Bajwa K, Szabo E, Kjellstrand CM: A prospective study of risk factors and decision making in discontinuation of dialysis. *Arch Intern Med* 1996;**156:**2571–2577. Table produced with NCSS; used with permission.

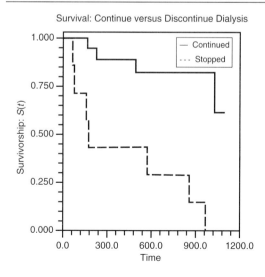

Figure 9–5. Kaplan–Meier survival curve for sample of 25 patients from the 235 patients. (Used, with permission, from Bajwa K, Szabo E, Kjellstrand CM: A prospective study of risk factors and decision making in discontinuation of dialysis. *Arch Intern Med* 1996;**156:**2571–2577. Figure produced with NCSS; used with permission.)

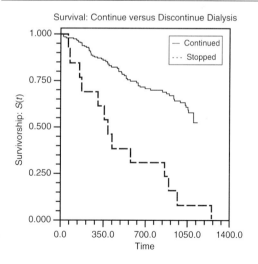

Figure 9–6. Kaplan–Meier survival curve comparing patients who continued versus those who stopped dialysis. (Used, with permission, from Bajwa K, Szabo E, Kjellstrand CM: A prospective study of risk factors and decision making in discontinuation of dialysis. *Arch Intern Med* 1996;**156:**2571–2577. Figure produced with NCSS; used with permission.)

dialysis with those for patients who stopped (Bajwa et al, 1996).

As seen in Figure 9–6, the survival curve for patients continuing dialysis is above the curve for patients who stopped, indicating that a higher proportion of patients in the former group survived at any point in time. Variation in samples may be expected to occur, however, simply by chance, and a reasonable question is whether the difference between the two patient groups is greater than expected by chance. To test this hypothesis, we need methods to compare survival distributions. If no censored observations occur, the **Wilcoxon rank sum test** introduced in Chapter 6 is appropriate for comparing the ranks of survival time. The independent-groups t test is not appropriate because survival times are not normally distributed; they tend to be positively skewed (extremely so, in some cases). If some observations are censored, however, other procedures must be used.

Several methods may be used to compare survival curves when censored observations occur. At one time, a larger number of procedures appeared in the medical literature than is the case now. Most articles report a comparison of survival curves using the logrank statistic. Another statistic that is reported with some frequency is the Mantel–Haenszel chi-square statistic. This method has the added advantage of being applicable in situations other than comparing survival curves.

The computations for all of the methods are very time-consuming, and computer programs are readily available. We discuss the logrank and Mantel–Haenszel methods in detail. Both methods are straightforward, if computationally onerous, and are useful in helping us understand the logic behind the method. Within the context of the logrank statistic, we illustrate the hazard ratio, a useful descriptive statistic for comparing two groups at risk. Then we briefly describe some of the other methods and how they differ in their logic and approach.

9.5.1 The Logrank Test

Several forms of the logrank statistic have been published by different biostatisticians, so it is called by several different names in the literature: the Mantel logrank statistic, the Cox–Mantel logrank statistic, and simply the logrank statistic. The **logrank test** compares the number of observed deaths in each group with the number of deaths that would be expected from the number of deaths in the combined groups, that is, if group membership did not matter. An approximate **chi-square test** is used to test the significance of a mathematical expression involving the observed and expected number of deaths.

To facilitate the illustration of the logrank statistic, we first discuss an example in which survival is examined by intervals of time. We grouped the data for the entire sample of 235 dialysis patients into 180-day time intervals (Table 9–7).

The steps for calculating the logrank statistic follow.

1. The second and third columns contain the number of patients in each group (those who continued and those who stopped dialysis, respectively) who were at risk of dying during the time interval. Thus, at 0 to 180 days, all patients in each sample, 222 who continued dialysis and 13 who stopped, were at risk. At 181–360 days, patients who previously died or were censored (not having been in the study that long) are subtracted to obtain the number of patients still at risk, resulting in 202 and 9, respectively, still

Table 9–7. Illustration of calculations for the logrank statistic using entire sample of 235 dialysis patients.

Time Period	Number of Patients at Risk			Number of Observed Deaths			Number of Expected Deaths[a]		
	Continued	Stopped	Total	Continued	Stopped	Total	Continued	Stopped	Total
0–180	222	13	235	13	4	17	16.06	0.94	17
181–360	202	9	211	16	2	18	17.23	0.77	18
361–540	125	7	132	13	2	15	14.20	0.80	15
541–720	100	5	105	7	1	8	7.62	0.38	8
721–900	80	4	84	5	2	7	6.67	0.33	7
901–1080	71	2	73	8	1	9	8.75	0.25	9
1081–1260	12	1	13	1	1	2	1.85	0.15	2
Totals				63	13	76	72.38	3.62	76

Calculations of the logrank statistic

O − E	(O − E)^2	(O − E)^2/E	Sum
−9.38164	88.0151728	1.21598754	25.541
9.3816402	88.0151728	24.324605	

[a]Expected deaths are the total number of observed deaths times the proportion at risk in each population.
Source: Data, used with permission, from Bajwa K, Szabo E, Kjellstrand CM: A prospective study of risk factors and decision making in discontinuation of dialysis. *Arch Intern Med* 1996;**156:**2571–2577. Table produced with Microsoft Excel; used with permission.

at risk. In column 4, the total number at risk in the combined samples is given; that is, the sum of columns 2 and 3. This calculation continues through all periods.

2. In the fifth through the seventh columns, the number of patients in each group who died during that interval and the total number of deaths are listed. Thus, at 0–180 days, 13 patients who continued dialysis and 4 patients who stopped died. This calculation continues through all periods.

3. The last three columns contain the *expected* number of deaths for each group and the total at each period. The expected number of deaths for a given group is found by multiplying the total number of deaths in a given period by the proportion of patients in that group. For example, at 0–180 days, 17 deaths are noted; so $17 \times (222/235)$ is the number of deaths expected to occur among the patients who continued dialysis, and $17 \times (13/235)$ is the number of deaths expected to occur among the patients who stopped dialysis. This calculation continues through all periods.

4. The totals are calculated for each column. The following expression can be used to test the null hypothesis that the survival distributions are the same in the two groups:

$$\chi^2 = \frac{(O_1 - E_1)^2}{E_1} + \frac{(O_2 - E_2)^2}{E_2}$$

where O_1 is the total number of observed losses in group 1, E_1 is the total number of expected failures in group 1, and so forth. The statistic χ^2 follows an approximate chi-square distribution with 1 degree of freedom. In our example, the calculation is

$$\chi^2 = \frac{(63 - 72.38)^2}{72.38} + \frac{(13 - 3.62)^2}{3.62}$$
$$= 1.216 + 24.325$$
$$= 25.541$$

Consulting the chi-square distribution with 1 degree of freedom in Table A–5 indicates that the area above 25.541 is less than 0.001. We therefore conclude that a statistically significant difference exists in the distributions of survival times for patients who remained on dialysis versus those who stopped treatment.

Computer programs that calculate the logrank statistic do so without dividing the deaths, or failures, into periods. Instead, they calculate the observed and expected number of failures at each time that a patient dies or is censored (because he or she has been in the study for only that length of time). We reproduce the procedure for the sample of 25 patients in Table 9–8.

The procedure is exactly as we illustrated earlier: At each time an event (death or censoring) occurs, the number of patients at risk, the number of deaths, and the expected number of deaths are calculated. To illustrate, look at the line represented by the patient who

died at 576 days. At this time, 12 of the 18 patients who continued dialysis are still in the study, compared with only 3 of the 7 who stopped, for a total of 15 patients. The death is noted in the sixth column. The expected number of deaths in the continuation group is found by multiplying the number of deaths, 1, by the proportion at risk, 12 of a total of 15 patients at that time: $1 \times (12/15) = 0.8$. For the group that stopped, the expected number of deaths is $1 \times (3/15) = 0.2$.

After all the observed and expected numbers of deaths are recorded, the totals are found, and the calculation of the logrank statistic is done in the same manner as we described earlier. The value of the logrank statistic for this sample of 25 patients is 11.21 and again is significant. Use the CD-ROM and find the value of the logrank statistic for this sample. Is it in close agreement with our calculations?

9.5.2 The Hazard Ratio

One benefit of calculating the logrank statistic is that the **hazard ratio** can easily be calculated from the information given in Table 9–7. It is estimated by O_1/E_1 divided by O_2/E_2. In our example, the hazard ratio, or risk of death, in those who stopped dialysis compared with those who continued is

$$\text{Hazard ratio} = \frac{13/3.62}{63/72.38} = \frac{3.59}{0.87} = 4.13$$

Note that we reversed the groups and placed the group that discontinued dialysis in the numerator because it is the group at greater risk. The hazard ratio of 4.13 can be interpreted in a similar manner as the odds ratio: The risk of death at any time in the group that stops dialysis is approximately 4 times greater than the risk in the group that continues dialysis. Using the hazard ratio assumes that the hazard or risk of death is the same throughout the time of the study.

9.5.3 The Mantel–Haenszel Chi-Square Statistic

Another method for comparing survival distributions is an estimate of the odds ratio developed by Mantel and Haenszel that follows (approximately) a chi-square distribution with 1 degree of freedom. The **Mantel–Haenszel test** combines a series of 2×2 tables formed at different survival times into an overall test of significance of the survival curves.

We again use data from Presenting Problem 1 to illustrate the calculation of the Mantel–Haenszel statistic (see Table 9–9). The first step is to select the time intervals for which 2×2 tables will be formed; we use the 180-day intervals as before. For each time interval, the number of patients who were still alive and the number who died are the rows, and the number of patients in each group are the columns of the 2×2 tables.

As with the logrank test, the Mantel–Haenszel test is fairly onerous to compute. The first step estimates

Table 9–8. Illustration of calculations for the logrank statistic for sample of 25 dialysis patients.

Time of Event[a]	Number of Patients at Risk			Number of Observed Deaths			Number of Expected Deaths[b]		
	Continued	Stopped	Total	Continued	Stopped	Total	Continued	Stopped	Total
63	18	7	25	0	1	1	0.72	0.28	1
76	18	6	24	0	1	1	0.75	0.25	1
158	18	5	23	0	1	1	0.78	0.22	1
166	17	5	22	1	0	1	0.77	0.23	1
174	17	4	21	0	1	1	0.81	0.19	1
228	16	4	20	1	0	1	0.80	0.20	1
296	15	4	19	0	0	0	0.00	0.00	0
346	14	4	18	0	0	0	0.00	0.00	0
357	13	4	17	0	0	0	0.00	0.00	0
497	12	4	16	1	0	1	0.75	0.25	1
576	12	3	15	0	1	1	0.80	0.20	1
619	11	3	14	0	0	0	0.00	0.00	0
632	10	3	13	0	0	0	0.00	0.00	0
643	9	3	12	0	0	0	0.00	0.00	0
650	8	3	11	0	0	0	0.00	0.00	0
695	7	3	10	0	0	0	0.00	0.00	0
828	6	3	9	0	0	0	0.00	0.00	0
860	6	2	8	0	1	1	0.75	0.25	1
969	6	1	7	0	1	1	0.86	0.14	1
1016	6	0	6	0	0	0	0.00	0.00	0
1022	5	0	5	0	0	0	0.00	0.00	0
1031	4	1	5	1	0	1	0.80	0.20	1
1059	3	0	3	0	0	0	0.00	0.00	0
1064	2	0	2	0	0	0	0.00	0.00	0
1097	1	0	1	0	0	0	0.00	0.00	0
Totals				4	7	11	8.59	2.41	11

Calculations of the logrank statistic

$O - E$	$(O - E)^2$	$(O - E)^2/E$	Sum
−4.59	21.0864882	2.4541995	11.211
4.59	21.0864882	8.7568568	

[a]Shaded observations correspond to patients who stopped dialysis.
[b]Expected deaths are the total number of observed deaths times the proportion at risk in each population.
Source: Data, used with permission, from Bajwa K, Szabo E, Kjellstrand CM: A prospective study of risk factors and decision making in discontinuation of dialysis. *Arch Intern Med* 1996;**156**:2571–2577. Table produced with Microsoft Excel; used with permission.

a pooled odds ratio, which is useful for descriptive purposes but is not needed for the statistical test itself. The estimate is

$$OR = \frac{\Sigma(a \times d/n)}{\Sigma(b \times c/n)}$$

where a, b, c, d, and n are defined as they were in the 2×2 table in Table 6–11. The numerator and denominator are calculated in the columns under the heading "Odds Ratio." The sum of the terms in the numerator is 11.40 and in the denominator is 2.02. The estimate of the odds ratio using the Mantel–Haenszel approach is therefore 11.40/2.02 = 5.65. The hypothesis to be tested is whether 5.65 differs from 1.

The Mantel–Haenszel chi-square test is an approximate test. The formula and details of its calculations for the dialysis example are given in Table 9–9. The totals for rows and columns for each 2×2 table are calculated. The Mantel–Haenszel statistic focuses on cell (1, 1) of the table and calculates its expected value and

the variance of the expected value for each 2×2 table. For example, at 361–540 days, among the 125 patients who continued dialysis and who lived or were in the study at least 361 days, 112 remained alive and 13 died in that period. Among the seven patients who stopped dialysis and lived at least 361 days, five remained alive and two died. The expected values are found in the same manner as in the chi-square test discussed in Chapter 6. For example, the expected value of cell (1, 1) in this period is the row total times the column total divided by the grand total:

$$E(a_i) = \frac{\text{Row total} \times \text{Column total}}{\text{Grand total}}$$
$$= \frac{125 \times 117}{132} = 110.80$$

In addition, the variance of cell (1, 1) is calculated. Using the notation from Table 6–11, the estimated variance is

Table 9–9. Illustration of calculations for the Mantel–Haenszel chi-square statistic using the entire sample of 235 dialysis patients.

Time Period	Status	2 × 2 Table			Odds Ratio		Observed	Expected	Variance
		Continued	Stopped	Total	ad/n	bc/n	a_i	$E(a_i)$	$V(a_i)$
0–180	Lived	209	9	218	3.56	0.50	209	205.94	0.83
	Died	13	4	17					
	Total	222	13	235					
181–360	Lived	186	7	193	1.76	0.53	186	184.77	0.68
	Died	16	2	18					
	Total	202	9	211					
361–540	Lived	112	5	117	1.70	0.49	112	110.80	0.67
	Died	13	2	15					
	Total	125	7	132					
541–720	Lived	93	4	97	0.89	0.27	93	92.38	0.34
	Died	7	1	8					
	Total	100	5	105					
721–900	Lived	75	2	77	1.79	0.12	75	73.33	0.29
	Died	5	2	7					
	Total	80	4	84					
901–1080	Lived	63	1	64	0.86	0.11	63	62.25	0.21
	Died	8	1	9					
	Total	71	2	73					
1081–1260	Lived	11	0	11	0.85	0.00	11	10.15	0.13
	Died	1	1	2					
	Total	12	1	13					
	Sums				**11.40**	**2.02**	**749**	**739.62**	**3.15**
							Odds ratio		**5.65**
							Mantel–Haenszel chi-square		**27.92**

Source: Data, used with permission, from Bajwa K, Szabo E, Kjellstrand CM: A prospective study of risk factors and decision making in discontinuation of dialysis. *Arch Intern Med* 1996;**156:**2571–2577. Table produced with Microsoft Excel; used with permission.

$$V(a_i) = \left[\frac{(a + c)(b + d)(a + b)(c + d)}{(n)(n)(n - 1)} \right]$$

For this period, the variance is

$$\frac{[125 \times 7 \times 117 \times 15]}{[132 \times 132 \times 131]} = 0.67$$

After the expected value and the variance are found for each 2 × 2 table, these values are added, along with the number of observed patients in cell (1, 1) in each table. The three sums are 749, 739.62, and 3.15, as you can see in Table 9–9. The Mantel–Haenszel test is the squared difference between the sum of the observed number minus the sum of the expected number, all divided by the sum of the variances:

$$\text{Mantel–Haenszel} = \frac{[|\Sigma a_i - \Sigma E(a_i)|]^2}{\Sigma V(a_i)}$$

$$= \frac{[|749 - 739.62|]^2}{3.15} = 27.92$$

This value is somewhat larger than the value we found for the logrank test, but not terribly so. The Mantel–Haenszel statistic is very useful because it can be used to compare any distributions, not simply survival curves.

9.5.4 Summary of Procedures to Compare Survival Distributions

The logrank and Mantel–Haenszel statistics are used with a great deal of frequency in the medical literature. Several other methods are seen on occasion, however. Peto and Peto developed an alternative approach to the logrank test, which is sometimes referred to in journal articles as well. The logrank procedure gives all calculations the same weight, regardless of the time at which a death occurs. In contrast, the Peto logrank test weights the terms (observed minus expected) by the number of patients at risk at that time. This results in a weighted average that gives more weight to early deaths when the number of patients at risk is large. Some biostatisticians choose this method because they believe that calculations based on larger sample sizes should receive more weight than calculations based on smaller sample sizes that occur later in time. If the pattern of deaths is similar over time, the Peto logrank statistic and the logrank statistic illustrated earlier generally lead to the same conclusion. If, however, a higher proportion of deaths occurs during one interval, such as sometimes occurs early in the survival curve, the Peto logrank test and the logrank test may differ.

Little information is available to guide investigators in deciding which procedure is appropriate in any given application. In addition, readers of journal articles sometimes cannot determine which procedure actually was used. It is unfortunate that many of the statistical procedures used to compare survival distributions are called by a variety of names. Part of the confusion has occurred because the same biostatisticians (eg, Mantel, Gehan, Cox, Peto and Peto, Haenszel) are active researchers and have developed a number of statistical tests. Another source of confusion is that research on biostatistical methods for analyzing survival data is still underway; as a result, the Mantel procedure and the Peto logrank procedure were only recently shown to be equivalent.

The Mantel–Haenszel chi-square test is sometimes referred to as the logrank test in some texts, and although it is technically different, it generally leads to the same conclusion. This statistic actually may be considered an extension of the logrank test because it can be used in more general situations. For example, the Mantel–Haenszel chi-square test can be used to combine two or more 2×2 tables in other situations, such as a 2×2 table for men and a 2×2 table for women. This procedure is similar to other methods to control for confounding factors, topics discussed in Chapter 10.

To summarize, all logrank tests, regardless of what they are called, and the Mantel–Haenszel chi-square test may be considered similar procedures. The Gehan and Wilcoxon tests, however, are conceptually different. The **Gehan, or generalized Wilcoxon, test** is an extension of the Wilcoxon rank sum test illustrated in Chapter 6; however, it has been modified so that it can be used with censored observations (Gehan, 1965). This test is also referred to in the literature as the Breslow test or the generalized Kruskal–Wallis test for comparison of more than two

samples (Kalbfleisch and Prentice, 1980). Unfortunately, no one has yet developed a simple approximation, such as converting original observations to ranks and calculating the t statistic for ranks. As with the Peto logrank test, the generalized Wilcoxon test uses the number of patients at risk as weights. The generalized Wilcoxon test therefore counts losses that occur early in the survival distribution more heavily than losses that occur late because sample sizes are larger in early months relative to late months.

Another difference between these two families of tests is that the logrank statistic assumes that the ratio of hazard rates in the two groups stays the same throughout the period of interest. When a constant hazard ratio cannot be assumed, the generalized Wilcoxon procedure is preferred. The procedure is also preferable when data come from a distribution called the Weibell distribution, whereas the logrank procedures are better with exponential distributions. In the special situation in which the hazard rates are proportional, a method called **Cox's proportional hazard model** can be used; it is seen with some regularity in evaluating potential risk factors related to survival or a morbid event; this method is discussed in Chapter 10.

As you can see, the issue is complex and illustrates the advisability of consulting a statistician if performing a survival analysis. Readers who want more information are referred to the Lee (1992) text, which is possibly the most comprehensive text available. An introductory text devoted to survival analysis is that by Kleinbaum (1996). Other texts that discuss survival methods include books by Altman (1991a), Breslow and Day (1987; 1993), Collett (1994), Fisher and van Belle (1993), Fleiss (1981; 1999), and Schlesselman (1982).

Many of the statistical computer programs provide several test statistics for survival, but they generally provide at least one from the Gehan/Wilcoxon family and one from the logrank group. NCSS gives four statistics, the Peto/Wilcoxon and Gehan's Wilcoxon test, the logrank test, and the Cox–Mantel test. BMDP also employs the Cox–Mantel method. NCSS also computes the Mantel–Haenszel chi-square; it is a separate procedure and requires that the data file be reorganized as done in Table 9–9. SPSS provides the Gehan statistic with the actuarial, or life table, analysis procedure. In the Kaplan–Meier method, SPSS gives the Breslow test, the logrank test we discussed earlier, and another procedure developed by Tarone and Ware (1997). JMP gives two tests: the Wilcoxon test and the logrank test. SYSTAT provides the Breslow–Gehan test, the logrank test, and the test by Tarone and Ware.

9.6 THE HAZARD FUNCTION IN SURVIVAL ANALYSIS

In the introduction to this chapter, we stated that calculating mean survival is generally not useful, and we subsequently illustrated how its value depends on the time when the data are analyzed. Estimates of mean survival that are reasonable can be obtained, however, when the sample size is fairly large. This procedure depends on the **hazard function,** which is the probability that a person dies in time interval i to $i + 1$, given that the person has survived until time i. The hazard function is also called the conditional failure rate; in epidemiology, the term *force of mortality* is used.

Although the **exponential probability distribution** was not discussed in Chapter 4 when we introduced other probability distributions, such as the normal, binomial, and Poisson distributions, many survival curves follow an exponential distribution. It is a continuous distribution that involves the natural logarithm, ln, and it depends on a constant rate (which determines the shape of the curve) and on time. It provides a model for describing processes such as radioactive decay.

If an exponential distribution is a reasonable assumption for the shape of a survival curve, then the following formula can be used to estimate the hazard rate, symbolized by the letter H, when censored observations occur:

$$H = \frac{d}{\Sigma f + \Sigma c}$$

where d is the number of deaths, Σf is the sum of failure times, and Σc is the sum of censored times.

If you refer again to Table 9–6, note that the NCSS computer program calculates both the hazard function and its standard error as part of the Kaplan–Meier analysis. For the sample of 18 patients who continued dialysis, the estimated hazard function is 0.4855. When the assumption of an exponential distribution with a constant failure rate is not tenable, other forms of the hazard function based on different probability distributions are used. Details on using the hazard function are given in the comprehensive text on survival analysis by Lee (1992).

9.7 INTERPRETING SURVIVAL CURVES FROM THE LITERATURE

In the study described in Presenting Problem 2, the authors presented 20-year survival information for 1698 patients who underwent coronary bypass surgery between 1968 and 1975 (Lawrie et al, 1991). They provided survival curves for a number of subgroups; groups defined by the vessel involved are displayed in Figure 9–7. The authors use the expected survival for age- and sex-adjusted population from the 1970 U. S. census to provide a baseline comparison in this figure. The curves themselves

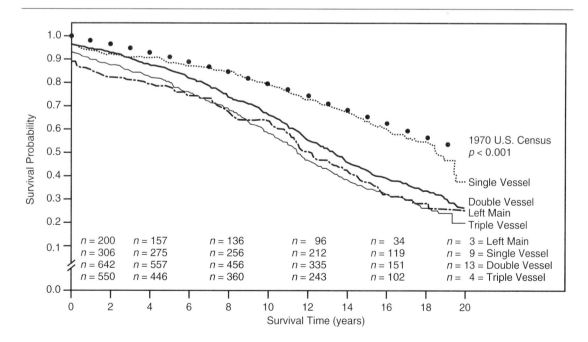

Figure 9–7. Survival probabilities for 1698 patients according to the extent of coronary artery disease before operation. (Reproduced, with permission, from Figure 3 in Lawrie GM, Morris GC, Earle N: Long-term results of coronary bypass surgery. *Ann Surg* 1991;**213:**377–385.)

were calculated using the Kaplan–Meier method. The source of the statistical test for the P value given in the table is not completely clear; the investigators stated they used chi-square tests and analysis of variance but did not specify how they compared the survival curves.

What conclusions are possible from Figure 9–7? Clearly, survival was best for patients whose disease was restricted to a single vessel; the survival for this group was the same as for the age- and sex-adjusted reference population for several years (between 7 and 14 years after surgery). The highest mortality rate was observed among patients with left main vessel or triple-vessel disease; the median survival for these two groups was approximately 12 years.

This study also reported that age at operation, diabetes mellitus, systolic hypertension, and a history of stroke, as well as the extent of coronary disease, were significant predictors of survival. Total serum cholesterol level was not a risk factor for early mortality. It should be emphasized that the current practice of coronary artery bypass surgery differs in several respects from the methods employed in this study. Saphenous vein was used exclusively in this study, whereas now at least one internal mammary bypass is performed in most patients. Newer cardiovascular drugs, including beta-blockers and calcium channel blockers, are currently in common use but were not used in most of these study patients at the time of their surgery. Improved techniques in current use are expected to contribute to more favorable long-term results.

The investigators in the study described in Presenting Problem 3 (Crook et al, 1997) reported on a group of 207 men followed prospectively after treatment for prostate carcinoma with radiotherapy. The patients were treated between January 1990 and February 1994. Follow-up included systematic transrectal ultrasound-guided biopsies and measurements of serum prostate-specific antigen (PSA) levels. The median duration of follow-up for the patients at the time of analysis was 36 months, with a range from 12 to 70 months. Failures were observed in 68 patients. The investigators wanted to look at the relationship between patient outcome and both the stage of the tumor at diagnosis and pretreatment PSA levels. Time-dependent variables, survival, and time to failure were examined using the Kaplan–Meier product limit method. All outcomes were calculated from the time the patient completed radiotherapy. The curves were compared using the logrank test. This study is an example in which the outcome is not necessarily patient survival but is instead the failure of treatment, which may occur in several different ways. For example, patients were categorized by whether they had a local, distant, or chemical failure. The investigators examined the relationship between multiple variables and the time until failure using the Cox proportional hazard model; we return to this study when we discuss this method in Chapter 10.

The authors presented six different survival curves:

1. Overall survival by tumor stage
2. Disease-free survival by tumor stage
3. Time to any failure by pretreatment PSA level (divided into six categories)
4. Time to local failure
5. Time to distant failure
6. Time to any failure by the lowest (nadir) posttreatment PSA

We reproduced two of the figures using the NCSS computer program and the data provided by the authors. Figure 9–8 shows the disease-free survival curves for patients categorized by their tumor stage (T classification) using the NCSS computer program. The curves for T1b–c and T2a are very similar and, in fact, cross several times. The survival rate was very high in these two groups for the first 2 years following treatment. Even without a statistical test, it appears that the survival pattern for patients with these tumor stages follows similar survival curves. The situation is different for those with stages T2b–c and T3–4. Survival rates in these two stages are considerably lower. Both curves demonstrate a fairly steady decrease in disease-free survival over time.

Table 9–10 gives the results of the statistical tests comparing the survival curves using the NCSS computer program. You can see that the values for

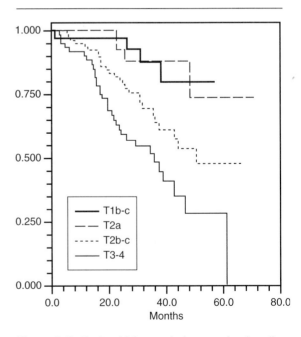

Figure 9–8. Kaplan–Meier survival curve showing disease-free survival by tumor state. (Used, with permission, from Crook JM et al: Radiotherapy for localized prostate carcinoma. *Cancer* 1997;**79**:328–336. Figure produced with NCSS; used with permission.)

Table 9–10. Statistical tests for survival curves by tumor stages.

Gehan–Wilcoxon Section

Tumor Stage Value	Failed Count	Censored Count	Total Count	Sum	Mean
T1b–c	4	30	34	1231.00	36.2059
T2a	4	30	34	1255.00	36.9118
T2b–c	27	52	79	−15.00	−0.1899
T3–4	33	27	60	−2471.00	−41.1833
Chi-square = 25.94	df = 3	Probability = 0.000010			

Peto–Wilcoxon Section

Tumor Stage Value	Failed Count	Censored Count	Total Count	Sum	Mean
T1b–c	4	30	34	−7.02	−0.2066
T2a	4	30	34	−7.28	−0.2141
T2b–c	27	52	79	0.37	0.0047
T3–4	33	27	60	13.93	0.2322
Chi-square = 27.98	df = 3	Probability = 0.000004			

Logrank Section

Tumor Stage Value	Failed Count	Censored Count	Total Count	Sum	Mean
T1b–c	4	30	34	−8.55	−0.2514
T2a	4	30	34	−8.74	−0.2571
T2b–c	27	52	79	0.66	0.0084
T3–4	33	27	60	16.63	0.2771
Chi-square = 27.70	df = 3	Probability = 0.000004			

Source: Data, used with permission, from Crook JM et al: Radiotherapy for localized prostate carcinoma. *Cancer* 1997;**79**:328–336. Output produced with NCSS; used with permission.

the three procedures are in close agreement: the Gehan–Wilcoxon chi-square is 25.94, the Peto–Wilcoxon is 27.98, and the logrank is 27.70. All are highly significant and substantiate our tentative conclusion that the curves, certainly for tumor stages T2b–c and T3–4, are significantly lower, indicating earlier deaths in patients with these two tumor stages. We can use the filter procedure in NCSS or SPSS to select a subset of the cases to learn if the curves for patients with tumor stages T2b–c and T3–4 differ. Selecting only the patients with stages T2b–c and T3–4 gives a chi-square value for the logrank statistic of 6.81 with a *P* value of 0.009. We suggest you replicate these analyses using the CD-ROM.

Figure 9–9 shows the six survival curves for the patients categorized according to their pretreatment PSA levels using the NCSS computer program. The investigators formed these six categories of PSA level: 0–5, 5.1–10, 10.1–15, 15.1–20, 20.1–50, and >50.

Is the pattern of survival what you would expect; that is, that patients with lower pretreatment PSA values survive longer, on average? What would you advise a patient with a PSA level of 3? It appears that such a patient has a very good chance of survival to 5 or 6 years, although it is important to remember that the curves are based on a small number of patients. The problem associated with small samples is exacerbated when the subjects are divided into groups. What would you tell a patient who inquires about survival if he has a pretreatment PSA level greater than 15?

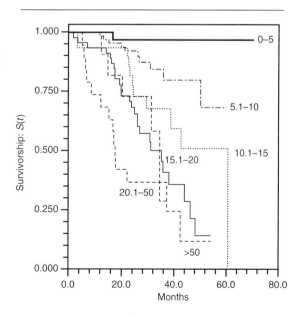

Figure 9–9. Kaplan–Meier survival curve showing time to any failure by pretreatment PSA level group. (Used, with permission, from Crook JM et al: Radiotherapy for localized prostate carcinoma. *Cancer* 1997;**79**:328–336. Figure produced with NCSS; used with permission.)

Use the CD-ROM to determine the logrank statistic for survival by pretreatment PSA. We produced the output in Table 9–11.

9.8 THE INTENTION-TO-TREAT PRINCIPLE

In the method section of journal articles that report clinical trial results, investigators often state that they analyzed the data on an **intention-to-treat** basis. For instance, Presenting Problem 6 in Chapter 3 described a study evaluating antenatal administration of thyrotropin-releasing hormone to improve pulmonary outcome in preterm infants (Ballard et al, 1998). The study consisted of 996 women in active labor who were randomized to receive an injection of thyrotropin-releasing hormone or normal saline. The primary outcome was infant death on or before the 28th day after delivery or chronic lung disease, defined as the need for oxygen therapy for 21 of the first 28 days of life.

In the method section, the researchers state: "All analyses were based on the intention-to-treat principle...." This statement means that the results for each patient who entered the trial were included in the analysis of the group to which the patient was randomized, regardless of any subsequent events. In Ballard and coworkers' study, 18 women in the treatment group (3.7%) and 7 in the placebo group (1.4%) withdrew from the trial because of side effects. These patients, however, were included in the analysis.

Analyzing data on an intention-to-treat basis is appropriate for several reasons. First is the issue of dropouts, as in the study by Ballard and coworkers. Although the percentage of patients dropping out of this study was relatively small, more than twice as many patients dropped out of the treatment group than from the control group. Is it possible that the patients who dropped out of the treatment group had

some characteristics that, independent of the treatment, could affect the outcome? Suppose, for instance, that the women who dropped out of the study had gestations of fewer than 26 weeks. Women with gestations of fewer than 26 weeks are more likely to have infants with respiratory distress. If these patients are omitted from the analysis, the results may appear to be better for the early-gestation group than they should; that is, the results are biased. Although there is no indication that this occurred in the study by Ballard and coworkers, it is easy to see how such events could affect the conclusions, and these investigators were correct to analyze the data on the intention-to-treat basis.

The intention-to-treat principle is also important in studies in which patients cross over from one treatment group to another. For example, the classic Coronary Artery Surgery Study (CASS, 1983) was a randomized trial of coronary bypass surgery. Patients were assigned to medical treatment or surgical intervention to evaluate the effect of treatment on outcomes for patients with coronary artery disease. As in many studies that compare a conservative treatment with a more aggressive intervention, some patients in the CASS study who were randomized to medical treatment subsequently underwent surgery. And, some patients randomized to surgery were treated medically instead.

The problem with studies in which patients cross over from one treatment to another is that we do not know why the crossover occurred. Did some of the patients originally assigned to medical treatment improve so that they became candidates for surgery? If so, this could cause results in the surgery group to appear better than they really were (because "healthier" patients were removed from the medical group and transferred to the surgery group). On the other hand, perhaps the condition of the patients originally assigned to medical treatment worsened to such a de-

Table 9–11. Statistics comparing time to any failure by pretreatment PSA group.

Survival Analysis for Months of Survival

		Total	Number of Events	Number Censored	Percent Censored
GPPREPSA	1.0 to 5.0	34	1	33	97.06
GPPREPSA	5.1 to 10.0	66	10	56	84.85
GPPREPSA	10.1 to 15.0	31	11	20	64.52
GPPREPSA	15.1 to 20.0	11	5	6	54.55
GPPREPSA	20.1 to 50	46	26	20	43.48
GPPREPSA	> 50.0	19	15	4	21.05
Overall		207	68	139	67.15

Test Statistics for Equality of Survival Distributions for PSA Pretreatment Groups

	Statistic	df	Significance
Logrank	64.73	5	0.0000
Breslow	56.64	5	0.0000
Tarone–Ware	60.41	5	0.0000

Source: Data, used with permission, from Crook JM et al: Radiotherapy for localized prostate carcinoma. *Cancer* 1997;**79**:328–336. Produced with SPSS; used with permission.

gree that the patient or family insisted on having surgery. If so, this could cause the surgery group results to appear worse than they really were (because "sicker" patients were transferred from the medical to the surgical group). The point is, we do not know why the patients crossed over, and neither do the investigators.

In the past, some investigators presented with such a situation analyzed the patients by the group they were in at the end of the study. Other researchers omitted from the analysis any patients who crossed over. It should be easy to see why both of these approaches are potentially biased. The best approach, one recommended by biostatisticians and advocates of **evidence-based medicine,** is to perform all analyses on the original groups to which the patients were randomized. The CASS study occurred several years ago, and no consensus existed at that time on the best way to analyze the findings. The CASS investigators therefore performed the analyses in several ways: by the original group (intention-to-treat), by the final groups of the study, and by eliminating all crossovers from the analysis. All of these methods gave the same result, namely that no difference in survival occurred, although later studies showed differences in quality-of-life indicators.

The intention-to-treat principle applies to studies other than those with survival as the outcome. We included the topic here, however, because it is so pertinent to survival studies. Gillings and Koch (1991) provide a comprehensive and very readable discussion. We briefly mention the issue again in Chapter 13 in the discussion of study biases.

9.9 SUMMARY

Special methods are needed to analyze data from studies of survival time because censored observations occur when patients enter at different times and remain in a study for different periods. Otherwise, investigators would have to wait until all subjects were in the study for a given period before analyzing the data. In medicine, survival curves are commonly drawn by using one of two methods: the Kaplan–Meier product limit method and, less frequently, the actuarial (life table) method. The quality of survival studies published in the medical literature was reviewed by Altman and associates (1995). They found that almost half of the papers did not summarize the length of follow-up or clearly define all endpoints. They suggested some guidelines for presenting survival analyses in medical journals.

We illustrated the Kaplan–Meier and actuarial methods for the length of survival time among patients who were receiving hemodialysis in a study reported by Bajwa and colleagues (1996). The Kaplan–Meier method calculates survival each time a patient dies. The actuarial method divides the time into intervals and calculates survival at each interval. If many observations are made, the actuarial method is simpler to calculate; but with the widespread use of computers, Kaplan–Meier curves are increasingly being used.

The presence of censored observations also requires special methods for comparing two or more survival distributions. We illustrated the two most commonly used methods, the logrank and the Mantel–Haenszel chi-square test, again using dialysis data. We noted the confusion that results because the statistics used to compare survival are approximations and can be calculated in several different ways; they are also called by several different names in the literature. Although we used the observations on hemodialysis to illustrate survival analysis, we pointed out that survival analysis methods are applicable in a variety of situations, not simply in studies examining mortality. The Mantel–Haenszel test is quite versatile and can be applied to any set of 2×2 tables.

We again used the data from Bajwa and colleagues (1996) to illustrate the calculation and interpretation of the logrank and Mantel–Haenszel statistics. We concluded that the survival rate was greater in those patients who continued dialysis. The investigators also reported the results of analysis of comorbid conditions, such as cardiac disease, stroke, peripheral vascular disease, and malignancy. They found that the sum of major comorbid disease was twice as high in the patients who discontinued dialysis ($P = 0.05$), but no individual comorbidity factor reached statistical significance. Patients who discontinued dialysis were older and were more likely to have lost their spouse through death or divorce and to live in a nursing home. Physical discomfort, classified in four grades from none to severe, and the Karnovsky scale, a measure of physical activity, were also associated with the decision to discontinue dialysis. Psychologic variables were not predictive. Although independent predictors of discontinuation were identified, no reliable predictive model could be created.

We discussed two examples of survival analysis from the published literature. In the study described in Presenting Problem 2, Lawrie and colleagues (1991) compared survival in patients who had coronary artery bypass surgery 15–20 years ago. Although surgical methods have changed since these patients had surgery, it is useful to have such complete long-term follow-up on patients. Published results on treatment failure for men with prostate carcinoma treated with radiotherapy were examined in Presenting Problem 3 (Crook et al, 1997). This study found that treatment failure and survival are related to the initial tumor stage and the pretreatment PSA level: patients with T classifications of T1b, T1c, or T2a and those with lower PSA levels had relatively long survival times.

We concluded the chapter with a discussion of the important principle of intention-to-treat, whereby pa-

Table 9–12. Survival of kidney in patients having a transplant; 1978–1979 data.

Patient	Date of Transplant	Months in Study
1	1-11-1978	2
2	1-18-1978	23
3	1-29-1978	23
4	4-4-1978	1
5	4-19-1978	20
6	5-10-1978	19
7	5-14-1978	3
8	5-21-1978	5
9	6-6-1978	17
10	6-17-1978	18
11	6-21-1978	18
12	7-22-1978	3
13	9-27-1978	15
14	10-5-1978	3
15	10-22-1978	14
16	11-15-1978	13
17	12-6-1978	12
18	12-12-1978	12
19	2-1-1979	10
20	2-16-1979	10
21	4-8-1979	8
22	4-11-1979	8
23	4-18-1979	8
24	6-26-1979	1
25	7-3-1979	5
26	7-12-1979	5
27	7-18-1979	1
28	8-23-1979	4
29	10-16-1979	2
30	12-12-1979	1
31	12-24-1979	1

Source: Data courtesy of Dr. A. Birtch.

Table 9–13. Survival of kidneys in patients having a transplant; 1984 data.

Patient	Date of Transplant	Months in Study
1	2-8-1984	22
2	2-22-1984	22
3	2-25-1984	22
4	2-29-1984	8
5	3-12-1984	21
6	3-22-1984	1
7	4-26-1984	20
8	5-2-1984	19
9	5-9-1984	19
10	6-6-1984	18
11	7-11-1984	17
12	7-20-1984	17
13	8-18-1984	16
14	9-5-1984	15
15	9-15-1984	15
16	10-3-1984	14
17	11-9-1984	13
18	11-27-1984	6
19	12-5-1984	12
20	12-6-1984	12
21	12-19-1984	12

Source: Data courtesy of Dr. A. Birtch.

tients are analyzed in the group to which they were originally assigned. We described some of the problems in interpreting the results when this principle is not adhered to, and we pointed out the applicability of the intention-to-treat principle to any study, regardless of whether the outcome is survival or another variable.

EXERCISES

1. A renal transplant surgeon compared two groups of patients who received kidney transplants.[1] One group underwent transplantation in 1978 and 1979 and received azathioprine to retard rejection of the transplanted organ. The other group was transplanted in 1984 and was treated with cyclosporine, a newer immunomodulatory substance. Data are given on these two groups in Tables 9–12 and 9–13.

   a. Perform the calculations for Kaplan–Meier survival curves. We suggest you use the CD-ROM and the file called "Birtch."

   b. Draw the survival curves. Do you think the survival curves are significantly different?

   c. Perform the logrank test, and interpret the results.

2. Camitta and colleagues (1979) studied 110 patients with severe aplastic anemia. Patients ($n = 47$) who had human leukocyte antigen (HLA)-matched siblings entered the bone marrow transplantation group of the study. Patients who did not have marrow donors were randomly assigned to one of three treatments to evaluate the role of androgens in marrow transplantation: oral androgen (PO, $n = 27$), intramuscular androgen (IM, $n = 23$), and no androgen (NO, $n = 13$). Follow-up of the patients ranged from 9 to 45 months. Survival distributions were evaluated using the Kaplan–Meier method and the logrank test. Survival curves are given in Figures 9–10 and 9–11.

   a. What conclusion can you draw about the use of androgens from Figure 9–10?

   b. Figure 9–11 illustrates survival in transplanted versus nontransplanted patients, the latter being all androgen groups combined. What conclusion can you draw?

   c. From Figure 9–11, what is the median survival in patients given a marrow transplant? In patients not given a marrow transplant?

   d. In interpreting the results shown in Figure 9–11, the authors stated:

---

[1]Data kindly provided by Dr. Alan Birtch, Southern Illinois University School of Medicine, Department of Surgery.

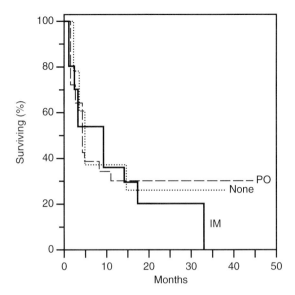

Figure 9–10. Comparison of survival in patients receiving androgen. (Reproduced, with permission, from Camitta BM et al: A prospective study of androgens and bone marrow transplantation for treatment of severe aplastic anemia. *Blood* 1979;**53**:504–514.)

The estimated probability of surviving 6 months is 0.70 for transplanted patients (95% confidence limits 0.57–0.83) and 0.35 for nontransplanted patients (95% confidence limits 0.24–0.48). Thirty-three patients in the transplantation arm and 22 in the nontransplantation arm survived at least 6 months. The distributions of survival times beyond 6 months did not significantly differ between these two groups (P = 0.27), which indicates that the variation in overall survival occurs primarily during the first 6 months.

How do you interpret the 95% confidence limits at 6 months? What is an alternative explanation for why the survival distributions do not differ significantly beyond 6 months?

e. What do the small dots in Figure 9–11 designate?

3. Moertel and colleagues (1985) performed a double-blind, randomized trial of high-dose vitamin C versus placebo in the treatment of advanced colorectal cancer in patients who had not ever received chemotherapy. In addition to analyzing survival as an outcome, the investigators used the Kaplan–Meier method and the logrank statistic to analyze progression of the disease. Progression was defined as any of the following: an increase of more than 50% in the product of the perpendicular diameters of any area of known malignancy, new area of malignancy, substantial worsening of symptoms or performance status, or weight loss of 10% or more. The results of their analysis are reproduced in Figure 9–12.

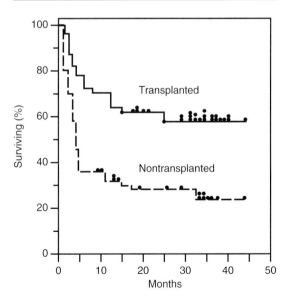

Figure 9–11. Comparison of patients with and without bone marrow transplantations. (Reproduced, with permission, from Camitta BM et al: A prospective study of androgens and bone marrow transplantation for treatment of severe aplastic anemia. *Blood* 1979;**53**:504–514.)

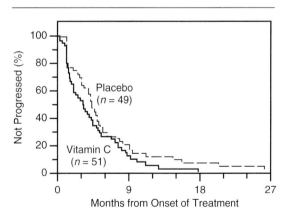

Figure 9–12. Comparison of disease progression in patients with colorectal cancer receiving vitamin C versus placebo. (Reproduced, with permission, from Moertel CG et al: High-dose vitamin C versus placebo in the treatment of patients with advanced cancer who have had no prior chemotherapy: A randomized double-blind comparison. *N Engl J Med* 1985;**312**:137–141.)

a. What conclusion can be drawn from the figure?

b. What is the median time to disease progression in each group?

c. Do you think the analysis of survival times found a statistically significant difference?

4. Use the data from Bajwa and colleagues (1996) to compare survival for patients treated using continuous ambulatory peritoneal dialysis with that for those treated using traditional hemodialysis procedures.

a. Which treatment resulted in longer survival times? Was the longer survival sustained over a long period?

b. What is the value of the logrank statistic? What do you conclude from this value?

c. What are the potential biases in drawing conclusions about treatment method in this study?

5. Refer to Figure 9–8, illustrating the survival curves for the patients categorized by the stage of their tumor (Crook et al, 1997). Is it possible to find the median survival for any of these groups? If so, what is the median survival time for any of these groups?

6. Refer to the MRFIT study discussed in Chapter 8 and used as a group exercise in that chapter. Refer to Figure 2 in the study: cumulative coronary heart disease and total mortality rates for the two groups. What statistical method is optimal for determining whether the two groups differed in either of these outcomes?

Statistical Methods for Multiple Variables

10

PRESENTING PROBLEMS

Presenting Problem 1. We examined data from the study by Henderson and colleagues (1997) in Chapter 5 to illustrate the McNemar test. Recall that the purpose of this study was to gain insights into depression in the elderly. The researchers examined the outcome of depressive states 3–4 years after initial diagnosis to identify factors associated with persistence of depressive symptoms and to test the hypothesis that depressive symptoms in the elderly are a risk factor for dementia or cognitive decline. Please refer to Chapter 5 for more details of the study. One of the statistical methods used by Henderson and colleagues was multiple regression. We will use their analysis to illustrate many of the concepts about multiple regression. Table 3 from the article is reproduced in Section 10.2.3, and data are in the file on the CD-ROM entitled, "Henderson."

Presenting Problem 2. Blood flow through an artery measured as peak systolic velocity (PSV) increases with narrowing of the artery. The well-known relationship between area of the arterial vessels and velocity of blood flow is important in the use of carotid Doppler measurements for grading stenosis of the artery.

Alexandrov and collaborators (1997) wanted to know if the measurement of PSV in the carotid artery measured by carotid Doppler examination correlates with angiographic measurement of carotid artery stenosis. In a large multicenter study undertaken previously, a retrospective analysis of PSV data comparing angiographic measurement of carotid stenosis for 1011 symptomatic patients showed only moderate sensitivity and specificity with the ultrasound method (varying from 61% to 71%) in grading carotid stenosis. No relationship existed between PSV data and risk of stroke.

Alexandrov and collaborators therefore designed a prospective study of 40 patients referred for evaluation of stroke, transient ischemic attack, or carotid bruit. Each patient underwent imaging of each carotid artery bifurcation by both color-coded duplex ultrasound and intraarterial digital subtraction angiography. Eighty bifurcations were imaged in these 40 patients. By angiography, 25 vessels (31%) were normal, 5 vessels (6%) were occluded, and 50 vessels

(63%) had mild to severe stenosis. PSV measurements by ultrasound never exceeded 140 cm/s in normal vessels but increased proportionally with increasing degree of carotid stenosis. The maximum PSV of 550 cm/s occurred at 70–96% stenosis and decreased to 0 cm/s at complete occlusion. We use this study to illustrate polynomial regression. We reproduced two figures from their study using data in the file, "Alexandrov," on the CD-ROM.

Presenting Problem 3. Soderstrom and coinvestigators (1997) wanted to develop a model to identify trauma patients who are likely to have a blood alcohol concentration (BAC) in excess of 50 mg/dL. They evaluated data from a clinical trauma registry and toxicology database at a level I trauma center. Such patients might be candidates for alcohol and drug abuse and dependence treatment and intervention programs.

Data, including BAC, were available on 11,062 patients. Approximately 71% were male and 65% were Caucasian. The mean age was 35 years with a standard deviation of 17 years. Type of injury was classified as unintentional, typically accidental (78.2%), or intentional, including suicide attempts (21.8%). Of these patients, 3180 (28.7%) had alcohol detected in the blood, and 91.2% of those patients had a BAC in excess of 50 mg/dL. Among the patients with a BAC > 50, percentages of men and Caucasians did not differ appreciably from the entire sample; however, the percentage of intentional injuries in this group was higher (28.9%). We use a random sample of data provided by the investigators to illustrate the calculation and interpretation of the logistic model, the statistical method they used to develop their predictive model. Data are in a file called "Soderstrom" on the CD-ROM.

Presenting Problem 4. In the previous chapter we used a study by Crook and colleagues (1997) to illustrate the Kaplan–Meier survival analysis method. These investigators studied the correlation between both the pretreatment prostate-specific antigen (PSA) and posttreatment nadir PSA levels in men with localized prostate cancer who were treated using external beam radiation therapy. The Gleason histologic scoring system was used to classify tumors on a scale of 2 to 10. A low score indicates a well-differentiated tumor, a medium score a moderately differentiated tumor, and a high score a poorly differentiated tumor. Tumors were also classified using the TNM (tumor, node, metastasis) staging system, called the T classification. A T1 tumor is a nonpalpable tumor identified by biopsy. A T2 tumor is palpable on digital rectal examination and limited to the prostate gland. T3 and T4 tumors have invaded adjacent prostate structures, such as the bladder neck or seminal vesicle. The investigators wanted to determine the factors associated with treatment failure, and we use observations from their study to describe an application of the Cox proportional hazard model. Data on the patients are given in the file entitled "Crook" on the CD-ROM.

Presenting Problem 5. The use of central venous catheters to administer parenteral nutrition, fluids, or drugs is a common medical practice. Catheter-related bloodstream infections (CR-BSI) are a serious complication estimated to occur in about 200,000 patients each year. Many studies have suggested that impregnation of the catheter with the antiseptic chlorhexidine/silver sulfadiazine reduces bacterial colonization, but only one study has shown a significant reduction in the incidence of bloodstream infections.

It is difficult for physicians to interpret the literature when studies report conflicting results about the benefits of a clinical intervention or practice. As you now know, studies frequently fail to find significance because of low power associated with small sample sizes. Traditionally, conflicting results in medicine are dealt with by reviewing many studies published in the literature and summarizing their strengths and weaknesses in what are commonly called review articles. Veenstra and colleagues (1999), however, used a more structured method to combine the results of several studies in a statistical manner. They applied meta-analysis to 11 randomized, controlled clinical trials, comparing the incidence of bloodstream infection in impregnated catheters versus nonimpregnated catheters, so that overall conclusions regarding efficacy of the practice could be drawn. Section 10.6 summarizes the results.

10.1 PURPOSE OF THE CHAPTER

The purpose of this chapter is to present a conceptual framework that applies to almost all the statistical procedures discussed so far in this text. We also describe some of the more advanced techniques used in medicine.

10.1.1 A Conceptual Framework

The previous chapters illustrated statistical techniques that are appropriate when the number of observations on each subject in a study is limited. For example, a t test is used when two groups of subjects are studied and the measure of interest is a single numerical variable—such as in Presenting Problem 1 in Chapter 6, which described operating room times for patients who underwent either a vaginal or an abdominal procedure for pelvic reconstruction (Benson et al, 1996). When the outcome of interest is nominal, the chi-square test can be used—such as in Good and colleagues' study of sleep-disordered breathing (Chapter 6, Presenting Problem 3). Regression analysis is used to predict one numerical measure from another, such as in the study predicting insulin sensitivity in hyperthyroid women (Gonzalo et al, 1996; Chapter 7, Presenting Problem 2).

Alternatively, each of these examples can be viewed conceptually as involving a set of subjects with two observations on each subject: (1) for the t test, one numerical variable, time in the operating room, and one nominal (or group membership) variable, the surgical procedure; (2) for the chi-square test, two nominal variables, normal or elevated desaturation index and discharge to home or an extended-care facility; (3) for regression, two numerical variables, insulin sensitivity and body mass index. The advantage of this perspective will become apparent as we discuss the more advanced techniques necessary when many variables are included in a study.

To practice viewing research questions from a conceptual perspective, let us reconsider the problem of determining whether differences exist in immune function in women who have low, moderate, or high levels of social adjustment. Here, again, the problem may be seen as involving a set of subjects with two observations per subject: one numerical variable, immune function (as measured by natural killer cell activity), and one ordinal (or group membership) variable, social adjustment, with three values. If only two values were included for social adjustment, the t test would be used. With more than two groups, however, one-way analysis of variance (ANOVA) is appropriate (Irwin et al, 1987; Chapter 7 Presenting Problem 1).

Many problems in medicine have more than two observations per subject because of the complexity involved in studying disease in humans. In fact, many of the presenting problems used in this text have multiple observations, although we chose to simplify the problems by examining only selected variables. One method involving more than two observations per subject has already been discussed: two-way ANOVA. Recall that in Presenting Problem 2 in Chapter 7 insulin sensitivity was examined in overweight and normal weight women with and without hyperthyroid disease (Gonzalo et al, 1996). For this analysis, the investigators classified women according to two nominal variables (weight status and thyroid status, both measured as normal or higher than normal) and one numerical variable, insulin sensitivity. (Although both weight and thyroid level are actually numerical measures, the investigators transformed them into nominal variables by dividing the values into two categories.)

If the term **independent variable** is used to designate the group membership variables (eg, vaginal or abdominal surgical procedure), or the X variable (eg, blood pressure measured by a finger device), and the term **dependent** is used to designate the variables whose means are compared (eg, operating room times), or the Y variable (eg, blood pressure measured by the cuff device), the observations can be summarized as in Table 10–1. For the sake of simplicity, this summary omits ordinal variables. When independent variables are measured on an ordinal scale, they are often treated as if they were nominal (eg, using "high" versus "low" Apgar scores to predict infant survival during the first months of life). When dependent variables are ordinal (eg, examining level of functional capacity in rheumatoid arthritis categorized as class 1–class 4 from age at onset), one of the nonparametric methods or chi-square is often used, depending on the scale of the independent variable.

Data from several of the presenting problems are available on the CD-ROM, and we invite you to replicate the analyses as you go through this chapter.

10.1.2 Introduction to Methods for Multiple Variables

Statistical techniques involving multiple variables are used increasingly in medical research, and several of them are illustrated in this chapter. The multiple-regression model, in which several independent variables are used to explain or predict the values of a single numerical response, is presented first, partly because it is a natural extension of the regression model for one independent variable illustrated in Chapter 8. More importantly, however, all the other advanced methods except meta-analysis can be viewed as modifications or extensions of the multiple-regression model. All except meta-analysis involve more than two observations per subject and are concerned with explanation or prediction.

The goal in this chapter is to present the logic of the different methods listed in Table 10–2 and to illustrate how they are used and interpreted in medical research. Although the models are sometimes given in equation form, we will not perform any calculations. These methods are generally not mentioned in traditional introductory texts, and most people who take statistics courses do not learn about them until their third or fourth course. These methods are being used more frequently in medicine, however, partly because of the increased involvement of statisticians in medical research and partly because of the availability of complex statistical computer programs (Altman, 1991b). In truth, few of these methods would be used very much in any field were it not for computers because of the time-consuming and complicated computations involved. To read the literature with confidence, especially studies designed to identify prognostic or risk factors, physicians must therefore have a reasonable acquaintance with the methods described in this chapter. Few of the available elementary books discuss multivariate methods. One that is directed toward statisticians is nevertheless quite readable (Chatfield, 1988); others intended for readers of the medical literature include Katz (1999) and Norman and Streiner (1996). The introductory text by Kleinbaum (1994) is devoted to logistic regression analysis.

Before we examine the advanced methods, however, a comment on terminology is necessary. Some statisticians reserve the term "multivariate" to refer to situations that involve more than one dependent (or response) variable. Using this definition, the study of de-

Table 10–1. Summary of conceptual framework[a] for questions involving two variables.

Independent Variable	Dependent Variable	Method
Nominal	Nominal	Chi-square
Nominal (binary)	Numerical	t test[a]
Nominal (more than two values)	Numerical	One-way ANOVA[a]
Nominal	Numerical (censored)	Actuarial methods
Numerical	Numerical	Regression[b]

Abbreviation: ANOVA = analysis of variance.
[a]Assuming the necessary assumptions (eg, normality, independence, etc) are met.
[b]Correlation is appropriate when neither variable is designated as independent or dependent.

Table 10–2. Summary of conceptual framework[a] for questions involving two or more independent (explanatory) variables.

Independent Variables	Dependent Variable	Method
Nominal	Nominal	Log-linear
Nominal and numerical	Nominal (dichotomous)	Logistic regression
Nominal and numerical	Nominal (two or more values)	Discriminant analysis[a]
Nominal	Numerical	ANOVA[a]
Numerical	Numerical	Multiple regression[a]
Numerical and nominal	Numerical (censored)	Cox regression
Nominal with confounding factors	Numerical	ANCOVA[a]
Nominal with confounding factors	Nominal	Mantel–Haenszel
Numerical only	—	Factor analysis[a] and cluster analysis[a]

Abbreviations: ANOVA = analysis of variance; ANCOVA = analysis of covariance.
[a]Certain assumptions (eg, multivariate normality, independence, etc) are needed to use these methods.

pression in the elderly (Henderson et al, 1997) would not be classified as multivariate because, even though several risk factors were evaluated, the only response variable was depression score at the time of the second measurement (wave 2). By this strict definition, multiple regression and most of the other methods discussed in this chapter would not be classified as multivariate techniques. Other statisticians, ourselves included, use the term "multivariate" more freely to refer to methods that examine the simultaneous effect of multiple independent variables. By this definition, all the techniques discussed in this chapter (with the possible exception of some meta-analyses) are classified as multivariate.

10.2 MULTIPLE REGRESSION

10.2.1 Review of Regression

Simple linear regression (Chapter 8) is used when investigators wish to predict the value of a response (dependent) variable, denoted Y, from an explanatory (independent) variable X. The regression model is

$$Y = a + bX$$

For simplicity of notation, note that in this chapter, we use Y to denote the dependent variable, even though Y', the predicted value, is actually given by this equation. We also use a and b, the sample estimates, instead of the population parameters, β_0 and β_1.

With only one explanatory variable, the simple regression model has a geometric interpretation, in which a is the intercept and b is the slope. More generally, however, b is called the **regression coefficient,** and the t test may be used to see whether a significant relationship exists between X and Y by testing whether b is different from zero (see Chapter 8). For example, using data from Gonzalo and colleagues (1996), we found a regression equation to predict insulin sensitivity from body mass index (BMI) in women to be

$$Y = 1.58 - 0.043 \times BMI$$

This regression line intersects the Y-axis at 1.58 and has a negative slope equal to -0.043, indicating that insulin sensitivity decreases by 0.043 with each increase of 1 in BMI. If the regression coefficient is found to be significant (as it is in this example), the equation can be used to predict a woman's insulin sensitivity in the future from her BMI. For example, if a woman's BMI is 30 g, the insulin sensitivity is predicted to be

$$Y = 1.58 - 0.043 \times 30$$
$$= 1.58 - 1.29 = 0.29$$

The actual value for a woman with a BMI of 30 probably differs from this value somewhat; the idea is

that, on the average, women with a BMI of 30 have an insulin sensitivity of 0.29. The standard error introduced in Chapter 8 can be used to find confidence limits for the prediction of an individual person's insulin sensitivity.

10.2.2 Multiple Regression

The extension of simple regression to two or more independent variables is straightforward. For example, if four independent variables are being studied, the **multiple regression** model is

$$Y = a + b_1 X_1 + b_2 X_2 + b_3 X_3 + b_4 X_4$$

where X_1 is the first independent variable and b_1 is the regression coefficient associated with it, X_2 is the second independent variable and b_2 is the regression coefficient associated with it, and so on. The formulas for a and b were given in Chapter 8, but we do not give the formulas in multiple regression because they become more complex as the number of independent variables increases; and no one calculates them by hand, in any case.

Any arithmetic equation in the form of the previous equation is called a **linear combination;** thus, the response variable Y can be expressed as a (linear) combination of the explanatory variables. Note that a linear combination is really just a weighted average that gives a single number (or index) after the X's are multiplied by their associated b's and the bX products are added. Thus, a linear combination is an efficient way to summarize the value of several variables as one value.

As in simple regression, the dependent (or response) variable Y is a numerical measure. The traditional multiple-regression model calls for the independent variables to be numerical measures as well; however, nominal independent variables may be used, as discussed in the next section, but nominal dependent variables may not be. To summarize, the appropriate technique used with numerical independent variables and a numerical dependent variable is multiple-regression analysis, as indicated in Table 10–2.

10.2.3 Interpreting the Multiple Regression Equation

Henderson and colleagues (1997) (Presenting Problem 1) presented the regression equation for predicting a person's depression score at the follow-up interview (designated as wave 2) 3–6 years following an initial interview (designated as wave 1). We reproduced their findings in Table 10–3.

Let us examine the regression equation to predict depression score in greater detail. The regression coefficients in Table 10–3 were obtained by the investigators using a computer program. Recall from Chapter 8 that the regression coefficients are determined so that the differences between the predicted and actual values of the dependent variable are minimized (actually the

Table 10–3. Regression results for predicting depression at wave 2.

Predictor Variable[a]	b	Beta[b]	P	R^2	R^2 Change
Depression Score					
Wave 1	0.267	0.231	0.000	0.182	0.182
Sociodemographic					
Age	−0.014	−0.024	0.538	0.187	0.005
Sex	0.165	0.034	0.370		
Psychologic Health					
Neuroticism, wave 1	0.067	0.077	0.056	0.0237	0.050
Past history of depression	0.320	0.136	0.000		
Physical Health					
ADL, wave 1	−0.154	−0.103	0.033	0.411	0.174
ADL, wave 2	0.275	0.283	0.012		
ADL^2, wave 2	−0.013	−0.150	0.076		
Number of current symptoms, wave 2	0.115	0.117	0.009		
Number of medical conditions, wave 2	0.309	0.226	0.000		
BP, systolic, wave 2	−0.010	−0.092	0.010		
Global health rating change	0.284	0.079	0.028		
Sensory impairment change	−0.045	−0.064	0.073		
Social support/inactivity					
Social support—friends, wave 2	−1.650	−0.095	0.015	0.442	0.031
Social support—visits, wave 2	−1.229	−0.087	0.032		
Activity level, wave 2	0.061	0.095	0.025		
Services (community residents only), wave 2	0.207[c]	0.135[c]	0.001[c]	0.438[c]	0.015[c]

Abbreviation: BP = blood pressure.

[a]Only those variables are shown that were included in the final model.

[b]Standardized beta value, controlling for all other variables in the regression, except service use. Based on community and institutional residents.

[c]Regression limited to community sample only; coefficients for other variables vary only very slightly from those obtained with regression on the full sample.

Source: Table 3 from the article was modified with the addition of unstandardized regression coefficients; used, with permission, from Henderson AS et al: The course of depression in the elderly: A longitudinal community-based study in Australia. *Psychol Med* 1997;**27**:119–129.)

sum of the squared differences). The regression coefficients can be used to predict the depression score at the follow-up interview by multiplying a given patient's value for each independent variable X by the corresponding regression coefficient b and then summing to obtain the predicted depression score.

The first variable is a numerical variable, the depression score at the beginning of the study, termed wave 1. The regression coefficient, b, of 0.267 is multiplied by the subject's depression score at wave 1, indicating that higher depression scores at wave 1 are associated with higher depression scores at wave 2, which certainly makes sense. The second variable, age, is also numerical; the negative regression coefficient of −0.014 indicates that older ages are associated with lower depression scores, indicating less depression, although the P value is large.

The third variable, sex, is a binary variable having two values. Typically, binary variables are coded with either a 0 or a 1; in the Henderson example, females have a 0 code for sex, and males have a 1. This procedure, called **dummy coding,** allows investigators to include nominal variables in a regression equation in a straightforward manner. Nominal variables with dummy coding are sometimes referred to as dummy or indicator variables. The dummy variables are interpreted as follows: A subject who is male has the code for males, 1, multiplied by the regression coefficient for sex, 0.165, resulting in an additional 0.165 points being added to his depression score. The decision of which value is assigned 1 and which is assigned 0 is an arbitrary decision made by the researcher but can be chosen to facilitate interpretations of interest to the researcher.

Next, variables related to psychologic health are entered into the regression equation. They both have positive coefficients, indicating that subjects who were considered neurotic at wave 1 or who had a past history of depression had higher depression scores at wave 2, again a conclusion that seems reasonable. The variables in the next block are related to physical health. Interestingly, some of the coefficients are positive and others are negative, indicating that the physical health variables are not measuring a unidimensional factor. The coefficients for friends and social visits are negative, indicating that subjects with more friends and social visits had lower depression scores, again, a logical finding. On the other hand, the relationship is positive for both activity level (higher scores indicate greater inactivity) and community services (higher scores indicated greater use).

Multiple regression measures only the linear relationship between the independent variables and the dependent variable, just as in simple regression. For example, the regression equation in this study assumes that the increase in depression score for people between the ages of 75 and 80 is the same as the increase in depression score for people between the ages of 80 and 85. If investigators suspect that the relationship between a given independent variable and the dependent measure is not linear, they may include squared terms (eg, age × age) or the logarithm of age (eg, ln[age]) in the regression equation, depending on the nature of the suspected curvilinear relationship. Notice that Henderson and colleagues included the square of the variable activities of daily living, ADL^2, at wave 2 in the regression because their preliminary investigation of the relationships indicated that the relationship between ADL at wave 2 and depression was not linear.

Regression coefficients are interpreted differently in multiple regression than in simple regression. In simple regression, the regression coefficient b indicates the amount the predicted value of Y changes each time X increases by 1 unit. In multiple regression, a given regression coefficient indicates how much the predicted value of Y changes each time X increases by 1 unit, *holding the values of all other variables in the regression equation constant.* For example, the predicted depression score at wave 2 is increased by 0.267 point for each point the person scored on the depression scale at wave 1, assuming all other variables are held constant. This feature of multiple regression makes it an ideal method to control for baseline differences, as we discuss in Section 10.3.

10.2.4 Statistical Tests for the Regression Coefficient

Table 10–3 also gives the P value associated with each regression coefficient. Both the t test and the F test can be used to determine whether each regression coefficient is different from zero, or the t distribution can be used to form confidence intervals for each regression coefficient. Remember that even though the P values for depression score at wave 1, past history

of depression, and number of medical conditions are reported as 0.000, there is always some probability, even if it is very small. Sometimes authors report 0.000 because computer programs, printing only a limited number of decimal places, often report the probability in this way. Many statisticians believe, and we agree, that it is more accurate to report $P < 0.001$.

10.2.5 Standardized Regression Coefficients

Some authors present regression coefficients that can be used with individual subjects to obtain predicted Y values. But the size of the regression coefficients cannot be used to decide which independent variables are the most important, because their size is also related to the scale on which the variables are measured, just as in simple regression. For example, in Henderson and colleagues' study, the variable sex was coded 1 if male and 0 if female, and the variable age was coded as the number of years of age at the time of the first data collection. Then, if gender and age were equally important in predicting subsequent depression, the regression coefficient for sex would be much larger than the regression coefficient for age so that the same amount would be added to the prediction for each variable. These regression coefficients are sometimes called *unstandardized;* the only conclusion that can be drawn from them is that their positive or negative sign typically describes the direction of the relationship or the correlation between them and the dependent variable Y.

One way to eliminate the effect of scale is to *standardize* the regression coefficients. Standardization can be done by subtracting the mean value of X and dividing by the standard deviation before analysis, so that all variables have a mean of 0 and a standard deviation of 1. Then it is possible to compare the magnitudes of the regression coefficients and draw conclusions about which explanatory variables play an important role. (It is also possible to calculate the standardized regression coefficients after the regression equation using the value of b and the standard deviations of the independent variable X and the dependent variable Y.[1]) The larger the standardized coefficient, the larger the value of the t statistic. **Standardized regression coefficients** are often referred to as beta (β) coefficients. The major disadvantage of standardized regression coefficients is that they cannot readily be used to predict outcome values.

Table 10–3 contains the standardized regression coefficients for the significant variables used to pre-

---

[1]The standardized coefficient = the unstandardized coefficient multiplied by the standard deviation of the X variable and divided by the standard deviation of the Y variable: $\beta_j = b_j (SD_X/SD_Y)$.

dict depression at wave 2 in Henderson and colleagues' study. In fact, these investigators reported the standardized coefficients in the journal article; we added the unstandardized coefficients to the table to facilitate our discussion of regression coefficients. Using the standardized coefficients in Table 10–3, can you determine which variable, age or sex, has more influence in predicting subsequent depression? If you chose sex, you are correct, because the absolute value of its beta coefficient is larger, 0.034, compared with –0.024 for age.

10.2.6 Multiple *R*

Multiple *R* is the multiple-regression analogue of the Pearson product moment correlation coefficient *r*. It is also called the coefficient of multiple determination, but most authors use the shorter term. As an example, suppose the depression score is calculated for each person in the study by Henderson and colleagues; then, the correlation between the predicted depression score and the actual depression score is calculated. This correlation is the multiple *R*. If the multiple *R* is squared (R^2), it measures how much of the variation in the actual depression score is accounted for by knowing the information included in the regression equation. The term R^2 is interpreted in exactly the way r^2 is in simple correlation and regression, with 0 indicating no variance accounted for and 1.00 indicating 100% of the variance accounted for. Recall that in simple regression, the correlation between the actual value *Y* of the dependent variable and the predicted value, denoted *Y'*, is the same as the correlation between the dependent variable and the independent variable; that is, $r_{Y'Y} = r_{XY}$. Thus, *R* and R^2 in multiple regression play the same role as *r* and r^2 in simple regression. The statistical test for *R* and R^2, however, uses the *F* distribution instead of the *t* distribution.

The computations are time-consuming, and fortunately, computers do them for us. In the study by Henderson and colleagues, $R^2 = 0.438$ after all variables are entered into the regression equation, indicating that almost half of the variability in depression score is accounted for by knowing the patient's depression score at baseline, age, sex, and so on. Because R^2 is less than 1, we know that factors other than those included in the study also play a role in determining a person's level of depression. Studies in medicine rarely have R^2 values in excess of 0.50, because many variables play a role in predicting patient response to a therapy or intervention.

10.2.7 Stepwise Multiple Regression

The primary purpose of Henderson and colleagues in their study of depression in the elderly was explanation; they used multiple regression analysis to determine variables that help explain certain health outcomes. Had these investigators been principally interested in using the regression equation for prediction of outcomes for future subjects, they might have included in their final regression equation only the variables that added to prediction in a statistically significant way. This practice has the obvious advantage of requiring less data collection for future applications of the equation.

Deciding on the variables that provide the best prediction is a process sometimes referred to as **model building.** Selecting the number of variables can be accomplished in several ways. In one approach, all variables are introduced into the regression equation; then, the variables that do not have significant regression coefficients are eliminated from the equation. Using this approach, in Table 10–3 age, sex, neuroticism, ADL squared, and change in sensory impairment are eliminated from the equation. The regression equation is then recalculated using only the variables retained because the regression coefficients have different values when some variables are removed from the analysis.

Computer programs may also be used to select an optimal set of explanatory variables. One such procedure is called **forward selection.** Forward selection begins with one variable in the regression equation; then, additional variables are added one at a time until all statistically significant variables are included in the equation. The first variable in the regression equation is the *X* variable that has the highest correlation with the response variable *Y*. The next *X* variable considered for the regression equation is the one that increases R^2 by the largest amount. If the increment in R^2 is statistically significant by the *F* test, it is included in the regression equation. This step-by-step procedure continues until no *X* variables remain that produce a significant increase in R^2. The values for the regression coefficients are calculated, and the regression equation resulting from this forward selection procedure can be used to predict outcomes for future subjects.

A similar **backward elimination** procedure can also be used; in it, all variables are initially included in the regression equation. Instead of using *t* tests to determine which variables are significant predictors, however, the single *X* variable that reduces R^2 by the smallest increment is removed from the equation. If the resulting decrease is not statistically significant, that variable is permanently removed from the equation. Next, the remaining *X* variables are examined to see which produces the next smallest decrease in R^2. This procedure continues until the removal of an *X* variable from the regression equation causes a significant reduction in R^2. That *X* variable is retained in the equation, and the regression coefficients are calculated.

When features of both the forward selection and the backward elimination procedures are used together, the method is called **stepwise regression** (stepwise selection). Stepwise selection begins in the same manner as forward selection. After each addition of a new X variable to the equation, however, all previously entered X variables are checked to see whether they maintain their level of significance. Previously entered X variables are retained in the regression equation only if their removal would cause a significant reduction in R^2. The forward versus backward versus stepwise procedures have subtle advantages related to the correlations among the independent variables that cannot be covered in this text. They do not generally produce identical regression equations, but conceptually, all approaches determine a "parsimonious" equation using a subset of explanatory variables.

Some statistical programs examine all possible combinations of predictor values and determine the one that produces the overall highest R^2; however, we do not recommend this procedure. A more appealing approach can be used when investigators want to build a model in a logical way. They may group variables according to their function and add them to the regression equation as a group or block; this process is often called **hierarchical regression.** Henderson and colleagues essentially used hierarchical regression in the prediction of depression score at wave 2: the sociodemographic variables, age and sex, were added to the equation at the same time, as were the psychologic health variables, the physical health variables, and the social support/inactivity variables. The last column in Table 10–3 reports the R^2 change for the separate blocks of variables. Which block increases R^2 the most, after the initial introduction of the variable, baseline depression score? The physical health variables do so, increasing R^2 by 0.174, or over 17%. The advantage of a logical approach to building a regression model is that, in general, the results tend to be more stable and reliable and are more likely to be replicated in similar studies.

10.2.8 Polynomial Regression

Polynomial regression is a special case of multiple regression in which each term in the equation is a power of X. Polynomial regression provides a way to fit a regression model to curvilinear relationships and is an alternative to transforming the data to a linear scale. For example, the following equation can be used to predict a quadratic relationship:

$$Y = b_0 + b_1 X + b_2 X^2$$

If analysis of the residuals fails to indicate an adequate fit, a cubic term, a fourth-power term, and so on, can also be included until an adequate fit is obtained.

Alexandrov and collaborators (1997) reported a study on the reliability of peak systolic velocity (PSV) criteria for grading carotid stenosis. They compared measurement of PSV in the carotid artery using the Doppler technique with two angiographic methods of measuring carotid stenosis (the North American or NASCET [N] method and the common carotid [C] method). They investigated the fit provided by a linear equation, a quadratic equation, and a cubic equation and found that a quadratic equation based on the carotid method provided the best fit or prediction of PSV. The regression equation is

$$Y = 80.185 + 0.21096X + 0.048872X^2$$

where Y is peak systolic velocity and X is the measurement of angiographic stenosis using the carotid method. Thus, a stenosis of 60% predicts a PSV as follows:

$$\begin{aligned}
Y &= 80.185 + (0.21096 \times 60) + [0.048872 \times (60)^2] \\
&= 80.185 + 12.7 + 175.9 \\
&= 268.8
\end{aligned}$$

A scatterplot of the prediction of PSV using the carotid method is given in Figure 10–1.

Draw a vertical line from 60 on the X-axis to the regression line, and then draw a horizontal line to the Y-axis. The predicted PSV occurs where the line crosses the Y-axis; it should be approximately 270. Do you agree that a quadratic curve fits the data better than a straight line? Do you think that a linear equation would provide an adequate fit if the three observations with a zero angiographic reading were removed from the analysis?

10.2.9 Missing Observations

When studies involve several variables, some observations on some subjects may be missing. Controlling the problem of missing data is easier in studies in which information is collected prospectively; it is much more difficult when information is obtained from already existing records, such as patient charts. Two important factors are whether a small percentage or a large percentage of the observations is missing and whether missing observations are randomly missing or missing because of some causal factor.

For example, suppose a researcher designs a case–control study to examine the effect of leg length inequality on the incidence of loosening of the femoral component after total hip replacement. Cases are patients who developed loosening of the femoral component, and controls are patients who did not. In reviewing the records of routine follow-up, the researcher found that leg length inequality was measured in some patients by using weight-bearing anterior–posterior (AP) hip and lower-extremity films, whereas other patients had measurements taken using non-weight-bearing films. The type of film ordered during follow-up may well be related to whether the patient complained of hip pain, however; that is, patients with symptoms were more likely to have received the weight-bearing films, and patients without symptoms were more likely to have had the routine

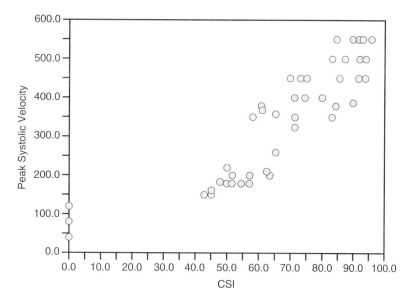

Figure 10–1. Curvilinear relationship between carotid stenosis index (CSI) and peak systolic velocity. (Produced, with permission, from Alexandrov AV et al: Correlation of peak systolic velocity and angiographic measurement of carotid stenosis revisited. *Stroke* 1997;**28**:339–342. Figure produced with NCSS; used with permission.)

non-weight-bearing films. A researcher investigating this question must not base the leg length inequality measures on weight-bearing films only, because controls are less likely than cases to have weight-bearing film measures in their records. In this situation, the missing leg length information occurred because of symptoms and not randomly.

The potential for missing observations increases in studies involving multiple variables. Depending on the cause of the missing observations, solutions include dropping subjects who have missing observations from the study, deleting variables that have missing values from the study, or substituting some value for the missing data, such as the mean across all other subjects. Investigators in this situation should seek advice from a statistician on the best way to handle the problem.

10.2.10 Cross Validation

The statistical procedures for all regression models are based on correlations among the variables, which, in turn, are related to the amount of variation in the variables included in the study. Some of the observed variation in any variable, however, occurs simply by chance; and the same degree of variation does not occur if another sample is selected and the study is replicated. The mathematical procedures for determining the regression equation cannot distinguish between real and chance variation. If the equation is to be used to predict scores for future subjects, it should therefore be validated on a second sample, a process called **cross validation.** Cross validating the regres-

sion equation gives a realistic evaluation of the usefulness of the prediction it provides.

Alternatively, one can estimate the magnitude of R or R^2 in another sample without actually performing the cross validation. This R^2 is smaller than the R^2 for the original sample because the mathematical formula used to obtain the estimate removes the chance variation. For this reason, the formula is called a formula for *shrinkage*. Many computer programs provide both R^2 for the sample used in the analysis as well as R^2 adjusted for shrinkage, often referred to as the adjusted R^2.

10.2.11 Sample Size Requirements

The only easy way for determining how large a sample is needed in multiple regression or any multivariate technique is to use a computer program. Some rules of thumb, however, may be used for guidance. A common recommendation by statisticians calls for ten times as many subjects as the number of independent variables. For example, this rule of thumb prescribes a minimum of 70 subjects for a study predicting the outcome from six independent variables. Having a large ratio of subjects to variables decreases problems that may arise because assumptions are not met. Assumptions about normality are complicated, depending on whether the independent variables are viewed as fixed or random (as in fixed-effects model or random-effects model in ANOVA), and they are beyond the scope of this text. To ensure that estimates of regression coefficients and multiple R and

R^2 are accurate representatives of actual population values, we suggest that investigators should never perform regression unless at least five times as many subjects are included as there are variables.

A more accurate estimate is found by using a computer power program. We used the PASS power program to find the power of a study using 17 predictor variables, such as the one by Henderson and colleagues (1997). We posed the question: How many subjects are needed to test whether a given variable increases R^2 by 0.05, given that 16 variables are already in the regression equation and they collectively provide an R^2 of 0.50? The output from the program is shown in Box 10–1. The power table indicates that a sample of 100 gives power of 0.855, assuming an α or P value of 0.05. The accompanying graph shows the power curve for different sample sizes and different values of α. As you can see, the sample of 595 subjects in the study by Henderson and colleagues was more than adequate for the regression model.

10.3 ANALYSIS OF COVARIANCE

Analysis of covariance (ANCOVA) is the statistical technique used to control for the influence of a

---

Box 10–1. Results from power analysis.

Multiple-Regression Power Analysis

Power	N	α	β	Independent Variables Tested		Independent Variables Controlled	
				Count	R^2	Count	R^2
0.628	50	0.050	0.372	1	0.050	16	0.500
0.909	100	0.050	0.091	1	0.050	16	0.500
0.982	150	0.050	0.018	1	0.050	16	0.500
0.997	200	0.050	0.003	1	0.050	16	0.500
0.999	250	0.050	0.001	1	0.050	16	0.500
1.000	300	0.050	0.000	1	0.050	16	0.500

Summary Statements

A sample size of 50 achieves 37% power to detect an R-Squared of 0.050 attributed to 1 independent variable(s) using an F-Test with a significance level (α) of 0.010. The variables tested are adjusted for an additional 16 independent variable(s) with an R-Squared of 0.500.

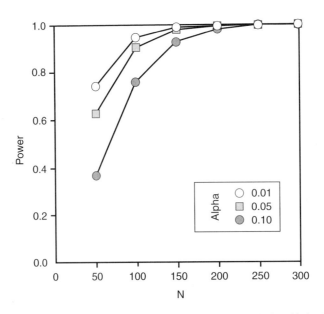

Data, used with permission, from Henderson AS et al: The course of depression in the elderly: A longitudinal community-based study in Australia 1997;**27**:119–129. Output produced using PASS. Used with permission.

confounding variable. **Confounding variables** occur most often when subjects cannot be assigned at random to different groups, that is, when the groups of interest already exist. Recall the study by Gonzalo and colleagues (1996) (Chapters 7 and 8, Presenting Problems 2 and 4, respectively) to predict insulin sensitivity from body mass index (BMI). Gonzalo and colleagues wanted to control for age of the women and did so by adding age to the regression equation. When BMI alone is used to predict insulin sensitivity (IS) in hyperthyroid women, the regression equation is

$$IS = 2.336 - 0.077 \times BMI$$

where IS is the insulin sensitivity level. Using this equation, a hyperthyroid woman's insulin sensitivity level is predicted to decrease by 0.077 for each increase of 1 in BMI. For instance, a woman with a BMI of 25 has a predicted insulin sensitivity of 0.411. What would happen, however, if age were also related to insulin sensitivity? A way to control for the possible confounding effect of age is to include that variable in the regression equation. The equation with age included is

$$IS = 2.291 - 0.0045 \times Age - 0.068 \times BMI$$

Using this equation, a hyperthyroid woman's insulin sensitivity level is predicted to decrease by 0.068 for each increase of 1 in BMI, *holding age constant* or *independent of age*. A 30-year-old woman with a BMI of 25 has a predicted insulin sensitivity of 0.456, whereas a 60-year-old woman with the same BMI of 25 has a predicted insulin sensitivity of 0.321.

A more traditional use of ANCOVA is illustrated by a study of the negative influence of smoking on the cardiovascular system. Investigators wanted to know whether smokers have more ventricular wall motion abnormalities than nonsmokers (Hartz et al, 1984). They might use a *t* test to determine whether the mean number of wall motion abnormalities different in these two groups. The investigators know, however, that wall motion abnormalities are also related to the degree of coronary stenosis, and smokers generally have a greater degree of coronary stenosis. Thus, any difference observed in the mean number of wall abnormalities between smokers and nonsmokers may really be a difference in the amount of coronary stenosis between these two groups of patients.

This situation is illustrated in the graph of hypothetical data in Figure 10–2; in the figure, the relationship between occlusion scores and wall motion abnormalities appears to be the same for smokers and nonsmokers. Nonsmokers, however, have both lower occlusion scores and lower numbers of wall motion abnormalities; smokers have higher occlusion scores and higher numbers of wall motion abnormalities.

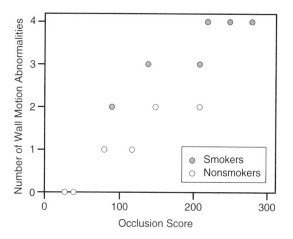

Figure 10–2. Relationship between degree of coronary stenosis and ventricular wall motion abnormalities in smokers and nonsmokers (hypothetical data).

The question is whether the difference in wall motion abnormalities is due to smoking, to occlusion, or to both.

In this study, the investigators must control for the degree of coronary stenosis so that it does not confound (or confuse) the relationship between smoking and wall motion abnormalities. Useful methods to control for confounding variables are analysis of covariance (ANCOVA) and the Mantel–Haenszel chi-square procedure. Table 10–2 specifies ANCOVA when the dependent variable is numerical (eg, wall motion) and the independent measures are grouping variables on a nominal scale (eg, smoking versus nonsmoking), and confounding variables occur (eg, degree of coronary occlusion). If the dependent measure is also nominal, such as whether a patient has survived to a given time, the Mantel–Haenszel chi-square discussed in Chapter 9 can be used to control for the effect of a confounding (nuisance) variable. ANCOVA can be performed by using the methods of ANOVA; however, most medical studies use one of the regression methods discussed in this chapter.

If ANCOVA is used in this example, the occlusion score is called the **covariate,** and the mean number of wall motion abnormalities in smokers and nonsmokers is said to be *adjusted for* the occlusion score (or degree of coronary stenosis). Put another way, ANCOVA simulates the Y outcome observed if the value of X is held constant, that is, if all the patients had the same degree of coronary stenosis. This adjustment is achieved by calculating a regression equation to predict mean number of wall motion abnormalities from the covariate, degree of coronary stenosis, and from a dummy variable coded 1 if the subject is a member of the group (ie, a smoker) and 0 otherwise. For example, the regression equation determined for the hypothetical observations in Figure 10–2 is

$$Y = -0.19 + 0.01 \times \text{Occlusion score} + 1.28 \text{ if a smoker}$$

The equation illustrates that smokers have a larger number of predicted wall motion abnormalities, because 1.28 is added to the equation if the subject is a smoker. The equation can be used to obtain the mean number of wall motion abnormalities in each group, adjusted for degree of coronary stenosis.

If the relationship between coronary stenosis and ventricular motion is ignored, the mean number of wall motion abnormalities, calculated from the observations in Figure 10–2, is 3.33 for smokers and 1.00 for nonsmokers. If, however, ANCOVA is used to control for degree of coronary stenosis, the adjusted mean wall motion is 2.81 for smokers and 1.53 for nonsmokers, a difference of 1.28, represented by the regression coefficient for the dummy variable for smoking. In ANCOVA, the adjusted Y mean for a given group is obtained by (1) finding the difference between the group's mean on the covariate variable X, denoted $\bar{X}_j$, and the grand mean $\bar{\bar{X}}$; (2) multiplying the difference by the regression coefficient; and (3) subtracting this product from the unadjusted $\bar{Y}$ mean. Thus, for group j, the adjusted mean is

$$\text{Adjusted } \bar{Y}_j = \text{Unadjusted } \bar{Y}_j - b(\bar{X}_j - \bar{\bar{X}})$$

(See Exercise 1.)

This result is consistent with our knowledge that coronary stenosis alone has some effect on abnormality of wall motion; the unadjusted means contain this effect as well as any effect from smoking. Controlling for the effect of coronary stenosis therefore results in a smaller difference in number of wall motion abnormalities, a difference related only to smoking.

Figure 10–3 illustrates schematically the way ANCOVA adjusts the mean of the dependent variable if the covariate is important. Using unadjusted means is analogous to using a separate regression line for each group. For example, the mean value of Y for group 1 is found by using the regression line drawn through the group 1 observations to project the mean value $\bar{X}_1$ onto the Y-axis, denoted $\bar{Y}_1$ in Figure 10–3. Similarly, the mean of group 2 is found at $\bar{Y}_2$ by using the regression line to project the mean $\bar{X}_2$ in that group. The Y means in each group *adjusted for the covariate* (stenosis), however, are analogous to the projections based on the overall mean value of the covariate; that is, as though the two groups had the same mean value for the covariate. The adjusted means for groups 1 and 2, Adj. $\bar{Y}_1$ and Adj. $\bar{Y}_2$, are illustrated by the dotted line projections of $\bar{X}$ from each separate regression line in Figure 10–3.

ANCOVA assumes that the relationship between

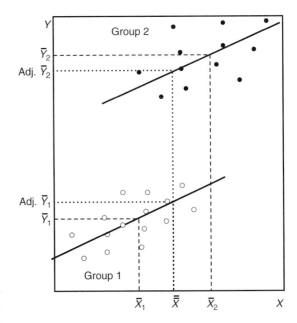

Figure 10–3. Illustration of means adjusted using analysis of covariance.

the covariate (X variable) and the dependent variable (Y) is the same in both groups, that is, that any relationship between coronary stenosis and wall motion abnormality is the same for smokers and nonsmokers. This assumption is equivalent to requiring that the regression slopes be the same in both groups; geometrically, ANCOVA asks whether a difference exists between the intercepts, assuming the slopes are equal.

ANCOVA is an appropriate statistical method in many situations that occur in medical research. For example, age is a variable that affects almost everything studied in medicine; if preexisting groups in a study have different age distributions, investigators must adjust for age before comparing the groups on other variables, just as Gonzalo and colleagues recognized. The methods illustrated in Chapter 3 to adjust mortality rates for characteristics such as age and birth weight are used when information is available on groups of individuals; when information is available on individuals themselves, ANCOVA is used.

Before leaving this section, we point out some important aspects of ANCOVA. First, although only two groups were included in the example, ANCOVA can be used to adjust for the effect of a confounding variable in more than two groups. In addition, it is possible to adjust for more than one confounding variable in the same study, and the confounding variables may be either nominal or numerical. Thus, it is easy to see why the multiple regression model for analysis of covariance provides an ideal method to incorporate confounding variables.

Finally, ANCOVA can be considered as a special case of the more general question of comparing two regression lines (discussed in Chapter 8). In ANCOVA, we assume that the slopes are equal, and attention is focused on the intercept. We can also perform the more global test of both slope and intercept, however, by using multiple regression. In Presenting Problem 4 in Chapter 8 on insulin sensitivity (Gonzalo et al, 1996), interest focused on comparing the regression lines predicting insulin activity from body mass index (BMI) in women who had normal versus elevated thyroid levels. ANCOVA can be used for this comparison using dummy coding. If we let X be BMI, Y be insulin sensitivity level, and Z be a dummy variable, where $Z = 1$ if the woman is hyperthyroid and $Z = 0$ for controls, then the multiple-regression model for testing whether the two regression lines are the same (coincident) is

$$Y = a + b_1X + b_2Z + b_3XZ$$

The regression lines have equal slopes and are parallel when b_3 is 0, that is, no interaction between the independent variable X and the group membership variable Z. The regression lines have equal intercepts and equal slopes (are coincident) if both b_2 and b_3 are 0; thus, the model becomes the simple regression equation $Y = a + bX$. The statistical test for b_2 and b_3 is the t test discussed in Section 10.2.4.

10.4 PREDICTING NOMINAL OR CATEGORICAL OUTCOMES

In the regression model discussed in the previous section, the outcome or dependent Y variable is measured on a numerical scale. When the outcome is measured on a nominal scale, other approaches must be used. Table 10–2 indicates that three methods can be used to analyze problems with several independent variables when the dependent variable is nominal. First we discuss logistic regression, a method that is being used a great deal more frequently in the health field. One reason for the popularity of logistic regression is that many outcomes in health are nominal, actually binary, variables; that is, they either occur or do not occur. The second reason is that the regression coefficients obtained in logistic regression can be transformed into odds ratios. So, in essence, logistic regression provides a way to obtain an odds ratio for a given risk factor that controls for, or is adjusted for, confounding variables; in other words, we can do analysis of covariance with logistic regression as well as with multiple linear regression.

The other two methods are discriminant analysis and log-linear analysis. Discriminant analysis is used less and less, partly because of the increasing use of logistic regression. Nevertheless, it still appears in the medical literature, so we briefly describe it with

an example. Log-linear analysis, on the other hand, is rarely used in the health field. We postpone the discussion of these two methods to Section 10.7, where we discuss several methods that appear only occasionally in the medical literature.

10.4.1 Logistic Regression

Logistic regression is commonly used when the independent variables include both numerical and nominal measures and the outcome variable is binary (dichotomous). Logistic regression can also be used when the outcome has more than two values (Hosmer and Lemeshow, 1989), but its most frequent use is as in Presenting Problem 3, which illustrates the use of logistic regression to identify trauma patients who are alcohol-positive, a yes-or-no outcome. Soderstrom and his coinvestigators (1997) wanted to develop a model to help emergency department staff identify the patients most likely to have blood alcohol concentrations (BAC) in excess of 50 mg/dL at the time of admission. The logistic model gives the probability that the outcome, such as high BAC, occurs as an exponential function of the independent variables. For example, with three independent variables, the model is

$$p_x = \frac{1}{1 + \exp[-(b_0 + b_1X_1 + b_2X_2 + b_3X_3)]}$$

where b_0 is the intercept, b_1, b_2, and b_3 are the regression coefficients, and exp indicates that the base of the natural logarithm (2.718) is taken to the power shown in parentheses. The equation can be derived by specifying the variables to be included in the equation or by using a variable selection method similar to the ones for multiple regression. A chi-square test (instead of the t or F test) is used to determine whether a variable adds significantly to the prediction.

In the study described in Presenting Problem 3, the variables used by the investigators to predict blood alcohol concentrations included the variables listed in Table 10–4. The authors kindly provided us with a random sample of the subjects analyzed in their study. The investigators coded the values of the independent variables as 0 and 1, a method useful both for dummy variables in multiple regression and for variables in logistic regression. This practice makes it easy to interpret the odds ratio. In addition, if a goal is to develop a score, as is the case in the study by Soderstrom and coinvestigators, the coefficient associated with a given variable needs to be included in the score only if the patient has a 1 on that variable. For instance, if patients are more likely to have BAC ≥ 50 mg/dL on weekends, the score associated with day of week is not included if the injury occurs on a weekday.

The investigators calculated logistic regression equations for each of four groups: males with intentional injury, males with unintentional injury, fe-

Table 10–4. Variables, codes, and frequencies for variables.[a]

	Value	Frequency
Age		
39 or younger	0	3514
40 or older	1	1534
Time of Day		
6 PM–6 AM	0	2601
6 AM–6 PM	1	2447
Day of week		
Monday–Thursday	0	2642
Friday–Sunday	1	2406
Sex		
Female	0	1457
Male	1	3591
Race		
Non-Caucasian	0	1758
Caucasian	1	3290
Injury Type		
Unintentional	0	3966
Intentional	1	1082
Blood Alcohol Concentration		
<50 mg/dL	0	4067
≥50 mg/dL	1	1465

[a]Not all totals are the same because of missing data on some variables.
Source: Data, used with permission, from Soderstrom CA et al: Predictive model to identify trauma patients with blood alcohol concentrations ≥ 50 mg/dL. *J Trauma* 1997;**42:**67–73.

males with intentional injury, and females with unintentional injury. The results of the analysis on males who were injured unintentionally are given in Table 10–5.

We need to know which value is coded 1 and which 0 in order to interpret the results. For example, time of day has a negative regression coefficient. The hours of 6 AM–6 PM are coded as 1, so a male coming to the emergency department with unintentional injuries in the daytime is *less* likely to have BAC ≥ 50 mg/dL than a male with unintentional injuries at night. The age variable is not significant ($P > 0.268$). Interpreting the equation for the other variables indicates that males with unintentional injuries who come to the emergency department at night and on weekends and are Caucasian are more likely to have elevated blood alcohol levels.

The logistic equation can be used to find the probability for any given individual. For instance, let us find the probability that a 27-year-old Caucasian man who comes to the emergency department at 2 PM on Thursday has BAC ≥ 50 mg/dL. The regression coefficients from Table 10–5 are

$$-0.80 - (1.84 \times \text{Daytime}) + (0.66 \times \text{Weekday}) + (0.28 \times \text{Race}) - (0.11 \times \text{Age})$$

and we evaluate it as follows:

$$-0.80 - (1.84 \text{ if daytime}) + (0.66 \text{ if Fri.–Sun.}) + (0.28 \text{ if Caucasian}) - (0.11 \text{ if 40 or older})$$
$$= -0.80 - 1.84 + 0.28$$
$$= -2.36$$

Substituting −2.36 in the equation for the probability:

$$p_x = \frac{1}{1 + \exp[-(b_0 + b_1X_1 + b_2X_2 + b_3X_3)]}$$
$$= \frac{1}{1 + \exp[-(-2.36)]} = \frac{1}{1 + 10.59} = 0.0863$$

Therefore, the chance that this man has a high BAC is less than 1 in 10. See Exercise 3 to determine the likelihood of a high BAC if the same man came to the emergency department on a Saturday night.

One advantage of using logistic regression is that it requires no assumptions about the distribution of the independent variables. Another is that the regression coefficient can be interpreted in terms of relative risks in cohort studies or odds ratios in case–control studies. In other words, the relative risk of an elevated BAC in males with unintentional trauma during the day is exp (−1.845) = 0.158. The relative risk for night is the reciprocal, 1/0.158 = 6.33; therefore, males with unintentional injuries who come to the ER at night are more than six times more likely to have BAC ≥ 50 mg/dL than males coming during the day.

How can readers easily tell which odds ratios are statistically significant? Recall from Chapter 8 that if the 95% confidence interval does not include 1, we can be 95% sure that the factor associated with the odds ratio either is a significant risk or provides a significant level of protection. Do any of the independent variables in Table 10–5 have a 95% confidence interval for the odds ratio that contains 1? Did you already know without looking that it would be age because the age variable is not statistically significant?

Before leaving the topic of logistic regression, it is worthwhile to inspect the classification table in Table 10–5. This table gives the actual and the predicted number of males with unintentional injuries who had normal versus elevated BAC. The logistic equation tends to underpredict those with elevated concentrations: 470 males are predicted versus the 682 who actually had BAC ≥ 50 mg/dL. Overall, the prediction using the logistic equation correctly classified 76.62% of these males. Although this sounds rather impressive, it is important to compare this percentage with the baseline: 74.12% of the time we would be correct if we simply predicted a male to have normal BAC. Can you recall an appropriate way to compensate for or take the baseline into consideration? Although computer programs typically do not provide the kappa statistic, discussed in Chapter 5, it provides a way to evaluate the percentage correctly classified (see Exercise 4).

Table 10–5. Logistic regression report for men with unintentional injury.[a]

Filter	sex=1; injtype=0
Response	BAC50

Parameter Estimation Section

Variable	Regression Coefficient	Standard Error	χ^2	Probability Level	Last R^2
Intercept	−0.7960357	0.1188189	44.88	0.000000	0.016780
Daytime	−1.8445640	0.1062133	301.60	0.000000	0.102879
Weekday	0.6622602	0.0975930	46.05	0.000000	0.017208
Race	0.2780667	0.1125357	6.11	0.013477	0.002316
Age 40	−0.1198371	0.1082209	1.23	0.268148	0.000466

Odds Ratio Estimation Section

Variable	Regression Coefficient	Standard Error	Odds Ratio	Lower 95% Confidence Limit	Upper 95% Confidence Limit
Intercept	−0.796036	0.118819			
Daytime	−1.844564	0.106213	0.158094	0.128383	0.194682
Weekday	0.662260	0.097593	1.939170	1.601565	2.347942
Race	0.278067	0.112536	1.320574	1.059186	1.646468
Age 40	−0.119837	0.108221	0.887065	0.717526	1.096663

Model Summary Section

Model R^2	Model df	Model χ^2	Model Probability
0.141881	4	434.84	0.000000

Classification Table

Actual		Predicted 0	Predicted 1	Total
0	Count	1751.00	202.00	1953.00
	Row percent	89.66	10.34	100.00
	Column percent	80.88	42.98	74.12
1	Count	414.00	268.00	682.00
	Row percent	60.70	39.30	100.00
	Column percent	19.12	57.02	25.88
Total	Count	2165.00	470.00	2635.00
	Row percent	82.16	17.84	
	Column percent	100.00	100.00	

Percent correctly classified = 76.62

[a]Results from logistic regression for men with unintentional injury.
Source: Data, used with permission, from Soderstrom CA et al: Predictive model to identify trauma patients with blood alcohol concentrations ≥50 mg/dL. *J Trauma* 1997;**42:**67–73. Output produced using NCSS; used with permission.

10.5 PREDICTING A CENSORED OUTCOME: PROPORTIONAL HAZARD MODEL

In Chapter 9, we found that special methods must be used when an outcome has not yet been observed for all subjects in the study sample. Studies of survival naturally fall into this category; investigators usually cannot wait until all patients in the study die before presenting information on survival. From an analysis perspective, the problem is one of **censored observations,** a situation in which subjects have been observed unequal lengths of time and the outcome is not yet known for all of them.

We examined methods for comparing duration of survival of two or more groups of patients in which the groups are formed on the basis of one variable. But many times in clinical trials or cohort studies, investigators wish to look at the simultaneous effect of several variables on length of survival. For example, in the study described in Presenting Problem 4, Crook and her colleagues (1997) wanted to evaluate the relationship of pretreatment prostate-specific antigen (PSA) and posttreatment nadir PSA on the failure pattern of radiotherapy for treating localized prostate carcinoma. They categorized failures as biochemical, local, and distant. They analyzed data from a cohort study of 207 patients, but only 68 had a failure due to any cause in the 70 months during which the study was underway. These 68 observations on failure were therefore censored. The independent variables they examined included the Gleason score, the T classification, whether the patient had received hormonal treatment, the PSA before treatment, and the lowest PSA following treatment.

Table 10–2 indicates that the regression technique developed by Cox (1972) is appropriate when time-dependent censored observations are included. This technique is called the **Cox regression,** or **proportional hazard, model.** In essence this model allows the covariates (independent variables) in the regression equation to vary with time. The dependent variable is the survival time of the jth patient, denoted Y_j. Both numerical and nominal independent variables may be used in the model.

The Cox regression coefficients can be used to determine the relative risk or odds ratio (introduced in Chapter 3) associated with each independent variable and the outcome variable, adjusted for the effect of all other variables in the equation, as we will see in the analysis of Presenting Problem 5. Thus, instead of giving adjusted means, as ANCOVA does in regression, the Cox model gives adjusted relative risks. We can also use a variety of methods to select the independent variables that add significantly to the prediction of the outcome, as in multiple regression; however, a chi-square test (instead of the F test) is used to test for significance.

The Cox proportional hazard model involves a complicated exponential equation (Cox, 1972). Although we will not go into detail about the mathematics involved in this model, its use is so common in medicine that at least a minimal understanding of the process is worth the effort. Our primary focus, however, is on the application and interpretation of the Cox model; we accomplish this by illustrating its use with the data from Presenting Problem 4.

10.5.1 Understanding the Cox Model

Recall from Chapter 9 that the survival function gives the probability that a person will survive the next interval of time, given that he or she has survived up until that time. The hazard function, also defined in Chapter 9, is in some ways the opposite: it is the probability that a person will die (or that there will be a failure) in the next interval of time, given that he or she has survived until the beginning of the interval. The hazard function plays a key role in the Cox model.

For the readers who want to look at the details, the Cox model examines two pieces of information: the amount of time since the event first happened to a person, and the person's observations on the dependent variables. Using the Crook example, the amount of time might be 3 years, and the observations would be the patient's Gleason score, T classification, whether he had been treated with hormones, and the two PSA scores (pretreatment and lowest posttreatment). In the Cox model, the length of time is evaluated using the hazard function, and the linear combination of the independent values (like the linear combination we obtain when we use multiple regression) is the exponent of the natural logarithm, e. For example, for the Crook study, the model is written as

$$h(t, X_1, X_2 \ldots X_5) = h_0(t)e^{b_1 X_1 + b_2 X_2 + \cdots + b_5 X_5}$$

In words, the model is saying that the probability of dying in the next time interval, given that the patient has lived until this time and has the given values for Gleason score, T classification, and so on, can be found by multiplying the baseline hazard (h_0) by the natural log raised to the power of the linear combination of the independent variables. If we take the antilog of the linear combination, we multiply rather than add the values of the covariates. In this model, the covariates have a multiplicative, or proportional, effect on the probability of dying—thus, the term "proportional hazard" model.

10.5.2 An Example of the Cox Model

In the study described in Presenting Problem 4, Crook and her colleagues (1997) used the Cox proportional hazard model to examine the relationship between pretreatment PSA and posttreatment PSA nadir and treatment failure in men with prostate carcinoma following treatment with radiotherapy. Failure was categorized as chemical, local, or distant. The investigators wanted to control for possible confounding variables, including the Gleason score, the T classification, both measures of severity, and whether the patient received hormones prior to the radiotherapy. The outcome is a censored variable, the amount of time before the treatment fails, so the Cox proportional hazard model is the appropriate statistical method. We use the results of analysis using SPSS, given in Table 10–6, to point out some salient features of the method.

Both numerical and nominal variables can be used as independent variables in the Cox model. If the variables are nominal, it is necessary to tell the computer program so they can be properly analyzed. SPSS prints this information. PRERTHOR, pretreatment hormone therapy, is recoded so that 0 = no and 1 = yes. Prior to doing the analysis, we recoded the Gleason score into a variable called GSCORE with two values: 0 for Gleason scores 2–6 and 1 for Gleason scores 7–10. The T classification variable, TUMSTAGE, was recoded by the computer program using dummy variable coding. Note that for four values of TUMSTAGE, only three variables are needed, with the three more advanced stages compared with the lowest stage, T1b–2.

Among the 207 men in the study, 68 had experienced a failure by the time the data were analyzed. The authors reported a median follow-up of 36 months with a range of 12 to 70 months. The log likelihood statistic (LL) is used to evaluate the significance of the overall model; smaller values indicate that the data fit the model better. The change in the log likelihood associated with the initial (full) model in which no independent variables are included in the equation and the log likelihood after the variables are

Table 10–6. Results from Cox proportional hazard model using both pretreatment and posttreatment variables.

Indicator Parameter Coding

	Value	Frequency			
PRERTHOR					
	1.00	44	0.000		
	2.00	163	1.000		
GSCORE	Recoded Gleason score				
	2–6	168	0.000		
	7–10	39	1.000		
TUMSTAGE	Tumor stage				
	T1b–2	34	0.000	0.000	0.000
	T2a	34	1.000	0.000	0.000
	T2b–c	79	0.000	1.000	0.000
	T3–4	60	0.000	0.000	1.000

207 Total cases read

Dependent Variable: TIMEANYF

	Events	Censored
	68	139 (67.1%)

Beginning block number 0.   Initial log likelihood function
–2 Log likelihood   649.655
Beginning block number 1.   Method: Enter
Variable(s) Entered at step number 1.
      GSCORE   Recoded Gleason score
      TUMSTAGE   Tumor stage
      PRERTHOR
      PRERXPSA
      NADIRPSA

Coefficients converged after seven iterations.

–2 Log likelihood   576.950

	χ^2	df	Significance
Overall (score)	274.737	7	0.0000
Change (–2LL) from			
Previous block	72.706	7	0.0000
Previous step	72.706	7	0.0000

Variables in the equation

Variable	B	SE	Wald	df	Significance	R
GSCORE	0.4420	0.2843	2.4172	1	0.1200	0.0253
TUMSTAGE			14.3608	3	0.0025	0.1134
TUMSTAGE (1)	–0.0224	0.7077	0.0010	1	0.9747	0.0000
TUMSTAGE (2)	0.8044	0.5506	2.1342	1	0.1440	0.0144
TUMSTAGE (3)	1.5075	0.5548	7.3828	1	0.0066	0.0910
PRERTHOR	–0.1348	0.3168	0.1811	1	0.6704	0.0000
PRERXPSA	0.0040	0.0029	1.8907	1	0.1691	0.0000
NADIRPSA	0.0769	0.0115	44.7491	1	0.0000	0.2565

Variable	Exp (B)	95% CI for Exp (B)	
		Lower	Upper
GSCORE	1.5558	0.8912	2.7161
TUMSTAGE (1)	0.9778	0.2443	3.9140
TUMSTAGE (2)	2.2353	0.7597	6.5770
TUMSTAGE (3)	4.5156	1.5221	13.3962
PRERTHOR	0.8739	0.4697	1.6260
PRERXPSA	1.0040	0.9983	1.0098
NADIRPSA	1.0799	1.0559	1.1045

Abbreviations: df = degrees of freedom; *SE* = standard error; CI = confidence interval; Wald = statistic used by SPSS to test the significance of variances.
Source: Data, used with permission, from Crook JM et al: Radiotherapy for localized prostate carcinoma. *Cancer* 1997;**79**:328–336. Output produced using SPSS 10.0, a registered trademark of SPSS, Inc; used with permission.

entered is calculated. In this example, the change is 72.706 (highlighted in Table 10–6), and it is the basis of the chi-square statistic used to determine the significance of the model. The significance is reported, as often occurs with computer programs, as 0.0000.

In addition to testing the overall model, it is possible to test each independent variable to see if it adds significantly to the prediction of failure. Were any of the potentially confounding variables significant? The significance of TUMSTAGE requires some explanation. The variable itself is significant, with $P = 0.0025$ (highlighted in the printout). The TUMSTAGE(3) variable (which indicates the patient has T3–4 stage tumor), however, is the one that really matters because it is the only significant stage ($P = 0.0066$). Note that Gleason score and hormone therapy were not significant. Was either of the PSA values important in predicting failure? It appears that the pretreatment PSA is not significant, but the lowest PSA (NADIRPSA) reached following treatment has a very low P value.

As in logistic regression, the regression coefficients in the Cox model can be interpreted in terms of relative risks or odds ratios (by finding the antilog) if they are based on independent binary variables, such as hormone therapy. For this reason, many researchers divide independent variables into two categories, as we did with Gleason score, even though this practice can be risky if the correct cutpoint is not selected. The T classification variable was recoded as three dummy variables to facilitate interpretation in terms of odds ratios for each stage. The odds ratios are listed under the column titled "Exp (B)" in Table 10–6. Using the T3–4 stage (TUMSTAGE(3)) as an illustration, the antilog of the regression coefficient, 1.5075, is exp (1.5075) = 4.5156. Note that the 95% confidence interval goes from approximately 1.52 to 13.40; because this interval does not contain 1, the odds ratio is statistically significant (consistent with the P value).

Crook and colleagues (1997) also computed the Cox model using only the variables known prior to treatment (see Exercise 8).

10.5.3 Importance of the Cox Model

The Cox model is very useful in medicine, and it is easy to see why it is being used with increasing frequency. It provides the only valid method of predicting a time-dependent outcome, and many health-related outcomes are related to time. If the independent variables are divided into two categories (dichotomized), the exponential of the regression coefficient, exp (b), is the odds ratio, a useful way to interpret the risk associated with any specific factor. In addition, the Cox model provides a method for producing survival curves that are adjusted for confounding variables. The Cox model can be extended to the case of multiple events for a subject, but that topic is beyond our scope. Investigators who have repeated measures in a time-to-survival study are encouraged to consult a statistician.

10.6 META-ANALYSIS

Meta-analysis is a way to combine results of several independent studies on a specific topic. Meta-analysis is different from the methods discussed in the preceding sections because its purpose is not to identify risk factors or to predict outcomes for individual patients; rather, this technique is applicable to any research question. We briefly introduced meta-analysis in Chapter 2. Because we could not talk about it in detail until the basics of statistical tests (confidence limits, P values, etc) were explained, we included it in this chapter. It is an important technique increasingly used for studies in health and it can be looked on as an extension of multivariate analysis.

The idea of summarizing a set of studies in the medical literature is not new; review articles have long had an important role in helping practicing physicians keep up to date and make sense of the many studies on any given topic. Meta-analysis takes the review article a step further by using statistical procedures to combine the results from different studies. Glass (1977) developed the technique because many research projects are designed to answer similar questions, but they do not always come to similar conclusions. The problem for the practitioner is to determine which study to believe, a problem unfortunately too familiar to readers of medical research reports. A concise review of some of the early meta-analysis applications in medicine is given by L'Abbé, Detsky, and O'Rourke (1987).

Sacks and colleagues (1987) reviewed meta-analyses of clinical trials and concluded that meta-analysis has four purposes: (1) to increase statistical power by increasing the sample size, (2) to resolve uncertainty when reports do not agree, (3) to improve estimates of effect size, and (4) to answer questions not posed at the beginning of the study. Purpose 3 requires some expansion because the concept of effect size is central to meta-analysis. Cohen (1988) developed this concept and defined **effect size** as the "*degree to which the phenomenon is present in the population.*" An effect size may be thought of as an index of how much difference exists between two groups—generally, a treatment group and a control group. The effect size is based on means if the outcome is numerical, on proportions or odds ratios if the outcome is nominal, or on correlations if the outcome is an association. The effect sizes themselves are statistically combined in meta-analysis.

The use of meta-analysis in the medical literature continues to grow. Altman (1991b) reported the results of a MEDLINE search and found the number of papers referring to meta-analysis increased from fewer than 50 in 1988 or any earlier year to approximately 250 in 1989. Several of the Patient Outcomes Research Team projects (Raskin and Maklan, 1991) performed a comprehensive meta-analysis to establish a baseline for patient outcome studies.

The investigators in Presenting Problem 5 used meta-analysis to evaluate the efficacy of impregnating central venous catheters with an antiseptic. They examined the literature, using manual and computerized searches, for publications containing the words "chlorhexidine," "antiseptic," and "catheter" and found 215 studies. Of these, 24 were comparative studies in humans. Nine studies were eliminated because they were not randomized, and another two were excluded based on the criteria for defining catheter colonization and catheter-related bloodstream infection. Ten studies examined both outcomes, two examined only catheter colonization, and one reported only catheter-related bloodstream infection.

Two authors independently read and evaluated each article. They reviewed the sample size, patient population, type of catheter, catheterization site, other interventions, duration of catheterization, reports of adverse events, and several other variables describing the incidence of colonization and catheter-related bloodstream infection. The authors also evaluated the appropriateness of randomization, the extent of blinding, and the description of eligible subjects. Discrepancies between the reviewers were resolved by a third author. Some basic information about the studies evaluated in this meta-analysis is given in Table 10–7.

The authors of the meta-analysis article calculated the odds ratios and 95% confidence intervals for each study and used a statistical method to determine summary odds ratios over all the studies. These odds ratios and intervals for the outcome of catheter-related bloodstream infection are illustrated in Figure 10–4. This figure illustrates the typical way findings from meta-analysis studies are presented. Generally the results from each study are shown, and the summary or combined results are given at the bottom of the figure. When the summary statistic is the odds ratio, a line representing the value of 1 is drawn to make it easy to see which of the studies have a significant outcome.

From the data in Table 10–7 and Figure 10–4, it appears that only one study (of the 11) reported a statistically significant outcome because only one has a confidence interval that does not contain 1. The entire confidence interval in Maki and associates' study (1997) is less than 1, indicating that these investigators found a protective effect when using the treated catheters. Of interest is the summary odds ratio, which illustrates that by pooling the results from 11 studies, treating the catheters appears to be beneficial. Several of the studies had relatively small sam-

ple sizes, however, and the failure to find a significant difference may be due to low power. Using meta-analysis to combine the results from these studies can provide insight on this issue.

A meta-analysis does not simply add the means or proportions across studies to determine an "average" mean or proportion. Although several different methods can be used to combine results, they all use the same principle of determining an effect size in each study and then combining the effect sizes in some manner. The methods for combining the effect sizes include the z approximation for comparing two proportions (Chapter 6); the t test for comparing two means (Chapter 6); the P values for the comparisons, and the odds ratio as shown in Veenstra and colleagues' study (1999). The values corresponding to the effect size in each study are the numbers combined in the meta-analysis to provide a pooled (overall) P value or confidence interval for the combined studies. The most commonly used method for reporting meta-analyses in the medical literature is the odds ratio with confidence intervals.

In addition to being potentially useful when published studies reach conflicting conclusions, meta-analysis can help raise issues to be addressed in future clinical trials. The procedure is not, however, without its critics (Thompson and Pocock, 1991), and readers should be aware of some of the potential problems in its use. To evaluate meta-analysis, LeLorier and associates (1997) compared the results of a series of large randomized, controlled trials with relevant previously published meta-analyses. Their results were mixed: They found that meta-analysis accurately predicted the outcome in only 65% of the studies; however, the difference between the trial results and the meta-analysis results was statistically significant in only 12% of the comparisons. Ioannidis and colleagues (1998) determined that the discrepancies in the conclusions were attributable to different disease risks, different study protocols, varying quality of the studies, and possible publication bias (discussed in a following section). These reports serve as a useful reminder that well-designed clinical trials remain a critical source of information.

Studies designed in dissimilar manners should not be combined. In performing a meta-analysis, investigators should use clear and well-accepted criteria for deciding whether studies should be included in the analysis, and these criteria should be stated in the published meta-analysis.

Most meta-analyses are based on the published literature, and some people believe it is easier to publish studies with "significant" results than studies that show no difference. This potential problem is called publication bias. Researchers can take at least three important steps to reduce publication bias. First, they can search for unpublished data, typically done by contacting the authors of published articles. Veenstra and his colleagues (1999) did this and contacted the manufacturer

Table 10–7. Characteristics of studies comparing antiseptic-impregnated with control catheters.

Study, y[a]	Number of Catheter Lumens	Patient Population	Catheter Exchange[b]	Number of Catheters (Number of Patients)		Catheter Duration Mean, d		Outcome Definitions	
				Treatment Group	Control Group	Treatment Group	Control Group	Catheter Colonization[c]	Catheter-Related Bloodstream Infection[d]
Tennenberg et al, 1997	2,3	Hospital	No	137 (137)	145 (145)	5.1	5.3	SQ (IV, SC, >15 CFU)	SO (IV, SC, site), CS, NS
Maki et al, 1997	3	ICU	Yes	208 (72)	195 (86)	6.0	6.0	SQ (IV, >15 CFU)	SO (>15 CFU, IV, hub, inf)[e]
van Heerden et al, 1996[f]	3	ICU	No	28 (28)	26 (26)	6.6	6.8	SQ (IV, >15 CFU)	NR
Hannan et al, 1996	3	ICU	NR	68 (NR)	60 (NR)	7	8	SQ (IV, >10^3 CFU)[g]	SQ (IV, >10^3 CFU), NS
Bach et al, 1994[f]	3	ICU	No	14 (14)	12 (12)	7.0	7.0	QN (IV, >10^3 CFU)	NR
Bach et al, 1996[f]	2, 3	Surgical	No	116 (116)	117 (117)	7.7	7.7	QN (IV, >10^3 CFU)	SO (IV)
Heard et al, 1998[f]	3	SICU	Yes	151 (107)	157 (104)	8.5	9	SQ (IV, SC, >14 CFU)	SO (IV, SC, >4 CFU)
Collin, in press	1, 2, 3	ED/ICU	Yes	98 (58)	139 (61)	9.0	7.3	SQ (IV, SC, >15 CFU)	SO (IV, SC)
Ciresi et al, 1996[f]	3	TPN	Yes	124 (92)	127 (99)	9.6	9.1	SQ (IV, SC, >15 CFU)	SO (IV, SC)
Pemberton et al, 1996	3	TPN	No	32 (32)	40 (40)	10	11	NR	SO (IV), res, NS
Ramsay et al, 1994[e]	3	Hospital	No	199 (199)	189 (189)	10.9	10.9	SQ (IV, SC, >15 CFU)	SO (IV, SC)
Trazzera et al, 1995[e]	3	ICU/BMT	Yes	123 (99)	99 (82)	11.2	6.7	SQ (IV, >15 CFU)	SO (IV, >15 CFU)
George et al, 1997	3	Transplant	No	44 (NR)	35 (NR)	NR	NR	SQ (IV, >5 CFU)	SO (IV)

Abbreviations: NR = not reported; ICU = intensive care unit; SICU = surgical intensive care unit; TPN = total parenteral nutrition; BMT = bone marrow transplant; ED = emergency department; hospital, hospitalwide or a variety of settings; SQ = semiquantitative culture; QN = quantitative culture; CFU = colony-forming units; IV = intravascular catheter segment; SC = subcutaneous catheter segment; site = catheter insertion site; hub = catheter hub; inf = catheter infusate; SO = same organism isolated from blood and catheter; CS = clinical symptoms of systemic infection; res = resolution of symptoms on catheter removal; and NS = no other sources of infection.

[a]Readers should refer to the original article for these citations.

[b]Catheter exchange was performed using a guide wire.

[c]Catheter segments cultured and criteria for positive culture are given in parentheses.

[d]Catheter segment or site cultured and criteria for positive culture are given in parentheses.

[e]Organism identity was confirmed by restriction-fragment subtyping.

[f]Additional information was provided by author (personal communications, Jan 1998–Mar 1998).

[g]Culture method is reported as semiquantitative; criteria for culture growth suggest quantitative method.

Source: Table 1 from Veenstra DL et al: Efficacy of antiseptic-impregnated central venous catheters in preventing catheter-related bloodstream infection. *JAMA* 1999;**281:**261–267. Copyright © 1999, American Medical Association; used with permission.

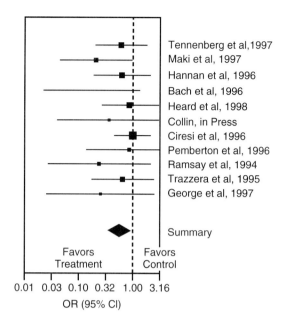

Tennenberg et al,1997
Maki et al, 1997
Hannan et al, 1996
Bach et al, 1996
Heard et al, 1998
Collin, in Press
Ciresi et al, 1996
Pemberton et al, 1996
Ramsay et al, 1994
Trazzera et al, 1995
George et al, 1997

Summary

Favors Treatment   Favors Control

0.01 0.03 0.10 0.32 1.00 3.16
OR (95% CI)

Figure 10–4. Analysis of catheter-related bloodstream infection in trials comparing chlorhexidine/silver sulfadiazine-impregnated central venous catheters with nonimpregnated catheters. The diamond indicates odds ratio (OR) and 95% confidence interval (CI). Studies are ordered by increasing mean duration of catheterization in the treatment group. The size of the squares is inversely proportional to the variance of the studies. (Reproduced, with permission, from Veenstra DL et al: Efficacy of antiseptic-impregnated central venous catheters in preventing catheter-related bloodstream infection. *JAMA* 1999; **281**:261–267. Copyright © 1999, American Medical Association.)

of the treated catheters as well but were unable to identify any unpublished data. Second, researchers can perform an analysis to see how sensitive the conclusions are to certain characteristics of the studies. For instance, Veenstra and colleagues assessed sources of heterogeneity or variation among the studies and reported that excluding these studies had no substantive effect on the conclusions. Third, investigators can estimate how many studies showing no difference would have to be done but not published to raise the pooled P value above the 0.05 level or produce a confidence interval that includes 1 so that the combined results would no longer be significant. The reader can have more confidence in the conclusions from a meta-analysis that finds a significant effect if a large number of unpublished negative studies would be required to repudiate the overall significance. The increasing use of computerized patient databases may lessen the effect of publication bias in future meta-analyses.

The Cochrane Collection is a large and growing database of meta-analyses that were done according to specific guidelines. Each meta-analysis contains a de-

scription and an assessment of the methods used in the articles that constitute the meta-analysis. Graphs such as Figure 10–4 are produced, and, if appropriate, graphs for subanalyses are presented. For instance, if both cohort studies and clinical trials have been done on a given topic, the Cochrane Collection presents a separate figure for each. The Cochrane Collection is available on CD-ROM or via the Internet for an annual fee. The Cochrane Web site states that:

> Cochrane reviews (the principal output of the Collaboration) are published electronically in successive issues of The Cochrane Database of Systematic Reviews. Preparation and maintenance of Cochrane reviews is the responsibility of international collaborative review groups. At the beginning of 1997, the existing and planned review groups (over 40) cover most of the important areas of health care. The members of these groups—researchers, health care professionals, consumers, and others—share an interest in generating reliable, up-to-date evidence relevant to the prevention, treatment, and rehabilitation of particular health problems or groups of problems. How can stroke and its effects be prevented and treated? What drugs should be used to prevent and treat malaria, tuberculosis, and other important infectious diseases? What strategies are effective in preventing brain and spinal cord injury and its consequences, and what rehabilitative measures can help those with residual disabilities?

No one has argued that meta-analyses should replace clinical trials. Veenstra and his colleagues (1999) conclude that a large trial may be warranted to confirm their findings. Despite their shortcomings, meta-analyses can provide guidance to clinicians when the literature contains several studies with conflicting results, especially when the studies have relatively small sample sizes. Furthermore, based on the increasingly large number of published meta-analyses, it appears that this method is here to stay. As with all types of studies, however, the methods used in a meta-analysis need to be carefully assessed before the results are accepted.

10.7 OTHER METHODS FOR MULTIPLE VARIABLES

To make this chapter as complete as possible, we briefly mention several other methods occasionally referred to in the medical literature: discriminant analysis, log-linear analysis, factor analysis, cluster analysis, multivariate analysis of variance (MANOVA), and canonical correlation. These methods tend to be more common in the psychiatric and behavioral sciences literature, but they are sometimes seen in the literature of other specialties as well. These methods all involve multiple measurements on each subject, but they have different purposes; that is, they are used to answer different research questions.

10.7.1 Discriminant Analysis

Logistic regression is used almost exclusively in the biologic sciences. A related technique, **discriminant analysis,** although used with less frequency in medicine, is a common technique in the social sciences. It is similar to logistic regression in that it is used to predict a nominal or categorical outcome. It differs from logistic regression, however, in that it assumes that the independent variables follow a multivariate normal distribution, so it must be used with caution if some X variables are nominal.

The procedure involves determining several discriminant functions, which are simply linear combinations of the independent variables that separate or discriminate among the groups defined by the outcome measure as much as possible. The number of discriminant functions needed is determined by a multivariate test statistic called Wilks' lambda. The discriminant functions' coefficients can be standardized and then interpreted in the same manner as in multiple regression to draw conclusions about which variables are important in discriminating among the groups.

Lord and colleagues (1991) examined the relationships between several sensory and motor factors and measures of postural stability in 95 individuals living in a facility for elderly persons who remain independent. One of their goals was to learn which measures of sensory and motor function were predictive of an individual's ability to maintain his or her balance. In this study, the outcome measures of balance were nominal variables with three categories: poor, moderate, and good. Discriminant analysis is useful when investigators want to evaluate several explanatory variables and the goal is to classify subjects into two or more categories or groups, such as that defined by poor, moderate, and good.

Although discriminant analysis is most often employed to explain or describe factors that distinguish among groups of interest, the procedure can also be used to classify future subjects. Classification involves determining a separate prediction equation corresponding to each group that gives the probability of belonging to that group, based on the explanatory variables. For classification of a future subject, a prediction is calculated for each group, and the individual is classified as belonging to the group he or she most closely resembles.

10.7.2 Log-Linear Analysis

Sports injuries arise from several different factors. Buckley (1988) investigated the risk that a player receives a concussion while playing college football by analyzing the games played by 49 college teams in the 8-year period 1975–1982. Although not explicitly stated, historical records were probably used in the study; however, the research question indicates that this study was cross-sectional. The hypothesis was that the variables of team (offense and defense), player position, situation (rushing and passing), and activity (blocking and tackling) had no effect on the occurrence of game-related concussions. The frequency of injury under each condition was determined by the investigator, and the raw frequencies were then adjusted to reflect the facts that a player is involved in the activity of blocking more often than tackling and that rushing plays occur more often than passing plays. The adjusted frequencies of game-related concussions by team, situation, and activity are given in Table 10–8.

Each independent variable in this research problem is measured on a categorical or nominal scale (team, player position, situation, and activity), as is the outcome variable (whether a concussion occurred). If only two variables are being analyzed, the chi-square method introduced in Chapter 6 can be used to determine whether a relationship exists between them; with three or more nominal or categorical variables, a statistical method called log-linear analysis is appropriate. **Log-linear analysis** may be interpreted as a regression model in which all the variables, both independent and dependent, are measured on a nominal scale. The technique is called log-linear because it involves using the logarithm of the observed frequencies in the contingency table.

Buckley (1988) concluded that the highest risk of concussion exists for an offensive player involved in a block on a rushing play. The second highest level of risk occurs for defensive players involved in a block during a rushing play. Furthermore, rushing plays result in the highest risk of injury, regardless of team or activity. The lowest risk occurs during passing plays for both offensive and defensive teams, regardless of whether they are blocking or tackling.

Log-linear analysis may also be used to analyze multidimensional contingency tables in situations in which no distinction exists between independent and dependent variables, that is, when investigators simply want to examine the relationship among a set of

Table 10–8. Adjusted frequency of game-related concussions by team, situation, and activity for National Athletic Injury/Illness Reporting System I/II college football.

Team	Situation	Activity	
		Tackle	**Block**
Offense	Rushing	41	274
	Passing	17	39
Defense	Rushing	109	197
	Passing	18	30

Source: Reproduced, with permission, from Table 4 in Buckley WE: Concussions in college football. *Am J Sports Med* 1988;**16**:51–56.

nominal measures. The fact that log-linear analysis does not require distinguishing between independent and dependent variables points to a major difference between it and other regression models—namely, that the regression coefficients are not interpreted in log-linear analysis.

10.7.3 Factor Analysis

Psychiatrists need to know how a patient scores on the Minnesota Multiphasic Personality Inventory (MMPI), a commonly used personality test, to decide how to counsel the patient. Similarly, the Medical Outcomes Study Short Form 36 (MOS-SF36) is a questionnaire commonly used to measure patient outcomes (Stewart et al, 1988; Ware and Davies, 1995). In examples such as these, tests with a large number of items are developed, patients or other subjects take the test, and scores on various items are combined to produce scores on the relevant factors.

Let us consider the MOS-SF36 because it is probably used more frequently than any other questionnaire to measure functional outcomes and quality of life. The questionnaire contains 36 items that are combined to produce a patient profile on eight concepts: physical functioning, role-physical, bodily pain, general health, vitality, social functioning, role-emotional, and mental health. The first four concepts are combined to give a measure of physical health, and the last four concepts are combined to give a measure of mental health. The developers used **factor analysis** to decide how to combine the questions to develop these concepts.

In a research problem in which factor analysis is appropriate, all variables are considered to be independent variables; in other words, there is no desire to predict one on the basis of others. Conceptually, factor analysis works as follows: First, a large number of people are measured on a set of items; a rule of thumb calls for at least ten times as many subjects as items. The second step involves calculating correlations. To illustrate, suppose 500 patients answered the 36 questions on the MOS-SF36. Factor analysis answers the question of whether some of the items group together in a logical way, such as items that measure the same underlying component of physical activity. If two items measure the same component, they can be expected to have higher correlations with each other than with other items.

In the third step, factor analysis manipulates the correlations among the items to produce linear combinations, similar to a regression equation without the dependent variable. The difference is that each linear combination, called a **factor,** is determined so that the first one accounts for the most variation among the items, the second factor accounts for the most residual variation after the first factor is taken into consideration, and so forth. Typically, a small number of factors account for enough of the variation

among subjects that it is possible to draw inferences about a patient's score on a given factor. For example, it is much more convenient to refer to scores for physical functioning, role-physical, bodily pain, and so on, than to refer to scores on the original 36 items. Thus, the fourth step involves determining how many factors are needed and how they should be interpreted.

Investigators who use factor analysis usually have an idea of what the important factors are, and they design the items accordingly. Many other issues are of concern in factor analysis, such as how to derive the linear combinations, how many factors to retain for interpretation, and how to interpret the factors. Using factor analysis, as well as the other multivariate techniques, requires considerable statistical skill.

10.7.4 Cluster Analysis

A statistical technique similar conceptually to factor analysis is **cluster analysis.** The difference is that cluster analysis attempts to find similarities among the subjects that were measured instead of among the measures that were made. The object in cluster analysis is to determine a classification or taxonomic scheme that accounts for variance among the subjects. Cluster analysis can also be thought of as similar to discriminant analysis, except that the investigator does not know to which group the subjects belong. As in factor analysis, all variables are considered to be independent variables.

Cluster analysis is frequently used in archeology and paleontology to determine if the existence of similarities in objects implies that they belong to the same taxon. Biologists use this technique to help determine classification keys, such as using leaves or flowers to determine appropriate species. Journalists and marketing analysts also use cluster analysis, referred to in these fields as Q-type factor analysis, as a way to classify readers and consumers into groups with common characteristics. Physicians have not used this technique to a great extent, except in areas of interdisciplinary research with one of these other fields.

10.7.5 Multivariate Analysis of Variance

Multivariate analysis of variance and canonical correlation are similar to each other in that they both involve *multiple dependent* variables as well as multiple independent variables; thus, they are not listed in Table 10–2. **Multivariate analysis of variance (MANOVA)** conceptually (although not computationally) is a simple extension of the ANOVA designs discussed in Chapter 7 to situations in which two or more dependent variables are included. As with ANOVA, MANOVA is appropriate when the independent variables are nominal or categorical and the outcomes are numerical. If the results from the MANOVA are statistically significant, using the multivariate statistic called Wilks' lambda, follow-up ANOVAs may be done to investigate the individual outcomes.

The motivation for doing MANOVA prior to univariate ANOVA is similar to the reason for performing univariate ANOVA prior to *t* tests: to eliminate doing many significance tests and increasing the likelihood that a chance difference is declared significant. In addition, MANOVA permits the statistician to look at complex relationships among the dependent variables. The results from MANOVA are often difficult to interpret, however, and it is used sparingly in the medical literature.

10.7.6 Canonical Correlation Analysis

Canonical correlation analysis also involves both multiple independent and multiple dependent variables. This method is appropriate when *both* the independent variables and the outcomes are numerical and the research question focuses on the relationship between the set of independent variables and the set of dependent variables. For example, suppose researchers wish to examine the overall relationship between indicators of health outcome (physical functioning, mental health, health perceptions, age, gender, etc) measured at the beginning of a study and the set of outcomes (physical functioning, mental health, social contacts, serious symptoms, etc) measured at the end of the study. Canonical correlation analysis forms a linear combination of the independent variables to predict not just a single outcome measure, but a linear combination of outcome measures. The two linear combinations of independent variables and dependent variables, each resulting in a single number (or index), are determined so the correlation between them is as large as possible. The correlation between the pair of linear combinations (or numbers or indices) is called the **canonical correlation.** Then, as in factor analysis, a second pair of linear combinations is derived from the residual variation after the effect of the first pair is removed, and the third pair from those remaining, and so on. Generally, the first two or three pairs of linear combinations account for sufficient variation, and they can be interpreted to gain insights about related factors or dimensions.

10.8 SUMMARY OF ADVANCED METHODS

The advanced methods presented in this chapter are used in approximately 8–10% of the articles in medical and surgical journals (Emerson and Colditz, 1983; Reznick et al, 1987; Altman, 1991b). We think their use is growing for a number of reasons, including increasing statistical knowledge by investigators, increased collaboration with statisticians in medical

studies, the growing concern by journal editors that poorly designed and analyzed studies not be published in their journals, and the widespread availability of statistical packages for computers. Unfortunately for the consumer of the medical literature, these methods are complex and not easy to understand, and they are not always described adequately. As with other complex statistical techniques, investigators should consult with a statistician if one of these advanced methods is planned. This chapter attempts to present these methods in a conceptually oriented way so that medical students and physicians can understand their purpose and the situations in which they are appropriate.

We illustrated concepts important in multiple regression to predict the depression score at 3–4 years later in a cohort of elderly men and women after an initial interview (Henderson et al, 1997). Depression was diagnosed in 30 of the participants at the initial evaluation and in 24 patients at the follow-up. Only 4 of these 24 had been diagnosed as depressed at the outset of the study. The best predictors of the number of depressive symptoms at the follow-up visit included the number of depressive symptoms at the initial visit, deterioration in health and in activities of daily living, poor current health, poor social support, and high levels of use of physician and nurse services. No relationship was found between increasing age and level of depressive symptoms or change in depressive symptoms, nor did symptoms of depression predict subsequent cognitive decline or development of dementia.

Alexandrov and his coinvestigators (1997), in their prospective study in patients with symptoms or signs of carotid artery disease, found a strong correlation between angiographic measurement and peak systolic velocity (PSV) when accessed in a single laboratory using carefully standardized equipment and criteria for interpretation of test data. The relationship between PSV and angiographic stenosis was curvilinear, regardless of the angiographic method. We discussed this study in the context of polynomial regression, in which higher-order terms, such as the square or the cube of the independent variable, improve the prediction. The PSV is an important criterion that should be used carefully with other imaging and flow data in the evaluation of patients with possible carotid artery disease.

Using data from Soderstrom and coinvestigators (1997), we developed a logistic equation to predict the probability that a man who goes to the emergency department with an unintentional injury has a blood alcohol concentration greater than 50 mg/dL. The authors were able to develop a very simple scoring system based on their analyses for men and women as well as for intentional and unintentional injury. They included only four variables: age ($\geq$40), race (Caucasian), day of trauma (weekend), time of day (night) to identify patients at low, medium, and high risk for having blood alcohol concentration >50 mg/dL. Scores of 0, 1, or 2 were assigned to these factors based on sex and whether the injury was intentional or unintentional.

We used observations from Crook and colleagues (1997) to illustrate the Cox proportional hazard model. This important model is used increasingly in medicine because it permits the prediction of a time-dependent outcome. We found that posttreatment nadir PSA level was the most significant independent predictor for any failure; however, the authors found that this was true for all subtypes of failures (chemical, local, distant) as well. When the model is based on only pretreatment variables, the pretreatment prostate-specific antigen (PSA) level was the dominant predictor, along with the T classification.

Veenstra and colleagues (1999) performed a meta-analysis and found that using central venous catheters impregnated with chlorhexidine and silver sulfadiazine can reduce the incidence of catheter colonization and catheter-related bloodstream infections in high-risk patients.

EXERCISES

1. Using the following formula, verify the adjusted mean number of ventricular wall motion abnormalities in smokers and nonsmokers from the hypothetical data in Section 10.3. That is,

$$\text{Adjusted } \overline{Y}_j = \text{Unadjusted } \overline{Y}_j - b(\overline{X}_j - \overline{\overline{X}})$$

2. Nelson and Ellenberg (1986) presented the results of a multivariate analysis of the risk factors for cerebral palsy. They studied 54,000 pregnancies over a 7-year period and collected data on more than 400 potential risk factors. Variables that related to cerebral palsy (CP) at the 0.05 level of significance using univariate (rather than multivariate) analyses or that were of interest on the basis of earlier reports were examined with multivariate techniques. The investigators used stepwise logistic regression at five different periods, beginning before pregnancy and extending through the child's first month of life. An excerpt from the methods section of the paper states:

> Each stage, from before pregnancy through the nursery period, was examined separately with use of the stepwise multiple logistic procedure. Then, in sequence, important factors from earlier stages were examined in conjunction with factors at the subsequent stage. At each stage, the inclusion of a variable required, in addition

to statistical significance, that it contribute an increase in R^2, a measure of predictive ability in a logistic model, of at least 5%.

Table 10–9 reproduces a table from the article.
   a. Why did the authors require a variable to increase R^2 by 5% before adding it to the regression equation?
   b. From Table 10–9, which stage was best predicted?
   c. Of all the variables, which is the most predictive of CP?
   d. Why do the 95% confidence intervals for the relative risk for many predictor variables contain 1 when the predictor variable was supposed to be significantly related to CP in order to be used in the regression equation?

3. Refer to the study by Soderstrom and coinvestigators (1997). Find the probability that a 27-year-old Caucasian man who comes to the emergency department on Saturday night has a BAC ≥ 50 mg/dL.

4. Refer to the study by Soderstrom and coinvestigators (1997). From Table 10–5, find the value of the kappa statistic for the agreement between the predicted and actual number of males with unintentional injuries who have a BAC ≥ 50 mg/dL when they come to the emergency department.

5. Bale and associates (1986) performed a study to consider the physique and anthropometric variables of athletes in relation to their type and amount of training and to examine these variables as potential predictors of distance running performance. Sixty runners were divided into three groups: (1) elite runners with 10-km runs in less than 30 min; (2) good runners with 10-km times between 30 and 35 min, and (3) average runners with 10-km times between 35 and 45 min. Anthropometric data included body density, percentage fat, percentage absolute fat, lean body mass, ponderal index, biceps and calf circumferences, humerus and femur widths, and various skinfold measures. The authors wanted to determine whether the anthropometric variables were able to differentiate between the groups of runners. What is the best method to use for this research question?

6. Ware and collaborators (1986; 1987) reported a study of the effects on health for patients in health maintenance organizations (HMO) and for patients in fee-for-service (FFS) plans. Within the FFS group, some patients were randomly assigned to receive free medical care and others shared in the costs. The health status of the adults was evaluated at the beginning and again at the end of the study. In addition, the number of days spent in bed because of poor

Table 10–9. Prediction of cerebral palsy.

Stage[a]	Prevalence of Antecedent in NCPP (%)	Predicted Risk[b] (%)	95% Confidence Limits	Percentage of CP Cases with Antecedent
Before pregnancy (R^2 = 0.0121)				
Maternal mental retardation[c]	0.4	2.3	0.9/5.5	2.7
Motor deficit in older sibling	1.2	1.4	0.7/2.9	4.4
Hyperthyroidism[c]	0.6	1.8	0.8/4.4	2.7
Maternal seizures[c]	0.4	1.6	0.6/4.4	2.7
Prior fetal deaths > 2	0.6	1.2	0.4/3.2	2.2
Pregnancy (R^2 = 0.0102)				
Severe proteinuria[c]	1.1	1.3	0.6/2.6	4.3
Third-trimester bleeding[c]	13.7	0.6	0.4/0.9	22.3
Thyroid and estrogen use	0.14	1.9	0.4/8.0	1.1
Asymptomatic heart disease	0.9	1.2	0.5/2.8	2.7
Incompetent cervix (rubella)[c]	0.3	1.5	0.5/5.0	1.6
Labor and delivery (R^2 = 0.0635)				
Gestational age ≤32 weeks	3.3	1.4	0.9/2.0	21.0
Lowest fetal heart rate ≤60 beats/min[c]	1.0	1.4	0.7/2.7	5.7
Breech presentation[c]	2.6	0.8	0.5/1.3	11.1
Chorionitis	2.3	0.7	0.4/1.2	10.1
Placental weight ≤325 g	8.7	0.5	0.4/0.8	25.6
Placental complications	3.2	0.6	0.4/1.0	11.2
Immediately post partum (R^2 = 0.0610)				
Birth weight ≤2000 g	1.7	1.6	1.0/2.6	22.2
Time to cry ≥5 min[c]	1.1	1.0	0.6/1.9	12.0
Moro's reflex asymmetric	4.5	0.4	0.3/0.7	18.8
White race	45.8	0.3	0.2/0.5	55.0
Microcephaly[c] (male sex)[c]	2.0	0.6	0.3/1.2	4.9
Nursery period (R^2 = 0.0876)				
Neonatal seizures[c]	0.3	9.6	6.0/15.2	12.2
Major non-CNS malformation[c]	6.8	0.8	0.6/1.2	21.7
Antibiotics, no infection[c]	9.2	0.7	0.5/1.0	20.8
Infection	1.2	1.2	0.7/2.3	7.5

Abbreviations: NCPP = Collaborative Perinatal Project of the National Institute of Neurological and Communicative Disorders and Stroke; CP = cerebral palsy; R^2 = the proportion of log-likelihood explained by the logistic regression, which is a measure of the predictive ability of the model; and CNS = central nervous system.
[a]R^2 represents the value attained when all the listed factors were included in the model.
[b]The risk of cerebral palsy is estimated from the multiple logisitic regression model for each stage, and for each antecedent assumes that only the antecedent of interest is present.
[c]Indicates the major predictors among children weighing 2500 g or more at birth. Factors in parentheses were important only among this group of children.
Source: Reproduced, with permission, from Table 1 in Nelson KB, Ellenberg JH: Antecedents of cerebral palsy. *N Engl J Med* 1986;**315**:81–86.

health was determined periodically throughout the study. These measures, recorded at the beginning of the study—along with information on the participant's age, gender, income, and the system of health care to which he or she was assigned (HMO, free FFS, or pay FFS)—were the independent variables used in the study. The dependent variables were the values of these same 13 measures at the end of the study. The results from a multiple-regression analysis to predict number of bed days are given in Table 10–10.

Table 10–10. Regression coefficients and t test values for predicting bed-days in RAND study.

Explanatory Variables and Other Measures (X)	Dependent-Variable Equation	
	Coefficient (b)	t Test
Intercept	0.613	22.36
FFS freeplan	−0.017	−2.17
FFS payplan	−0.014	−2.18
Personal functioning	−0.0002	−1.35
Mental health	−0.00006	0.25
Health perceptions	−0.002	−5.17
Age	−0.0001	−0.54
Male	−0.026	−4.58
Income	−0.021	−1.65
Three-year term	0.002	0.44
Took physical	−0.003	−0.56
Income · freeplan	0.021	0.86
Income · payplan	0.0002	0.01
Health · freeplan	0.0002	0.33
Health · payplan	0.0006	1.47
Health · income	0.001	1.88
Health · term3	0.0007	1.79
Health · income · freeplan	−0.0034	−2.13
Health · income · payplan	0.0018	1.42
Bed-day00	0.105	6.15
Sample size	1568	
R^2	0.12	
Residual standard error	0.01	

Abbreviation: FFS = fee for service.
Source: Reproduced, with permission, from Ware JE et al: *Health Outcomes for Adults in Prepaid and Fee-for-Service Systems of Care.* (R–3459–HHS.) Santa Monica, CA: The RAND Corporation, 1987, p. 59.

Table 10–11. Values for prediction equation.

Variable	Value
Personal functioning	80
Mental heatlh	80
Health perceptions	75
Age	70
Income	10 (from a formula used in the RAND study)
Three-year term*	Yes
Took physical*	Yes
Bed-day00	14

*Indicates a dummy variable with 1 = yes and 0 = no.

Use the regression equation to predict the number of bed-days during a 30-day period for a 70-year-old woman in the FFS pay plan who has the values on the independent variables shown in Table 10–11 (asterisks designate dummy variables given a value of 1 if yes and 0 if no).

7. Nathan and colleagues (1984) evaluated the clinical information provided in the glycosylated hemoglobin assay by comparing it with practitioners' estimates of glucose control. Their 10-week study included 216 patients with diabetes. They reported a multiple-regression equation to predict physicians' estimates of blood glucose level; the equation included urine test results, insulin use, nocturia, and polydipsia, and it had a multiple correlation coefficient of $R = 0.39$. When the result of random blood glucose testing was added to the regression equation, R increased to 0.58. What is the increase in percentage of variation accounted for in physicians' estimates with information on glucose testing, and how should this finding be interpreted?

8. Table 10–12 contains the results from an analysis of the data from Crook and colleagues (1997) using only information known before treatment was given.
   a. Is the overall Cox model significant when based on pretreatment variables only? What level of significance is reported?
   b. Were any of the potentially confounding variables significant?
   c. Confirm the value of the odds ratios associated with the TUMSTAGE(3) variable of T classifications, and interpret the confidence interval.
   d. What are the major differences in this analysis compared with the one that included posttreatment variables as well?

9. Hindmarsh and Brook (1996) examined the final height of 16 short children who were treated with growth hormone. They studied several variables they thought might predict height in these children, such as the mother's height, the father's height, the child's chronologic and bone age, dose of the growth hormone during the first year, age at the start of therapy, and the peak response to an insulin-induced hypoglycemia test. All anthropometric indices were expressed as standard deviation scores; these scores express height in terms of standard deviations from the mean in a norm group. For example, a height score of −2.00 indicates the child is 2 standard deviations below the mean height for his or her age group.

Data are given in Table 10–13 and in a file entitled "Hindmarsh" on the CD-ROM.
   a. Use the data to perform a stepwise regression and interpret the results. We reproduced a portion of the output in Table 10–14.
   b. What variable entered the equation on the

Table 10–12. Cox proportional hazard model using only pretreatment variables.

−2 Log Likelihood	610.312		

	χ^2	df	Significance
Overall (score)	51.483	6	0.0000
Change (−2LL) from			
Previous block	39.344	6	0.0000
Previous step	39.344	6	0.0000

Variables in the Equation

Variable	B	SE	Wald	df	Significance	R
GSCORE	0.2999	0.2818	1.1321	1	0.2873	0.0000
TUMSTAGE			12.1032	3	0.0070	0.0969
TUMSTAGE (1)	−0.0263	0.7075	0.0014	1	0.9703	0.0000
TUMSTAGE (2)	1.0141	0.5419	3.5014	1	0.0613	0.0481
TUMSTAGE (3)	1.4588	0.5535	6.9458	1	0.0084	0.0873
PRERTHOR	0.1332	0.3262	0.1668	1	0.6830	0.0000
PRERXPSA	0.0080	0.0027	9.0391	1	0.0026	0.1041

		95% CI for Exp (B)	
Variable	Exp (B)	Lower	Upper
GSCORE	1.3497	0.7768	2.3450
TUMSTAGE (1)	0.9740	0.2434	3.8979
TUMSTAGE (2)	2.7568	0.9530	7.9746
TUMSTAGE (3)	4.3008	1.4534	12.7264
PRERTHOR	1.1425	0.6028	2.1654
PRERXPSA	1.0080	1.0028	1.0133

Abbreviations: df = degree of freedom; *SE* = standard error; CI = confidence interval; Wald = statistic used by SPSS to test the significance of variables.
Source: Data, used with permission of the author and publisher, from Crook JM et al: Radiotherapy for localized prostate carcinoma. *Cancer* 1997;**79:**328–336. Output produced using SPSS 10.0, a registered trademark of SPSS, Inc. Used with permission.

Table 10–13. Case summaries.[a]

	Final Height SDS	Age	Dose	Father's Height	Mother's Height	Height SDS Chronologic Age	Height SDS Bone Age
1	−2.18	6.652	20.00	−2.14	−2.20	−3.07	−1.75
2	−2.15	10.383	16.00	−2.78	−0.15	−2.20	−2.43
3	−1.65	10.565	16.00	−1.91	−1.87	−2.62	−0.90
4	−1.18	10.104	15.00	0.84	−1.63	−2.43	−2.06
5	−1.31	11.145	14.00	−1.80	−0.70	−1.92	−1.49
6	−1.35	9.682	14.00	0.09	0.38	−1.38	−0.54
7	−1.18	9.863	16.00	−0.26	−1.70	−2.08	−1.32
8	−2.51	9.463	15.00	−3.62	−0.75	−2.36	−0.45
9	−1.61	7.704	19.00	−2.11	−1.25	−1.98	1.23
10	−2.15	5.858	25.00	1.31	0.23	−2.43	−1.95
11	0.80	5.153	22.00	−0.14	−1.83	−2.36	−0.39
12	−0.20	6.986	21.00	−0.14	−1.83	−2.09	−0.98
13	0.20	8.967	17.00	−0.14	−1.83	−1.38	−0.19
14	−0.71	6.970	21.00	0.50	1.63	−1.09	0.49
15	−1.71	6.515	13.00	0.84	−0.10	−1.98	−0.18
16	−2.32	7.548	21.00	−2.89	−0.20	−3.30	−2.25
Total *N*	16	16	16	16	16	16	16

[a]Limited to first 100 cases.
Abbreviation: SDS = standard deviation score.
Source: Data, used with permission, from Hindmarsh PC, Brook CGD: Final height of short normal children treated with growth hormone. *Lancet* 1996;**348:**13–16. Table produced using SPSS 10.0; used with permission.

Table 10–14. Results from stepwise multiple regression to predict final height in standard deviation scores.[a]

Model		Unstandardized Coefficients		Standardized Coefficients		
		B	**SE**	**β**	**t**	**Significance**
1	(Constant)	−1.055	0.248		−4.261	0.001
	Father's height	0.302	0.142	0.494	2.126	0.052
2	(Constant)	−1.335	0.284		−4.705	0.000
	Father's height	0.337	0.135	0.552	2.503	0.026
	Mother's height	−0.343	0.200	−0.378	−1.715	0.110
3	(Constant)	0.205	0.734		0.280	0.785
	Father's height	0.211	0.131	0.345	1.612	0.133
	Mother's height	−0.478	0.185	−0.527	−2.581	0.024
	Height SDS chronologic age	0.820	0.368	0.505	2.230	0.046
4	(Constant)	−1.110	0.927		−1.198	0.256
	Father's height	0.128	0.124	0.210	1.035	0.323
	Mother's height	−0.559	0.170	−0.617	−3.284	0.007
	Height SDS chronologic age	1.132	0.363	0.697	3.116	0.010
	Dose	0.104	0.052	0.385	2.009	0.070
5	(Constant)	−1.138	0.929		−1.225	0.244
	Mother's height	−0.575	0.170	−0.634	−3.381	0.005
	Height SDS chronologic age	1.325	0.313	0.816	4.229	0.001
	Dose	0.121	0.049	0.451	2.487	0.029

Abbreviations: SE = standard error; SDS = standard deviation scores.
[a]Dependent variable: final height SDS.
[b]*Note:* Because the sample size is small, we set probability for variables to enter the regression equation at 0.15 and for variables to be removed at 0.20.
Source: Data, used with permission, from Hindmarsh PC, Brook CGD: Final height of short normal children treated with growth hormone. *Lancet* 1996;**348**:13–16. Stepwise regression results produced using SPSS; used with permission.

first iteration (model 1)? Why do you think it entered first?

c. What variables are in the equation at the final model? Which of these variables makes the greatest contribution to the prediction of final height?

d. Why do you think the variable that entered the equation first is not in the final model?

e. Using the regression equation, what is the predicted height of the first child? How close is this to the child's actual final height (in SDS scores)?

11   Methods of Evidence-Based Medicine

PRESENTING PROBLEMS

Presenting Problem 1. A 27-year-old woman with a pregnancy of 17 weeks gestation and a 5-year history of insulin-dependent diabetes mellitus comes for obstetric evaluation. (The control of her serum glucose level during the first trimester of her pregnancy has been poor, with fasting values often >200 mg/dL.) She is apprehensive about the outcome of her pregnancy, because she has heard that women with poor control of diabetes during their pregnancy have a high risk of a malformed fetus. Based on your review of the literature, you find that women with poorly controlled diabetes have a risk of fetal malformation of 20–30%. She had a maternal serum α-fetoprotein test that was interpreted as abnormally high. Should she now undergo an ultrasound examination by an experienced ultrasonographer? Greene and Benacerraf (1991) reported 56% sensitivity and 99.5% specificity for ultrasonography and 34% sensitivity and 86% specificity for maternal serum α-fetoprotein determinations in the detection of fetal malformations. You may wish to consult articles by Wenstrom and colleagues (1998) and by Haddow and coworkers (1998) to continue research on the usefulness of α-fetoprotein in detecting abnormalities.

Presenting Problem 2. The electrocardiogram (ECG) is a valuable tool in the clinical prediction of an acute myocardial infarction (MI). In patients with ST segment elevation and chest pain typical of an acute MI, the chance that the patient has experienced an acute MI is greater than 90%. In patients with left bundle-branch block (LBBB) that precludes detection of ST segment elevation, however, the ECG has limited usefulness in the diagnosis of acute MI. Recently, an algorithm based on ST segment changes in patients with acute MI in the presence of LBBB showed a **sensitivity** of 78% for the diagnosis of an MI. A **true-positive rate** of 78% means that a substantial proportion of patients (22%) with LBBB who presented with acute MI would have a **false-negative test** result and possibly be denied acute reperfusion therapy.

Shlipak and his colleagues (1999) conducted a historical cohort study of patients with acute cardiopulmonary symptoms who had LBBB to evaluate further the diagnostic test characteristics and clinical utility of this ECG algorithm for patients with suspected MI. They used their results to develop a **decision tree** for estimating the outcome for three different clinical approaches to these patients: (1) treat all such patients with thrombolysis, (2) treat none of them with thrombolysis, and (3) use the ECG algorithm as a screening test for thrombolysis.

Eighty-three patients with LBBB who presented 103 times with symptoms suggestive of MI were studied. Nine individual ECG predictors of acute MI were evaluated. None of the nine predictors effectively distinguished the 30% of patients with MI from those with other diagnoses. The ECG algorithm had a sensitivity of only 10%. The decision analysis estimated that 92.9% of patients with LBBB and chest pain would survive if all received thrombolytic therapy, whereas only 91.8% would survive if treated according to the ECG algorithm. Data summarizing some of their findings are given in Section 11.3. We use some of these findings to illustrate sensitivity and specificity.

Presenting Problem 3. A major challenge of obstetric practice is the recognition of pregnancies with an elevated risk of adverse perinatal outcome. Maulik and colleagues (1991) applied Doppler ultrasound technology to the study of the hemodynamic condition of the fetal circulatory system. Preliminary studies have demonstrated that changes in the umbilical artery blood flow can be associated with various pregnancy complications and can be used to predict adverse perinatal outcome. Several descriptive indices based on peak systolic and end-diastolic values of the Doppler waveform have been developed to measure umbilical artery flow. Although the systolic–diastolic ratio is the index widely used in the United States, the authors wished to compare the diagnostic validity of four Doppler indices in predicting adverse perinatal outcome in a high-risk population of 350 pregnant women with gestational ages from 34 to 36 weeks. A Doppler examination was performed once on each patient. The perinatal outcome was considered abnormal when any one or combination of the following parameters was present: small for gestational age (< 10th percentile), Apgar score < 7 at 5 min, umbilical arterial pH < 7.10, fetal distress, fetal scalp pH < 7.2, presence of thick meconium, or admission to the neonatal intensive care unit. They used **receiver operating characteristic (ROC) curves** to evaluate the diagnostic value of the four indices of umbilical artery blood flow.

Presenting Problem 4. Steinberg and associates (1986) of the Office of Medical Practice Evaluation at the Johns Hopkins Hospital in Baltimore point out that the efficacy of a given diagnostic test in medical practice is most often reported in terms of sensitivity and specificity, but the clinician's perception of the efficacy of a test determines when the test is used and how results are interpreted. They therefore studied physicians' perceptions of the value of the liver–spleen scan (LSS) in the detection of liver metastases.

The investigators interviewed 42 physicians who had ordered 62 scans to evaluate the possible presence of a liver metastasis. The physicians' estimates of the sensitivity and specificity of the LSS for detecting metastases as well as estimates of likelihood ratios (ratios of true-positives to false-positives) for predicting various scan results were calculated from interviews in which each physician was asked to estimate the probability that an LSS would be normal or abnormal in a series of patients with known pathologic conditions. This cross-sectional study found wide variability in the physicians' perceptions of the sensitivity and specificity of the LSS in detecting liver metastases. The **likelihood ratios** for scans showing a focal defect suggested that some physicians believed that a focal defect was unequivocally diagnostic of a liver metastasis; that is, no false-positive results occurred.

In clinical medicine, treatment decisions are profoundly affected by the physician's interpretation of a test result. Physicians' understanding of a test's sensitivity and specificity undoubtedly reduces the magnitude of errors of inference that may adversely influence patient treatment. Solomon and collaborators (1998) report on several techniques that are helpful in allowing physicians to improve their interpretation and use of diagnostic tests.

11.1 PURPOSE OF THE CHAPTER

"Decision making" is a term that applies to the actions people take many times each day. Many decisions—such as what time to get up in the morning, where and what to eat for lunch, and where to park the car—are often made with little thought or planning. Others—such as how to prepare for a major examination, whether or not to purchase a new car and, if so, what make and model—require some planning and may even include a conscious outlining of the steps involved. This and the following chapters address the second type of decision making as applied to problems within the context of medicine. These problems include evaluating the accuracy of diagnostic procedures, interpreting the results of a positive or negative procedure in a specific patient, **modeling** complex patient problems, and selecting the most appropriate approach to the problem. These topics are very important in using and applying **evidence-based medicine;** they are broadly defined as methods in **medical decision making** or **analysis.** They are applications of probabilistic and statistical principles to *individual patients,* although they are not usually covered in introductory biostatistics textbooks.

We decided to include this material for several reasons. The reviews of journal articles indicate that 2% of articles in psychiatry (Hokanson et al, 1986b) and 7% of articles in surgery (Reznick et al, 1987) and family practice (Fromm and Snyder, 1986) use the methods discussed in this chapter and the next. More importantly, medical decision making is becoming an increasingly important area of research in medicine for evaluating patient outcomes and informing health policy. Thus, more and more quality assurance articles deal with topics such as evaluating new diagnostic procedures, determining the most cost-effective approach for dealing with certain diseases or conditions, and evaluating options available for treatment of a specific patient. These methods also form the basis for cost–benefit analysis, which most leaders in medicine expect to be an area of continuing emphasis.

Finally and most important, correct application of the principles of evidence-based medicine helps clinicians make better diagnostic and management decisions. Physicians and other health care providers who read the medical literature and wish to evaluate new procedures and recommended therapies for patient care need to understand the basic principles discussed in this chapter.

For these reasons, this chapter departs from previous ones in which the emphasis was on understanding the logic of and basis for statistical procedures, leaving the details of calculations to computer programs. People who make decisions about patients must be able to perform the calculations outlined in this chapter. For other perspectives, you may also want to consult resources that discuss the basic concepts involved in medical decision making (eg, Davidoff, 1999; Doubilet, 1988; Eraker et al, 1986; Ingelfinger et al, 1993; Kassirer and Koppelman, 1991; Sackett et al, 1998; Sox, 1988).

We begin the presentation with a discussion of the threshold model of decision making, which provides a unified way of deciding whether to perform a diagnostic procedure; we use Presenting Problem 1 to illustrate the model. Next, the concepts of sensitivity and specificity are defined and illustrated with Presenting Problem 2 on using an ECG to identify patients suspected of having a myocardial infarction. The way sensitivity and specificity are used to make decisions about individual patients is illustrated, again using Presenting Problem 1. Four different methods that lead to equivalent results are presented. Then, an extension of the diagnostic testing problem in which the test results are numbers, not simply positive or negative, is given using the ROC curves in Presenting Problem 3. Presenting Problem 4 is used to illustrate how physicians can revise probabilities more accurately.

11.2 EVALUATING DIAGNOSTIC PROCEDURES WITH THE THRESHOLD MODEL

Consider the patient described in Presenting Problem 1, the 27-year-old woman whose pregnancy is at 17 weeks gestation, who has poorly controlled diabetes mellitus and is concerned about malformations to the fetus. Before deciding whether to order a diagnostic test, the physician must first consider the probability that the fetus has abnormalities. This probability may simply be the **prevalence** of a particular disease if a screening test is being considered. If a history and a physical examination have been performed, the prevalence is adjusted, upward or downward, according to the patient's characteristics (eg, age, gender, and race), symptoms, and signs. Physicians sometimes use the term "index of suspicion" for the probability of a given disease prior to performing a diagnostic procedure; it is also called the **prior probability.** It may also be considered in the context of a threshold model (Pauker and Kassirer, 1980).

The **threshold model** is illustrated in Figure 11–1A. The physician's estimate that the patient has the disease, from information available without using the diagnostic test, is called the probability of disease. It helps to think of the probability of disease as a line that extends from 0 to 1. According to Pauker and Kassirer, the **testing threshold,** T_t, is the point on the probability line at which no difference exists between the value of not treating the patient and performing the test. Similarly, the **treatment threshold,** T_{rx}, is the point on the probability line at which no difference exists between the value of performing the test and treating the patient without doing a test. The points at which the thresholds occur depend on several factors: the risk of the diagnostic test, the benefit of the treatment to patients who have the disease, the risk of the treatment to patients with and without the disease, and the accuracy of the test.

Figure 11–1B illustrates the situation in which the test is quite accurate and has very little risk to the patient. In this situation, the physician is likely to test at a lower probability of disease as well as at a high probability of disease. Figure 11–1C illustrates the opposite situation, in which the test has low accuracy or is risky to the patient. In this case, the test is less likely to be performed. Pauker and Kassirer further

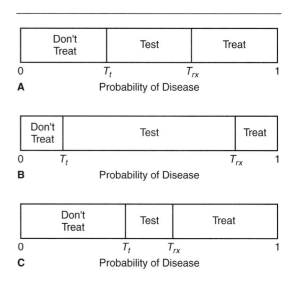

Figure 11–1. Threshold model of decision making. **A:** Threshold model. **B:** Accurate or low-risk test. **C:** Inaccurate or high-risk test. (Adapted and reproduced, with permission, from Pauker SG, Kassirer JP: The threshold approach to clinical decision making. *N Engl J Med* 1980;**302:**1109–1117.)

show that the test and treatment thresholds can be determined for a diagnostic procedure if the risk of the test, the risk and the benefit of the treatment, and the accuracy of the test are known. Although such an analysis is beyond the scope of this text, the statistical method to determine the accuracy of the test can and will be presented. After completing this chapter, you may wish to consult the original article by Pauker and Kassirer (1980).

11.3 MEASURING THE ACCURACY OF DIAGNOSTIC PROCEDURES

The accuracy of a diagnostic test or procedure has two aspects. The first is the test's ability to detect the condition it is testing for, thus being positive in patients who actually have the condition; this is called the **sensitivity** of the test. If a test has high sensitivity, it has a low **false-negative** rate; that is, the test does not falsely give a negative result in many patients who have the disease. Sensitivity can be defined in many equivalent ways: the probability of a positive test result in patients who have the condition; the proportion of patients with the condition who test positive; the **true-positive** rate. Some people use aids such as *positivity in disease* or *sensitive to disease* to help them remember the definition of sensitivity.

The second aspect of accuracy is the test's ability to identify those patients who do *not* have the condition, called the **specificity** of the test. If the specificity of a test is high, the test has a low **false-positive** rate; that is, the test does not falsely give a positive result in many patients without the disease. Specificity can also be defined in many equivalent ways: the probability of a negative test result in patients who do not have the condition; the proportion of patients without the condition who test negative; 1 minus the false-positive rate. The phrases for remembering the definition of specificity are *negative in health* or *specific to health*.

Sensitivity and specificity of a diagnostic procedure are commonly determined by administering the test to two groups: a group of patients known to have the disease (or condition) and another group known not to have the disease (or condition). The sensitivity is then calculated as the proportion (or percentage) of patients known to have the disease who test positive; specificity is the proportion of patients known to be free of the disease who test negative. Of course, we do not always have a **gold standard** immediately available or one totally free from error. Sometimes, we must wait for autopsy results for definitive classification of the patient's condition, as with Alzheimer's disease.

In Presenting Problem 2, Shlipak and colleagues (1999) wanted to evaluate the accuracy of several ECG findings in identifying patients with an MI. They identified 83 patients who had presented 103 times between 1994 and 1997 with chest pain. It was subsequently found that 31 presentations were with an MI and 72 were without. The investigators reviewed the ECG findings and noted the features present; information is given in Table 11–1.

Let us use the information associated with ST segment elevation $\geq$ 5 mm in discordant leads to develop a 2 $\times$ 2 table from which we can calculate sensitivity

and specificity of this finding. Table 11–2 illustrates the basic setup for the 2 $\times$ 2 table method. Traditionally, the columns represent the disease (or condition), using D^+ and D^- to denote the presence and absence of disease (presentation with MI, in this example). The rows represent the tests, using T^+ and T^- for positive and negative test results, respectively (ST segment elevation $\geq$ 5 mm or < 5 mm). **True-positive** (TP) results go in the upper left cell, the T^+D^+ cell. False-positives (FP) occur when the test is positive but no ST segment elevation is present, the upper right T^+D^- cell. Similarly, **true-negatives** (TN) occur when the test is negative in patient presentations that do not have an MI, the T^-D^- cell in the lower right; and false-negatives (FN) are in the lower left T^-D^+ cell corresponding to a negative test in patient presentations with an MI.

In Shlipak and colleagues' study, 31 patient presentations were positive for an MI; therefore, 31 goes at the bottom of the first column, headed by D^+. Seventy-two patient presentations were without an MI, and this is the total of the second (D^-) column. Because 6 ECGs had an ST elevation $\geq$ 5 mm in discordant leads among the 31 presentations with MI, 6 goes in the T^+D^+ (true-positive) cell of the table, leaving 25 of the 31 samples as false-negatives. Among the 72 presentations without MI, 59 did not have the defined ST elevation, so 59 is placed in the true-negative cell (T^-D^-). The remaining 13 presentations are called false-positives and are placed in the T^+D^- cell of the table. Table 11–3 shows the completed table.

Table 11–1. Number of patients having the specified electrocardiogram criteria for acute myocardial infarction among the 31 patients with MI and the 72 without.

ECG Characteristic	Number of Positive Tests Presentations with MI	Number of Negative Tests Presentations without MI
ST elevation $\geq$1 mm in concordant leads[a]	2	72
ST depression $\geq$1 mm in leads V_1, V_2, V_3[a]	1	72
ST elevation $\geq$5 mm in discordant leads[a]	6	59

Abbreviation: MI = myocardial infarction.
[a]Criteria used with algorithm.
Source: Information used, with permission, from Shlipak MG et al: Should the electrocardiogram be used to guide therapy for patients with left bundle-branch block and suspected myocardial infarction? *JAMA* 1999;**281**:714–719.

Table 11–2. Basic setup for 2 $\times$ 2 table.

Test	Disease	
	Positive D⁺	Negative D⁻
Positive T⁺	TP (true-positive)	FP (false-positive)
Negative T⁻	FN (false-negative)	TN (true-negative)

Table 11–3. 2 $\times$ 2 table for evaluating sensitivity and specificity of test for ST elevation.

Lab Finding	MI	
	Present	Absent
ST elevation $\geq$ 5 mm	(TP) 6	(FP) 13
ST elevation < 5 mm	(FN) 25	(TN) 59
	31	72

Abbreviations: TP = true-positive; FP = false-positive; FN = false-negative; TN = true-negative.

Using Table 11–3, we can calculate sensitivity and specificity of the ECG criterion for development of an MI. Try it before reading further. (The sensitivity of an ST elevation ≥ 5 mm in discordant leads is the proportion of presentations with MI that exhibit this criterion, 6 of 31, or 19%. The specificity is the proportion of presentations without MI that do not have the ST elevation, 59 of 72, or 82%.)

11.4 USING SENSITIVITY & SPECIFICITY TO REVISE PROBABILITIES

The values of sensitivity and specificity cannot be used alone to determine the value of a diagnostic test in a specific patient; instead, they are combined with a clinician's index of suspicion (or the prior probability) that the patient has the disease to determine the probability of disease (or nondisease) given knowledge of the test result. Note that a physician's index of suspicion is not always based on probabilities determined by experiments or observations; sometimes, it must simply be a best guess, which is simply an estimate lying somewhere between the prevalence of the disease being investigated in this particular patient population and certainty. A physician's best guess generally begins with baseline prevalence and then is revised upward (or downward) based on clinical signs and symptoms. Some vagueness is acceptable in the initial estimate of the index of suspicion; in the next chapter, we discuss a technique called *sensitivity analysis* for evaluating the effect of the initial estimate on the final decision.

Some clinicians learn how to manipulate the index of suspicion (or prior probability) quite well; others have more difficulty with this concept. We present four different methods because some people prefer one method to another. We personally find the first method, using a 2×2 table, to be the easiest in terms of probabilities. The likelihood ratio method is superior if you can think in terms of odds, and it is important for physicians to understand because it is used in evidence-based medicine. You can use the method that makes the most sense to you or is the easiest to remember and apply.

11.4.1 The 2×2 Table Method

In Presenting Problem 1, a decision must be reached on whether to order ultrasonography for the 27-year-old pregnant woman. This decision depends on three pieces of information: (1) the probability of fetal malformation (index of suspicion) prior to performing any tests; (2) the accuracy of ultrasonography in detecting abnormalities among pregnant women who are subsequently shown to have abnormal fetuses (sensitivity); and (3) the frequency of a negative result for the procedure in pregnant women who subsequently have normal infants (specificity).

What is your index of suspicion for fetal malformation in this patient both before and after the maternal serum α-fetoprotein (MSAFP) test? Consider that this condition is fairly rare in pregnant women of this age. The patient has had poor control of her diabetes, however, a situation that makes fetal abnormalities more likely. A reasonable prior probability of fetal malformation in a woman like this one is 20–30%; let us use 20% for this example.

How did this probability change with the positive MSAFP test? How will it change if ultrasonography is performed and interpreted as abnormal? If it is negative? Answers to these questions help us determine the testing threshold and indicate whether ultrasound should be performed. First, we must know how sensitive and specific the MSAFP test is for fetal anomalies and use this information to revise the probability considering that the test was abnormally high. These new probabilities are called the **predictive values of a positive test,** or the **posterior probabilities.** Then we must repeat the process with ultrasound; that is, determine its sensitivity and specificity and use the information to revise the probability after interpreting the MSAFP test.

The first step in the 2×2 table method for determining predictive values of a diagnostic test includes the information reflecting the physician's best guess that the patient has the disease before the test is done, which is the index of suspicion (or prior probability) of disease. Many people find it easier to work with whole numbers rather than percentages when evaluating diagnostic procedures. Another way of saying that the fetus has a 20% chance of having anomalies is to say that 200 out of 1000 patients like this one would have abnormal fetuses. In Table 11–4, this number (200) is written at the bottom of the D^+ column. Similarly, 800 patients out of 1000 would not have a fetus with anomalies, and this number is written at the bottom of the D^- column.

The second step is to fill in the cells of the table by using the information on the test's sensitivity and specificity. Table 11–4 shows that the true-positive rate, or sensitivity, corresponds to the T^+D^+ cell (labeled TP). Greene and Benacerraf (1991) reported 34% sensitivity and 86% specificity for the MSAFP test for predicting fetal abnormalities. Thirty-four

Table 11–4. Step one: Adding the prior probabilities to the 2×2 table.

Test	Disease	
	D^+	D^-
T^+	(TP)	(FP)
T^-	(FN)	(TN)
	200	800

Abbreviations: TP = true-positive; FP = false-positive; FN = false-negative; TN = true-negative.

percent of the 200 patients with fetal malformations, or 68 patients, are therefore true-positives, and 100% − 34% = 66%, or 132, are false-negatives (Table 11–5). Using the same reasoning, we find that a test that is 86% specific results in 688 true-negatives in the 800 patients without fetal abnormalities, and 800 − 688 = 112 false-positives occur.

The third step is to add across the rows. From row 1, we see that 68 + 112 = 180 women like this patient would have a positive MSAFP test (Table 11–6). Similarly, 820 women would have a negative test.

The fourth step involves the calculations for predictive values. From Table 11–6, of the 180 women with a positive test, 68 actually have abnormal fetuses, giving a result of 37.8%. Similarly, 688 of the 820 women with a negative test do not have abnormal fetuses, giving a result of 83.9%. The percentage 37.8% is called the **predictive value of a positive test,** abbreviated PV^+, and gives the percentage of patients with a positive test result who actually have the condition (or the probability of fetal anomalies, given a positive MSAFP test). The percentage 83.9% is called the **predictive value of a negative test,** abbreviated PV^-, and gives the probability that the patient does not have the condition when the test is negative. Two other probabilities can be estimated from this table as well, although they do not have specific names: 112/180 = 0.622 is the probability that the patient does not have the condition, even though the test is positive; and 132/820 = 0.161 is the probability that the patient does have the condition, even though the test is negative.

To summarize so far, the MSAFP test is not very sensitive and is moderately specific for detecting fetal malformations when used at this stage of gestation. When it is used with a woman who has an increased risk due to poor diabetic control, the MSAFP test provides only a moderate amount of information. When positive, it increases the probability of fetal malformation from 20% to almost 38%; and when negative, it only slightly increases the probability of no fetal malformation from 80% to approximately 84%. Thus, in general, tests that have high sensitivity

Table 11–6. Step 3: Completed 2 × 2 table for calculating predictive values.

A. Completed Table

Test	Disease		
	D⁺	**D⁻**	
T⁺	(TP) 68	(FP) 112	180
T⁻	(FN) 132	(TN) 688	820
	200	800	1000

B. Step 4

Predictive value of a positive test	$PV^+ = TP/(TP + FP) = 68/180$ $= 0.378$
Predictive value of a negative test	$PV^- = TN/(TN + FN) = 688/820$ $= 0.839$

Abbreviations: TP = true-positive; FP = false-positive; FN = false-negative; TN = true-negative.

are useful for ruling out a disease in patients when the test is negative. A positive test does not tell us much, however, partly because of its low specificity.

Now we repeat the previous reasoning for the ultrasound examination. Presenting Problem 1 indicates that the woman's MSAFP test was positive; therefore, from Table 11–6, we know that the probability of fetal anomalies with a positive MSAFP test is 37.8%, or approximately 38%. When a second diagnostic test is performed, the results of the first test determine the prior probability. Based on the positive MSAFP test, 38%, or 380 out of 1000 women, are therefore likely to have an abnormal fetus, and 620 are not. These numbers are the column totals in Table 11–7. Ultrasound was shown to be 56% sensitive and 99.5% specific for fetal malformations; applying these statistics gives (0.56)(380), or 212.8, true-positives and (0.995)(620), or 616.9, true-negatives. Subtraction gives 167.2 false-negatives and 3.1 false-positives. After adding the rows, the predictive value of a positive ultrasound examination is 212.8/215.9, or 98.6%, and the predictive value of a negative ultrasound is 78.7% (see Table 11–7).

Greene and Benacerraf (1991) concluded that the MSAFP is of minimal utility in a high-risk population that is examined by an experienced sonographer. To see why, consider the predictive value of ultrasound used without the MSAFP test; that is, with a 20% prior probability of fetal malformation. The positive predictive value of ultrasound is 96.6%, and the negative predictive value is 90.0%. We suggest you confirm these calculations to be sure we are correct.

To summarize, a positive ultrasound examination following a positive MSAFP is highly (98.6%) predictive of fetal anomalies. A negative ultrasound following a positive MSAFP indicates a fetus without

Table 11–5. Step 2: Using sensitivity and specificity to determine number of true-positives, false-negatives, true-negatives, and false-positives in 2 × 2 table.

Test	Disease	
	D⁺	**D⁻**
T⁺	(TP) 68	(FP) 112
T⁻	(FN) 132	(TN) 688
	200	800

Abbreviations: TP = true-positive; FP = false-positive; FN = false-negative; TN = true-negative.

Table 11–7. Completed 2 × 2 table for ultrasound examination from Presenting Problem 1.

A. Completed Table

Test	Disease D⁺	Disease D⁻	
T⁺	(TP) 212.8	(FP) 3.1	215.9
T⁻	(FN) 167.2	(TN) 616.9	784.1
	380	620	1000.9

B. Step 4

Predictive value of a positive test	PV⁺ = TP/(TP + FP) = 212.8/215.9 = 0.986
Predictive value of a negative test	PV⁻ = TN/(TN + FN) = 616.9/784.1 = 0.787

Abbreviations: TP = true-positive; FP = false-positive; FN = false-negative; TN = true-negative.

abnormalities in almost 80% of similar situations. Omitting the initial MSAFP test has little effect on these percentages, lending support to the argument that MSAFP has little value if ultrasound is to be performed anyway.

11.4.2 The Likelihood Ratio

An alternative method for revising prior probabilities uses a quantity called the likelihood ratio and works with prior **odds** rather than prior probabilities. The likelihood ratio is being used with increasing frequency in the medical literature, especially within the context of evidence-based medicine. Even if you decide not to use this particular approach to revising probabilities, you need to know how to use the likelihood ratio. Because it makes calculating predictive values very simple, many people prefer it after becoming familiar with it.

The **likelihood ratio** expresses the odds that the test result occurs in patients with the disease versus the odds that the test result occurs in patients without the disease. Thus, a positive test has one likelihood ratio and a negative test another. For a positive test, the likelihood ratio is the odds of a positive test in patients with the disease, or the sensitivity, versus a positive test in patients without the disease, or the false-positive rate. Thus, we find the likelihood ratio by dividing the true-positive rate by the false-positive rate.

The likelihood ratio is multiplied by the prior, or **pretest odds,** to obtain the **posttest odds** of a positive test. Thus,

Pretest odds × Likelihood ratio = Posttest odds

In Presenting Problem 1, the sensitivity of the MSAFP test for fetal anomalies is assumed to be 34%, and the specificity is 86%; so the false-positive rate is $100\% - 86\% = 14\%$. The likelihood ratio (LR) for a positive test is therefore

$$LR = \frac{0.34}{0.14} = 2.43$$

To use the likelihood ratio, we must convert the prior probability into prior odds. The prior probability MSAFP test is 0.20, and the odds are found by dividing the prior probability by 1 minus the prior probability. We obtain

$$
\begin{aligned}
\text{Pretest odds} &= \frac{\text{Prior probability}}{1 - \text{Prior probability}} \\
&= \frac{0.20}{1 - 0.20} \\
&= \frac{0.20}{0.80} = 0.25
\end{aligned}
$$

It helps to keep in mind that the probability is like a proportion: It is the number of times a given outcome occurs divided by all the occurrences. If we take a sample of blood from a patient five times, and the sample is positive one time, we can think of the probability as being 1 in 5, or 0.20. The odds, on the other hand, is a ratio: It is the number of times a given outcome occurs divided by the number of times that specific outcome does not occur. With the blood sample example, the odds of a positive sample is 1 to 4, or $1/(5 - 1)$.

Continuing with the MSAFP example, we multiply the pretest odds by the likelihood ratio to obtain the posttest odds:

Posttest odds = 0.25 × 2.43 = 0.607

Because the posttest odds are really 0.607 to 1, although the "to 1" part does not appear in the preceding formula, these odds can be used by clinicians simply as they are. Or they can be reconverted to a probability by dividing the odds by 1 plus the odds. That is,

$$
\begin{aligned}
\text{Posterior probability} &= \frac{\text{Posttest odds}}{1 + \text{Posttest odds}} \\
&= \frac{0.607}{1 + 0.607} = 0.378
\end{aligned}
$$

The posterior probability is, of course, the predictive value of a positive test and is the same result we found with previous methods.

Most journal articles that present likelihood ratios use the LR as just defined, which is actually the likelihood ratio for a positive test. The evidence-based medicine literature sometimes uses the notation of ⁺LR to distinguish it from the LR for a negative test, generally denoted by ⁻LR. The negative likelihood ratio, as defined in the literature, can be used to find the odds of disease, even if the test is negative. It is the ratio of false-negatives to true-negatives (FN/TN).

To illustrate the use of the negative likelihood ratio, let us find the probability of fetal anomalies if the MSAFP test is negative. The ⁻LR in this example is 0.66 (1 minus sensitivity) divided by 0.86 (true-negatives), or 0.767. Multiplying the ⁻LR by the prior odds of the disease gives $0.767 \times 0.25 = 0.192$, the posttest odds of disease with a negative test. We can again convert the odds to a probability by dividing 0.192 by 1 + 0.192 to obtain 0.161, or 16.1%. This value tells us that a woman such as our patient, about whom our index of suspicion is 20%, has a posttest probability of fetal anomaly, even with a negative test, of approximately 16%. This result is consistent with the predictive value of a negative test of 84% (Section 11.4.1). So, another way to interpret the ⁻LR is that it is analogous to 1 minus PV⁻.

Absolutely nothing is wrong with thinking in terms of odds instead of probabilities. If you are comfortable using odds instead of probabilities, the calculations are really quite streamlined. One way to facilitate conversion between probability and odds is to recognize the simple pattern that results. We list some common probabilities in Table 11–8, along with the odds and the action to take with the likelihood ratio to find the posttest odds.

To use the information in Table 11–8, note that the odds in column 2 are < 1 when the probability is < 0.50, are equal to 1 when the probability is 0.50, and are > 1 when the probability is > 0.50. The last column shows that we divide the likelihood ratio to obtain the posttest odds when the prior probability is < 0.50 and multiply when it is > 0.50. To illustrate, suppose your index of suspicion, prior to ordering a diagnostic procedure, is about 25%. A probability of 0.25 gives 1 to 3 odds, so the likelihood ratio is divided by 3. If your index of suspicion is 75%, the odds are 3 to 1, and the likelihood ratio is multiplied by 3. Once the posttest odds are found, columns 2 and 1 can be used to convert back to probabilities.

A major advantage of the likelihood ratio method is the need to remember only one number, the ratio, instead of two numbers, sensitivity and specificity. Sackett and colleagues (1991) indicate that likelihood

ratios are much more stable (or robust) for indicating changes in prevalence than are sensitivity and specificity; these authors also give the likelihood ratios for some common symptoms, signs, and diagnostic tests.

A nomogram published by Fagan (1975) makes the likelihood ratio somewhat simpler to use. In this nomogram, reproduced in Figure 11–2, the pretest and posttest odds are converted to prior and posterior probabilities, eliminating the need to perform this extra calculation.

To use the nomogram, place a straightedge at the point of the prior probability, denoted $P(D)$, on the right side of the graph and the likelihood ratio in the center of the graph; the revised probability, or predictive value $P(D|T)$, is then read from the left-hand side of the graph. In our example, the prior percentage of 20 and the likelihood ratio of 2.43 result in a revised percentage near 40, consistent with the previous calculations.

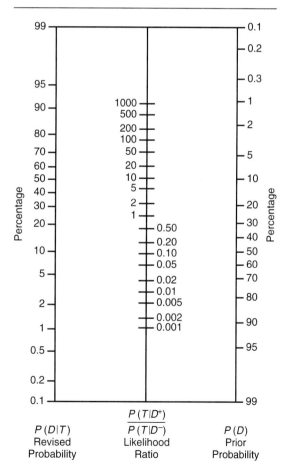

Figure 11–2. Nomogram for using Bayes' theorem. (Adapted and reproduced, with permission, from Fagan TJ: Nomogram for Bayes' theorem. (Letter.) *N Engl J Med* 1975;**293**:257.)

Table 11–8. Conversion table for changing probabilities to odds and action to take with likelihood ratio to obtain posttest odds.

Prior Probability	Prior Odds	Posttest Odds = Likelihood Ratio
0.10	1 to 9	÷ by 9
0.20	1 to 4	÷ by 4
0.25	1 to 3	÷ by 3
0.33	1 to 2	÷ by 2
0.50	1 to 1	× by 1
0.66	2 to 1	× by 2
0.75	3 to 1	× by 3
0.80	4 to 1	× by 4
0.90	9 to 1	× by 9

11.4.3 The Decision Tree Method

Using Presenting Problem 1 again, we illustrate the **decision tree** method for revising the initial probability, a 20% chance of fetal malformation in this example. Trees are useful for diagramming a series of events, and they can easily be extended to more complex examples. Figure 11–3 illustrates that prior to ordering a test, the patient can be in one of two conditions: with the disease (or condition) or without the disease (or condition). These alternatives are represented by the branches, with one labeled D^+, indicating a disease present and the other labeled D^-, representing no disease.

In the second step, the prior probabilities are included on the tree. Figure 11–4 shows the 20% best guess that this woman's fetus has anomalies, written above the D^+ branch. The chance that the fetus is normal, 80% (found by subtracting 20% from 100%), is written above the D^- line.

Figure 11–5 illustrates the third step in determining the predictive values for a diagnostic test. The test can be either positive or negative, regardless of the patient's true condition. These situations are denoted by T^+ for a positive test and T^- for a negative test and are illustrated in the decision tree by the two branches connected to both the D^+ and D^- branches.

In the fourth and fifth steps, information on sensitivity and specificity of the test is added to the tree. In the fourth step, we concentrate on the 20% of the time a malformation is present, the D^+ branch; an MSAFP test is positive in approximately 34% of these patients. Figure 11–6 shows the 34% sensitivity of the test written on the T^+ line. In 66% of the cases (100% – 34%), therefore, the test is negative, written on the T^- line. This information is then combined to obtain the numbers at the end of the lines: The result for 34% of the 20% of the women with abnormal fetuses, or (20%)(34%) = 6.8%, is written at the end of the D^+T^+ branch; the result (20%)(66%) = 13.2% for women with abnormal fetuses who have a negative test is written at the end of the D^+T^- branch.

In the fifth step, we concentrate on the 80% of the women who have a normal fetus (Figure 11–7). If the test is 86% specific in the patient population of interest, we expect 86% of those without abnormal fetuses to have a negative test, written on the T^- line. The remain-

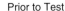
Prior to Test

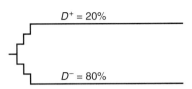

$D^+ = 20\%$

$D^- = 80\%$

Figure 11–4. Step 2: Decision tree with prior probabilities on branches.

ing 14% are false-positives, written on the T^+ line. Multiplying the percentages gives 11.2% at the end of the D^-T^+ branch and 68.8% at the end of the D^-T^- branch.

The tree for the entire situation at this point is shown in Figure 11–8. Note that the percentages at the ends of the four branches add to 100%.

The next step is to reverse the tree so that it more accurately describes the situation confronting the physician: The physician does not know if any fetal abnormalities are present; the result of the MSAFP test is all the information given. Figure 11–9 shows that the tree is reversed by putting the *test* first and then drawing a conclusion about whether the disease is likely from the test results.

To complete the reversed tree, we transfer the numbers from the ends of the branches on the first tree to the ends of the branches on the reversed tree (Figure 11–10). Thus, the D^+T^+ 6.8% goes to the T^+D^+ line; the D^+T^- 13.2% goes to the T^-D^+ line; the D^-T^+ 11.2% goes to the T^+D^- line; and the D^-T^- 68.8% goes to the T^-D^- line. Finally, working backward in the reversed tree, we add the numbers at the ends of the branches to obtain the percentages of patients in whom positive and negative tests are found. Figure 11–11 illustrates that in this clinical problem, a positive test is expected in 18% of the patients (6.8% + 11.2%). Similarly, a negative test is expected in 82% of the patients (13.2% + 68.8%).

The answers to the key questions (or the predictive values) can now be determined. If this woman has a positive MSAFP test, the revised probability that her fetus is abnormal is found by dividing 6.8% by 18%, giving a 37.8% chance. If the test is negative, the chance that the fetus is normal is given by 68.8% divided by 82%, or a 83.9% chance. The decision tree can also be used to determine the probability that a patient with this symptom complex who has a positive test has a normal fetus, which is 62.2% (11.2% divided by 18%). Similarly, 16.1% (13.2% divided by 82%) of those with a negative test actually have a fetus with malformations. These conclusions are, of course, exactly the same as the conclusions reached by using the 2×2 table method.

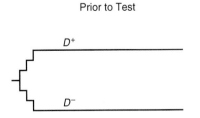

Prior to Test

D^+

D^-

Figure 11–3. Step 1: Decision prior to ordering diagnostic test.

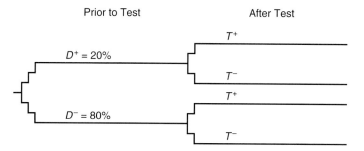

Figure 11–5. Step 3: Decision tree with test result branches.

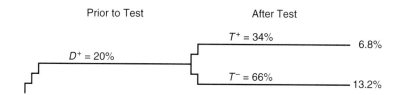

Figure 11–6. Step 4: Decision tree with sensitivity information included on D^+ branch.

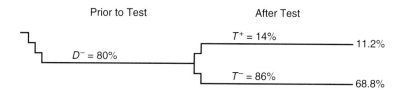

Figure 11–7. Step 5: Decision tree with specificity information included on D^- branch.

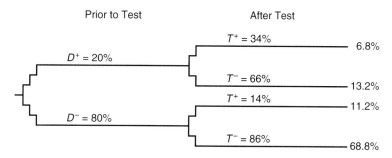

Figure 11–8. End of step 5: Decision tree with test result information.

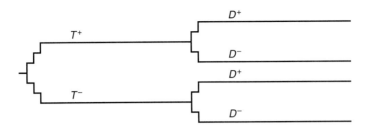

Figure 11–9. Step 6: Reversing tree to correspond with situation facing physicians.

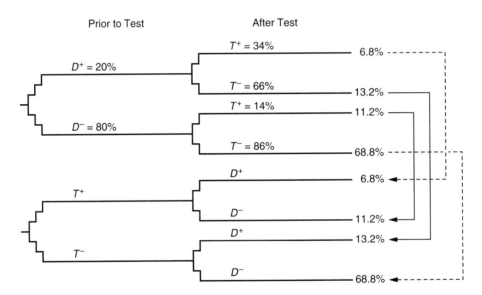

Figure 11–10. Step 7: Transferring numbers to reversed tree.

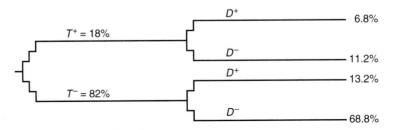

Figure 11–11. Final reversed decision tree.

11.4.4 Bayes' Theorem

A final method for calculating the predictive value of a positive test involves the use of a mathematical formula. Bayes' theorem is not new; it was developed in the 18th century by an English clergyman and mathematician, Thomas Bayes, but was not published until after his death. It had little influence at the time, but two centuries later it became the basis for a different way to approach statistical inference, called Bayesian statistics. In the early clinical epidemiology literature, Bayes' theorem was used almost exclusively for revising probabilities. The two methods discussed first, however, the 2×2 table and likelihood ratio, are now seen with greater frequency than Bayes' theorem. Nonetheless, because it is referred to on occasion, it is worth knowing its purpose.

The formula for Bayes' theorem gives the predictive value of a positive test, or the chance that a patient with a positive test has the disease. The symbol P stands for the probability that an event will happen (see Chapter 4), and $P(D'|T')$ is the probability that the disease is present, given that the test is positive. As we discussed in Chapter 4, this probability is a **conditional probability** in which the event of the disease being present is dependent, or conditional, on having a positive test result. The formula, known as **Bayes' theorem,** can be rewritten from the form we used in Chapter 4, as follows:

$$P(D^+ | T^+) = \frac{P(T^+ | D^+) \, P(D^+)}{P(T^+ | D^+) \, P(D^+) + P(T^+ | D^-) \, P(D^-)}$$

This formula specifies the probability of disease, given the occurrence of a positive test. The two probabilities in the numerator are (1) the probability that a test is positive, given that the disease is present (or the sensitivity of the test) and (2) the best guess (or prior probability) that the patient has the disease to begin with. The denominator is simply the probability that a positive test occurs at all, $P(T^+)$, which can occur in one of two ways: a positive test when the disease is present, and a positive test when the disease is not present. The first product in the denominator is the same as the numerator. The second product in the denominator is the probability of a positive test, given that the disease is not present, multiplied (or weighted) by the probability that the disease is not present. The first quantity in this term is simply the false-positive rate, and the second can be thought of as 1 minus the probability that the disease is present.

Rewriting Bayes' theorem in terms of sensitivity and specificity, we obtain

$$\frac{\text{Sensitivity} \times \text{Prior probability}}{\begin{array}{c}(\text{Sensitivity} \times \text{Prior probability}) \\ + \, [(\text{False-positive rate} \times (1 - \text{Prior probability})]\end{array}}$$

We again use Presenting Problem 1 to illustrate the use of Bayes' formula. Recall that the prior probabil-

ity of a fetus with malformation is 0.20, and sensitivity and specificity of the MSAFP test for malformation are 34% and 86%, respectively. Most people find it easier to work with decimals than with percentages in Bayes' theorem. In the numerator, the sensitivity times the probability of disease is (0.34)(0.20). In the denominator, that quantity is repeated and added to the false-positive rate, 0.14, times 1 minus the probability of malformation, 0.80. Thus, we have

$$P(D^+ | T^+) = \frac{0.34 \times 0.20}{(0.34 \times 0.20) + (0.14 \times 0.80)}$$
$$= \frac{0.068}{0.068 + 0.112} = 0.378$$

This result, of course, is exactly the same as the result obtained with the 2×2 table and the decision tree methods.

A similar formula may be derived for the predictive value of a negative test:

$$P(D^- | T^-) = \frac{P(T^- | D^-) P(D^-)}{P(T^- | D^-) P(D^-) + P(T^- | D^+) P(D^+)}$$

Written in terms of sensitivity, specificity, and prior probability, the formula is

$$\frac{\text{Specificity} \times (1 - \text{Prior probability})}{\begin{array}{c}[\text{Specificity} \times (1 - \text{Prior probability})] \\ + \, (\text{False-positive rate} \times \text{Prior probability})\end{array}}$$

Calculation of the predictive value using Bayes' theorem for a negative test in the MSAFP example is left as an exercise.

11.4.5 Summary of Methods

We illustrated four equivalent methods for revising the probability that a patient has a disease based on the results of a diagnostic test. This process assumes that the prior probability of the disease, the accuracy and risks associated with the test, and the risks and benefits of treatment interact in such a way as to position the problem between the testing threshold and the treatment threshold. Illustrating all four methods gives you an opportunity to choose the approach that makes the most sense to you and is easiest to understand and remember. We personally find the 2×2 table approach the easiest, but all of the other methods also appear in the literature, the likelihood ratio with increasing frequency, especially within the context of evidence-based medicine. We will use the decision tree approach again in the next chapter to model more complex problems.

It is important to recognize that the values for the sensitivity and specificity of diagnostic procedures assume the procedures are interpreted without error. For example, variation is inherent in determining the value of many laboratory tests. As mentioned in

Chapter 3, the coefficient of variation is used as a measure of the replicability of assay measurements. In Chapter 5 we discussed the concepts of intrarater and interrater reliability, including the statistic kappa to measure interjudge agreement. Variability in test determination or in test interpretation is ignored in calculating values for sensitivity, specificity, and the predictive values of tests.

Before leaving this section, we include some final comments regarding the use of these methods in clinical medicine. Fairly typical in medicine is the situation in which a very sensitive test (95–99%) is used to detect the presence of a disease with low prevalence (or prior probability); that is, the test is used in a screening capacity. By itself, these tests have little diagnostic meaning. When used indiscriminately to screen for diseases that have low prevalence (eg, 1 in 1000), the rate of false positivity is high. Tests with these statistical characteristics become more helpful in making a diagnosis when used in conjunction with clinical findings that suggest the possibility of the suspected disease. To summarize, when the prior probability is very low, even a very sensitive and specific test increases the posttest probability only to a moderate level. For this reason, a positive result based on a very sensitive test is often followed by a very specific test, such as following a positive antinuclear antibody test (ANA) for systemic lupus erythematosus with the anti-DNA antibody procedure.

As another example of a test with high sensitivity for a particular disease, consider the serum calcium level. It is a good screening test because it is almost always elevated in patients with primary hyperparathyroidism; meaning, it rarely "misses" a person with primary hyperparathyroidism. Serum calcium level is not specific for this disease, however, because other conditions, such as malignancy, sarcoidosis, multiple myeloma, or vitamin D intoxication, may also be associated with an elevated serum calcium. A more specific test, such as radioimmunoassay for parathyroid hormone, may therefore be ordered after finding an elevated level of serum calcium. The posterior probability calculated by using the serum calcium test becomes the new index of suspicion (prior probability) for analyzing the effect of the radioimmunoassay.

The diagnosis of AIDS in low-risk populations provides an example of the important role played by prior probability. Some states in the United States required premarital testing for the HIV antibody in couples applying for a marriage license. The enzyme-linked immunosorbent assay (ELISA) test is highly sensitive and specific; some estimates range as high as 99% for each. The prevalence of HIV antibody in a low-risk population, such as people getting married in a Midwestern community, however, is very low; estimates range from 1 in 1000 to 1 in 10,000. How useful is a positive test in such situations? For the higher estimate of 1 in 1000 for the prevalence and

99% sensitivity and specificity, 99% of the people with the antibody test positive (99% × 1 = 0.99 person), as do 1% of the 999 people without the antibody (9.99 people). Among those with a positive ELISA test (0.99 + 9.99 = 10.98 people), therefore, less than 1 person is truly positive (the positive predictive value is actually about 9% for these numbers).

The previous examples illustrate three important points:

1. To **rule out** a disease, we want to be sure that a negative result is really negative; therefore, not very many false-negatives should occur. A sensitive test is the best choice to obtain as few false-negatives as possible if factors such as cost and risk are similar; that is, high sensitivity helps rule out if the test is negative. As a handy acronym, if we abbreviate sensitivity by **SN,** and use a sensitive test to rule **OUT,** we have **SNOUT.**

2. To find evidence of a disease, we want a positive result to indicate a high probability that the patient has the disease; that is, a positive test result should really indicate disease. We therefore want few false-positives. The best method for achieving this is a highly specific test; that is, high specificity helps rule in if the test is positive. Again, if we abbreviate specificity by **SP,** and use a specific test to rule **IN,** we have **SPIN.**

3. To make accurate diagnoses, we must understand the role of prior probability of disease. If the prior probability of disease is extremely small, a positive result does not mean very much and should be followed by a test that is highly specific. The usefulness of a negative result depends on the sensitivity of the test.

11.5 ROC CURVES

The preceding procedures for revising the prior (pretest) probability of a disease or condition on the basis of information from a diagnostic test are applicable if the outcome of the test is simply positive or negative. Many tests, however, have values measured on a **numerical scale.** When test values are measured on a continuum, sensitivity and specificity levels depend on where the cutoff is set between positive and negative. This situation can be illustrated by two normal (gaussian) distributions of laboratory test values: one distribution for people who have the disease and one for people who do not have the disease. Figure 11–12 presents two hypothetical distributions corresponding to this situation in which the mean value for people with the disease is 75 and that for those without the disease is 45. If the cutoff point is placed at 60, about 10% of the people without the disease are incorrectly classified as abnormal (false-positive) because their test value is greater than 60, and about 10% of the people with the disease are incorrectly classified as normal (false-negative) because their

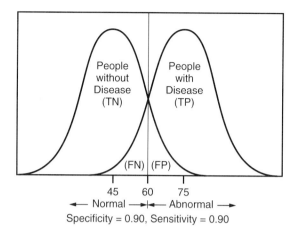

Figure 11–12. Two hypothetical distributions with cutoff at 60. *Abbreviations:* TN = true-negative; TP = true-positive; FN = false-negative; FP = false-positive.

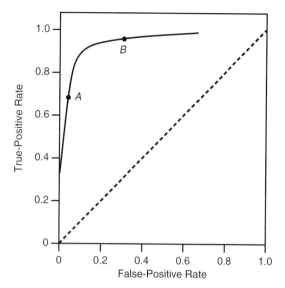

Figure 11–14. Receiver operating characteristic curve.

test value is less than 60. In other words, this test has a sensitivity of 90% and a specificity of 90%.

Suppose a physician decides to use a test with greater sensitivity, meaning that the physician prefers to have more false-positives than to miss people who really have the disease. Figure 11–13 illustrates what happens if the sensitivity is increased by lowering the cutoff point to 55 for a normal test. The sensitivity is increased, but at the cost of a lower specificity.

A more efficient way to display the relationship between sensitivity and specificity for tests that have continuous outcomes is with **receiver operating characteristic,** or **ROC, curves.** ROC curves were developed in the communications field as a

way to display signal-to-noise ratios. If we think of true-positives as being the correct signal from a diagnostic test and false-positives as being noise, we can see how this concept applies. The ROC curve is a plot of the sensitivity (or true-positive rate) to the false-positive rate. The dotted diagonal line in Figure 11–14 corresponds to a test that is positive or negative just by chance. The closer an ROC curve is to the upper left-hand corner of the graph, the more accurate it is, because the true-positive rate is 1 and the false-positive rate is 0. As the criterion for a positive test becomes more stringent, the point on the curve corresponding to sensitivity and specificity (point *A*) moves down and to the left (lower sensitivity, higher specificity); if less evidence is required for a positive test, the point on the curve corresponding to sensitivity and specificity (point *B*) moves up and to the right (higher sensitivity, lower specificity).

ROC curves are useful graphic methods for comparing two or more diagnostic tests. For example, in Presenting Problem 3, Maulik and colleagues (1991) compared four indices corresponding to umbilical arterial Doppler waveforms for their accuracy in predicting adverse perinatal outcome. These investigators' findings are reproduced in Figure 11–15. Comparing for the accuracy, three of the four indices were observed to be fairly interchangeable, but one, the PI (pulsatility index) was found to be far less accurate.

A statistical test can be performed to determine whether two ROC curves are significantly different. A commonly used procedure involves determining the area under each ROC curve and uses a modifica-

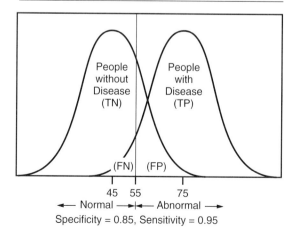

Figure 11–13. Two hypothetical distributions with cutoff at 55. *Abbreviations:* TN = true-negative; TP = true-positive; FN = false-negative; FP = false-positive.

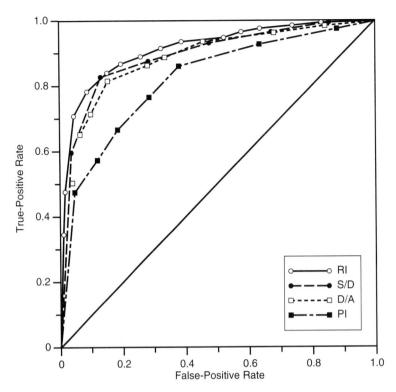

Figure 11–15. Receiver operating characteristic curves of umbilical arterial Doppler indices. Data points are measured values of indices. *Abbreviations:* RI = resistance index = (systolic − diastolic)/systolic; S/D = systolic-to-diastolic ratio; D/A = diastolic-to-average ratio; PI = pulsatility index = (systolic − diastolic)/average. (Used, with permission, from Figure 2 in Maulik et al: Comparative efficacy of umbilical arterial Doppler indices for predicting adverse perinatal outcome. *Am J Obstet Gynecol* 1991;**164**:1434–1440.)

tion of the Wilcoxon rank sum procedure to compare them (Hanley and McNeil, 1983).

11.6 ASSUMPTIONS IN USING SENSITIVITY & SPECIFICITY

The methods for revising probabilities described in this chapter are equivalent, and you should feel free to use the one you find easiest to understand and remember. All the methods are based on two assumptions: (1) The diseases or diagnoses being considered are mutually exclusive and include the actual diagnosis; and (2) the results of each diagnostic test are independent from the results of all other tests.

The first assumption is easy to meet if the diagnostic hypotheses are stated in terms of the probability of disease, $P(D^+)$, versus the probability of no disease, $P(D^-)$, as long as D^+ refers to a specific disease. Also, a more general form of Bayes' theorem can be used to consider the probability of several dif-

ferent diseases. For example, Sonnenberg and collaborators (1986) analyze the case of a 75-year-old woman who had suspected renal cell carcinoma and consider three diagnoses: renal cell carcinoma, transitional cell carcinoma, and benign lesion. In this situation, the authors assume that only these three conditions are possible and that only one of them is present.

The second assumption of mutually independent diagnostic tests is more difficult to meet. Two tests T_1 and T_2 for a given disease are independent if the result of T_1 does not influence the chances associated with the result of T_2. When applied to individual patients, independence means that if T_1 is positive in patient A, T_2 is no more likely to be positive in patient A than in any other patient in the population that patient A represents. Even though the second assumption is violated in many medical applications of decision analysis, the methods described in this chapter appear to be fairly robust, as we will see in the next chapter.

11.7 ILLUSTRATION OF PHYSICIANS' ABILITIES TO REVISE PROBABILITIES

Some people ask whether physicians really need to learn how to revise pretest probabilities or whether the correct interpretation does not become intuitive after some clinical experience. Although some physicians do learn intuitively how to revise the chance that a patient has a disease from the results of a diagnostic test, many apparently do not. One problem many people have, including physicians, is called the base-rate fallacy. Let us look at a classic example from Kahneman and Tversky (1972):

> Two cab companies operate in a given city, the Blue and the Green (according to the color of the cab they run). Eighty-five percent of the cabs in the city are Blue, and the remaining 15% are Green. A cab was involved in a hit-and-run accident at night. A witness later identified the cab as a Green cab. The court tested the witness' ability to distinguish between Blue and Green cabs under nighttime visibility conditions. It found the witness was able to identify each color correctly about 80% of the time, but confused it with the other color about 20% of the time. What do you think are the chances that the errant cab was indeed Green, as the witness claimed? (Kahneman and Tversky, 1972, p 13)

The answer is 0.41 (the problem is left as an exercise). Many people, however, answer 0.80, either ignoring the fact that only 15% of the cabs are Green, or not correctly using the information about the accuracy of the witness. Hopefully, the analogy to diagnostic tests is easy to see. Another researcher determined that physicians as well as the general public fall prey to the base-rate fallacy—and, in fact, determined that this fallacy is found in the recommendations for diagnostic testing in some medical textbooks (Bar-Hillel, 1980).

To illustrate how physicians are subject to the base-rate fallacy, let us examine Presenting Problem 4 in more detail. Although the diagnostic modality evaluated in the study is quickly becoming outdated with more advanced technologies, the methods the investigators used are applicable in evaluating any diagnostic procedure. In this study, physicians were asked to designate why they were ordering a liver–spleen scan (Steinberg et al, 1986). If liver metastasis was given as a reason, they were further asked to state (1) the pretest probability of liver metastasis—how likely they thought liver metastasis was in the patient; and (2) the probability that the liver–spleen scan would be normal, would show a focal defect, or would show a nonhomogeneous distribution of tracer without focal defect.

From the answers to these questions, the investigators worked backward to infer each physician's estimate of sensitivity and specificity of liver–spleen scans for liver metastasis. The authors then compared the physicians' probabilities on the second question with what they should have been according to the pretest probability given in question 1 and the inferred sensitivity and specificity. First of all, the investigators found that the physicians' estimates of sensitivity and specificity varied over a broad range, regardless of the definition of a positive scan. For example, when a positive scan was defined as showing a focal defect, estimates of sensitivity of the liver–spleen scan ranged from 0.10 to 1.00 in patients with underlying parenchymal disease, and from 0.20 to 1.00 in patients without underlying disease. Similarly, when a positive scan was defined as either focal defect or nonhomogeneous distribution of tracer without focal defect, the estimates of sensitivity ranged from 0.75 to 1.00 and from 0.50 to 1.00, respectively.

The investigators also found that a physician's stated posttest probability often did not agree with what the posttest probability should have been from the physician's inferred estimates of sensitivity and specificity. For example, 69% of the physicians' estimates differed by 0.01–0.24, and 19% differed by 0.25 or more.

As a result of their study, these investigators recommended that hospitals make available to physicians the performance capabilities (sensitivity and specificity) of liver–spleen scans and other diagnostic procedures. Furthermore, they recommended that physicians be given microcomputer assistance in estimating the effect of a diagnostic test on the probability of disease. Although these aims were laudable, we have not seen this come about in the time since this study was published. Instead we have seen a greater emphasis on improving resident and attending physicians' skills in interpreting diagnostic procedures as pressure to use them in a cost-effective manner continues.

Solomon and collaborators (1998) reviewed a number of articles describing various interventions aimed at improving clinicians' skills in diagnostic test interpretation. Some studies used lectures and dissemination of guidelines; some provided a utilization audit periodically, generally with charges for the procedures included; others used administrative procedures, such as eliminating standing laboratory orders or limiting the number of tests allowed each day. These studies reported variable results, and the authors of the review point out that the studies are often of poor quality. Our goal is to provide some tools to help you apply these concepts and perform the necessary calculations yourself. The techniques presented in the next chapter will continue the emphasis on methods of evidence-based medicine.

11.8 SUMMARY

Topics in this and the following chapters are departures from the topics considered in traditional introductory biostatistics textbooks. The increase in medical studies using methods in decision making and the growing emphasis on evidence-based medicine, however, indicate that practitioners should be familiar with the concepts. Equally important, the methods discussed in this chapter for calculating the probability of disease are ones that every clinician must be able to use in everyday patient care. These methods allow clinicians to integrate the results of published studies into their own practice of medicine. Many physicians need more insight into how these methods work, as illustrated in Presenting Problem 4. The analysis of physicians' interpretation of the liver–spleen scan in detecting liver metastases resulted in a broad range of physician estimates of the sensitivity and specificity of this test. The physicians' posttest probability of the disease state often did not agree with the inferred probability based on the physicians' estimates of sensitivity and specificity.

We presented four equivalent methods for determining how likely a disease (or condition) is in a given patient from the results of a diagnostic procedure. Three pieces of information are needed: (1) the probability of the disease or condition prior to any procedure, that is, the base rate (or prevalence); (2) the accuracy of the procedure in identifying the condition when it is present (sensitivity); and (3) the accuracy of the procedure in identifying the absence of the condition when it is indeed absent (specificity). We can draw an analogy with hypothesis testing: A false-positive is similar to a type I error, falsely declaring a significant difference; and sensitivity is like power, correctly detecting a difference when it is present. In Presenting Problem 1 the clinician used knowledge of the sensitivity and specificity of two tests, the MSAFP and fetal ultrasound, to determine their predictive value for the presence of fetal malformation in a pregnant diabetic woman. The MSAFP test had a low predictive value, approximately 38%, compared with ultrasound, approximately 97%. The analysis of these two tests supported the idea that the MSAFP has little value if ultrasound is available.

The methods in this chapter can also be used when test results are measured on a continuum. ROC curves were used to compare the diagnostic efficacy of Doppler waveform indices in detecting an increased risk in women with a high-risk pregnancy. The authors found that three of the four indices were close in terms of accuracy and clearly superior to the fourth.

The logic discussed in this chapter is applicable in many situations other than diagnostic testing. For example, the answer to each history question or the finding from each action of the physical examination may be interpreted in a similar manner. When the outcome from a procedure or inquiry is expressed as a numerical value, rather than as the positive or negative evaluation, ROC curves can be used to evaluate the ramifications of decisions.

Unfortunately, articles in the literature purporting to evaluate diagnostic procedures frequently do not contain the information needed for readers to interpret them correctly, and many contain misleading information. A common error is investigators presenting information related only to sensitivity and ignoring the performance of the procedure in patients without the condition. Misleading information results when investigators calculate predictive values by using the same subjects they used to determine sensitivity and specificity, ignoring the fact that predictive values change as the prior probability or prevalence changes. As readers, we can only assume they do not recognize the crucial role that prior probability (or prevalence) plays in interpreting the results of both positive and negative procedures.

Examples of more complex decision problems in medicine are discussed in the next chapter. Not many introductory texts discuss topics in medical decision making, partly because it is still relatively new and partly because much of the research in this field is interdisciplinary. A survey of the biostatistics curriculum in medical schools (Dawson-Saunders et al, 1987), however, found that these topics were taught at 87% of the medical schools. If you are interested in learning more about this growing field, consult the books by Weinstein and associates (1980), by Sox and colleagues (1988), and by Sackett and coworkers (1998), and the articles by Davidoff (1999) and by Greenhalgh (1997a). Although somewhat dated, the articles by Albert (1978) and by Griner and collaborators (1981) have good illustrations, as do those by Sox (1986) and Pauker and Kassirer (1987). Chapters 3 and 4 in the text on clinical epidemiology by Sackett and colleagues (1991) covers these topics.

Before leaving this chapter, we want to mention a very useful Web site:

http://araw.mede.uic.edu/~alansz/tools.html

It contains several computational aids for finding predictive values. One routine calculates predictive values for 2×2 tables. Check our Web site (www.clinicalbiostatistics.com) for any new information in this area.

EXERCISES

1. Suppose a 70-year-old woman comes to your office because of fatigue, pain in her hands and knees, and intermittent, sharp pains in her chest. Physical examination reveals an otherwise healthy female—the cardiopulmonary examination is normal, and no swelling is present in her joints. A possible diagnosis in this case is systemic lupus erythematosus (SLE). The question is whether to order an ANA (antinuclear antibody) test and, if so, how to interpret the results. Tan and coworkers (1982) reported that the ANA test is very sensitive to SLE, being positive 95% of the time when the disease is present. It is, however, only about 50% specific: Positive results are also obtained with connective tissue diseases other than SLE, and the occurrence of a positive ANA in the normal healthy population also increases with age.

   a. Assuming this patient has a baseline 2% chance of SLE, how will the results of an ANA test that is 95% sensitive and 50% specific for SLE change the probabilities of lupus if the test is positive? Negative?

   b. Suppose the woman has swelling of the joints in addition to her other symptoms of fatigue, joint pain, and intermittent, sharp chest pain. In this case, the probability of lupus is higher, perhaps 20%. Recalculate the probability of lupus if the test is positive and if it is negative.

2. Use Bayes' theorem and the likelihood ratio method to calculate the probability of no lupus when the ANA test is negative, using a pretest probability of lupus of 2%.

3. Given the information on Blue and Green cabs from Section 11.7, calculate the probability the errant cab was indeed Green.

4. A 43-year-old white male comes to your office for an insurance physical examination. Routine urinalysis reveals glucosuria. You recently learned of a newly developed test that produced positive results in 138 of 150 known diabetics and in 24 of 150 persons known not to have diabetes.

   a. What is the sensitivity of the new test?
   b. What is the specificity of the new test?
   c. What is the false-positive rate of the new test?
   d. Suppose a fasting blood sugar is obtained with known sensitivity and specificity of 0.80 and 0.96, respectively. If this test is applied to the same group that the new test used (150 persons with diabetes and 150 persons without diabetes), what is the predictive validity of a positive test?

   e. For the current patient, after the positive urinalysis, you think the chance that he has diabetes is about 90%. If the fasting blood sugar test is positive, what is the revised probability of disease?

5. Consider a 22-year-old woman who comes to your office with palpitations. Physical examination shows a healthy female with no detectable heart murmurs. In this situation, your guess is that this patient has a 25–30% chance of having mitral valve prolapse, from prevalence of the disease and physical findings for this particular patient. Echocardiograms are fairly sensitive for detecting mitral valve prolapse in patients who have it—approximately 90% sensitive. Echocardiograms are also quite specific, showing only about 5% false-positives; in other words, a negative result is correctly obtained in 95% of people who do not have mitral valve prolapse.

   a. How does a positive echocardiogram for this woman change your opinion of the 30% chance of mitral valve prolapse? That is, what is your best guess on mitral valve prolapse with a positive test?

   b. If the echocardiogram is negative, how sure can you be that this patient does not have mitral valve prolapse?

6. Borowitz and Glascoe (1986) reported a study to determine whether the language portion of the Denver Developmental Screening Test (DDST) is a sensitive screen of speech and language development in preschool-age children with suspected developmental problems. Seventy-one children were given the DDST plus the Preschool Language Scale (PLS), a well-accepted measure of language development, and the latter was used as the gold standard. On each test, children were assigned either a pass or a fail measurement. They were evaluated on three subtests measuring articulation and expressive and receptive abilities. The authors used the information given in Table 11–9.

   a. Comment on the information presented. Is this information adequate for evaluating the accuracy of the DDST? What are the sensitivity and specificity for the DDST?

   b. What statistical procedure was used to compare the results of the PLS and DDST? Was this test appropriate?

7. Assume a diagnostic test is 90% sensitive and 95% specific. Complete Table 11–10. What conclusions should be drawn from this chart?

8. Assume a patient comes to your office complaining of symptoms consistent with a myocardial infarction (MI). Based on your clinical ex-

Table 11–9. Evaluation of Denver Developmental Screening Test.

| Speech/ Language Deficit | Number (%) of Deficits Detected by[a] | | Z Value |
	Speech/ Language Screening	DDST Language Sector	
Any	65 (92)	30 (42)	−5.16[b]
Articulation	60 (84)	28 (39)	−4.49[b]
Expressive	56 (79)	30 (42)	−4.56[b]
Receptive	36 (51)	25 (34)	−1.24

Abbreviation: DDST = Denver Developmental Screening Test.
[a]$N = 71$.
[b]$P < 0.001$.
Source: Reproduced, with permission, from Table 1 in Borowitz KC, Glascoe P: Sensitivity of the Denver Developmental Screening Test in speech and language screening. *Pediatrics* 1986:**78:**1075–1078.

perience with similar patients, your index of suspicion for an MI is 80%. Use the information from Shlipak and associates (1999) and Table 11–1 to answer the following questions.

a. The ECG on this patient shows ST elevation ≥ 5 mm in discordant leads. What is the probability that the patient has an MI?

b. If the ECG does not exhibit ST elevation, what is the probability that the patient has an MI anyway?

c. What do these probabilities tell you?

d. What is the likelihood ratio for ST elevation ≥ 5 mm in discordant leads?

e. What are the pretest odds? The posttest odds?

9. The *Journal of the American Medical Association* frequently publishes a case study with com-

ments by a discussant. Weinstein (1998) was the discussant on a case involving a 45-year-old man with low back pain and a numb left foot. Table 1 in the article gives the sensitivity and specificity of several physical examination maneuvers for lumbar disk herniation based on a study by Deyo and colleagues (1992). Selected tests are listed in Table 11–11.

a. Which physical examination test is best to rule in lumbar disk hernia?

b. Which physical examination test is best to rule out lumbar disk hernia?

10. Group Exercise. Select a diagnostic problem of interest and perform a literature search to find published articles on the sensitivity and specificity of diagnostic procedures used with the problem.

a. What terminology is used for sensitivity and specificity? Are these terms used, or are results discussed in terms of false-positives and false-negatives?

b. Are actual numbers given or simply the values for sensitivity and specificity?

c. Does a well-accepted gold standard exist for the diagnosis? If not, did investigators provide information on the validity of the assessment used for the gold standard?

d. Did investigators discuss the reasons for false-positives? Were the selection criteria used for selecting persons with and without the disease appropriate?

e. Did authors cite predictive values for positive and negative tests? If so, why is this inappropriate?

11. Group Exercise. The CAGE questionnaire was designed as a screening device for alcoholism (Bush et al, 1987). The questionnaire consists of four questions:

a. Have you ever felt you should *Cut* down on your drinking?

b. Have people *Annoyed* you by criticizing your drinking?

c. Have you ever felt bad or *Guilty* about your drinking?

Table 11–10. Predictive values for a test with 90% sensitivity and 95% specificity.

Prevalence (%)	Predictive Value of a Positive Result	Predictive Value of a Negative Result
0.1		
1		
2		
5		
10		
20		
50		
80		

Table 11–11. Sensitivity and specificity of different maneuvers for lumbar disk herniation.

Maneuver	Sensitivity	Specificity
Ipsilateral straight-leg raising	0.80	0.40
Impaired ankle reflex	0.50	0.60
Ankle dorsiflexion weakness	0.35	0.70
Sensory loss	0.50	0.50

Source: Information used, with permission, from Deyo R et al: What can the history and physical examination tell us about low back pain? *JAMA* 1992;**268:**760–765; cited in Weinstein JN: Clinical crossroads: A 45-year-old man with low back pain and a numb left foot. *JAMA* 1998;**280:**730–736.

d. Have you ever had a drink first thing in the morning to steady your nerves or get rid of a hangover (*Eye*-opener)?

The questionnaire is scored by counting the number of questions to which the patient says yes. Buchsbaum and coworkers (1991) studied the predictive validity of CAGE scores. Obtain a copy of the article and calculate the predictive validity for 0, 1, 2, 3, and 4 positive answers. Draw an ROC curve for the questionnaire. Do you think this questionnaire is a good screening tool?

12

Clinical Decision Making

PRESENTING PROBLEMS

Presenting Problem 1. No consensus exists regarding the management of incidental intracranial saccular aneurysms. Because of their own good results, some experts advocate surgery; others point out that the prognosis is relatively benign even without surgery, especially for aneurysms smaller than 10 mm. The decision of whether to perform surgery depends on several factors and is complicated because rupture of an incidental aneurysm is a long-term risk, spread out over many years, whereas surgery represents an immediate risk. Some patients may prefer to avoid surgery, even at the cost of later excess risk; others may not.

Decision analysis was used by van Crevel and colleagues (1986) to evaluate the dilemma of whether surgery should be performed in patients with incidental intracranial saccular aneurysms. To approach the problem, they considered a fictitious 45-year-old woman with migraine (but otherwise healthy) who had been having attacks for the past 2 years. Her attacks were invariably right-sided and did not respond to medication. She had no family history of migraine. Because of the patient's clinical symptoms, the neurologist suspected an arteriovenous malformation and ordered four-vessel angiography, which showed an aneurysm of 7 mm on the left middle cerebral artery. Should the neurologist advise the patient to have preventive surgery? The decision is diagrammed in Section 12.1.2.

Presenting Problem 2. Decision analysis was used by Phillips and coworkers (1987) to estimate the clinical and economic implications of testing women during routine gynecologic visits to a physician for cervical infection caused by *Chlamydia trachomatis*. Infections caused by *C trachomatis* are among the most common sexually transmitted diseases in the United States. Severe consequences of *C trachomatis* infection include morbidity associated with urethritis, mucopurulent cervicitis, and salpingitis. Salpingitis can lead to infertility, ectopic pregnancy, and chronic pelvic pain. *Chlamydia trachomatis* has been implicated as the etiologic agent in 20–40% of patients with this condition. The prevalence of chlamydial infection is reported to be 4–9% in primary care practices and even higher in other settings: 6–23% in

family planning clinics, and 20–30% in clinics for patients with sexually transmitted diseases. The investigators examined the consequences of routine culture, of test by direct immunofluorescence or enzyme immunoassay (rapid tests), and of no test. They also calculated the costs associated with each strategy to determine a threshold prevalence of infection at which medical costs would be reduced by testing routinely for *C trachomatis*. The strategy is diagrammed in Section 12.3.

Presenting Problem 3. The fecal occult blood test, such as the Hemoccult test, is a simple, inexpensive screening test for colorectal cancer in asymptomatic patients. Major drawbacks with this procedure are the number of cancers missed (false-negatives) and the number of false-positive results. Several procedures have been recommended in the literature as appropriate for follow-up to a positive Hemoccult. Many of the recommended procedures call for sigmoidoscopy, barium enema, repeat Hemoccult, and colonoscopy, but the recommended order of these procedures varies widely. Brandeau and Eddy (1987) evaluated 22 protocols for doing a workup on a typical asymptomatic patient who has a positive fecal occult blood test by using information on the prevalences of cancers, adenomas, and other conditions in such patients; the natural history of colorectal cancer; the effectiveness of screening tests; risks; and costs. They determined the number of cancers and polyps each protocol would be expected to identify and the cost involved. They also found the marginal costs and effectiveness of the best protocols from both the patient's and a societal perspective. Selected results from their analysis are given in Section 12.4.

Presenting Problem 4. Invasive carcinoma of the cervix occurs in about 15,000 women each year in the United States. About 40% ultimately die of the disease. Cervical carcinoma in situ is diagnosed in about 56,000 women annually, resulting in approximately 4800 deaths. Papanicolaou (Pap) smears play an important role in the early detection of cervical cancer at a stage when it is almost always asymptotic.

Although the American Cancer Society recommends annual Pap smears for at least 3 years beginning at the onset of sexual activity or 18 years of age, then less often at the discretion of the physician, only 12–15% of women undergo this procedure. The Pap smear is considered to be a cost-effective tool, but certainly imperfect—it has a sensitivity rate of only 75–85%. New technologies have improved the sensitivity of Pap testing but at an increased cost per test. Brown and Garber (1999) assessed the cost-effectiveness of three new technologies in the prevention of cervical cancer morbidity and mortality.

12.1 THE DECISION PROCESS

This chapter extends the topic of using evidence-based medicine to aid decision making (introduced in Chapter 11) to cover more complex problems. The challenge in many clinical situations is to compare two options for solving a problem. For example, in Presenting Problem 1, the problem is whether to operate on a patient with an incidental aneurysm. Surgery is termed the *active option.* The active option often carries with it an increased benefit if it is successful; however, increased risks and costs are also associated with surgery. The *passive option* is not to perform surgery.

Both active and passive options can have positive or negative outcomes. Thus, the surgery option is positive if successful but negative if death or disability results; the passive option is positive if no rupture occurs but negative if one does, especially if the rupture is followed by disability or death. The physician's role is to decide which outcome is more likely and then, balancing this probability with the risks and the benefits of the options, discuss the options with the patient and determine an approach. The increasing emphasis on controlling the costs associated with medical care and concerns regarding litigation have caused the profession to examine this process in more detail. Presenting Problem 3 on screening for colorectal cancer and Presenting Problem 4 on screening for cervical cancer are two examples of the way costs and benefits can be analyzed to provide useful information to busy clinicians.

12.1.1 Purpose of the Chapter

The methods discussed in this chapter are applicable to decisions about individual patients, such as whether to perform surgery, and to health policy decisions, such as whether to recommend screening of the general population. We use the problem of deciding whether to perform surgery on a patient with an incidental aneurysm, described in Presenting Problem 1, to illustrate some of the components of medical decision making. Presenting Problem 2 illustrates the use of decision analysis in screening. We illustrate the creative application of decision analysis as a method for evaluating a set of suggested proposals for follow-up to a positive Hemoccult test in an asymptomatic patient (Presenting Problem 3).

Finally, we discuss a decision problem that incorporates the frequency and timing of screening as a variable in the decision process (Presenting Problem 4). Our discussion provides only a brief introduction to this rapidly growing field, and the calculations we perform illustrate specific aspects of the process; as usual, we assume you will use computer programs to perform the actual applications. For further details, consult the texts by Ingelfinger and associates (1993), Sackett and collaborators (1998), and Weinstein and colleagues (1980).

12.1.2 Components of Making a Decision

12.1.2.a. Defining the Problem, Alternative Actions, and Possible Outcomes: Decision analysis can be applied to any problem in which a choice is possible among different alternative actions. Recall from Chapter 11 that Pauker and Kassirer (1980) developed the threshold model as one way of deciding whether to treat a patient, perform a diagnostic procedure, or do nothing. Any decision has two major components: specifying the alternative actions and determining the possible outcomes from each alternative action. Figure 12–1 illustrates both components. The alternative actions are to operate or not to operate; and if no operation is performed, to determine whether the aneurysm subsequently ruptures, causing subarachnoid hemorrhage. The outcomes are death, disability, or recovery after a rupture; no rupture; and death, disability, or success following surgery. These components represent the branches on the decision tree.

The point at which a branch occurs is called a *node;* note that in Figure 12–1, nodes are identified by either a square or a circle. The square denotes a decision node, that is, the point at which the decision is under the control of the decision maker; thus, whether to operate is a decision over which the physician and the patient have control. The circle denotes chance nodes, or points at which the results occur by chance; thus, whether the aneurysm ruptures without surgery is a chance outcome of the decision not to operate.

12.1.2.b. Determining Probabilities: The next step in developing a decision tree is to assign a probability to each branch leading from each chance node. For example, what is the probability of aneurysm rupture if no surgery is performed? What is the probability of death with surgery? Of disability with surgery? Of success with surgery? If the aneurysm does rupture, what is the probability of a good outcome (recovery) versus a poor outcome (disability or death)?

12.1.2.c. Deciding on the Value of the Outcomes: The final step in defining a decision problem requires *assigning a value,* or *utility,* to each outcome. With some decision problems, the outcome is cost, and dollar amounts can be used as the utility of each outcome. For example, in Presenting Problem 1, some way must be found to quantify the outcomes of

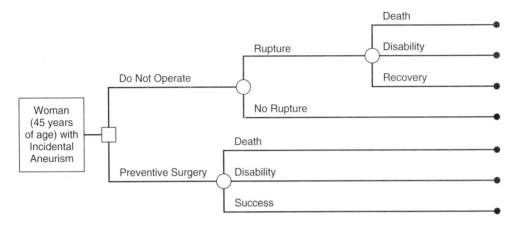

Figure 12–1. Decision tree for management and outcome in incidental aneurysms. (Reproduced, with permission, from van Crevel H et al: Decision analysis of the management of incidental intracranial saccular aneurysms. *Neurology* 1986;**36:**1335–1339.)

death, disability, and so on. The actual analysis of the decision tree involves combining the probabilities of each action with the utility of each so that the optimal decision can be made at the decision nodes. Each step and the analysis of the aneurysm problem are illustrated in the next section.

12.2 MAKING A DECISION FOR AN INDIVIDUAL PATIENT

To decide whether to perform surgery on a 45-year-old woman with a 7-mm aneurysm on the left middle cerebral artery, the investigators in Presenting Problem 1 defined the decision alternatives and possible outcomes as illustrated in Figure 12–1. This step is the *art* of any decision analysis. The investigators define "recovery" as the patient being able to function at her present, presurgery level, although minor symptoms or signs may be present; "disability" means that she cannot function at her present level.

12.2.1 Determining the Probability of Each Branch

To determine the probabilities for the decision tree, the investigators surveyed the medical literature and found they needed to take the following information into consideration.

1. The risk of rupture depends on the life expectancy or age of the patient, and the size of the aneurysm influences the risk of rupture, with smaller aneurysms carrying a lower risk. The risk of rupture over a patient's lifetime is approximately $1 - (1 - R)^L$, where R is the annual risk and L is the life expectancy. For a 45-year-old woman with a 7-mm aneurysm, the annual risk (R) of rupture without surgery is about 1%, and the life expectancy (L) is approximately 35 years; therefore, the lifetime risk is approximately 0.29.

2. The mortality from subarachnoid hemorrhage is high, about 55%.

3. Serious morbidity after subarachnoid hemorrhage (hemiparesis, dysphasia, or mental deterioration) is also high, estimated at 15%.

4. Surgical mortality and morbidity for incidental aneurysm are much lower than for ruptured aneurysms, estimated at 2% and 6%, respectively.

5. The attitude of the patient toward short-term and long-term risks must be considered. Operation carries an immediate risk, whereas a rupture, if it occurs, appears on average after about one-half of the patient's life expectancy has elapsed.

In Figure 12–2, the preceding probabilities are added to the branches of the decision tree. (The expected utilities listed in the figure are discussed in Section 12.2.3.) For example, because the probability of rupture without surgery is estimated as 0.29, the probability of no rupture is $1 - 0.29 = 0.71$. Similarly, the probability of success following surgery is found by subtracting from 1 the probabilities of death and disability, that is, $1 - 0.02 - 0.06 = 0.92$.

12.2.2 Determining the Utility of Each Outcome

12.2.2.a. Objective versus Subjective Outcomes: Outcomes based on objective probabilities, such as costs, numbers of years of life, or other variables that have an inherent numeric value, can be used as the utilities for a decision. When outcomes are based on **subjective probabilities,** as in our example, investigators must find a way to give them a

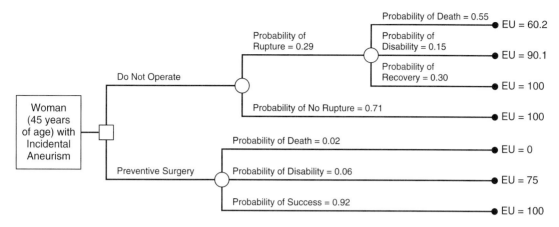

Figure 12–2. Decision tree for aneurysms with probabilities and utilities included. *Abbreviation:* EU = expected utility. (Adapted and reproduced, with permission, from van Crevel H et al: Decision analysis of the management of incidental intracranial saccular aneurysms. *Neurology* 1986;**36**:1335–1339.)

value. This process is known as assigning a utility to each outcome.

The scale used for utilities is arbitrary, although a scale from 0 for least desirable outcome to 1 or 100 for most desirable outcome is frequently used. The investigators in Presenting Problem 1 developed a scale for the utility of each outcome, ranging from 0 for death to 100 for perfect health. They decided that disability following surgery should be valued at 75. Although this value is not completely arbitrary, other individuals might assign different values for disability. For example, some people feel that having a serious disability is a terrible outcome, almost as bad as dying, and they might give this outcome a utility of 10 or 20 rather than 75. For this reason, the term "subjective utilities" is sometimes used to describe the utilities determined in this kind of situation.

12.2.2.b. An Example of Determining Subjective Utilities: Subjective utilities can be obtained informally, as just described, or by a more rigorous process called a lottery technique. This technique involves a process called **game theory.**

To illustrate, suppose we ask you to play a game in which you can choose a prize of $50 or you can play the game with a 50–50 chance of winning $100 (and nothing if you lose). Here, the **expected value** of playing the game is 0.50 × $100 = $50, the same as the prize. Do you take the sure $50 or play the game? If you choose not to gamble and take $50 instead, then we ask whether you will play the game if the chance of winning increases from 50% to 60%, resulting in an expected value of $60, $10 more than the prize. If you still take $50, then we increase the chance to 70%, and so on, until it reaches a point at which you cannot decide whether to play the game or take the prize, called the point of indifference. This is

the value you attach to playing this game. We say you are risk-averse when you refuse to gamble even when the odds are in your favor, that is, when the expected value of the game is more than the prize.

Suppose now that a colleague plays the game and chooses the $50 prize when the chance of winning $100 is 50–50. Then, we ask whether the colleague will still play if the chance of winning $100 is only 40%, and so on, until the point of indifference is reached. We describe your colleague as risk-seeking when he or she is willing to gamble even when the odds are unfavorable and the expected value of the game is less than the prize.

12.2.2.c. The Subjective Utilities in the Aneurysm Example: A similar process can be used to determine the values of survival, death, and disability. The patient or decision maker is given a set of alternative scenarios and asked to choose between them. In the aneurysm example, a patient is asked to choose between the option of living 10 years with mental deterioration and the option of undergoing a procedure resulting 50% of the time in disability-free survival for 10 years and 50% of the time in immediate death. This set of scenarios is systematically varied until the patient's point of indifference is reached, and this point is used to determine how much the patient values life with disability.

The determination of utilities for the outcomes that follow a rupture is more difficult. The same values could be used (ie, 0 for death, 75 for disability, and 100 for recovery); however, this technique ignores the number of years the patient lives prior to the rupture of the aneurysm. As an alternative, a lottery procedure can be used to determine the value the patient assigns to death and to disability after a period of survival. The authors assumed the patient was somewhat risk-averse and used a procedure called **discounting** to determine the utility of each outcome at some later date, assuming no operation is performed. A utility of 100 is still used for no rupture and for recovery following a rupture. Disability following a rupture at some time in the future is considered more positive, however, than disability following immediate surgery and is given a utility of 90.1. Similarly, death following a future rupture is preferred to death immediately following surgery and is given a utility of 60.2. These utilities are appended to the ends of the branches of the decision tree in Figure 12–2.

12.2.3 Analyzing the Decision Tree

The decision tree is analyzed by a process known as **calculating the expected utilities,** or folding back the tree. Folding back the tree begins with the outcomes and works backward through the tree to the point where a decision must be made. In our example, the first step is to determine the expected utility (EU) of the outcomes related to a ruptured aneurysm without an operation, obtained by multiplying the probability of each outcome by the utility for that outcome and summing the relevant products. In words, we add the probability of death times the utility of death, the probability of disability times the utility of disability, and the probability of recovery times the utility of recovery:

$$EU \text{ (Rupture without operation)} = (0.55 \times 60.2)$$
$$+ (0.15 \times 90.1) + (0.30 \times 100)$$
$$= 33.1 + 13.5 + 30 = 76.6$$

The result, 76.6, indicates the average value over all outcomes from the decision not to perform surgery in patients who subsequently have a rupture. Because the utility scale in this example is arbitrary, the value of 76.6 must be compared with values of 100 for no rupture and 0 for surgery with perioperative death.

This process is repeated for each chance node, one step at a time, back through the tree. Continuing with the example, the expected utility of not operating is the probability of rupture times the utility associated with this outcome, just found to be 76.6, plus the probability of no rupture times the utility; that is,

$$EU \text{ (No operation)} = (0.29 \times 76.6) + (0.71 \times 100) = 93.3$$

Similarly, the expected value of preventive surgery is

$$EU \text{ (Surgery)} = (0.02 \times 0) + (0.06 \times 75) + (0.92 \times 100)$$
$$= 96.5$$

The expected utilities are added to the decision tree in Figure 12–3. The expected utility of surgery is 96.5 (based on 100) for a woman who lives and dies according to life table chances, compared with 93.3 for nonsurgical management. Surgery therefore reduces the loss of utility caused by an incidental aneurysm from 6.7 (100 − 93.3) to 3.5 (100 − 96.5); with a life expectancy of 35 years, this reduction translates into 2.3 fewer years (6.7% × 35 years) with conservative management and 1.2 fewer years (3.5% × 35 years) with surgical management, on the average.

The optimal decision (performing surgery, in this example) is the one with the largest expected value, and the decision maker's choice appears relatively easy because of the increased survival of 1.2 years with surgery. When the expected utility of two decisions is very close, the situation is called a toss-up,

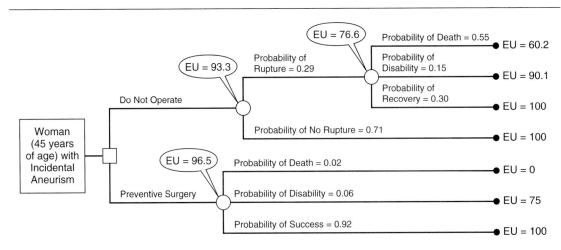

Figure 12–3. Decision tree for aneurysms with completed analysis. *Abbreviation:* EU = expected utility. (Adapted and reproduced, with permission, from van Crevel H et al: Decision analysis of the management of incidental intracranial saccular aneurysms. *Neurology* 1986;**36**:1335–1339.)

and considerations such as the estimates used in the analysis become more important. In fact, some of you may have been uncomfortable with the numbers used in the decision analysis and may have speculated on the effect different numbers would have on the decision. The final step in the analysis is therefore to determine how the decision changes if some of the values in the analysis change. This process shows how robust the decision is, that is, how applicable it is in situations other than the specific one included in the analysis.

12.2.4 Evaluating the Decision: Sensitivity Analysis

Accurate probabilities for each branch in a decision tree are frequently difficult to obtain from the literature. Investigators often have to use estimates made for related situations. For example, in Presenting Problem 1, the authors state that annual risk of rupture of an incidental aneurysm is not precisely known. Some studies have shown that a first rupture occurs at a rate of about 1% a year, and this is the value used in the decision analysis. The investigators want to know, however, whether the decision is the same if the rate is either more or less than 1%. Similarly, the decision depends on the probability of mortality from subarachnoid hemorrhage, estimated at 0.55 in the preceding analysis; and again, the investigators want to know whether the decision changes if that probability changes. The procedure for evaluating the way the decision changes as a function of changing probabilities and utilities is called **sensitivity analysis.**

To illustrate the logic involved in performing a sensitivity analysis, we determine the risk of aneurysm rupture that changes the optimal choice of treatment from surgical to conservative management. From Figure 12–3, the expected utility when the probability of rupture is 0.29 is 93.3; we want to know what the probability of rupture must be for the expected utility to be the same as for preventive surgery, that is, for it to be 96.5. Letting X stand for the probability of rupture, we need to solve the following equation for X:

$$76.6X + 100(1 - X) = 96.5$$
$$76.6X + 100 - 100X = 96.5$$
$$76.6X - 100X = 96.5 - 100$$
$$-23.4X = -3.5 \quad \text{or} \quad X = 0.15$$

Thus, when the probability of rupture is 0.15 instead of 0.29, the decision is a toss-up because the expected utilities of the two options, conservative treatment and preventive surgery, are the same. Working backward in the formula for lifetime risk equal to 0.15 [ie, solving $1 - (1 - R)^{35} = 0.15$ for R] gives an annual risk equal to 0.00463, or slightly less than 0.5%. The decision to perform preventive surgery therefore remains the same until the annual risk for someone with a 35-year life expectancy decreases to half the value used in the decision analysis.

Although our illustration of sensitivity analysis varied only one component, risk of rupture, it is possible to perform an analysis to determine the sensitivity of the final decision to other assumptions used in the decision. In addition, it is possible to determine the sensitivity of two or more assumptions simultaneously. Most statisticians and researchers in decision analysis recommend that all published reports of a decision analysis include a sensitivity analysis.

The authors of the decision analysis on management of incidental aneurysms performed a sensitivity analysis to determine whether the decision was stable. They found that the decision does not change as long as the probabilities are within the following ranges: annual risk of rupture, 0.5–2%; mortality from rupture, 50–60%; disability after rupture, 10–20%; surgical mortality, 1–4%; surgical morbidity, 4–10%; and disability utility, 62.5–87.5. They also gave information on the decrease in benefits from surgery with older patients. For example, with surgical mortality of 2% and morbidity of 4%, the break-even value of surgical management is a life expectancy of 12 years; that is, surgery is beneficial only to patients who have 12 or more years of life expectancy.

This example illustrates the use of decision trees for making a decision regarding a particular patient, a 45-year-old woman with a 7-mm aneurysm. The same tree can be used with another patient; but the lifetime probability of rupture must be adjusted for the patient's age, and different utilities are needed to reflect the patient's values. Trees for decisions that do not depend on the specific features of any given patient are also possible, as we will see in the next section.

12.3 MAKING A DECISION ON HEALTH POLICY

The investigators in Presenting Problem 2 used decision analysis to calculate the economic implications of strategies for treating women seeking routine gynecologic care. The strategies they analyzed included routine culture for *C trachomatis*, a routine test with direct immunofluorescence or enzyme immunoassay (rapid tests), and no test. The decision tree for this problem is given in Figure 12–4, and it illustrates the use of subtrees, a helpful technique when trees become complex, with repetitive branches.

12.3.1 Designing the Decision Tree

The basic tree considers three options: rapid test, culture, or no test. In each situation, the patient either does or does not have a chlamydial infection. The bracket in Figure 12–4 for the rapid test and culture

Decision Tree

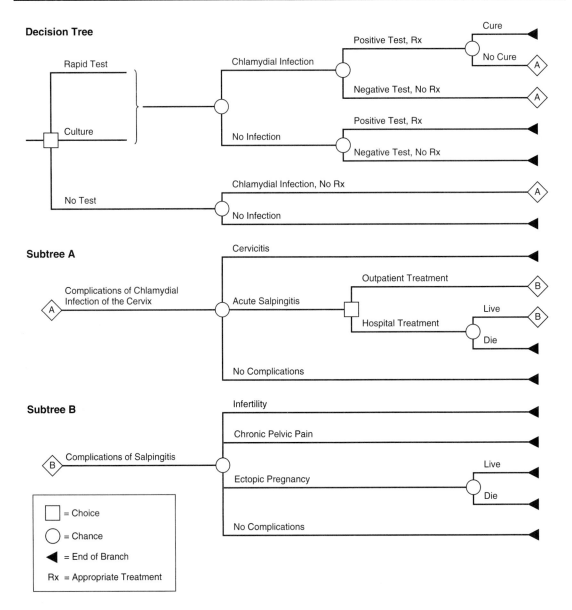

Figure 12–4. Decision tree for screening strategies for *Chlamydia trachomatis* infection. (Adapted and reproduced, with permission, from Phillips RS et al: Should tests for *Chlamydia trachomatis* cervical infection be done during routine gynecologic visits? An analysis of the costs of alternative strategies. *Ann Intern Med* 1987;**107**:188–194.)

branches indicates that all subsequent branches are the same and only one repetition is illustrated. In the no-test branch with infection, as in all other branches leading to untreated or uncured infection, the reader is directed to subtree A (illustrated in the middle portion of Figure 12–4), which contains the ramifications of chlamydial infection of the cervix: cervicitis, acute salpingitis, and no complications. A patient with acute salpingitis may be hospitalized or treated as an outpatient. The reader is referred to subtree B, which contains the complications of this condition:

infertility, chronic pelvic pain, ectopic pregnancy, or none. Note that the decision tree in Figure 12–4 shows many possible outcomes.

The decision model was designed for women without symptoms or signs of acute salpingitis, urethritis, or mucopurulent cervicitis and for women without gonorrhea, because these patients should receive therapy with antibiotics active against chlamydial infection. Pregnant women were also excluded because their complications from the infection differ from those in nonpregnant women.

This particular decision problem provides a good illustration of how judgments are involved in the process of determining the branches for the tree. For example, an additional strategy in this example is to treat the patients without first performing a culture. A letter to the editor from Ingelfinger (1988) discussing this decision tree suggested the strategy of giving all patients a prescription for nystatin to be filled if they develop vaginitis. Another possible branch in this decision problem addresses complications from treating women who do not have a chlamydial infection. In this decision analysis, the risk of complications from treating the false-positive patients is quite small; but in other situations, it would be an important branch to include on the tree.

12.3.2 Determining the Probabilities

Because the decision tree is so complex, the probabilities and other assumptions used in the analysis are listed by the authors rather than being shown graphically. They are as follows:

1. Sensitivity and specificity of cultures were 0.75 and 1.00, respectively; for the two rapid tests (direct immunofluorescence test and enzyme immunoassay), sensitivity = 0.60 and specificity = 0.98.

2. Patients with a positive test would be treated as recommended by the Centers for Disease Control and Prevention (CDC), with a cure rate of 90%. A complication of vaginitis occurs in 15% of patients with a positive test.

3. For each patient with a positive test, one partner would also be treated.

4. Patients with acute salpingitis would be treated with a regimen recommended by the CDC, with two follow-up visits and a follow-up culture; 21% are expected to be hospitalized for treatment.

5. An estimated 32% of women with undetected *C trachomatis* cervical infections seek medical attention for related problems within 1 year; the estimate is 15% for acute salpingitis and 17% for symptomatic cervicitis.

6. Estimates of risks for adverse sequelae from acute salpingitis within 10 years are infertility in 18%, chronic pelvic pain in 15%, and ectopic pregnancy in 5%.

7. Risk of death is 0.0025 for patients hospitalized with salpingitis and 0.00009 for patients with ectopic pregnancy.

8. An estimated 50% of women would attempt pregnancy after an episode of salpingitis and be at risk for ectopic pregnancy; 50% who experience infertility would seek medical evaluation. All women with chronic pelvic pain seek medical care.

9. Direct costs included culture, $40; rapid tests, $15. Estimates of outpatient care and hospitalization were obtained from insurance records.

10. Indirect costs included lost wages, lost house hold management, and lost lifetime earnings in the event of death.

12.3.3 Stating Results of the Decision Analysis

Using the previous estimates for probabilities and utilities of the appropriate branches, the authors found that using a rapid test and subsequently treating women who have positive results would be cost-efficient if the prevalence of infection is 7% or greater. Routine cultures would result in lower costs than no test if the prevalence of infection is 14% or greater.

The authors performed a sensitivity analysis to see how the three different strategies compare, varying the previously mentioned factors over a reasonable range. They found that the rapid test strategy resulted in costs lower than the culture strategy unless the prevalence of infection exceeds 42%. The factors most important in influencing the decision for rapid tests were the estimate of acute salpingitis resulting from untreated chlamydial infection, the costs of the tests, and the probability of adverse sequelae occurring after treatment of cervical infection. For example, if the risk for salpingitis is increased from 15% to 20%, the threshold prevalence of infection before treatment is recommended drops from 7% to 5%. A lower cost of the rapid tests also resulted in a lower threshold of infection required for cost-effectiveness. Similarly, if the culture costs only half as much, it would be the test of choice, with a prevalence of 7%. The estimates of sensitivity and specificity had a minimal effect on the decision: If the sensitivity decreases from 80% to 60%, the threshold increases to 9%; if the specificity decreases from 98% to 95%, the threshold increases to 8%. The results of the sensitivity analysis related to the costs of the tests are presented graphically in Figure 12–5. The graph clearly illustrates the 7% and 14% thresholds and shows that no testing is cost-effective when the prevalence is less than 7%.

From their analysis, the investigators recommend a rapid test for routine testing of women seeking gynecologic care, because the prevalence of infection reported among women seen in office practices exceeds the 7% threshold. At this level of prevalence, only about 69% of the patients with a positive test have the infection, and about a third of the patients with positive tests have false-positive results. They do not recommend follow-up of a positive rapid test with a culture because of insensitivity of the culture procedure with use of a cervical swab. Any decision to implement such a plan in another setting would, of course, depend on the prevalence of infection and the cost of rapid tests in that setting. For example, if the prevalence of chlamydial infection were less than 7%, the cost of rapid tests would need to be correspondingly less than $15 to justify screening of all women.

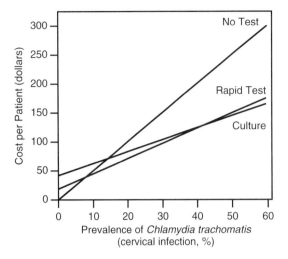

Figure 12–5. Sensitivity analysis of screening strategy to prevalence of *Chlamydia trachomatis*. (Adapted and reproduced, with permission, from Phillips RS et al: Should tests for *Chlamydia trachomatis* cervical infection be done during routine gynecologic visits? An analysis of the costs of alternative strategies. *Ann Intern Med* 1987;**107:**188–194.)

12.4 USING DECISION ANALYSIS TO COMPARE DIFFERENT METHODS

The topic of screening for colorectal cancer receives considerable attention in the medical literature. Some researchers conclude that screening asymptomatic persons is not justified (Ransohoff and Lang, 1991), but others conclude it is optional (Eddy, 1990). Organizations also vary in their recommendations. The American Cancer Society endorses screening of persons over the age of 50, but the U. S. Prevention Services Task Force and the Canadian Periodic Health Examination Task Force do not recommend screening for persons not at risk.

No consensus exists about which diagnostic tool is the best for follow-up in an asymptomatic patient who has a positive Hemoccult screening test. Among the available diagnostic procedures are rigid and flexible sigmoidoscopy, colonoscopy, and a barium enema. An ideal diagnostic protocol would combine these tests so that all cancers could be found without undue costs, risks, or discomfort to the patient. The ideal does not exist, however, because none of the tests is perfect; and as more tests are done, the costs and risks increase accordingly.

Several protocols have been recommended in the literature, and the range of procedures used in actual practice varies widely. Brandeau and Eddy (1987) therefore designed a decision analysis study to determine the most cost-effective protocol. They examined 22 protocols: 7 recommended in the literature and 15 that could be justified on a logical basis. We discuss 7 of the 22 protocols in this section; they are reproduced in Figure 12–6. Four protocols are from the literature

(protocols 1, 2, 3, 4) and three approaches were generated by the authors (protocols A, B, C).

12.4.1 Protocols Evaluated

In addition to evaluating several protocols recommended in the literature, the investigators were interested in some specific research questions. One question of interest was whether a negative barium enema should be followed by a colonoscopy; this question considers the difference between barium enema and colonoscopy (protocol A) and barium enema alone (protocol B). A second question was whether preceding a colonoscopy with a barium enema has any value if colonoscopy is eventually used in all cases; thus, protocol C (colonoscopy alone) was also evaluated.

A summary of the seven protocols follows.

1. Sigmoidoscopy: Sigmoidoscopy, if negative, is followed by barium enema. If it is positive, it is followed by colonoscopy.

2. Rigid Sigmoidoscopy: Rigid sigmoidoscopy, if negative, is followed by repeat Hemoccult. If the repeat Hemoccult is positive, both a barium enema and colonoscopy are done, in that order.

3. Repeat Hemoccult: Repeat Hemoccult, if positive, is followed by both sigmoidoscopy (type not indicated) and barium enema, in that order.

4. Flexible Sigmoidoscopy: Flexible sigmoidoscopy, if positive, is followed by colonoscopy. If it is negative, it is followed by barium enema, which is followed by colonoscopy if positive. If barium enema is negative, it is followed by repeat Hemoccult. If repeat Hemoccult is positive, it is followed by colonoscopy. If colonoscopy is negative, it is followed by upper gastrointestinal (GI) series.

A. Barium Enema (& Colonoscopy): Barium enema is always followed by colonoscopy. If colonoscopy is negative, it is followed by repeat barium enema. If repeat barium enema is positive, it is followed by second colonoscopy.

B. Barium Enema: Barium enema is followed by colonoscopy only if positive. If colonoscopy is negative, it is followed by repeat barium enema. If repeat barium enema is positive, it is followed by second colonoscopy.

C. Colonoscopy: Colonoscopy is followed by barium enema only if negative. If barium enema is positive, it is followed by second colonoscopy.

12.4.2 Assumptions Made in the Analysis

12.4.2.a. Estimating Patient Conditions: A decision problem of this scope required the investigators to estimate the proportion of Hemoccult-positive patients who have cancer, polyps, and miscellaneous bleeding and who are true false-positives having no bleeding. From information in the medical literature, they assumed that 8% of the patients with a positive Hemoccult had cancer, 40% had polyps, 36% had miscellaneous bleeding, and 16% had no bleeding.

Hendrix and Sabe: Indications for Use of the Barium Enema

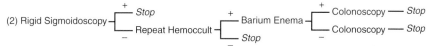

Hardcastle et al: Hemoccult Screening in Nottingham, England

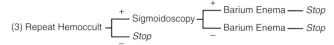

Miller and Knight: Hemoccult Screening at Mather AFB, Florida

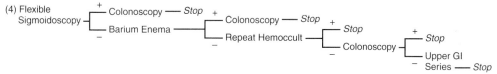

Stroehlein et al: Diagnostic Approach to Evaluating Cause of a Positive Fecal Occult Blood Test

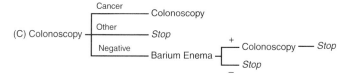

Figure 12–6. Workups proposed for follow-up of asymptomatic patients with positive fecal occult blood test. (Adapted and reproduced, with permission, from Brandeau ML, Eddy DM: The workup of the asymptomatic patient with a positive fecal occult blood test. *Med Decis Making* 1987;**7**:32–46.)

12.4.2.b. Determining the Characteristics of the Procedures: Several characteristics of the procedures must be taken into consideration in the design of a decision strategy. Rigid sigmoidoscopy, flexible sigmoidoscopy, barium enema study, and colonoscopy can search different regions of the bowel, and they have different accuracies for detecting cancer and polyps; these accuracies can also depend on the results of the tests that precede them. For example, colonoscopy and flexible sigmoidoscopy are thought to be more accurate if they follow a barium enema, because the barium enema results can

guide the endoscopist's search for abnormal lesions. These tests also have different diagnostic ability because all but the barium enema permit a biopsy at the time of the examination. The tests also cause different amounts of discomfort, have different complication rates, and are associated with different costs. Again, the literature was consulted to obtain information regarding these characteristics.

1. Rigid Sigmoidoscopy: Approximately 40–45% of colonic cancers occur within the reach (18–20 cm) of a rigid sigmoidoscope. Within this range, the sensitivity for detecting cancer and polyps is estimated to be 40–60% and 35–50%, respectively. Many patients experience discomfort, and colonic perforation occurs in 1 in 10,000 procedures. The cost of this procedure varies from $25 to $150; an estimate of $49 was used in the analysis.

2. Flexible Sigmoidoscopy: Within a range of 50–55 cm, the sensitivity of flexible sigmoidoscopy is 60–90%. Patients tolerate this procedure better than rigid sigmoidoscopy, and the complication rate is about the same. Cost is approximately $105.

3. Colonoscopy: A colonoscopy can examine the entire colon. Its sensitivity is estimated as 80–90%, increasing to 90–98% if preceded by a barium enema. Complication rates are higher, with bleeding in 18 of 10,000 cases and, when combined with barium enema, perforation in 3 of 1000 cases. It is also more expensive, costing $400-$800; a cost of $680 was used in the analysis.

4. Barium Enema: A barium enema has a sensitivity for cancer and polyps of 40–60%; this value can be increased with careful patient preparation to 95% for cancer and 92% for polyps larger than 5 mm. False-positive results occur about 5% of the time. Colonic perforation occurs in 2 of 10,000 patients, and an unmeasured risk from radiation occurs. The cost, with air contrast, is about $175.

5. Repeat Hemoccult: A repeat Hemoccult has sensitivity for both cancer and polyps of about 55%. Its cost is minimal, about $8.

6. Upper GI Series: This procedure has about 5% sensitivity for detecting miscellaneous bleeding and 0 sensitivity for cancer and polyps. Cost is about $150.

12.4.3 The Decision Tree

A decision tree was developed to evaluate each of the protocols. Figure 12–7 shows the tree for protocol

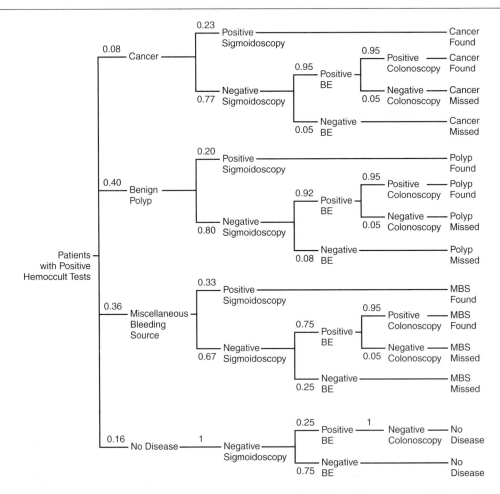

Figure 12–7. Example of decision tree for protocol 1. *Abbreviations:* BE = barium enema; MBS = multiple bleeding sources. (Redrawn and reproduced, with permission, from Brandeau ML, Eddy DM: The workup of the asymptomatic patient with a positive fecal occult blood test. *Med Decis Making* 1987;**7**:32–46.)

1 (sigmoidoscopy), in which a rigid sigmoidoscopy is followed by an air contrast barium enema if negative, which in turn is followed by a colonoscopy if positive.

The probabilities of cancer, polyps, bleeding, and no bleeding were discussed earlier. The other probabilities in Figure 12–7 were estimated from a review of the literature by the authors. For example, the probability is 0.23 that the sigmoidoscopy will find a cancer; that is, sensitivity is 50% for detecting the 45% of cancers in the range of a sigmoidoscope. Similarly, if the sigmoidoscopy fails to detect cancer in a patient with cancer, an air contrast barium enema is positive 95% of the time, and a positive barium enema leads to a positive colonoscopy 95% of the time. Thus, the probability that cancer is found by using this protocol, if cancer is present, is 0.23 (the probability of a positive sigmoidoscopy) plus 0.77 × 0.95 × 0.95 (the probability of negative sigmoidoscopy followed by positive barium enema and positive colonoscopy), or 0.23 + 0.69 = 0.92, or 92%. This protocol therefore misses a cancer in 8% of the patients. Similarly, the probability of finding polyps when present is 0.20 + (0.80 × 0.92 × 0.95) = 0.90, or 90%; and this process is continued for the remainder of the branches of the tree.

12.4.4 Results of the Decision Analysis

The investigators developed a similar decision tree for each of the protocols evaluated in their study. Using a computer program, they evaluated each tree to determine the effectiveness of the protocol in detecting cancer and polyps. The fraction of cancers found, cancers and polyps found, and the average cost per patient are given in Table 12–1. In general, the relationship between the cost of a protocol and its effectiveness in detecting lesions is positive. The procedure that detects the most cancers and polyps is protocol A, barium enema and colonoscopy; however, it puts patients through a great deal of discomfort and is the most costly ($876). Protocol C, colonoscopy alone, does almost as well, and it costs $110 less.

The authors could not designate one protocol as the very best; however, they could determine which strategies were better in a relative sense. The authors prepared a graph comparing the fraction of cancers and precancerous lesions found for the average cost per patient in all 22 protocols they evaluated. The protocols appearing along the line connecting protocols 3 (repeat Hemoccult) and A (barium enema and colonoscopy) are said to dominate over protocols below the line because they detect more lesions for the same cost. The graph for all 22 protocols is reproduced in Figure 12–8; the 7 we discussed are identified on the graph. Four of the seven strategies are on the line and are relatively better than the other three: protocols 3 (repeat Hemoccult), A (barium enema

Table 12–1. Selected results from fecal occult blood study.

Protocol[a]	Fraction Found		Average Cost per Patient
	Cancers	Cancers and Polyps	
1. Sigmoidoscopy	0.886	0.860	$522
2. Rigid sigmoid-oscopy	0.627	0.598	430
3. Repeat Hemoccult	0.607	0.580	149
4. Flexible sig-moidoscopy	0.896	0.870	797
A. Barium enema and colonoscopy	0.988	0.970	876
B. Barium enema	0.967	0.941	687
C. Colonoscopy	0.981	0.960	766

[a]See Figure 12–6 for a complete description of each protocol; this table lists the first step only.
Source: Adapted and reproduced, with permission, from Table 3 in Brandeau ML, Eddy DM: The workup of the asymptomatic patient with a positive fecal occult blood test. *Med Decis Making* 1987;7:32–46.

and colonoscopy), B (barium enema), and C (colonoscopy). Figure 12–8 may be used to make recommendations about the protocols. For example, protocol 2 (rigid sigmoidoscopy) should not be used because it detects only 2% more lesions than protocol 3 (repeat Hemoccult) but costs about $250 more.

12.4.5 Conclusions from the Decision Analysis

From the results of the decision analysis of the 22 different protocols they analyzed, the investigators drew several conclusions. Performing a barium enema prior to sigmoidoscopy or colonoscopy increases the overall sensitivity for cancers and precancerous lesions by about only 0.3%, with an average cost increase of about $45. Furthermore, using a barium enema as a screening procedure and following it with a colonoscopy only if it is positive (protocol B) produces a $165 reduction in cost with only a 2% reduction in the number of lesions found. These conclusions are generally the same even if the sensitivity of colonoscopy without a preceding barium enema is reduced from 90% to 80%. For physicians who do not have access to colonoscopy, however, the most effective workup is to perform a barium enema and follow it with flexible sigmoidoscopy in all patients. Overall, the effectiveness of workups with sigmoidoscopy ranged from 60% to 93%, compared with 91% to 97% for workups with colonoscopy.

Four of the seven protocols in the literature and the American Cancer Society recommend repeat Hemoccults. The analysis shows, however, that a repeat Hemoccult is not advantageous. This test has a false-

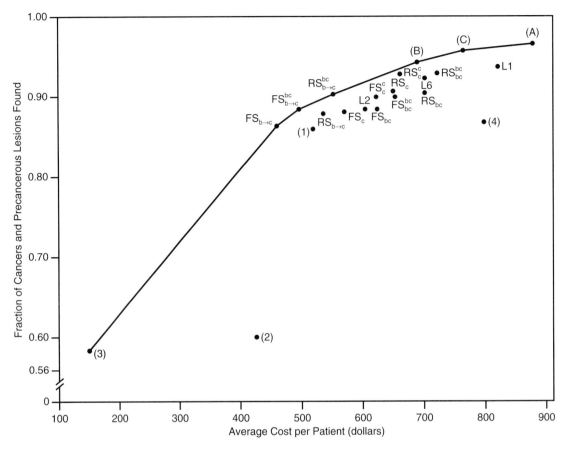

Figure 12–8. Information on cost and effectiveness of all protocols. *Abbreviations:* RS = rigid sigmoidoscopy; FS = flexible sigmoidoscopy; A = barium enema (& colonoscopy); B = barium enema; C = colonoscopy. The symbols $FS_{b \to c}$ and $FS_{b \to c}^{bc}$ and so on represent the additional 15 protocols evaluated by the investigators; we refer you to the original paper for their definition. (Adapted and reproduced, with permission, from Brandeau ML, Eddy DM: The workup of the asymptomatic patient with a positive fecal occult blood test. *Med Decis Making* 1987;**7**:32–46.)

negative rate of 45% for cancers and polyps. Although a repeat Hemoccult may provide a cost-effective way of eliminating some patients with initial false-positive Hemoccults, too many cancers are missed (false-negative results) with these protocols.

12.5 USING DECISION ANALYSIS TO EVALUATE TIMING & METHODS

In Presenting Problem 4, Brown and Garber (1999) evaluated the cost-effectiveness (CE) of three new technologies to improve the sensitivity of detecting cancer screening compared with the Pap smears that are the standard of care. The Pap smear is considered to be a cost-effective tool, but it has a low sensitivity rate for a screening test, only about

75–85%. Several new technologies have been developed that are reported to improve the sensitivity of Pap testing; however, the new technologies increase the cost of each test.

The investigators began by conducting a MEDLINE search for articles published between 1987 and 1997 on the use of AutoPap 300 QC, Papnet, and ThinPrep 2000 in the detection of cervical cytopathologic abnormalities. They also conducted hand searches of three specific cytopathology journals and obtained data from the manufacturers of the three new technologies. They used the estimates of the sensitivity or true-positive rate (TP) and the cost for each test in a mathematical model to calculate the lifetime costs and health effects associated with these screening strategies. The four screening strategies they evaluated were:

1. Pap smear with rescreening of a 10% random sample
2. ThinPrep with rescreening of a 10% random sample
3. Pap smear with AutoPap-assisted rescreening of all results that were within normal limits
4. Pap smear with Papnet-assisted rescreening of all results that were within normal limits

They investigated these four technologies for annual, biennial, triennial, and quadrennial screening examinations.

The investigators used a theoretical cohort of women and assumed that screening starts at 20 years of age, life expectancy is 78.27 years, and unscreened women have about a 2.5% lifetime chance of developing cervical cancer and a 1.2% chance of dying from the disease. All CE ratios are expressed as screening costs in U. S. dollars per year of life saved (YLS) by using a given technology or method. A relatively low CE ratio for a given intervention represents a good value. The CE ratio for each test was calculated for annual, biennial, triennial, and quadrennial screening frequencies.

The result of the CE analysis is reproduced in Table 12–2. The cost of the three new technologies increased the cost per woman screened by $30 to $257. For instance, for annual screening, the cost associated with Pap smear and AutoPap-assisted rescreen compared with the cost of Pap smear alone was $2089 – $1955, or $134. When the new technologies were compared with Pap smear alone, life expectancy increased by 5 hours to 1.6 days per woman screened depending on the technology and frequency of screening.

The final column of Table 12–2 gives the incremental cost per year of life saved. The least expensive is Pap smear screening every 4 years. Pap smear with Papnet-assisted rescreen is always the most expensive, although it is associated with the greatest increase in days of life. ThinPrep with 10% random rescreen was always dominated, meaning that this approach produced less health benefit at higher cost—thus, it would never be chosen as the best approach.

Figure 12–9 reproduces the figure in the article and illustrates the results of the cost-effectiveness analysis. Expressing the outcome in cost per year of life saved provides an interpretation that can be used to compare the cost and benefit of screening for one procedure versus another. This information can be especially useful when available resources require that decisions be made among screening for different diseases.

Another index used in the literature that evaluates cost-effectiveness and cost-benefit is the QALY, or quality-adjusted life year. QALYs are found by multiplying the utility, such as the ones found in Presenting Problem 1, by the number of years the patient is expected to live.

12.6 EXTENSIONS OF DECISION THEORY

Medical decision making is a rapidly evolving field, with results of new decision analyses being published with increasing frequency. Growth in the number of new methods being developed for this area is also significant. Three will be discussed here: multiple-testing strategies, Markov models, and artificial intelligence.

12.6.1 Multiple-Testing Strategies

For many clinical problems, protocols specify the combination of two diagnostic tests for reaching a treatment decision. In some situations, the two tests are administered at the same time, as in testing a patient with severe chest pain for a myocardial infarction (MI) by performing serial electrocardiograms (ECG) and cardiac enzyme measurements. Here, the physician may decide against a diagnosis of MI if either the ECG or the cardiac enzymes is normal. If both are abnormal in the characteristic pattern, however, MI is the most likely diagnosis.

In other clinical situations, two tests are administered in series; that is, the result of the first test is used to determine whether the second test should be done, as in patients with a possible diagnosis of primary hyperparathyroidism. Generally, the first test is a measurement of the patient's serum calcium level. If it is elevated, the second step is to measure the patient's level of parathyroid hormone (PTH), which is inappropriately high in patients with primary hyperparathyroidism. If the serum calcium level is normal, additional testing is unnecessary.

Hershey and coworkers (1987) evaluated situations for which two tests are recommended. They were interested in whether, in some circumstances, either parallel or series testing is always preferable to a using single test alone. For example, two types of clinical decisions involve parallel testing: Use test 1 and test 2 at the same time and treat only if *both* are positive, as with the MI example; or use test 1 and test 2 at the same time and treat if *either* is positive. For example, two tests are likely to be ordered for a patient with low back pain who is suspected of having a vertebral compression fracture caused by osteoporosis: a plain film of the lumbar spine to determine if a compression fracture is present (either acute or chronic) and a bone density test to determine the severity of bone loss. An abnormality on either test would be reason to treat for osteoporosis. Similarly, two decision approaches involve series testing: Perform test 1 and, if positive, perform test 2, as in the hyperparathyroid example; or perform test 1 and, if negative, perform test 2. As an example of this last situation, a patient who is suspected of having peptic ulcer disease may have an upper GI x-ray film first because it is less invasive than an endoscopy. If the upper GI film is negative, but the clinician's index of

Table 12–2. Cost-effectiveness of conventional and ThinPrep-, AutoPap-, and Papnet-enhanced cervical screening strategies, for screening women aged 20–65 years.

Screening Strategy	Lifetime Costs per Woman Screened		Lifetime Health Effects per Woman Screened				Incremental Cost per Year of Life Saved, $[b]
	Number of Screenings	Health Care Costs[a]	Developing Cervical Cancer (%)	Dying from Cervical Cancer (%)	Additional Days of Life		
Quadrennial							
Pap smear with 10% random rescreen	12	446	0.33	0.10	23.91		6814
ThinPrep with 10% random rescreen	12	505	0.28	0.09	25.07		Dominated
Pap smear with AutoPap-assisted rescreen	12	476	0.27	0.08	25.32		7777
Pap smear with Papnet-assisted rescreen	12	508	0.26	0.08	25.47		75406
Triennial							
Pap smear with 10% random rescreen	16	614	0.28	0.09	24.93		8996
ThinPrep with 10% random rescreen	16	695	0.25	0.07	25.73		Dominated
Pap smear with AutoPap-assisted rescreen	16	657	0.24	0.07	25.89		16259
Pap smear with Papnet-assisted rescreen	16	700	0.23	0.07	26.00		146783
Biennial							
Pap smear with 10% random rescreen	23	939	0.24	0.08	25.72		13334
ThinPrep with 10% random rescreen	23	1059	0.22	0.07	26.19		Dominated
Pap smear with AutoPap-assisted rescreen	23	1005	0.22	0.07	26.29		42666
Pap smear with Papnet-assisted rescreen	23	1068	0.22	0.07	26.35		343444
Annual							
Pap smear with 10% random rescreen	46	1955	0.20	0.06	26.56		26882
ThinPrep with 10% random rescreen	46	2194	0.19	0.06	26.80		Dominated
Pap smear with AutoPap-assisted rescreen	46	2089	0.19	0.06	26.86		166474
Pap smear with Papnet-assisted rescreen	46	2212	0.18	0.06	26.90		1069661

[a]In 1996 US dollars; all costs and benefits discounted at 3% per year. Pap indicates Papanicolaou.
[b]In 1996 US dollars compared with immediately less effective and nondominated alternative strategy within the same screening frequency.
Source: Reprinted, with permission, from Table 3 from Brown AD, Garber AM: Cost-effectiveness of three methods to enhance the sensitivity of Papanicolaou testing. *JAMA* 1999;**281**:347–353. Copyright © 1999, American Medical Association.

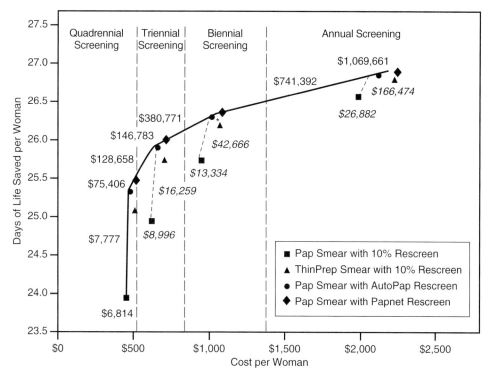

Figure 12–9. Cost-effectiveness of different technologies in average-risk women for screening intervals of 1–4 years. The solid lines apply when it is possible to vary both the technology and the frequency; dashed lines apply when the screening interval cannot be varied. Screening begins at age 20 years and continues to age 65. Numbers adjacent to the solid line are cost-effectiveness ratios in dollars per year of life saved for the two options being compared. Points below and to the right of lines represent dominated alternatives. (Reproduced, with permission, from Brown AD, Garber AM: Cost-effectiveness of three methods to enhance the sensitivity of Papanicolaou testing. *JAMA* 1999;**281**:347–353. Copyright © 1999, American Medical Association.)

suspicion is still high, an endoscopy is likely to be done.

The authors compared the decisions with parallel and series testing with the decisions made using test 1 only and using test 2 only. They determined mathematically that two tests, whether in parallel or in series, are never preferable to a single test over all ranges of prevalence (pretest probability or index of suspicion). In other words, for some pretest probabilities, single testing is always the approach of choice—generally, when the physician's index of suspicion is in the midrange of disease probabilities. Above this range, the either-test-positive criterion is better; and below this range, the both-tests-positive criterion is better. In the range of intermediate pretest probabilities, however, the best strategy is to perform only one test and act on the basis of the results of that test. Their work eloquently demonstrates the crucial role of the index of suspicion and why it is important for clinicians to be able to revise posttest probabilities.

12.6.2 Markov Models

One of the criticisms of decision analysis is that many decisions must be simplified if we are to use the methods available. For example, consider the question of how to treat patients who have incidental aneurysms in Presenting Problem 1. A patient with an aneurysm may develop a subarachnoid hemorrhage in any given year, or the aneurysm may remain without complications. If a hemorrhage occurs, the patient may be left with serious disability, or the patient may recover. The risks of both a rupture and a disability following rupture depend on the age of the patient. The investigators in Presenting Problem 1 took these issues into consideration by including the patient's life expectancy as part of the calculation of risk.

Another way to analyze this problem is to use a technique called a Markov process, which permits patients to move back and forth from one state of health to another. To illustrate the logic involved in the Markov process, suppose that a million hypothetical patients, each with an incidental aneurysm, were followed through time. During any given year, a patient in the aneurysm state could move to the aneurysm rupture state and then on to the disability state, the recovery state, or the death state. After recovering, a patient could decide to have surgery or not to have surgery and could move to the aneurysm state again in the future. The chance that a patient moves from one health state to another is called the transition probability for that state. The Markov model involves computing the transition probabilities so that they can be used in a decision analysis; they allow investigators to determine the expected survival for any of the million patients.

For example, for the 45-year-old woman with a 7-mm aneurysm, the investigators can determine the probability that she stays in the aneurysm state during the next year as well as the probabilities that she moves to the disability state or the death state. If she remains in the aneurysm state for this next year, then they can calculate the probabilities for the year following, and so on. From these probabilities, the physician and patient can make an informed decision regarding therapy. When computer programs are used for the calculations, the Markov model is a useful method for analyzing complex problems that evolve and change over time.

12.6.3 Artificial Intelligence

Artificial intelligence (AI) is a field of computer science concerned with designing computer programs that understand language, reason, and solve problems—in other words, computerized decision trees. Most AI programs in medicine determine diagnoses and make recommendations for therapy (Clancey and Shortliffe, 1984). Some of the programs are known as consultation or expert programs because they provide expert advice on how to handle a patient problem. These systems use clinical algorithms (protocols) in making decisions about how to manage a particular problem. Usually, the protocols are in the form of a decision tree that follows the simple branching logic illustrated in the presenting problems.

Expert physicians designed many of the original AI systems for use by paramedical personnel; recently, these systems have also been used to supplement and extend medical education. Some of the more complex programs are linked to laser disks so that sound and visual information are included in the program. It remains to be seen how large a role AI systems will play in medicine in the future, but some believe that the primary challenges to tomorrow's physician will be in the area of management, with AI computer programs being used to aid in most diagnostic decisions. If you are interested in this topic, you may wish to consult some recent articles published in *Artificial Intelligence in Medicine* or some texts related to decision making in medicine: *Expertise in Context: Human and Machine* by Feltovich and collaborators (1997) and *Readings in Medical Artificial Intelligence,* edited by Clancey and Shortliffe (1984).

12.7 COMPUTER PROGRAMS FOR DECISION ANALYSIS

Several computer programs have been written for researchers who wish to model clinical decision-making problems. These programs are generally single-purpose programs and are not included in the general statistical analysis programs illustrated in earlier chapters in this book.

Decision Analysis by TreeAge (DATA) software is a decision analysis program that lets the researcher build decision trees interactively on the computer screen. Once the tree is developed, TreeAge performs the calculations for the expected utilities to determine the optimal pathway for the decision. It also performs sensitivity analysis. The information from Presenting Problem 1 on management of intracranial aneurysm in a 45-year-old woman is used to illustrate the computer output from TreeAge in Figure 12–10. The expected values of the two main branches, 93.2 and 96.5, are within rounding error of the values we calculated. The researcher who uses computers to model decision problems is able to model complex problems, update or alter them as needed, and perform a variety of sensitivity analyses with relative ease.

12.8 SUMMARY

In Chapter 11, we introduced the idea of using probabilities to make decisions about individual patients from information provided by diagnostic procedures. In this chapter, we extended these simple applications to more complex situations. A diagnostic procedure is often part of a complex decision, and the methods discussed in the previous chapter can be used to determine appropriate probabilities for branches of the decision tree. These methods allow research findings to be integrated into the decisions physicians must make in diagnosing and managing diseases and conditions.

The problem of deciding whether to perform preventive surgery or manage conservatively a 45-year-old woman with an incidental intracranial saccular aneurysm was used to illustrate the process of developing a decision tree and determining the optimal decision. Although the analysis indicated that surgical management was the optimal decision for this patient, this decision depends on the assumptions made in de-

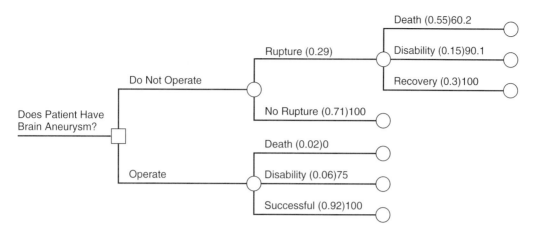

Figure 12–10. Illustration of a decision tree, using data on management of intracranial aneurysm in a 45-year-old woman from Presenting Problem 1. (Used, with permission, from van Crevel H et al: Decision analysis of the management of incidental intracranial saccular aneurysms. *Neurology* 1986;**36**:1335–1339. Decision Analysis by TreeAge (DATA) is a registered trademark of TreeAge Software, Inc.; used with permission.)

signing the tree and the patient's own preferences. It is important to keep in mind that the subjective utilities used in an example such as this one do not apply to all patients. A procedure called sensitivity analysis can be performed to determine which assumptions are important and how changes in the probabilities used in the decision analysis will change the decision.

The methods discussed in this chapter also apply to determining the most efficient approach for dealing with a problem. Because increasing attention is being focused on the cost of medical care, we think increasing numbers of articles dealing with decision analysis will be published in the literature. Decision analysis can help decision makers who must choose between committing resources to one program or another. We reviewed a study on screening women for *Chlamydia trachomatis* infection to illustrate a decision analysis dealing with clinical and economic implications of implementing a routine test. The conclusion was that using a rapid test reduces overall costs if the prevalence of infection is 7% or more. If prevalence of infection is 14% or greater, the more expensive but also more accurate procedure of obtaining a culture can be justified. As is appropriate for all problems like this one, the authors correctly pointed out that the best approach for any one clinic depends on several factors, including local costs of the tests, expertise of persons performing the tests, and prevalence of infection.

We also reviewed a novel but effective application of decision analysis to evaluating protocols recommended by experts but not subjected to clinical trial. The protocols outlined the steps to take in doing workups for asymptomatic patients who have a posi-

tive fecal occult blood test. This problem is important and clinically relevant and made even more timely with the recommendations of the American Cancer Society on routine screening for colorectal cancer. The authors of the report considered 22 protocols and subjected each to a decision analysis to determine the ones that were most effective in finding cancers and precancerous lesions for a given cost. As in many decision problems, the investigators had to search the literature to obtain estimates of sensitivity, specificity, risks, and costs of various diagnostic procedures as well as prevalence of colorectal cancer. Although the literature is not always complete or consistent, the growing use of computerized databases makes more and better information available all the time. This example also illustrates a familiar result in medicine, that no single answer is correct for the question of which protocol is best. The authors found that the numbers of detected lesions increase as the costs associated with the protocols increase. From the assumptions of the analysis, however, some recommended approaches were not among the optimal ones and hence should not be used.

Finally, we described a study that compares the standard of care, the Pap smear, to three new technologies and varies the frequency of screening. The investigators were hoping to find a cost-effective method to improve the poor sensitivity of the Pap smear. They found that screening every 3 years with AutoPap or Papnet used to rescreen all Pap smear results within normal limits actually produces more life years at lower costs than biennial Pap smears alone. The investigators discuss the sensitivity of their conclusions to the cost of the new technologies; the con-

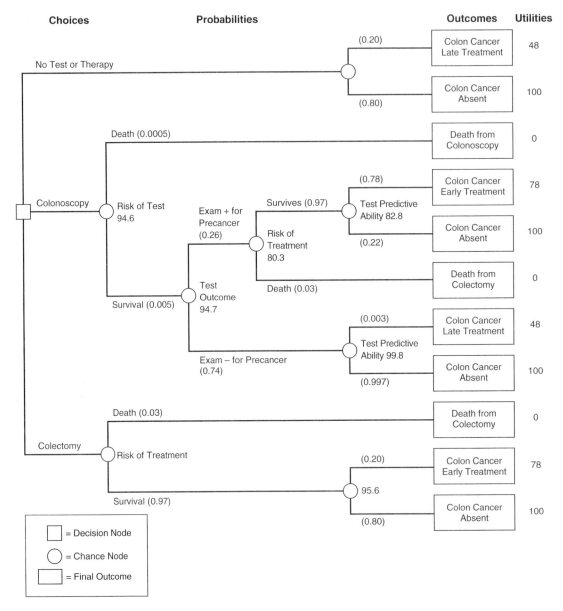

Figure 12–11. Decision tree for ulcerative colitis. (Adapted and reproduced, with permission, from Gage TP: Managing the cancer risk in chronic ulcerative colitis. A decision-analytic approach. *J Clin Gastroenterol* 1986;**8**:50–57.)

clusions from the study could change if these technologies become less expensive in the future.

In summary, we note that several published articles (Kassirer et al, 1987; Pauker and Kassirer, 1987; Raiffa, 1997) and texts (Eddy, 1996; Locket, 1997) discuss the role of decision analysis in medicine, and you may wish to consult these resources for a broader discussion of the issues. One advantage of performing a well-defined analysis of a medical decision problem is that the process itself

forces explicit consideration of all factors that affect the decision.

EXERCISES

1. An interesting phenomenon called reversal sometimes occurs when we try to determine a person's subjective utilities. For example, would you be willing to gamble with a 50–50 chance of winning $100 versus accepting a $50 prize? What about a gamble with a 50–50 chance of winning $100,000 versus a $50,000 prize? Or a gamble with a 50–50 chance of winning $1 versus a $0.50 prize? Did you reverse your preference, even though the expected value of the gamble is the same as the prize in each example? Can you think of ways this phenomenon could affect a patient's preference for surgery versus medical management?

2. Refer to Figure 12–5. At what prevalence of infection does performing a culture become cost-effective?

3. Confirm that the predictive value of a positive rapid test for *C trachomatis* infection is only 69% with 7% prevalence.

4. A decision analysis for managing ulcerative colitis points out that patients with this condition are at high risk of developing colon cancer (Gage, 1986). The analysis compares the decisions of colectomy versus colonoscopy versus no test or therapy. The decision tree developed for this problem is shown in Figure 12–11. The author used information from the literature for the data listed on the tree. The utilities are 5-year survival probabilities (multiplied by 100).

   a. What is the probability of colon cancer used in the analysis?

   b. The author gave a range of published values for sensitivity and specificity of colonoscopy with biopsy but did not state the precise values used in the analysis. Can you tell what sensitivity and specificity were used in the analysis?

   c. The expected utility of the colonoscopy arm is calculated as 94.6. Calculate the expected utility of the no-test-or-therapy arm and the colectomy arm. What is the procedure with the highest expected utility, that is, what is the recommended decision?

5. The occurrence of adverse effects from the combination vaccine against diphtheria, pertussis, and tetanus toxoids (DPT) has led some physicians to delay the initial administration of this childhood vaccination. Funkhouser and collaborators (1987) performed a complex decision analysis to evaluate the effect of delaying the recommended initial dose of DTP from 2, 4, and 6 months to 8, 10, and 12 months of age, respectively. The model for this decision is shown in Figure 12–12.

   a. Which variables in the decision tree are probably the most important in determining the decision? That is, which variables should be considered in a sensitivity analysis of the decision to maintain or to change the schedule?

b. The investigators calculated the expected numbers of different outcomes under the current vaccination schedule and the proposed schedule. They presented the results in terms of a base case scenario in which pertussis incidence in the 7–12-month age group is assumed to be 7.6 per 100,000 in children under 2 months of age, 17.7 in children age 2–6 months, 6.2 in children age 7–12 months, and 9.7 in children age 13–47 months. The results are given in Table 12–3. From this analysis, which schedule is better for minimizing the total number of cases of pertussis, the current schedule or the proposed schedule?

c. Which schedule is better from the perspective of minimizing the adverse effects from the vaccine?

6. **Group Exercise.** Several clinical trials have shown that adjuvant chemotherapy used postoperatively in women with breast cancer but with no positive axillary nodes results in moderate decreases in recurrence of the cancer. A decision analysis of the efficacy and cost-effectiveness of adjuvant chemotherapy for node-negative breast cancer was published by Hillner and Smith (1991). The conclusion from the analysis was that the benefit from chemotherapy increases quality-adjusted life expectancy at costs comparable to those for other widely accepted therapies; increases were an average of 5.1 months for a 45-year-old woman and 4.0 months for a 60-year-old woman. The authors also concluded, however, that the benefit may be too small for some women to choose chemotherapy. Focusing on the same issue, Levine and colleagues (1992) developed a bedside decision instrument to elicit patient preferences concerning adjuvant chemotherapy. Obtain copies of the articles by Hillner and Smith and by Levine and colleagues from your medical library.

   a. Figure 1 from the Hillner and Smith article illustrates an abbreviated version of a Markov model used to study movements from one state of health to another. Refer to the figure and the description of the basic model in the methods section of the paper, discuss the assumptions used in modeling the decision, and evaluate how reasonable and comprehensive they are.

   b. Hillner and Smith also performed a sensitivity analysis for 45-year-old women. What do these graphs indicate about the relationship between benefit of treatment, cost of treatment, the annual probability of recurrence, and the relative efficacy of chemotherapy?

   c. How did Hillner and Smith determine quality-adjusted survival? What was the source

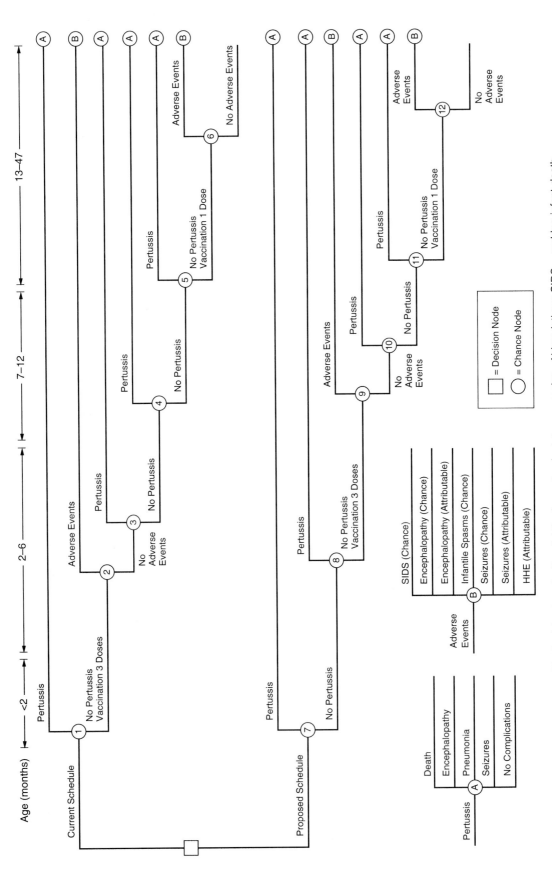

Figure 12-12. Decision tree for the diphtheria, pertussis, tetanus vaccine. *Abbreviations:* SIDS = sudden infant death syndrome; HHE = hypotonic-hyporesponsive episode. (Adapted and reproduced, with permission, from Funkhouser AW et al: Estimated effects of a delay in the recommended vaccination schedule for diphtheria and tetanus toxoids and pertussis vaccine. *JAMA* 1987;**257**:1341–1346.)

Table 12–3. Results of DPT analysis.

Outcome	Under Current Schedule	Under Proposed Schedule	Difference in Outcomes from Current Schedule No. (% Change)
Pertussis			
With death	11	11	0 (0)
With encephalopathy	5	7	2 (+40)
With seizures	33	52	19 (+58)
With pneumonia	266	360	94 (+35)
Uncomplicated	1,205	1,726	521 (+43)
Total	1,520	2,156	636 (+42)
Attributable events			
Encephalopathy	105	105	0 (0)
Seizures	8,447	8,447	0 (0)
Hypotonic–hyporesponsive episodes	8,447	8,447	0 (0)
Total	16,999	16,999	0 (0)
Chance events			
Death	423	70	−353 (−83)
Encephalopathy	20	22	2 (+10)
Infantile spasms	18	4	−14 (−78)
Seizures	2,478	3,789	1311 (+53)
Total	2,939	3,885	946 (+32)
None	3,678,541	3,676,963	−1578 (−0.04)
Total[a]	3,699,999	3,700,003	—

[a]These totals are not equal to 3,700,000 owing to rounding.
Source: Reproduced, with permission, from Centers for Disease Control and from Table 3 in Funkhouser AW et al: Estimated effects of a delay in the recommended vaccination schedule for diphtheria and tetanus toxoids and pertussis vaccine. *JAMA* 1987;**257:**1341–1346.

for the numbers in their Table 1? Is there a better source for this information?

d. Why did Levine and colleagues administer the questionnaire to a group of normal women to elicit patient preferences? How do you interpret the reported value for kappa ($\kappa = 0.84$)?

e. Discuss the pros and cons of using this questionnaire with women with node-negative breast cancer and of using similar instruments for patients with other diseases. What are some possible advantages? Disadvantages? Would you use this instrument or a similar one with your patients?

13

Reading the Medical Literature

13.1 PURPOSE OF THE CHAPTER

This final chapter has several purposes. Most importantly, it ties together concepts and skills presented in previous chapters and applies these concepts very specifically to reading medical journal articles. Throughout the text, we have attempted to illustrate the strengths and weaknesses of some of the studies discussed, but this chapter focuses specifically on those attributes of a study that indicate whether we, as readers of the medical literature, can use the results with confidence. The chapter begins with a brief summary of major types of medical studies. Next, we examine the anatomy of a typical journal article in detail, and we discuss the contents of each component—abstract or summary, introduction, methods, results, discussion, and conclusions. In this examination, we also point out common shortcomings, sources of bias, and threats to the validity of studies.

As a clinician you need to read the literature for many different reasons. Some articles are of interest because you want only to be aware of advances in a field. In these instances, you may decide to skim the article with little interest in how the study was designed and carried out. In such cases, it may be possible to depend on experts in the field who write review articles to provide a relatively superficial level of information. On other occasions, however, you want to know whether the conclusions of the study are valid, perhaps so that they can be used to determine patient care or to plan a research project. In these situations, you need to read and evaluate the article with a critical eye in order to detect poorly done studies that arrive at unwarranted conclusions.

To assist readers in their critical reviews, we present a checklist for evaluating the validity of a journal article. The checklist notes some of the characteristics of a well-designed and well-written article. The checklist is based on our experiences with medical students, journal clubs, and interactions with physician colleagues. It also reflects the opinions expressed in an article describing how journal editors and statisticians can interact to improve the quality of published medical research (Marks et al, 1988). As we reported in Chapter 1, a number of authors have found that only a minority of published studies meet the criteria for scientific adequacy. The checklist should assist you in using your time most effectively, that is, allowing you to differentiate valid articles from poorly done studies so that you can concentrate on the more productive ones.

13.2 REVIEW OF MAJOR STUDY DESIGNS

Chapter 2 introduced the major types of study designs used in medical research, broadly divided into **experimental studies** (including **clinical trials**); **observational studies** (cohort, case–control, cross-sectional/surveys, case–series); and meta-analyses. Each design has certain advantages over the others as well as some specific disadvantages; they are briefly summarized in the following paragraphs. (A more detailed discussion is presented in Chapter 2.)

Clinical trials provide the strongest evidence for causation because they are experiments and, as such, are subject to the least number of problems or biases. Trials with randomized controls are the study type of choice when the objective is to evaluate the effectiveness of a treatment or a procedure. Drawbacks to using clinical trials include their expense and the generally long time needed to complete them.

Cohort studies are the best observational study design for investigating the causes of a condition, the course of a disease, or **risk factors.** Causation cannot be proved with cohort studies, though, because they do not involve interventions. Because they are **longitudinal studies,** however, they incorporate the correct time sequence to provide strong evidence for possible causes and effects. In addition, in cohort studies that are **prospective,** as opposed to **historical,** investigators can control many sources of bias. Cohort studies have disadvantages, of course. If they take a long time to complete, they are frequently weakened by patient attrition. They are also expensive to carry out if the disease or outcome of interest is rare (so that a large number of subjects needs to be followed) or requires a long time to develop.

Case–control studies are an efficient way to study rare diseases, examine conditions that take a long time to develop, or investigate a preliminary hypothesis. They are the quickest and generally the least expensive studies to design and carry out. Case–control studies also are the most vulnerable to possible biases, however, and they depend entirely on high-quality existing records. A major issue in case–control studies is the selection of an appropriate control group. Some statisticians have recommended the use of two control groups: one similar in some ways to the cases (such as having been hospitalized or treated during the same period) and another made up of healthy subjects.

Cross-sectional studies and **surveys** are best for determining the status of a disease or condition at a particular point in time; they are similar to case–control studies in being relatively quick and inexpensive to complete. Because cross-sectional studies provide only a snapshot in time, they may lead to misleading conclusions if interest focuses on a disease or other time-dependent process.

Case–series studies are the weakest kinds of observational studies and represent a description of typically unplanned observations; in fact, many would not call them studies at all. Their primary use is to provide insights for research questions to be addressed by subsequent, planned studies.

Studies that focus on outcomes can be experimental or observational. Clinical outcomes remain the major focus, but emphasis is increasingly placed on functional status and quality-of-life measures. It is important to use properly designed and evaluated methods to collect outcome data. **Evidence-based medicine** makes great use of outcome studies.

Meta-analysis may likewise focus on clinical trials or observational studies. Meta-analyses differ from the traditional review articles in that they attempt to evaluate the quality of the research and quantify the summary data. They are helpful when the available evidence is based on studies with small sample sizes or when studies come to conflicting conclusions. Meta-analyses do not, however, take the place of well-designed clinical trials.

13.3 THE ABSTRACT & INTRODUCTION SECTIONS OF A RESEARCH REPORT

Journal articles almost always include an abstract or summary of the article prior to the body of the article itself. Most of us are guilty of reading *only* the abstract on occasion, perhaps because we are in a great hurry or have only a cursory, tangential interest in the topic. This practice is unwise when it is important to know whether the conclusions stated in the article are justified and can be used to make decisions. This section discusses the abstract and introduction portions of a research report and outlines the information they should contain.

13.3.1 The Abstract

The major purposes of the abstract are (1) to tell readers enough about the article so they can decide whether to read it in its entirely and (2) to identify the focus of the study. The International Committee of Medical Journal Editors (1988, p. 323) has recommended that the abstract "state the purposes of the study or investigation, basic procedures (selection of study subjects or experimented animals; observational and analytic methods), main findings (specific data and their statistical significance, if possible) and the principal conclusions." An increasing number of journals, especially those we consider to be of high quality, now use structured abstracts in which authors succinctly provide the above-mentioned information in separate, easily identified paragraphs (Haynes et al, 1990).

We suggest asking two questions to decide whether to read the article: (1) If the study has been properly designed and analyzed, would the results be important and worth knowing? (2) If the results are statistically significant, does the magnitude of the change or effect also have clinical significance; if the results are not statistically significant, was the sample size sufficiently large to detect a meaningful difference or effect? If the answers to these questions are yes, then it is worthwhile to continue to read the report. Structured abstracts are a boon to the busy reader and frequently contain enough information to answer these two questions.

13.3.2 The Introduction or Abstract

At one time, the following topics were discussed (or should have been discussed) in the introduction section; however, with the advent of the structured abstract, many of these topics are now addressed directly in that section. The important issue is that the information be available and easy to identify.

13.3.2.a. Reason for the Study: The introduction section of a research report is usually fairly short. Generally, the authors briefly mention previous research that indicates the need for the present study. In some situations, the study is a natural outgrowth or the next logical step of previous studies. In other circumstances, previous studies have been inadequate in one way or another. The overall purpose of this information is twofold: to provide the necessary background information to place the present study in its proper context and to provide reasons for doing the present study. In some journals, the main justification for the study is given in the discussion section of the article instead of in the introduction.

13.3.2.b. Purpose of the Study: Regardless of the placement of background information on the study, the introduction section is where the investigators communicate the purpose of their study. The purpose of the study is frequently presented in the last paragraph or last sentences at the end of the introduction. The purpose should be stated clearly and succinctly, in a manner analogous to a 15-second summary of a patient case. For example, in the study described in Presenting Problem 1 in Chapter 5, Dennison and colleagues (1997, p. 15) do this very well; they stated their objective as follows:

> To evaluate, in a population-based sample of healthy children, fruit juice consumption and its effects on growth parameters during early childhood.

This statement concisely communicates the population of interest (healthy children), the focus of the study or independent variable (fruit juice consumption), and the outcome (effects on growth). As readers, we should be able to determine whether the purpose for the study was conceived prior to data collection or if it evolved after the authors viewed their data; the latter situation is much more likely to capitalize on chance findings. The lack of a clearly stated research question is the most common reason medical manuscripts are rejected by journal editors (Marks et al, 1988).

13.3.2.c. Population Included in the Study: In addition to stating the purpose of the study, the structured abstract or introduction section sometimes contains information on the study's location, the length of time covered by the study, and the study's subjects. Alternatively, this information may be contained in the methods sections. This information helps readers decide whether the location of the study and the type of subjects included in the study are applicable in the readers' own practice environment.

The time covered by a study gives important clues regarding the **validity** of the results. If the study on a particular therapy covers too long a period, patients entering at the beginning of the study may differ in important ways from those entering at the end. For example, major changes may have occurred in the way the disease in question is diagnosed, and patients entering near the end of the study may have had their disease diagnosed at an earlier stage than did patients who entered the study early (see **detection bias,** Section 13.4.3.e). If the purpose of the study is to examine sequelae of a condition or procedure, the period covered by the study must be sufficiently long to detect consequences.

13.4 THE METHOD SECTION OF A RESEARCH REPORT

The method section contains information about how the study was done. Simply knowing the study design provides a great deal of information, and this information is often given in a structured abstract. In addition, the method section contains information regarding subjects who participated in the study or, in animal or inanimate studies, information on the animals or materials. The procedures used should be described in sufficient detail that the reader knows how measurements were made. If methods are novel or re-quire interpretation, information should be given on the reliability of the assessments. The study outcomes should be specified along with the criteria used to assess them. The method section also should include information on the sample size for the study and on the statistical methods used to analyze the data; this information is often placed at the end of the method section. Each of these topics is discussed in detail in this section.

How well the study has been designed is of utmost importance. The most critical statistical errors, according to the statistical consultant to the *New England Journal of Medicine*, involve improper research design: "Whereas one can correct incorrect analytical techniques with a simple reanalysis of the data, an error in research design is almost always fatal to the study—one cannot correct for it subsequent to data collection" (Marks et al, 1988, p. 1004). Many statistical advances have occurred in recent years, especially in the methods used to design, conduct, and analyze clinical trials (Simon, 1991), and investigators should offer evidence that they have obtained expert advice.

13.4.1 Subjects in the Study
13.4.1.a. Methods for Choosing Subjects: Authors of journal articles should provide several critical pieces of information about the subjects included in their study so that we readers can judge the applicability of the study results. Of foremost importance is how the patients were selected for the study and, if the study is a clinical trial, how treatment assignments were made.

Randomized selection or assignment greatly enhances the generalizability of the results and avoids biases that otherwise may occur in patient selection (see Section 13.4.2). Some authors believe it is sufficient merely to state that subjects were randomly selected or treatments were randomly assigned, but most statisticians recommend that the type of randomization process be specified as well. Authors who report the randomization methods provide some assurance that randomization actually occurred, because some investigators have a faulty view of what constitutes randomization. For example, an investigator may believe that assigning patients to the treatment and the control on alternate days makes the assignment random. As we emphasized in Chapter 4, however, randomization involves one of the precise methods that ensure that each subject (or treatment) has a known probability of being selected.

13.4.1.b. Eligibility Criteria: The authors should present information to illustrate that major selection biases (discussed in Section 13.4.2) have been avoided, an aspect especially important in **nonrandomized trials.** The issue of which patients serve as controls was discussed in Chapter 2 in the context of case–control studies. In addition, the eligibility criteria for both inclusion and exclusion of subjects in the study must be specified in detail. We should be able to state, given any hypothetical subject, whether this person would be included in or excluded from the study. Woolson and Watt (1991, p. 507) gave the following information on patients included in their study:

> Patients were excluded if they had an allergy to aspirin or warfarin, had recently had a peptic ulcer or other bleeding diathesis, had taken any drug that affects platelet function within two weeks before the operation, or were expected to remain in bed for more than four days after the operation.

13.4.1.c. Patient Follow-Up: For similar reasons, sufficient information must be given regarding the procedures the investigators used to follow up patients, and they should state the numbers lost to follow-up. Some articles include this information under the results section instead of in the methods section. In their 10-year follow-up of Coronary Artery Surgery Study (CASS) study patients, Rogers and colleagues (1990, p. 1648) described follow-up this way:

> At the time of this report, mean duration of follow-up was 11 years (range, 9.0–13.1 years). Follow-up

was 99.7% complete (778 of 780) for obtaining data on vital status. (Two patients were lost to follow-up at 4.6 and 10.5 years, respectively.) For other variables, follow-up was less complete, usually because data were not obtained or were obtained outside the follow-up time period. For each variable, the number of patients followed up at each time interval is indicated in the tables and figures.

The description of follow-up and dropouts should be sufficiently detailed to permit the reader to draw a diagram of the information. Occasionally, an article presents such a diagram, as was done by Hébert and colleagues in their study of elderly residents in Canada (1997), reproduced in Figure 13–1. Such a diagram makes very clear the number of patients who were eligible, those who were not eligible because of specific reasons, the dropouts, and so on.

13.4.2 Bias Related to Subject Selection

Bias in studies should not happen; it is an error related to selecting subjects or procedures or to measur-

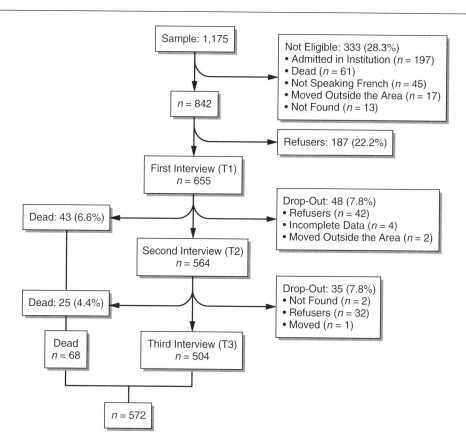

Figure 13–1. Flow of the subjects through the study, a representative sample of elderly people living at home in Sherbrooke, Canada, 1991–1993. (Reproduced, with permission, from Figure 1 in Hébert R et al: Incidence of functional decline and improvement in a community-dwelling very elderly population. *Am J Epidemiol* 1997;**145:**935–944.)

ing a characteristic. Biases are sometimes called **measurement errors** or **systematic errors** to distinguish them from **random error (random variation)**, which occurs any time a sample is selected from a population. This section discusses selection bias, a type of bias common in medical research.

Selection biases can occur in any study, but they are easier to control in clinical trials and cohort designs. It is important to be aware of selection biases, even though it is not always possible to predict exactly how their presence affects the conclusions. Sackett (1979) enumerated 35 different biases. We discuss some of the major ones that seem especially important to the clinician. If you are interested in a more detailed discussion, consult the article by Sackett and the text by Feinstein (1985), which devotes several chapters to the discussion of bias (especially Chapter 4, Section 2, and Chapters 15–17).

13.4.2.a. Prevalence or Incidence Bias: Prevalence (Neyman) bias occurs when a condition is characterized by early fatalities (some subjects die before they are diagnosed) or silent cases (cases in which the evidence of exposure disappears when the disease begins). Prevalence bias can result whenever a time gap occurs between exposure and selection of study subjects and the worst cases have died. A cohort study begun prior to the onset of disease is able to detect occurrences properly, but a case–control study that begins at a later date consists only of the people who did not die. This bias can be prevented in cohort studies and avoided in case–control studies by limiting eligibility for the study to newly diagnosed or incident cases. The practice of limiting eligibility is common in population-based case–control studies in cancer epidemiology. An article by Horwitz and colleagues (1990) discusses a creative approach to decreasing selection bias in cohort studies by using the same criteria for inclusion and exclusion as are used in clinical trials.

To illustrate prevalence or incidence bias, let us suppose that two groups of people are being studied: those with a risk factor for a given disease (eg, hypertension as a risk factor for stroke) and those without the risk factor. Suppose 1000 people with hypertension and 1000 people without hypertension have been followed for 10 years. At this point, we might have the situation shown in Table 13–1.

A cohort study begun 10 years ago would conclude correctly that patients with hypertension are more likely to develop cerebrovascular disease than patients without hypertension (300 to 100) and far more likely to die from it (250 to 20).

Suppose, however, a case–control study is undertaken at the end of the 10-year period without limiting eligibility to newly diagnosed cases of cerebrovascular disease. Then the situation illustrated in Table 13–2 occurs.

The **odds ratio** is calculated as $(50 \times 900)/(80 \times 700) = 0.80$, making it appears that hypertension is actually a protective factor for the disease! The bias introduced in an improperly designed case–control study of a disease that kills off one group faster than the other can lead to a conclusion exactly the opposite of the correct conclusion that would be obtained from a well-designed case–control study or a cohort study.

13.4.2.b. Admission Rate Bias: Admission rate bias (Berkson's fallacy) occurs when the study admission rates differ, which causes major distortions in risk ratios. As an example, admission rate bias can occur in studies of hospitalized patients when patients (cases) who have the risk factor are admitted to the hospital more frequently than either the cases without the risk factor or the controls with the risk factor.

This fallacy was first pointed out by Berkson (1946) in evaluating an earlier study that had concluded that tuberculosis might have a protective effect on cancer. This conclusion was reached after a case–control study found a negative association between tuberculosis and cancer: The frequency of tuberculosis among hospitalized cancer patients was less than the frequency of tuberculosis among the hospitalized control patients who did not have cancer. These counterintuitive results occurred because a smaller proportion of patients who had both cancer and tuberculosis were hospitalized and thus available for selection as cases in the study; chances are that patients with both diseases were more likely to die than patients with cancer or tuberculosis alone.

It is important to be aware of admission rate bias because many case–control studies reported in the

Table 13–1. Illustration of prevalence bias: Actual situation.

Patients	Number of Patients in 10-Year Cohort Study		
	Alive with Cerebrovascular Disease	Dead from Stroke	Alive with No Cerebrovascular Disease
With hypertension	50	250	700
Without hypertension	80	20	900

Table 13–2. Illustration of prevalence bias: Result with case–control design.

Patients	Number of Patients in Case–Control Study at End of 10 Years	
	With Cerebrovascular Disease	Without Cerebrovascular Disease
With hypertension	50	700
Without hypertension	80	900

medical literature use hospitalized patients as sources for both cases and controls. The only way to control for this bias is to include an unbiased control group, best accomplished by choosing controls from a wide variety of disease categories or from a population of healthy subjects. Some statisticians suggest using two control groups in studies in which admission bias is a potential problem.

13.4.2.c. Nonresponse Bias and the Volunteer Effect: Several steps can be taken to ensure the quality of surveys so as to reduce potential bias that occurs when subjects fail to respond to a survey. It is important that researchers not ask questions in a manner that biases or leads people to answer in any one direction; some public opinion polls are especially guilty of this problem. The sample of people who answer the questions should be randomly selected in an appropriate manner, and efforts should be made to follow up people who do not participate in the survey; otherwise, it is difficult to tell whether the responses are typical of those that would be received from all persons who were eligible to participate. Pilot testing is a critical step in the development of any high-quality survey procedure.

Survey researchers often make serious efforts to ensure a good response rate. With mailed questionnaires, it is common practice to follow up with at least one and sometimes two additional questionnaires to people who do not return the first one. On other occasions incentives are offered. For example, to increase the participation rate in their study on the availability of firearms and suicide, Kellerman and coworkers (1992) offered $10 compensation to people who agreed to be interviewed.

Bias that occurs when patients either volunteer or refuse to participate in studies is similar to nonresponse bias. This effect was studied in the nationwide Salk polio vaccine trials in 1954 by using two different study designs to evaluate the effectiveness of the vaccine (Meier, 1989). In some communities, children were randomly assigned to receive either the vaccine or a placebo injection. Some communities, however, refused to participate in a randomized trial; they agreed, instead, that second graders could be offered the vaccination and first and third graders could constitute the controls. In analysis of the data, researchers found that families who volunteered their children for participation in the nonrandomized study tended to be better educated and to have a higher income than families who refused to participate. They also tended to be absent from school with a higher frequency than nonparticipants.

Although in this example we might guess how absence from school could bias results, it is not always easy to determine how selection bias affects the outcome of the study; it may cause the experimental treatment to appear either better or worse than it should. Investigators should therefore reduce the potential for nonresponse bias as much as possible by using all possible means to increase the response rate and obtain the participation of most eligible patients. Using databases reduces response bias, but sometimes other sources of bias are present, that is, reasons that a specific group or selected information is underrepresented in the database.

13.4.2.d. Membership Bias: Membership bias is essentially a problem of preexisting groups. It also arises because one or more of the same characteristics that cause people to belong to the groups are related to the outcome of interest. For example, investigators have not been able to perform a clinical trial to examine the effects of smoking; some researchers have claimed it is not smoking itself that causes cancer but some other factor that simply happens to be more common in smokers. As readers of the medical literature, we need to be aware of membership bias because it cannot be prevented, and it makes the study of the effect of potential risk factors related to life-style very difficult.

A problem similar to membership bias is called the healthy worker effect; it was recognized in epidemiology when workers in a hazardous environment were unexpectedly found to have a higher survival rate than the general public. After further investigation, the cause of this incongruous finding was determined: Good health is a prerequisite in persons who are hired for work, but being healthy enough to work is not a requirement for persons in the general public.

13.4.2.e. Procedure Selection Bias: Procedure selection bias occurs when treatment assignments are made on the basis of certain characteristics of the patients, with the result that the treatment groups are not really similar. This bias frequently occurs in studies that are not randomized and is especially a problem in studies using historical controls. A good example is the comparison of a surgical versus a medical approach to a problem such as coronary artery disease. In early studies comparing surgical and medical treatment, patients were not randomized, and the evidence pointed to the conclusion that patients who received surgery were healthier than those treated medically; that is, only healthier patients were subjected to the risks associated with the surgery. The CASS study (1983), Presenting Problem 4 in Chapter 4, was undertaken in part to resolve these questions. It is important to be aware of procedure selection bias because many published studies describe a series of patients, some treated one way and some another way, and then proceed to make comparisons and draw inappropriate conclusions as a result.

13.4.3 Procedures Used in the Study and Common Procedural Biases

13.4.3.a. Terms and Measurements: The procedures used in the study are also described in the method section. Here authors provide definitions of measures used in the study, especially any operational definitions developed by the investigators. If unusual instruments or methods are used, the authors should provide a reference and a brief description. For example, Kaku and Lowenstein (1990, pp. 821–822), in Exercise 16 in Chapter 3, undertook a case–control study of the relationship between recreational drug use and stroke in young persons. They defined recreational drugs as

> those drugs used unlawfully for the maintenance of addiction or for their psychic effects (excluding marijuana and abused drugs that are commonly prescribed, such as sedative–hypnotics). Patients who stated they were abstinent for more than 1 year before admission or those for whom the chart lacked any information on drug abuse were not considered to be drug abusers.

We may or may not agree with this definition and the manner in which patients whose charts lacked information on drug use were classified as not being drug abusers. The authors' specification of how they handled the problem of missing data from the charts (and their notation of possible bias in the discussion section of the paper), however, makes it possible for us to form our own judgments.

The journal *Stroke* has the practice of presenting the abbreviations and acronyms used in the article in a box. This makes the abbreviations clear and also easy to refer to in reading other sections of the article. For example, in reporting their study of sleep-disordered breathing and stroke, Good and colleagues (1996, p. 253) presented a list of abbreviations at the top of the column that begins to describe the subjects and methods in the study. Good also defines terms explicitly, as in the following excerpt:

> The computerized analysis defines a desaturation event as a $\geq 4\%$ change in SaO_2 from baseline. A rise of 4% above the nadir of a desaturation event signals the end of that event.... [Desaturation index] was calculated by dividing the number of desaturation events by the total recording time.

Several biases may occur in the measurement of various patient characteristics and in the procedures used or evaluated in the study. Some of the more common biases are described in the following subsections.

13.4.3.b. Procedure Bias:
Procedure bias, discussed by Feinstein (1985), occurs when groups of subjects are not treated in the same manner. For example, the procedures used in an investigation may lead to detection of other problems in patients in the treatment group and make these problems appear to be more prevalent in this group. As another example, the patients in the treatment group may receive more attention and be followed up more vigorously than those in another group, thus stimulating greater compliance with the treatment regimen. The way to avoid this bias is by carrying out all maneuvers except the experimental factor in the same way in all groups and examining all outcomes using similar procedures and criteria.

13.4.3.c. Recall Bias:
Recall bias may occur when patients are asked to recall certain events, and subjects in one group are more likely to remember the event than those in the other group. For example, people take aspirin commonly and for many reasons, but patients diagnosed as having peptic ulcer disease may recall the ingestion of aspirin with greater accuracy than those without gastrointestinal problems. In the study of the relationship between juice consumption and growth, Dennison and associates (1997) asked parents to keep a daily journal of all the liquid consumed by their children; a properly maintained journal helps reduce recall bias.

13.4.3.d. Insensitive-Measure Bias:
Measuring instruments may not be able to detect the characteristic of interest or may not be properly calibrated. For example, routine x-ray films are an insensitive method for detecting osteoporosis because bone loss of approximately 30% must occur before a roentgenogram can detect it. Newer densitometry techniques are more sensitive and thus avoid insensitive-measure bias.

13.4.3.e. Detection Bias:
Detection bias can occur because a new diagnostic technique is introduced that is capable of detecting the condition of interest at an earlier stage. Survival for patients diagnosed with the new procedure inappropriately appears to be longer, merely because the condition was diagnosed earlier.

A spin-off of detection bias, called the Will Rogers phenomenon (because of his attention to human phenomena), was described by Feinstein and colleagues (1985). They found that a cohort of subjects with lung cancer first treated in 1953–1954 had lower 6-month survival rates for patients with each of the three main stages (localized, nodal involvement, and metastases) as well as for the total group than did a 1977 cohort treated at the same institutions. Newer imaging procedures were used with the later group; however, according to the old diagnostic classification, this group had a prognostically favorable zero-time shift in that their disease was diagnosed at an earlier stage. In addition, by detecting metastases in the 1977 group that were missed in the earlier group, the new technologic approaches resulted in stage migration; that is, members of the 1977 cohort were diagnosed as having a more advanced stage of the disease, whereas they would have been diagnosed as having earlier-stage disease in 1953–1954. The individuals who migrated from the earlier-stage group to the later-stage group tended to have the poorest survival in the earlier-stage group; so removing them resulted in an increase in survival rates in the earlier group. At the same time, these individuals, now assigned to the later-stage group, were better off than most other patients in this group, and their addition to the group resulted in an increased survival in the later-stage group as well. The authors stated that the 1953–1954 and 1977 cohorts actually had similar survival rates when patients in the 1977 group were classified according to the criteria that would have been in effect had there been no advances in diagnostic techniques.

13.4.3.f. Compliance Bias: Compliance bias occurs when patients find it easier or more pleasant to comply with one treatment than with another. For example, in the treatment of hypertension, a comparison of α-methyldopa versus hydrochlorothiazide may demonstrate inaccurate results because some patients do not take α-methyldopa owing to its unpleasant side effects, such as drowsiness, fatigue, or impotence in male patients.

13.4.4 Assessing Study Outcomes

13.4.4.a. Variation in Data: In many clinics, a nurse collects certain information about a patient (eg, height, weight, date of birth, blood pressure, pulse) and records it on the medical record before the patient is seen by a physician. Suppose a patient's blood pressure is recorded as 140/88 on the chart; the physician, taking the patient's blood pressure again as part of the physical examination, observes a reading of 148/96. Which blood pressure reading is correct? What factors might be responsible for the differences in the observation? We use blood pressure and other clinical information to examine sources of variation in data and ways to measure the reliability of observations. Two articles in the *Canadian Medical Association Journal* (McMaster University Health Sciences Centre, Department of Clinical Epidemiology and Biostatistics, 1980a; 1980b) discuss sources of clinical disagreement and ways disagreement can be minimized.

13.4.4.b. Factors that Contribute to Variation in Clinical Observations: Variation, or variability in measurements on the same subject, in clinical observations and measurements can be classified into three categories: (1) variation in the characteristic being measured, (2) variation introduced by the examiner, and (3) variation owing to the instrument or method used. It is especially important to control variation due to the second two factors as much as possible so that the reported results will generalize as intended.

Substantial variability may occur in the measurement of biologic characteristics. For example, a person's blood pressure is not the same from one time to another, and thus, blood pressure values vary. A patient's description of symptoms to two different physicians may vary because the patient may forget something. Medications and illness can also affect the way a patient behaves and what information he or she remembers to tell a nurse or physician.

Even when no change occurs in the subject, different observers may report different measurements. When examination of a characteristic requires visual acuity, such as the reading on a sphygmomanometer or the features on an x-ray film, differences may result from the varying visual abilities of the observers. Such differences can also play a role when hearing (detecting heart sounds) or feeling (palpating internal organs) is required. Some individuals are simply more skilled than others in history taking or performing certain examinations.

Variability also occurs when the characteristic being measured is a behavioral attribute. Two examples are measurements of functional status and measurements of pain; here the additional component of patient or observer interpretation can increase apparent variability. In addition, observers may tend to observe and record what they expect based on other information about the patient. These factors point out the need for a standardized protocol for data collection.

The instrument used in the examination can be another source of variation. For instance, mercury column sphygmomanometers are less inherently variable than aneroid models. In addition, the environment in which the examination takes place, including lighting and noise level, presence of other individuals, and room temperature, can produce apparent differences. Methods for measuring behavior-related characteristics such as functional status or pain usually consist of a set of questions answered by patients and hence are not as precise as instruments that measure physical characteristics.

Several steps can be taken to reduce variability. Taking a history when the patient is calm and not heavily medicated and checking with family members when the patient is incapacitated are both useful in minimizing errors that result from a patient's illness or the effects of medication. Collecting information and making observations in a proper environment is also a good strategy. Recognizing one's own strengths and weaknesses helps one evaluate the need for other opinions. **Blind assessment,** especially of subjective characteristics, guards against errors resulting from preconceptions. Repeating questionable aspects of the examination or asking a colleague to perform a key aspect (blindly, of course) reduces the possibility of error. Having well-defined operational guidelines for using classification scales helps people use them in a consistent manner. Ensuring that instruments are properly calibrated and correctly used eliminates many errors and thus reduces variation.

Authors of research reported in the *Lancet* studied variability in blood pressure readings of obese patients (Maxwell et al, 1982). They measured blood pressure in 1240 obese subjects by using the three cuff sizes available in clinical practice and found that regardless of arm circumference, recorded blood pressure rose with decreasing cuff size. When the cuff is too wide, measured blood pressure is often un-derestimated; when the cuff is too narrow, blood pressure is overestimated. The investigators com-pared blood pressure measurements in a large num-ber of moderately obese patients and found that when an appropriately large cuff was used, rather than the standard-size cuff, 37% of patients originally thought to be hypertensive were actually normotensive. This study highlights the practitioner's responsibility to consider carefully sources of error that may be intro-duced in measurement.

13.4.4.c. Ways to Measure Reliability: A com-mon strategy to ensure the **reliability** or reproducibil-ity of measurements, especially for research pur-poses, is to replicate the measurements and evaluate the degree of agreement. **Intrarater reliability** is ob-tained when one person measures the same item twice and the measurements are compared. When two or more persons measure the same item and their measurements are compared, an index of interob-server variability, called **interrater reliability,** is ob-tained. The index of reliability used depends on the type of measurement made.

Frequently in medicine, a practitioner must inter-pret whether a procedure indicates the presence of a disease or abnormality; that is, the observation is a yes-or-no outcome, which is a nominal measure. If it is desirable to determine the interrater reliability, an-other practitioner independently interprets the same procedure. Agreement between the two interpreta-tions can be evaluated using the kappa statistic, dis-cussed in Chapter 5.

Alternatively, some researchers control for varia-tion by having the same researcher repeat the task on some of the subjects. For instance, Shlipak and coworkers (1999, p. 715) studied features of the elec-trocardiogram (ECG) as predictors of myocardial in-farction. They stated:

> The scoring system derived by Sgarbossa et al de-fined the ECG finding as positive (suggestive of acute MI) if it scored 3 points or higher based on 3 criteria. To control for interobserver reliability, we used only the most senior electrocardiographer (G.T.E.) at our institution. His intraobserver reliabil-ity was tested in a random sample of 20% of the overall cohort whose ECGs were analyzed twice without his knowledge; his κ [kappa statistic of agreement] was 0.80 for the Sgarbossa et al criteria (positive vs negative findings).

Shlipak strengthened the measurement of reliability by having the electrocardiographer blind to the ECGs that were analyzed twice.

In many studies, the outcome is a numerical vari-able. For instance, suppose a clinician wants to deter-mine the reliability of measurements of the tracheal diameter in patients having chest roentgenograms. One approach is to measure a group of films and record the measurements. Then, some days or weeks later, measure the same films again without consult-ing the earlier figures. Because tracheal diameter is measured on a numerical scale, the statistic used to examine the relationship between two numerical characteristics is the correlation coefficient discussed in Chapter 8. The correlation between the two sets of tracheal diameter measurements therefore provides a measure of the reliability of the clinician's measure-ments.

Another aspect of reliability relates to the instru-ments' capacity to provide reproducible measure-ments. The coefficient of variation discussed in Chapter 3 is typically used to demonstrate the relia-bility of laboratory measurements or assays. If the in-strument is a paper scale or test used to measure behavioral or psychologic characteristics, some addi-tional ways are available for measuring reliability. The **internal consistency** reliability of the items on the instrument or scale indicates how strongly the items are related to one another; that is, whether they are measuring a single characteristic. Testing agen-cies that create examinations, such as the SAT or Na-tional Board USMLE Examinations, sometimes refer to the internal consistency reliability as Cronbach's alpha. An instrument's capacity to provide the same measurement on different occasions is called the **test–retest** reliability. Because it is difficult to ad-minister the same instrument to the same people on more than one occasion, testing agencies often use internal consistency reliability as an estimate of test–retest reliability. Reliability as measured in these ways can range from 0 to 1.00; an acceptable level of reliability is 0.80 or higher. Hodgson and Cutler (1997, p. 63), in their study of anticipatory dementia, used several instruments and reported the following:

> For purposes of the present study, we used a mea-sure of subjective memory functioning which is based on six questions developed for this study.... Scores on each of the six items were dichotomized and summed, resulting in a composite Memory As-sessment Index with a possible range from zero to six, with higher scores indicating a more positive as-sessment of memory. For the respondents in this study, the reliability coefficient (Cronbach's alpha) is 0.805.

In other words, if the instrument was used on the same subjects twice, the correlation between their scores is estimated to be approximately 0.80. More details about psychologic measurement can be found in classic texts on measurement, such as the one by Anastasi (1997).

13.4.4.d. Validity of Measurements: Note that kappa, the correlation coefficient, or other measures of reliability do not tell us anything about the **validity** of the measurements. "Validity" is a term for how well an instrument (or measurement procedure) measures what it purports to measure. The issue of validity motivates questions such as, how well do the Dukes' stages for colorectal cancer indicate the actual stage of cancer? Or, how accurate is the arthritis functional status scale for indicating a patient's level of activity? Or, how accurate is the National Board Examination in measuring students' knowledge of medicine? An issue related to validity is that instruments should be used to measure only those characteristics they were designed to measure.

Three commonly used measures of validity are content validity, criterion validity, and construct validity. For a test, **content validity** indicates the degree to which the items on the test are representative of the knowledge being tested. **Criterion validity** relates the measurement's capacity to predict another characteristic associated with the measure. For example, the criterion validity of the Dukes' stages is their ability to predict length of patient survival. The criterion may indicate either a concurrent or a future state. Ideally, criterion validity is established by comparing the measurement to a gold standard, if one exists. The third measure, **construct validity,** is somewhat indirect. It consists of demonstrating that the measure is related to other similar measures of the same characteristic and not related to other characteristics. It is generally established by using several instruments or tests on the same group of individuals and investigating the pattern of relationships among the measurements.

Hébert and colleagues (1997, pp. 936–937) used the Functional Autonomy Measurement System (SMAF) instrument to measure cognitive functioning and depression. They described the properties of this instrument as follows:

> Each item is scored on a four-point scale (0, independent; 1, needs supervision or stimulation; 2, needs help; 3, dependent) for a maximum score of 87. The SMAF must be administered by a trained health professional (nurse or social worker) who scores the individual after obtaining the information either by questioning the subject and proxies or by observing and even testing the subject. Reliability studies show mean . . . kappas of 0.75 for item scores and intraclass [alpha] correlation coefficients of 0.95 for total SMAF scores. Validity was tested by comparing the SMAF score with the nursing time required for care ($r = 0.88$) and discriminating disability scores between residents living in settings of different levels of care.

The high correlation between nursing time and score indicates that patients with higher (more dependent) scores required more nursing time, a reasonable expectation. Another indication of validity is higher disability scores among residents living in settings where they were provided with a high level of care and lower scores among residents who live independently.

13.4.4.e. Blinding: Another aspect of assessing the outcome is related to ways of increasing the objectivity and decreasing the subjectivity of the assessment. In studies involving the comparison of two treatments or procedures, the most effective method for achieving objective assessment is to have both patient and investigator be unaware of which method was used. If only the patient is unaware, the study is called **blind;** if both patient and investigator are unaware, it is called **double-blind.**

Ballard and colleagues (1998, p. 494) studied the effect of antenatal thyrotropin-releasing hormone in preventing lung disease in preterm infants in a randomized study. Experimental subjects were given the hormone, and controls were given placebo. The authors stated:

> The women were randomly assigned within centers to the treatment or placebo group in permuted blocks of four. The study was double-blinded, and only the pharmacies at the participating centers had the randomization schedule.

Blinding helps to reduce a priori biases on the part of both patient and physician. Patients who are aware of their treatment assignment may imagine certain side effects or expect specific benefits, and their expectations may influence the outcome. Similarly, investigators who know which treatment has been assigned to a given patient may be more watchful for certain side effects or benefits. Although we might suspect an investigator who is not blinded to be more favorable to the new treatment or procedure, just the opposite may happen; that is, the investigator may bend over backward to keep from being prejudiced by his or her knowledge and therefore may err in favor of the control.

Knowledge of treatment assignment may be somewhat less influential when the outcome is straightforward, as is true for mortality. With mortality, it is difficult to see how outcome assessment can be biased. Many examples exist in which the outcome appears to be objective, however, even though its evaluation contains subjective components. Many clinical studies attempt to ascribe reasons for mortality or morbidity, and judgment begins to play a role in these cases. For example, mortality is often an outcome of interest in studies involving organ transplantation, and investigators wish to differentiate between deaths from failure of the organ and deaths from an unrelated cause. If the patient dies in an automobile accident, for example, investigators can easily decide that the death is not due to organ rejection; but in most situations, the decision is not so easy.

The issue of blinding becomes more important as the outcome becomes less amenable to objective determination. As a follow-up to the Coronary Artery Surgery Study (Presenting Problem 4 in Chapter 4), Rogers and colleagues (1990) investigated several outcomes, including quality-of-life measures and mortality. Quality of life was evaluated by assessing such different outcomes as chest pain status; heart failure; activity limitation; employment status; recreational status; need for drugs; number of hospitalizations; and alteration of risk factors, such as smoking, blood pressure level, and cholesterol level. Some of these outcomes (eg, employment status, smoking cessation, and number of hospitalizations) can be measured in relatively objective ways. Others, however (eg, chest pain status, activity limitation, and recreational status), require subjective measures. Although patients cannot be blinded in a study like the CASS study, the subjective outcomes can be assessed by a person, such as another physician, a psychologist, or a physical therapist, who is blind to the treatment the patient received.

13.4.4.f. Data Quality and Monitoring: The method section is also the place where steps taken to ensure the accuracy of the data should be described. Increased variation and possibly incorrect conclusions can occur if the correct observation is made but is incorrectly recorded or coded. Dennison and colleagues (1997, p. 16) stated: "All questionnaire data were dual-entered and verified before being entered into a ... database." Dual or duplicate entry decreases the likelihood of errors because it is unusual for the same entry error to occur twice.

Multicenter studies provide additional data quality challenges. It is important that an accurate and complete protocol be developed to ensure that data are handled the same way in all centers. Gelber and colleagues (1997, p. 41) studied data collected from 63 centers in North America in setting normative values for cardiovascular autonomic nervous system tests. They reported that

> All site personnel were trained by a member of the Autonomic Nervous System (ANS) Reading Center in the use of the equipment and testing methodology. ... All data were analyzed at a single Autonomic Reading Center. The analysis program contains internal checks which alert the analyzing technician to any aberrant data points overlooked during the editing process and warns the technician when the results suggest that the test may have been performed improperly. The analysis of each study was reviewed by the director of the ANS Reading Center.

In addition to standardized training, the data entry process itself was monitored for potential errors.

13.4.5 Determining an Appropriate Sample Size

Specifying the sample size needed to detect a difference or an effect of a given magnitude is one of the most crucial pieces of information in the report of a medical study. Recall that missing a significant difference is called a **type II error,** and this error can happen when the sample size is too small. Freiman and collaborators (1978) reported that 50 out of 71 negative clinical trials published in the literature would have missed a 50% improvement because of their small sample size. The formulas for estimating sample sizes are illustrated in the chapters that discuss specific statistical methods, especially Chapters 5, 6, 7, 8, and 10.

Determination of sample size is referred to as power analysis or as determining the **power** of a study. An assessment of power is essential in negative studies, studies that fail to find an expected difference or relationship; we feel so strongly about this point that we recommend that readers disregard negative studies that do not provide information on power. The following examples illustrate the way authors generally present sample size information.

In their study of vaginal versus abdominal surgery to correct pelvic support defects, Benson and associates (1996, p. 1418) stated:

> On the basis of an estimate of an acceptable surgical cure rate of 90% and a clinically significant difference of 20% with power of 80% and an α level of 0.05, the calculated sample size necessary was 124 women (62 in each group).

This statement indicates that 62 women in each group would be sufficient to detect a difference if one procedure had a cure rate 20% less than the other.

Harper studied the use of paracervical block to diminish cramping associated with cryosurgery (1997, p. 706). She stated:

> To have a power of 80% to detect a difference of 20 mm on the visual analog scale at the 0.05 level of significance (assuming a standard deviation of 30 mm), the power analysis a priori showed that 35 women would be needed in each cohort. The first 35 women who met the inclusion and exclusion criteria for cryosurgery were treated in the usual manner with no anesthetic block given before cryosurgery. The variances of the actual responses were greater than anticipated in the a priori power analysis, leading to the subsequent enrollment of the next five women qualifying for the study for a total of 40 women in the usual treatment group. This increase in enrollment maintained the power of the study.

Thus, as a result of analysis of data, the investigator opted to increase the sample size to maintain power.

The effects of formaldehyde on the mucous membranes and lungs were studied by Horvath and associates (1988). One hundred nine workers and 254 control subjects were studied before and after their work shift. In the results and comment sections of their article, the authors stated that the differences between test and control groups on mean lung function parameters were not statistically significant.

> In part because of the large number of subjects studied, there was a high probability (power) of being able to detect 5% or 10% differences between these two groups.

This study may be an example in which investigators performed the power analysis after the study was completed and the data analyzed; they wish to assure readers that the sample was large enough to have found statistical significance had there actually been differences. Although it is preferable to address the question of sample size prior to undertaking a study, addressing the issue post hoc is better than not addressing it at all.

We repeatedly emphasized the need to perform a power analysis prior to beginning a study and have illustrated how to estimate power using statistical programs for that purpose. Investigators planning complicated studies or studies involving a number of variables are especially advised to contact a statistician for assistance.

13.4.6 Evaluating the Statistical Methods

Statistical methods are the primary focus of this text, and only a brief summary and some common problems are listed here. At the risk of oversimplification, the use of statistics in medicine can be summarized as follows: (1) to answer questions concerning differences; (2) to answer questions concerning associations; and (3) to control for confounding issues or to make predictions. If you can determine the type of question investigators are asking (from the stated purpose of the study) and the types and numbers of measures used in the study (**numerical, ordinal, nominal**), then the appropriate statistical procedure should be relatively easy to specify. Tables 10–1 and 10–2 in Chapter 10 and the flowcharts in Appendix C were developed to assist with this process. Some common biases in evaluating data are discussed in the next sections.

13.4.6.a. Fishing Expedition: A fishing expedition is the name given to studies in which the investigators do not have clear-cut research questions guiding the research. Instead, data are collected, and a search is carried out for results that are *significant.* The problem with this approach is that it capitalizes on chance occurrences and leads to conclusions that may not hold up if the study is replicated. Unfortunately, such studies are rarely repeated, and incorrect conclusions can remain a part of accepted wisdom.

13.4.6.b. Multiple Significance Tests: Multiple tests in statistics, just as in clinical medicine, result in increased chances of making a type I, or false-positive, error when the results from one test are interpreted as being independent of the results from another. For example, a **factorial design** for analysis of variance in a study involving four groups measured on three independent variables has the possibility of 18 comparisons (6 comparisons among the four groups on each of three variables), ignoring interactions. If each comparison is made for $P \leq 0.05$, the probability of finding one or more comparisons significant by chance is considerably greater than 0.05. The best way to guard against this bias is by performing the appropriate global test with analysis of variance prior to making individual group comparisons (Chapter 7) or using an appropriate method to analyze multiple variables (Chapter 10).

A similar problem can occur in a clinical trial if too many interim analyses are done. Sometimes it is important to analyze the data at certain stages during a trial to learn if one treatment is clearly superior or inferior. Many trials are stopped early when an interim analysis determines that one therapy is markedly superior to another. For instance, the Diabetes Control and Complications Trial (DCCT) was stopped early because an interim analysis clearly indicated that intensive diabetes therapy effectively delayed the onset of neuropathy in patients with insulin-dependent diabetes mellitus. In these situations, it is unethical to deny patients the superior treatment. Interim analyses should be planned as part of the design of the study, and the overall probability of a type I error (the α level) should be adjusted to compensate for the multiple comparisons.

13.4.6.c. Migration Bias: Migration bias occurs when patients who drop out of the study are also dropped from the analysis. The tendency to drop out of a study may be associated with the treatment (eg, its side effects), and dropping these subjects from the analysis can make a treatment appear more or less effective than it really is. Migration bias can also occur when patients cross over from the treatment arm to which they were assigned to another treatment. For example, in **crossover studies** comparing surgical and medical treatment for coronary artery disease, patients assigned to the medical arm of the study sometimes require subsequent surgical treatment for their condition. In such situations, the appropriate method is to analyze the patient according to his or her original group; this is referred to as analysis based on the **intention-to-treat** principle.

13.4.6.d. Entry Time Bias: Entry time bias may occur when time-related variables, such as survival or time to remission, are counted differently for different arms of the study. For example, consider a study comparing survival for patients randomized to a surgical versus a medical treatment in a clinical trial. Patients randomized to the medical treatment who die at any time after randomization are counted as treatment failures; the same rule must be followed with patients randomized to surgery, even if they die prior to the time surgery is performed. Otherwise, a bias exists in favor of the surgical treatment.

13.5 THE RESULTS SECTION OF A RESEARCH REPORT

The results section of a medical report contains just that: results of (or findings from) the research directed at questions posed in the introduction. Typically, authors present tables or graphs (or both) of quantitative data and also report the findings in the text. Findings generally consist of both **descriptive statistics** (means, standard deviations, risk ratios, etc) and results of **statistical tests** that were performed. Results of statistical tests are typically given as either *P* **values** or **confidence limits;** authors seldom give the value of the statistical test itself but, rather, give the *P* value associated with the statistical test. The two major aspects for readers evaluating the results section are the adequacy of information and the sufficiency of the evidence to withstand possible threats to the validity of the conclusions.

13.5.1 Assessing the Data Presented

Authors should provide adequate information about measurements made in the study. At a minimum, this information should include sample sizes and either means and standard deviations for numerical measures or proportions for nominal measures. For example, in describing the effects of a low-calorie, low-carbohydrate diet on abnormal pulmonary physiology in chronic hypercapnic respiratory patients, Tirlapur and Mir (1984, p. 990) specified in the method section that all data were presented as means plus or minus standard deviations, and that the paired *t* test was used to determine significance between the data before and after weight reduction. In the results section, they stated:

> The clinical characteristics of all the eight patients (four men and four women), together with the other data, are summarized. . . . Their age ranged from 49 to 69 years with a mean of 61.4 ± 6.1 years. The duration of chronic obstructive lung disease ranged from 5 to 15 years, with a mean of 10.0 ± 4.0 years. . . . The weight loss varied widely from patient to patient (mean 8.5 ± 3.6 kg), even though the dietary restrictions were supervised in the hospital in all patients. . . . The mean hematocrit fell significantly ($P \leq 0.02$) from 53.1 ± 6.6 to $49.6 \pm 5.1\%$. No correlation was observed between the reduction in the hematocrit and the weight loss or the improvement in hypoxemia.

This quotation illustrates several important points about reporting the results. Note that the authors provide adequate information for readers to draw conclusions about the patients in the study; that is, they specify range, mean, and standard deviation of age and duration of disease, and they give study information in the article. The weight loss results are clearly stated, as is the significant decrease in hematocrit, along with the *P* value that resulted. Because the authors previously specified that the paired *t* test was used for before-and-after comparisons, we know that $P < 0.02$ was from this test. Had the statistical test not been specified and only the *P* value given, sometimes called an "orphan *P,*" we would not know how the *P* value was obtained. This description has two shortcomings, however. First, the authors do not state which correlational methods they used. We can only assume, therefore, that the relationship between hema-

tocrit reduction and weight loss was evaluated using correct correlational procedures. Second, any negative finding could be a function of the small sample size; thus, a statement regarding power is essential.

In addition to presenting adequate information on the observations in the study, good medical reports use tables and graphs appropriately. As we outlined in Chapter 3, tables and graphs should be clearly labeled so that they can be interpreted without referring to the text of the article. Furthermore, they should be properly constructed, using the methods illustrated in Chapter 3.

13.5.2 Assuring the Validity of the Data

A good results section should have the following three characteristics. First, authors of medical reports should provide information about the baseline measures of the group (or groups) involved in the study. For example, consider the study by Lamas and colleagues (1992) that reported an increase in the number of persons using aspirin between 1987 and 1990. They used six enrollment periods in a randomized multicenter trial of the angiotensin-converting-enzyme inhibitor captopril to examine trends in aspirin use. The investigators presented data in Table 1 of their article about characteristics of patients in each of the six periods. This table is reproduced in Table 13–3. Tables like this one typically give information on the gender, age, previous medical history, and any important risk factors for subjects in the different groups. Lamas and his colleagues wanted to demonstrate that the six groups were similar on baseline characteristics; this was especially important because the six periods do not represent randomized groups of patients. Even with randomized studies, it is always a good idea to show that, in fact, the randomization worked and the groups were similar. Investigators often perform statistical tests to demonstrate the lack of significant difference on the baseline measures. If it turns out that the groups are not equivalent, it may be possible to make adjustments for any important differences by one of the covariance adjusting methods discussed in Chapter 10.

Second, readers should be alert for the problem of multiple comparisons in studies in which many statistical tests are performed. **Multiple comparisons** can occur because a group of subjects is measured at several points in time, for which repeated-measures analysis of variance should be used. They also occur when many study outcomes are of interest; investigators should use multivariate procedures in these situations. In addition, multiple comparisons result when investigators perform many subgroup comparisons, such as between men and women, among different age groups, or between groups defined by the absence or presence of a risk factor. Again, either multivariate methods or clearly stated a priori hypotheses are needed. If investigators find unexpected differences that were not part of the original hypotheses,

Table 13–3. Baseline characteristics of the study patients, according to 6-month enrollment period.[a]

Characteristic	1/87–6/87	7/87–12/87	1/88–6/88	7/88–12/88	1/89–6/89	7/89–1/90	P Value
Number enrolled in period	196	408	436	450	403	338	—
Mean age (yr)	57	59	59	59	60	60	0.058
Percentage of patients in group							
Male sex	85	81	86	84	81	79	0.092
Diabetes	23	26	18	22	21	22	0.086
Smoking	81	80	77	80	78	76	0.449
Angina	24	22	31	30	30	21	0.069
Hypertension	46	48	41	44	38	44	0.048
Previous MI	30	36	40	37	34	33	0.181
Previous CABG	10	9	13	13	14	9	0.104
Previous PTCA	4	2	3	4	4	6	0.129
Thrombolysis	25	27	28	34	40	40	<0.001

Abbreviations: MI = myocardial infarction; CABG = coronary-artery bypass grafting; PTCA = percutaneous transluminal coronary angioplasty.
[a]Values for thrombolysis refer to therapy for the index infarction. All the other data shown refer to characteristics before infarction. *P* values were obtained by a chi-square test for trend.
Source: Reproduced, with permission, from Table 1 in Lamas GA et al: Do the results of randomized clinical trials of cardiovascular drugs influence medical practice? *N Engl J Med* 1992;**327**:241–247.

these should be advanced as tentative conclusions only and should be the basis for further research.

Third, it is important to watch for inconsistencies between information presented in tables or graphs and information discussed in the text. Such inconsistencies may be the result of typographic errors, but sometimes they are signs that the authors have reanalyzed and rewritten the results or that the researchers were not very careful in their procedures. In any case, more than one inconsistency should alert us to watch for other problems in the study.

13.6 THE DISCUSSION & CONCLUSION SECTIONS OF A RESEARCH REPORT

The discussion and conclusion section(s) of a medical report may be one of the easier sections for clinicians to assess. The first and most important point to watch for is consistency among comments in the discussion, questions posed in the introduction, and data presented in the results. In addition, authors should address the consistency or lack of same between their findings and those of other published results. Careful readers will find that a surprisingly large number of published studies do not address the questions posed in their introduction. A good habit is to refer to the introduction and briefly review the purpose of the study just prior to reading the discussion and conclusion.

The second point to consider is whether the authors extrapolated beyond the data analyzed in the study. For example, are there recommendations concerning dosage levels not included in the study? Have conclusions been drawn that require a longer period of follow-up than that covered by the study? Have the results been generalized to groups of patients not represented by those included in the study?

Finally, note whether the investigators point out any shortcomings of the study, especially those that affect the conclusions drawn, and discuss research questions that have arisen from the study or that still remain unanswered. No one is in a better position to discuss these issues than the researchers who are intimately involved with the design and analysis of the study they have reported.

13.7 A CHECKLIST FOR READING THE LITERATURE

It is a rare article that meets all the criteria we have included in the following lists. Many articles do not even provide enough information to make a decision about some of the items in the checklist. Nevertheless, practitioners do not have time to read all the articles published, so they must make some choices about which ones are most important and best presented. Frequent readers of clinical trials may wish to consult two articles dealing specifically with published results of clinical trials (Pocock et al, 1987; Zelen, 1983); the companion to this book by Greenberg (1996) is recommended for suggestions in reading the epidemiologic literature. Greenhalgh (1997b) presents a collection of articles on various topics published in the *British Medical Journal,* and the *Journal of the American Medical Association* has published a series of excellent articles under the general title of "Users' Guides to the Medical Literature."

The following checklist is fairly exhaustive, and some readers may not want to use it unless they are reviewing an article for their own purposes or for a report. The items on the checklist are included in part as a reminder to the reader to look for these characteristics. Its primary purpose is to help clinicians decide whether a journal article is worth reading and, if so, what issues are important when deciding if the results are useful. The items in italics can often be found in a structured abstract. An asterisk (*) designates items that we believe are the most critical; these items are the ones readers should use when a less comprehensive checklist is desired.

13.7.1 Reading the Structured Abstract

*A. Is the topic of the study important and worth knowing about?

*B. What is the purpose of the study? Is the focus on a difference or a relationship? The purpose should be clearly stated; one should not have to guess.

C. What is the main outcome from the study? Does the outcome describe something measured on a numerical scale or something counted on a categorical scale? The outcome should be clearly stated.

D. Is the population of patients relevant to your practice—can you use these results in the care of your patients? The population in the study affects whether or not the results can be generalized.

*E. If statistically significant, do the results have clinical significance as well?

13.7.2 Reading the Introduction

If the article does not contain a structured abstract, the introduction section should include all of the above information plus the following information.

*A. What research has already been done on this topic and what outcomes were reported? The study should add new information.

13.7.3 Reading the Methods

*A. Is the appropriate study design used (clinical trial, cohort, case-control, cross-sectional, meta-analysis)?

B. Does the study cover an adequate period of time? Is the followup period long enough?

*C. Are the criteria for inclusion and exclusion of subjects clear? How do these criteria limit the applicability of the conclusions? The criteria also affect whether or not the results can be generalized.

D. Are standard measures used? Is a reference to any unusual measurement/procedure given if needed? Are the measures reliable/replicable?

E. What other outcomes (or dependent variables) and risk factors (or independent variables) are in the study? Are they clearly defined?

*F. Are statistical methods outlined? Are they appropriate? (The first question is easy to check; the second may be more difficult to answer.)

*G. Is there a statement about power—the number of patients that are needed to find the desired outcome? A statement about sample size is essential in a negative study.

H. In a clinical trial:
   1. How are subjects recruited?
   *2. Are subjects randomly assigned to the study groups? If not:
      a. How are patients selected for the study to avoid selection biases?
      b. If historical controls are used, are methods and criteria the same for the experimental group; are cases and controls compared on prognostic factors?
   *3. Is there a control group? If so, is it a good one?
   4. Are appropriate therapies included?
   5. Is the study blind? Double-blind? If not, should it be?
   6. How is compliance assured/evaluated?
   *7. If some cases are censored, is a survival method such as Kaplan-Meier or the Cox model used?

I. In a cohort study:
   *1. How are subjects recruited?
   2. Are subjects randomly selected from an eligible pool?
   *3. How rigorously are subjects followed? How many dropouts does the study have and who are they?
   *4. If some cases are censored, is a survival method such as Kaplan-Meier curves used?

J. In a case-control study:
   *1. Are subjects randomly selected from an eligible pool?
   2. Is the control group a good one (bias-free)?
   3. Are records reviewed independently by more than one person (thereby increasing the reliability of data)?

K. In a cross-sectional (survey, epidemiologic) study:
   1. Are the questions unbiased?
   *2. Are subjects randomly selected from an eligible pool?
   *3. What is the response rate?

L. In a meta-analysis:
   *1. How is the literature search conducted?
   2. Are the criteria for inclusion and exclusion of studies clearly stated?
   *3. Is an effort made to reduce publication bias (because negative studies are less likely to be published)?
   *4. Is there information on how many studies are needed to change the conclusion?

13.7.4 Reading the Results

*A. Do the reported findings answer the research questions?

*B. Are actual values reported—means, standard deviations, proportions—so that the magnitude of differences can be judged by the reader?

C. Are many *P* values reported, thus increasing the chance that some findings are bogus?

*D. Are groups similar on baseline measures? If not, how did investigators deal with these differences (confounding factors)?

E. Are the graphs and tables, and their legends, easy to read and understand?

*F. If the topic is a diagnostic procedure, is information on both sensitivity and specificity (false-positive rate) given? If predictive values are given, is the dependence on prevalence emphasized?

13.7.5 Reading the Conclusion and Discussion

*A. Are the research questions adequately discussed?

*B. Are the conclusions justified? Do the authors extrapolate more than they should, for example, beyond the length of time subjects were studied or to populations not included in the study?

C. Are the conclusions of the study discussed in the context of other relevant research?

D. Are shortcomings of the research addressed?

EXERCISES

For Questions 1–65, choose the single best answer.

1. Table 2 from Hodgson and Cutler (1997) is reproduced in Table 13–4. Which variable is most closely associated with anticipatory dementia?
   a. CES-D
   b. Psych symptoms
   c. Life satisfaction
   d. Health status

Questions 2–3

2. Henderson and colleagues (1997) studied a community sample of elderly subjects for a period of 3–4 years. One of their goals was to predict the level of depression, as measured by a depression score, at the end of the study period. Table 13–5 gives the list of measures used in their analysis. What type of statistical method was used to produce this information?
   a. Multiple regression
   b. Logistic regression
   c. Cox proportional hazard model
   d. Paired *t* tests
   e. Wilcoxon signed rank test

Table 13–4. Association between anticipatory dementia and well-being by sample group.

	Anticipatory Dementia	
	Adult Children (*n* = 25)	**Control** (*n* = 25)
CES-D		
r	0.352	0.266
P	0.085	0.200
Psych symptoms		
r	0.341	0.433
P	0.095	0.031
Life satisfaction		
r	−0.419	−0.283
P	0.037	0.171
Health status		
r	−0.173	−0.446
P	0.409	0.026

Abbreviation: CES-D = Center for Epidemiological Studies Depression Scale.
Source: Reproduced, with permission, from Hodgson LG, Cutler SJ: Anticipatory dementia and well-being. *Am J Alzheimer's Dis* 1997;**12**:62–66.

3. Which set of variables increased the prediction of depression score by the largest amount?
   a. Sociodemographic variables
   b. Age
   c. Psychologic health variables
   d. Physical health variables
   e. ADL at wave 2

4. Recall the analysis of mortality from selected diseases in England and Wales by Barker (1989) presented in Figure 3–9. The author stated that the trend in deaths from thyrotoxicosis rose to a peak in the 1930s and declined thereafter. Another graph from this investiga-tion is given in Figure 13–2. Based on this figure, which of the following statements is true?
   a. Iodine deficiency during childhood was not a problem among people born in Britain in the 1800s.
   b. Age-specific rates of thyrotoxicosis rose progressively beginning in 1836 and reached a peak in 1880.
   c. People who are iodine-deficient in youth are more able to adapt to increased iodine intake in later life.
   d. People exposed to increased levels of iodine during their adult years are more likely to develop thyrotoxicosis.

Questions 5–6: In a sample of 49 individuals, the mean total leukocyte count is found to be 7600 cells/mm^3, with a standard deviation of 1400 cells/mm^3.

5. If it is reasonable to assume that total leukocyte counts follow a normal distribution, then approximately 50% of the individuals will have a value

Table 13–5. Predictors of depression score at wave 2.

Predictor variable[a]	Beta[b]	P	R^2	R^2 change
Depression score, wave 1	0.231	0.000	0.182	0.182
Sociodemographic variables				
Age	−0.024	0.528	0.187	0.005
Sex	0.034	0.370		
Psychologic health variables				
Neuroticism, wave 1	0.077	0.056	0.237	0.050
Past history of depression or nervous breakdown, wave 2	0.136	0.000		
Physical health variables				
ADL, wave 1	−0.103	0.033	0.411	0.174
ADL, wave 2	0.283	0.012		
ADL squared, wave 2	−0.150	0.076		
Number current symptoms, wave 2	0.117	0.009		
Number medical conditions, wave 2	0.226	0.000		
Blood pressure: systolic, wave 2	−0.092	0.010		
Global health rating change between waves	0.079	0.028		
Sensory impairment change between waves	−0.064	0.073		
Social support/inactivity				
Social support—friends, wave 2	−0.095	0.015	0.442	0.031
Social support—social visits, wave 2	−0.087	0.032		
Activity level, wave 2	0.095	0.025		
Services (community residents only)				
Total services used, wave 2	0.135[c]	0.001[c]	0.438[c]	0.015[c]

[a]Only the variables shown were included in the final model.
[b]Standardized beta value, controlling for all other variables in the regression, except service use. Based on community and institutional residents.
[c]Regression limited to community sample only; coefficients for other variables vary only very slightly from those obtained with regression on the full sample.
Source: Reproduced, with permission, from Henderson AS et al: The course of depression in the elderly: A longitudinal community- based study in Australia. *Psychol Med* 1997;**27**:119–129.

    a. Between 6200 and 9000
    b. Between 7400 and 7800
    c. Below 6200 or above 9000
    d. Below 7600
    e. Above 9000
  6. Again assuming a normal distribution of total leukocyte counts, a randomly selected individual has a total leukocyte count lower than 4800 cells/mm^3
    a. 1% of the time
    b. 2.5% of the time
    c. 5% of the time
    d. 10% of the time
    e. 16.5% of the time
  7. If the correlation between two measures of functional status is 0.80, we can conclude that
    a. The value of one measure increases by 0.80 when the other measure increases by 1.

    b. 64% of the observations fall on the regression line.
    c. 80% of the observations fall on the regression line.
    d. 80% of the variation in one measure is accounted for by the other.
    e. 64% of the variation in one measure is accounted for by the other.

Questions 8–10: An evaluation of an antibiotic in the treatment of possible occult bacteremia was undertaken. Five hundred children with fever but no focal infection were randomly assigned to the antibiotic or to a placebo. A blood sample for culture was obtained prior to beginning therapy, and all patients were reevaluated after 48 hours.
  8. The design used in this study is best described as a
    a. Randomized clinical trial

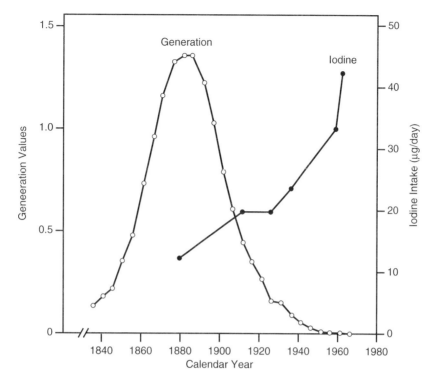

Figure 13–2. Relative mortality from thyrotoxicosis in successive generations of women in England and Wales according to year of birth, together with estimated per capita daily iodine intake from milk, meat, and fish. (Reproduced, with permission, from Figure 2 in Barker DJP: Rise and fall of Western diseases. *Nature* 1989;**338**:371–372.)

    b. Placebo-controlled trial
    c. Controlled clinical trial
    d. Cohort study
    e. Crossover study
9. The authors reported the proportion of children with major infectious morbidity among those with bacteremia was 13% in the placebo group and 10% in the antibiotic group. The 95% confidence interval for the difference in proportions was −2.6% to +8.6%. Thus, the most important conclusion is that
    a. The difference in major infectious morbidity between placebo and antibiotic is statistically significant.
    b. The proportion of children with major infectious morbidity is the same with placebo and antibiotic.
    c. No statistically significant difference exists in the proportions that received placebo and antibiotic.
    d. The study has low power to detect a difference owing to the small sample size, and no conclusions should be drawn until a larger study is done.
    e. Using a chi-square test to determine significance is preferable to determining a confidence interval for the difference.

10. What is the approximate number needed to treat to prevent one patient from developing occult bacteremia?
    a. 15
    b. 6.7 or 7
    c. 65
    d. 3
    e. 33.3 or 33

    Questions 11–12: A study of fluctuation in body weight and health outcomes using data on participants in the Framingham study was undertaken (Lissner et al, 1991). The investigators used body mass index (BMI) values (weight in kilograms divided by height squared in meters) from the first eight biennial examinations during the study plus the subject's recalled weight at age 25 to determine three measures for each subject: mean BMI, linear trend of BMI, and coefficient of variation. Refer to Figure 13–3 for a schematic drawing of these variables.
11. Using the terminology in Figure 13–3, the coefficient of determination is best described as
    a. The level minus the deviation
    b. The level divided by the deviation
    c. The deviation divided by the level
    d. The slope divided by the deviation
    e. The slope minus the level

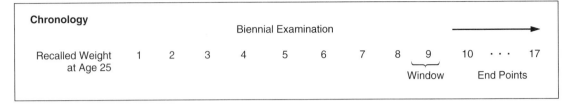

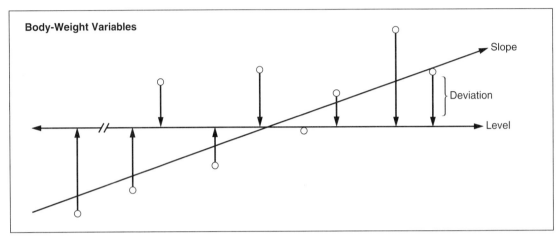

Figure 13–3. Chronology and schematic representation of body weight variables for a hypothetical subject. The chronology illustrates the timing of measurements of body weight (made at intervals of 2 years as part of the Framingham study) in relation to the occurrence of end points, with a 4-year interval (window) required between the measurement of weight at the eighth examination and the first end point included in the analysis. Weight was converted to body mass index (BMI), defined as the weight in kilograms divided by the square of the height in meters, which was used to calculate three key independent variables: a subject's mean BMI (level), the linear trend in BMI over time (slope), and the BMI's degree of variability from the mean (coefficient of variation). Determinations of the BMI are indicated by circles and arrows. (Reproduced, with permission, from Figure 1 in Lissner L et al: Variability of body weight and health outcomes in the Framingham population. *N Engl J Med* 1991;**324**:1839–1844.)

12. The statistical method most likely used to determine the slope was
    a. Correlation
    b. Simple linear regression
    c. Multiple regression
    d. Logistic regression
    e. Polynomial regression

Questions 13–16: Table 13–6 gives some of the results from the same study of fluctuation in body weight (Lissner et al, 1991). This table presents the regression coefficients and *P* values for level, slope, and coefficient of variation (CV) of BMI in predicting total mortality, morbidity and mortality from coronary heart disease, and morbidity from cancer for men and women separately.

13. The dependent variable best predicted for men was
    a. Total mortality
    b. Morbidity due to coronary heart disease (CHD)
    c. Mortality from CHD

    d. Morbidity due to cancer
    e. Impossible to determine

14. The measure of BMI most important in predicting outcomes for women was
    a. Level of BMI
    b. Slope of BMI
    c. CV of BMI
    d. Impossible to determine

15. The BMI variable with the widest 95% confidence interval is
    a. Level of BMI for morbidity due to CHD in men
    b. Slope of BMI for predicting total mortality in women
    c. CV of BMI for predicting morbidity due to cancer in women
    d. CV of BMI for predicting total mortality in men
    e. Impossible to determine

16. The legend to Table 13–6 says that these results are for a model that included five risk factors in addition to age and the three BMI variables. The main purpose for using this model is to

Table 13–6. Partial regression coefficients (β) and significance levels of selected independent variables, according to multivariate analysis in model C.[a]

Outcome	Level of BMI[b]		Slope of BMI		CV of BMI[c]	
	β	P value	β	P value	β	P value
Men						
Total mortality	+0.024	0.16	−2.52	0.0001	+9.24	0.0001
Morbidity due to CHD	+0.042	0.04	−2.24	0.0010	+10.89	0.0001
Mortality from CHD	+0.037	0.17	−3.16	0.0002	+12.42	0.0003
Morbidity due to cancer	+0.015	0.50	−1.46	0.0800	+5.42	0.0900
Women						
Total mortality	+0.024	0.09	−1.60	0.0002	+3.64	0.04
Morbidity due to CHD	+0.047	0.02	−1.13	0.0800	+4.92	0.07
Mortality from CHD	+0.057	0.01	−2.62	0.0004	+6.77	0.02
Morbidity due to cancer	+0.010	0.60	+0.14	0.8000	+0.67	0.80

[a]Model C included five risk factors for cardiovascular disease (smoking, serum cholesterol level, systolic blood pressure, glucose tolerance, and level of physical activity) in addition to age, level of the body mass index (BMI, the weight in kilograms divided by the square of the height in meters), slope of the BMI (defined as the change in the BMI per year from 25 years of age to the eighth examination), and the coefficient of variation (CV) of the BMI. CHD denotes coronary heart disease.
[b]Calculated as a mean value for each subject.
[c]Defined as the standard deviation of the BMI divided by the mean BMI.
Source: Reproduced, with permission, from Table 2 in Lissner L et al: Variability of body weight and health outcomes in the Framingham population. *N Engl J Med* 1991;**324**:1839–1844.

a. Include all relevant risk factors
b. Determine the effect of BMI variables controlling for risk factors
c. Determine if differences exist between men and women once risk factors are included
d. Determine if the risk factors are important

17. Table 1 from the study of glucose tolerance and insulin sensitivity in normal and overweight hyperthyroid women is reproduced below in Table 13–7 (Gonzalo et al, 1996). Which statistical procedure is best if the authors wanted to compare the baseline glucose (mmol/L) in the women to see if weight or thyroid level have an effect?
a. Correlation
b. Independent-groups *t* test
c. Paired *t* test
d. One-way ANOVA
e. Two-way ANOVA

18. If the relationship between two measures is linear and the coefficient of determination has a value near 1, a scatterplot of the observations
a. Is a horizontal straight line
b. Is a vertical straight line
c. Is a straight line that is neither horizontal nor vertical
d. Is a random scatter of points about the regression line
e. Has a positive slope

Questions 19–22: A study was undertaken to evaluate the use of computed tomography (CT) in the diagnosis of lumbar disk herniation. Eighty patients with lumbar disk herniation confirmed by surgery were evaluated with CT, as were 50 patients without herniation. The CT results were positive in 56 of the patients with herniation and in 10 of the patients without herniation.

Table 13–7. Clinical and metabolic details.[a,b]

Subjects	Age (years)	BMI (kg/m²)	Basal glucose (mmol/L)	Basal insulin (pmol/L)	KG (%/min)
NW-HT (*n* = 8)	39.4 ± 5.0 (20–62)	23.5 ± 0.6 (21.4 –25)	4.99 ± 0.26	84.8 ± 13.6	2.45 ± 0.41
OW-HT (*n* = 6)	42.7 ± 5.7 (23–60)	28.0 ± 0.7 (26–31.4)	5.05 ± 0.11	134 ± 23.6	1.84 ± 0.20
Total-HT (*n* = 14)	40.8 ± 3.7 (20–62)	25.4 ± 0.8 (21.4 –31.4)	5.02 ± 0.15	105.9 ± 13.9	2.19 ± 0.26
NW-C (*n* = 11)	42.8 ± 5.0 (22–66)	21.3 ± 0.9 (18–24)	4.81 ± 0.11	79.6 ± 7.0	2.35 ± 0.13
OW-C (*n* = 8)	45.0 ± 4.7 (26–62)	29.0 ± 0.8 (25.5–31.6)	5.0 ± 0.22	112.5 ± 20.5	2.65 ± 0.35
Total-C (*n* = 19)	43.7 ± 3.4 (22–66)	24.5 ± 1.0 (18–31.6)	4.89 ± 0.11	15.5 ± 1.6	2.47 ± 0.16

Abbreviations: BMI = body mass index; NW = normal weight; OW = overweight; HT = hyperthyroid patients; C = control subjects.
[a]Numbers in parentheses are range values.
[b]Data presented as mean plus or minus the standard error of the mean.
Source: Reproduced, with permission, from Table 1 in Gonzalo MA et al: Glucose tolerance, insulin secretion, insulin sensitivity and glucose effectiveness in normal and overweight hyperthyroid women. *Clin Endocrinol* 1996;**45**:689–697.

19. The sensitivity of CT for lumbar disk herniation in this study is
    a. 10/50, or 20%
    b. 24/80, or 30%
    c. 56/80, or 70%
    d. 40/50, or 80%
    e. 56/66, or 85%
20. The false-positive rate in this study is
    a. 10/50, or 20%
    b. 24/80, or 30%
    c. 56/80, or 70%
    d. 40/50, or 80%
    e. 56/66, or 85%
21. Computed tomography is used in a patient who has a 50–50 chance of having a herniated lumbar disk, according to the patient's history and physical examination. What are the chances of herniation if the CT is positive?
    a. 35/100, or 35%
    b. 50/100, or 50%
    c. 35/50, or 70%
    d. 40/55, or 73%
    e. 35/45, or 78%
22. The likelihood ratio is
    a. 0.28
    b. 0.875
    c. 1.0
    d. 3.5
    e. 7.0
23. In a placebo-controlled trial of the use of oral aspirin–dipyridamole to prevent arterial restenosis after coronary angioplasty, 38% of patients receiving the drug had restenosis, and 39% of patients receiving placebo had restenosis. In reporting this finding, the authors stated that $P > 0.05$, which means that
    a. Chances are greater than 1 in 20 that a difference would again be found if the study were repeated.
    b. The probability is less than 1 in 20 that a difference this large could occur by chance alone.
    c. The probability is greater than 1 in 20 that a difference this large could occur by chance alone.
    d. Treated patients were 5% less likely to have restenosis.
    e. The chance is 95% that the study is correct.
24. A study of the relationship between the concentration of lead in the blood and hemoglobin resulted in the following prediction equation: $Y = 15 - 0.1(X)$, where Y is the predicted hemoglobin and X is the concentration of lead in the blood. From the equation, the predicted hemoglobin for a person with blood lead concentration of 20 mg/dL is
    a. 13
    b. 14.8
    c. 14.9

d. 15
e. 20

Questions 25–26
25. D'Angio and colleagues (1995) studied a group of extremely premature infants to learn whether they have immunologic responses to tetanus toxoid and polio vaccines that are similar to the response of full-term infants. Figure 1 from their study contains the plots of the antitetanus titers before and after the vaccine was given (reproduced in Figure 13–4). The authors calculated the geometric means. Which statistical test is best to learn if the titer level increases in the preterm group after they were given the vaccine?
    a. One-group t test
    b. Paired t test
    c. Wilcoxon signed rank test
    d. Two independent-groups t test
    e. Wilcoxon rank sum test
26. Based on Figure 13–4, which is the appropriate conclusion?
    a. No difference exists between preterm and full-term infants before and after the vaccine.
    b. No difference exists between preterm and full-term infants before the vaccine, but a difference does occur after the vaccine.
    c. A difference exists between preterm and full-term infants before and after the vaccine.
    d. A difference exists between preterm and full-term infants before the vaccine but not after.

Questions 27–28: Figure 13–5 summarizes the gender-specific distribution of values on a laboratory test.
27. From Figure 13–5, we can conclude that
    a. Values on the laboratory test are lower in men than in women.
    b. The distribution of laboratory values in women is bimodal.
    c. Laboratory values were reported more often for women than for men in this study.
    d. Half of the men have laboratory values between 30 and 43.
    e. The standard deviation of laboratory values is equal in men and women.
28. The most appropriate statistical test to compare the distribution of laboratory values in men with that in women is
    a. Chi-square
    b. Paired t test
    c. Independent-groups t test
    d. Correlation
    e. Regression
29. A study was undertaken to evaluate any increased risk of breast cancer among women who use birth control pills. The relative risk was calculated. A type I error in this study consists of concluding

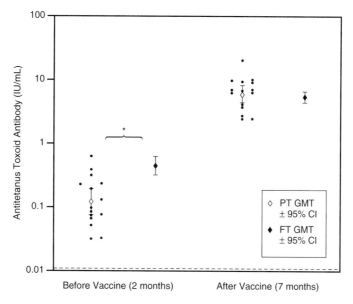

Figure 13–4. Antitetanus toxoid antibody levels. *Abbreviations:* PT = preterm; FT = full term; GMT = geometric mean titer. * indicates $P < 0.001$. (Reproduced, with permission, from Figure 1 in D'Angio CT et al: Immunologic response of extremely premature infants to tetanus, *Haemophilus influenzae,* and polio immunizations. *Pediatrics* 1995;**96**:18–22.)

a. A significant increase in the relative risk when the relative risk is actually 1
b. A significant increase in the relative risk when the relative risk is actually greater than 1
c. A significant increase in the relative risk when the relative risk is actually less than 1
d. No significant increase in the relative risk when the relative risk is actually 1
e. No significant increase in the relative risk when the relative risk is actually greater than 1

Questions 30–31

30. A graph of the lowest oxyhemoglobin percentage in the patients studied overnight in the study

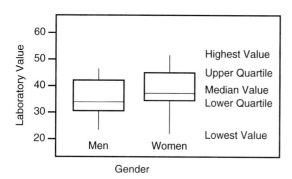

Figure 13–5. Gender-specific distributions of values on a laboratory test.

by Good and colleagues (1996) is given in Figure 1 from their article (see Figure 13–6). What is the best way to describe the distribution of these values?
a. Normal distribution
b. Chi-square distribution
c. Binomial distribution
d. Negatively skewed distribution
e. Positively skewed distribution

31. If the investigators wanted to compare oxyhemoglobin levels in patients who died within 12 months with the levels of oxyhemoglobin percentage in patients who survived, what method should they use?
a. *t* test for two independent groups
b. Wilcoxon rank sum test
c. Analysis of variance
d. Chi-square test
e. Kaplan–Meier curves

32. The scale used in measuring cholesterol is
a. Nominal
b. Ordinal
c. Interval
d. Discrete
e. Qualitative

33. The scale used in measuring presence or absence of a risk factor is
a. Binary
b. Ordinal
c. Interval
d. Continuous
e. Quantitative

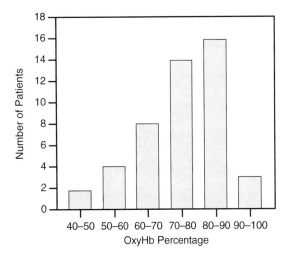

Figure 13–6. Distribution of lowest oxyhemoglobin (OxyHb) values for each patient during overnight oximetry. (Reproduced, with permission, from Figure 1 in Good DC et al: Sleep-disordered breathing and poor functional outcome after stroke. *Stroke* 1996;**27**:252–259.)

34. Which of the following sources is most likely to provide an accurate estimate of the prevalence of multiple sclerosis (MS) in a community?
  a. A survey of practicing physicians asking how many MS patients they are currently treating
  b. Information from hospital discharge summaries
  c. Data from autopsy reports
  d. A telephone survey of a sample of randomly selected homes in the community asking how many people living in the home have the disease
  e. Examination of the medical records of a representative sample of people living in the community

Questions 35–36: In an epidemiologic study of carbon-black workers, 500 workers with respiratory disease and 200 workers without respiratory disease were selected for study. The investigators obtained a history of exposure to carbon-black dust in both groups of workers. Among workers with respiratory disease, 250 gave a history of exposure to carbon-black dust; among the 200 workers without respiratory disease, 50 gave a history of exposure.

35. The odds ratio is
  a. 1.0
  b. 1.5
  c. 2.0
  d. 3.0
  e. Cannot be determined from the preceding information

36. This study is best described as a
  a. Case–control study
  b. Cohort study
  c. Cross-sectional study
  d. Controlled experiment
  e. Randomized clinical trial

37. A physician wishes to study whether a particular risk factor is associated with some disease. If, in reality, the presence of the risk factor leads to a relative risk of disease of 4.0, the physician wants to have a 95% chance of detecting an effect this large in the planned study. This statement is an illustration of specifying
  a. A null hypothesis
  b. A type I, or alpha, error
  c. A type II, or beta, error
  d. Statistical power
  e. An odds ratio

38. The most likely explanation for a lower crude annual mortality rate in a developing country than in a developed country is that the developing country has
  a. An incomplete record of deaths
  b. A younger age distribution
  c. An inaccurate census of the population
  d. A less stressful life-style
  e. Lower exposure to environmental hazards

Questions 39–40

39. The distribution of variation in heart rate to deep breathing and the Valsalva ratio from the study by Gelber and colleagues (1997) is given in Figure 1 in their article and is reproduced below in Figure 13–7. What is the best way to describe the distribution of these values?
  a. Normal distribution
  b. Chi-square distribution
  c. Binomial distribution
  d. Negatively skewed distribution
  e. Positively skewed distribution

40. What is the best method to find the normal range of values for the Valsalva ratio?
  a. The values determined by the mean ± 2 standard deviations
  b. The values determined by the mean ± 2 standard errors
  c. The values determined by the upper and lower 5% of the distribution
  d. The values determined by the upper and lower 2½% of the distribution
  e. The highest and lowest values defined by the whiskers on a box plot

41. A study of the exercise tolerance test for detecting coronary heart disease had the characteristics shown in Table 13–8. The authors concluded the exercise stress test has positive predictive value in excess of 75%. The error in this conclusion is that

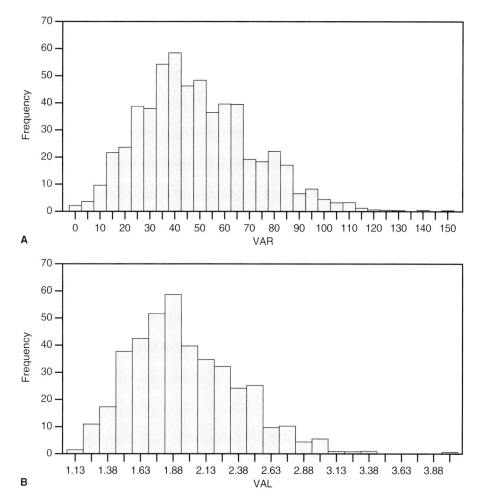

Figure 13–7. A: Distribution of normative values for heart rate variation to deep breathing (VAR) and **B:** Valsalva ratio (VAL) for the entire study population. (Reproduced, with permission, from Figure 1 in Gelber DA et al: Cardiovascular autonomic nervous system tests: Determination of normative values and effect of confounding variables. *J Auton Nerv Syst* 1997;**62**:40–44.)

a. Not enough patients are included in the study for precise estimates.
b. The sample sizes should be equal in these kinds of studies.
c. The positive predictive value is really 80%.
d. The prevalence of coronary heart disease (CHD) is assumed to be 33%.
e. No gold standard exists for D.

Table 13–8. Results of test.

	CHD Present	**CHD Absent**
Positive test	80	50
Negative test	20	150

Abbreviation: CHD = coronary heart disease.

Questions 42–44
42. Hébert and colleagues (1997) studied functional decline in a very elderly population of community-dwelling subjects. They used the Functional Autonomy Measurement System (SMAF) questionnaire to measure several indices of functioning. Figure 2 from their article displays box plots of scores for men and women at baseline and is reproduced in Figure 13–8. Based on the plots, men and women had the most similar scores on which measure?
a. ADL (adult daily living)
b. Mobility
c. Communication
d. Mental
e. IADL (instrumental activities of daily living)
f. Total score

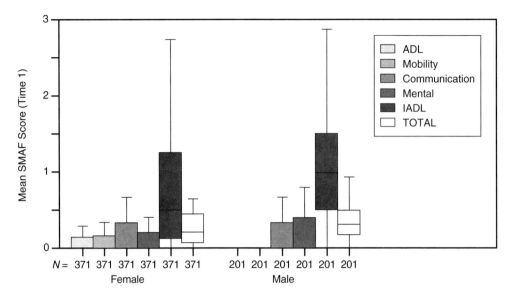

Figure 13–8. Box plots of the mean SMAF score and subscores at baseline (T1) according to sex, among a representative sample of elderly people living at home in Sherbrooke, Canada, 1991–1993. *Abbreviations:* SMAF = Functional Autonomy Measurement System; ADL = activities of daily living; IADL = instrumental activities of daily living. (Reproduced, with permission, from Figure 2 in Hébert R et al: Incidence of functional decline and improvement in a community-dwelling very elderly population. *Am J Epidemiol* 1997;**145**:935–944.)

g. Impossible to tell

43. Among men, which measure has the most symmetric distribution?

a. ADL (adult daily living)
b. Mobility
c. Communication
d. Mental
e. IADL (instrumental activities of daily living)
f. Total score
g. Impossible to tell

44. What is the median mental score for women?

a. 0
b. 0.15
c. 0.3
d. 0.7
e. Impossible to tell

Questions 45–46: Several studies have shown that men with a low blood cholesterol level as well as those with high levels have an increased risk of early death. A report in the March 21, 1993, *New York Times* described a study by Dr Carlos Iribarren at the University of Southern California on a cohort of 8000 Japanese-American men followed for 23 years. The purpose was to study further the link between low blood cholesterol levels and higher death rate. The men were divided into four groups: healthy men, men with chronic disorders of the stomach or liver, heavy smokers, and heavy drinkers. Within each group, subjects were stratified according to their cholesterol level. Among men with cholesterol levels below 189 mg/dL, death rates were higher in the chronic illness, heavy smoker, and heavy drinker groups but not in the group of healthy men.

45. This study highlights a potential threat that may have occurred in previous studies that suggested that low cholesterol is linked to higher death rates. The most likely threat in the previous studies is

a. Selection bias
b. Length of follow-up
c. A confounding variable
d. Inappropriate sample size

46. Using the guidelines in Table 10–2, select the most appropriate statistical method to analyze the data collected in this study.

a. Mantel–Haenszel chi-square
b. ANOVA
c. Multiple regression
d. Log-linear methods

Questions 47–48

47. Figure 2 in Dennison and colleagues (1997) shows the relationship between the age of children and daily consumption of fruit juice (see Figure 13–9). What is the best method to learn if a difference exists between 2-year-old and 5-year-old children?

Short Children Versus Juice Consumption

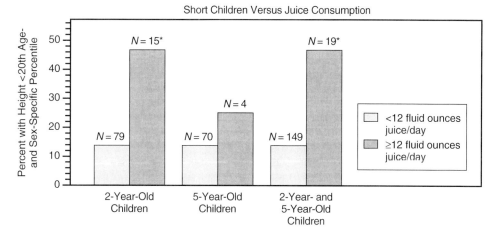

Figure 13-9. The prevalence of children with decreased stature (height less than 20th age- and sex-specific percentile) between children drinking less than 12 fl oz/day of fruit juice and children drinking ≥ 12 fl oz/day of fruit juice. * indicates Fisher's exact test *P* < 0.01. (Reproduced, with permission, from Figure 2 in Dennison BA et al: Excess fruit juice consumption by preschool-aged children is associated with short stature and obesity. *Pediatrics* 1997;**99**:15–22.)

a. Chi-square test
b. Fisher's exact test
c. Fisher's *z* distribution
d. Paired *t* test
e. Pearson correlation

48. What is the best way to describe the magnitude of the relationship between the age of children and daily consumption of fruit juice?
a. Kappa
b. Odds ratio
c. Pearson correlation
d. Spearman correlation
e. r^2

49. Birth weights of a population of infants at 40 weeks gestational age are approximately normally distributed, with a mean of 3000 g. Roughly 68% of such infants weigh between 2500 and 3500 g at birth. If a sample of 100 infants were studied, the standard error would be
a. 50
b. 100
c. 250
d. 500
e. None of the above

50. A significant positive correlation has been observed between alcohol consumption and the level of systolic blood pressure in men. From this correlation, we may conclude that
a. No association exists between alcohol consumption and systolic pressure.
b. Men who consume less alcohol are at lower risk for increased systolic pressure.
c. Men who consume less alcohol are at higher risk for increased systolic pressure.

d. High alcohol consumption can cause increased systolic pressure.
e. Low alcohol consumption can cause increased systolic pressure.

51. In a randomized trial of patients who received a cadaver renal transplant, 100 were treated with cyclosporin and 50 were treated with conventional immunosuppression therapy. The difference in treatments was not statistically significant at the 5% level. Therefore
a. This study has proven that cyclosporin is not effective.
b. Cyclosporin could be significant at the 1% level.
c. Cyclosporin could be significant at the 10% level.
d. The groups have been shown to be the same.
e. The treatments should not be compared because of the differences in the sample sizes.

52. The statistical method used to develop guidelines for diagnostic-related groups (DRGs) was
a. Survival analysis
b. *t* tests for independent groups
c. Multiple regression
d. Analysis of covariance
e. Correlation

53. Suppose the confidence limits for the mean of a variable are 8.55 and 8.65. These limits are
a. Less precise but have a higher confidence than 8.20 and 9.00
b. More precise but have a lower confidence than 8.20 and 9.00
c. Less precise but have a lower confidence than 8.20 and 9.00

d. More precise but have a higher confidence than 8.20 and 9.00

e. Indeterminate because the level of confidence is not specified

54. A senior medical student wants to plan her elective schedule. The probability of getting an elective in endocrinology is 0.8, and the probability of getting an elective in sports medicine is 0.5. The probability of getting both electives in the same semester is 0.4. What is the probability of getting into endocrinology or sports medicine or both?

   a. 0.4
   b. 0.5
   c. 0.8
   d. 0.9
   e. 1.7

55. A manager of a multispecialty clinic wants to determine the proportion of patients who are referred by their primary care physician to another physician within the group versus a physician outside the group. Every 100th patient chart is selected and reviewed for a letter from a physician other than the primary care physician. This procedure is best described as

   a. Random sampling
   b. Stratified sampling
   c. Quota sampling
   d. Representative sampling
   e. Systematic sampling

56. The probability is 0.6 that a medical student will receive his first choice of residency programs. Four senior medical students want to know the probability that they all will obtain their first choice. The solution to this problem is best found by using

   a. The binomial distribution
   b. The normal distribution
   c. The chi-square distribution
   d. The z test
   e. Correlation

57. The graph in Figure 13–10 gives the 5-year survival rates for patients with cancer at various sites. From this figure, we can conclude

   a. That breast and uterine corpus cancer are increasing at higher rates than other cancers
   b. That lung cancer is the slowest growing cancer
   c. That few patients are diagnosed with distant metastases
   d. That survival rates for patients with regional involvement are similar, regardless of the primary site of disease
   e. None of the above

Questions 58–59

58. Table 3 from Shlipak and colleagues (1999) provides diagnostic test characteristics of electro-

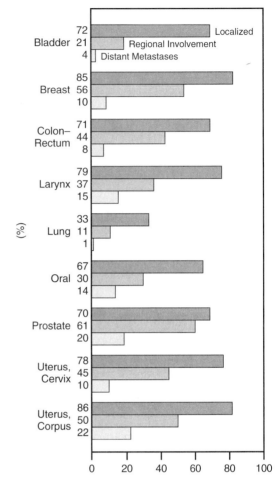

Figure 13–10. Five-year survival rates for patients with cancer. (Adapted and reproduced, with permission, from Rubin P [editor]: *Clinical Oncology: A Multidisciplinary Approach,* 6th ed. American Cancer Society, 1983.)

cardiographic criteria for determining myocardial infarction (MI) (see Table 13–9). Which of the following five features is the best single feature for ruling in MI?

   a. ST elevation ≥ 5 mm
   b. Overall ECG algorithm
   c. QRS notching
   d. RS complex in lead V_8
   e. Sign of Cabrera

59. Which of the following five features is the best single feature for ruling out MI?

   a. ST elevation ≥ 5 mm
   b. Overall ECG algorithm
   c. QRS notching
   d. RS complex in lead V_8
   e. Sign of Cabrera

Table 13–9. Diagnostic test characteristics of electrocardiographic criteria for acute myocardial infarction.[a]

ECG Characteristic	Sensitivity, % (95% CI)	Specificity, % (95% CI)	Positive Predictive Value (95% CI)	Negative Predictive Value (95% CI)
ST elevation ≥1 mm in concordant leads[b]	7 (1–21)	100 (95–100)	100 (16–100)	71 (61–80)
ST depression ≥1 mm in leads V_1, V_2, or V_3[b]	3 (0–17)	100 (95–100)	100 (2–100)	71 (61–79)
ST elevation ≥5 mm in discordant leads[b]	19 (7–37)	82 (71–90)	32 (13–57)	70 (59–80)
Overall ECG algorithm	10 (2–26)	100 (96–100)	100 (29–100)	72 (62–81)
QRS notching	39 (22–58)	57 (45–59)	28 (15–44)	68 (55–80)
RS complex in lead V_6	26 (12–45)	79 (68–88)	35 (16–57)	71 (60–81)
Sign of Cabrera	7 (1–21)	86 (76–93)	17 (2–48)	68 (58–78)
ST elevation ≥7 mm in discordant lead, or ≥2 mm depression in concordant lead	3 (0–17)	99 (93–100)	50 (1–100)	70 (60–79)
Positive T waves in lead with upright QRS complex	3 (0–17)	93 (85–98)	17 (0–64)	69 (59–78)
Sign of Chapman	3 (0–17)	92 (83–97)	14 (3–58)	68 (58–78)

Abbreviations: ECG = electrocardiogram; CI = confidence interval.
[a]Applies to patients with acute cardiopulmonary symptoms and left bundle-branch block among 31 patient presentations with myocardial infarction and 72 without.
[b]Criteria used in algorithm of Sgarbossa et al.
Source: Reproduced, with permission, from Table 3 from Shlipak MG et al: Should the electrocardiogram be used to guide therapy for patients with left bundle-branch block and suspected myocardial infarction? *JAMA* 1999;**281:**714–719.

60. A study was undertaken to compare treatment options in black and white patients who are diagnosed as having breast cancer. The 95% confidence interval for the odds ratio for blacks being more likely to be untreated than whites was 1.1 to 2.5. The statement that most accurately describes the meaning of these limits is that
 a. Ninety-five percent of the odds ratios fall within these limits.
 b. Black women are up to 2.5 times more likely than whites to be untreated.
 c. Ninety-five percent of the time blacks are more likely than whites to be untreated.
 d. Blacks are 95 times more likely than whites to receive no treatment for breast cancer.
 e. No difference exists in the treatment of black and white women.

Questions 61–63
61. In the study to identify risk factors for discontinuing dialysis, Bajwa and colleagues (1996) presented information on the sociodemographic characteristics of patients in the study (see Table 2 from Bajwa reproduced in Table 13–10). Which of these characteristics has the greatest statistical significance in identifying those who stopped versus those who continued on dialysis?
 a. Sex
 b. Age
 c. Marital status

 d. Treatment
 e. Education
62. What statistical technique can the investigators use to control for differences in any of the sociodemographic characteristics in the two groups that might confound the statistical analysis of mortality?
 a. Paired *t* test
 b. Analysis of variance
 c. Chi-square
 d. Regression
 e. Logistic regression
63. The results of the multivariate analysis to predict stopping dialysis from the study by Bajwa and colleagues (1996) is given in Table 13–11. All of the independent variables were coded as yes or no. The regression coefficient for severe pain is −1.20 and for comorbidity is 0.79. Why is the *P* value for comorbidity lower than the *P* value for severe pain?
 a. The standard error for comorbidity is smaller.
 b. The relationship between stopping dialysis and comorbidity is positive.
 c. The relative risk associated with comorbidity is higher.
 d. Comorbidity is a more objective measure.

Questions 64–65: Physicians wish to determine whether the emergency department (ED) at the local

Table 13–10. Sociodemographic data on all patients.[a]

Data	Stopped Dialysis	Other	P
Sex, F/M	7/6	86/136	0.43
Mean±SD age (years)	66 ± 10	54 ± 17	0.01
Race			
White	10	148	
Native American	1	21	0.76
Other	2	53	
Marital status			
Married or single	7	184	
Divorced or widowed	6	36	0.02
Treatment group			
CAPD	6	87	
ICD	7	135	0.77
Education			
Did not complete high school	5	76	
Completed high school	8	146	0.99
Lodging			
Nursing home	4	13	
Other	9	209	0.007
Location			
City	12	157	
Other	1	63	0.19
Income ($)			
≤10,000	3	55	
≥10,000	7	126	0.99
Occupation			
Work	1	65	
None	12	156	0.06
Outdoor activities			
Outdoor	3	117	
None	10	104	0.03
Church			
Religion	8	84	
None	5	137	0.10
Clubs			
Belongs	3	34	
None	10	187	0.48
Hobbies			
Hobbies	7	147	
None	6	74	0.53

Abbreviations: CAPD = continuous ambulatory peritoneal dialysis; ICD = in-center hemodialysis.
[a]Unless otherwise indicated, data are given as number of patients.
Source: Reproduced, with permission, from Table 2 from Bajwa K et al: A prospective study of risk factors and decision making in discontinuation of dialysis. *Arch Intern Med* 1996; **156:**2571–2577.

hospital is being overused by patients with minor health problems. A random sample of 5000 patients was selected and categorized by age and degree of severity of the problem that brought them to the ED; severity was measured on a scale of 1 to 3, with 3 being most severe; the results are given in Table 13–12.

64. The joint probability that a 3-year-old patient with a problem of high severity is selected for review is
　　a. 200/5000 = 0.04
　　b. 200/1600 = 0.125
　　c. 1600/5000 = 0.32
　　d. 1100/5000 = 0.22
　　e. 1600/5000 + 1100/5000 = 0.54

65. If a patient comes to the ED with a problem of low severity, how likely is it that the patient is older than 14 years of age?
　　a. 1700/5000 2200/5000 = 0.15
　　b. 600/2200 = 0.27
　　c. 1700/5000 = 0.34
　　d. 600/1700 = 0.35
　　e. 2200/5000 = 0.44

Questions 66–70: These questions constitute a set of extended matching items. For each of the situations outlined here, select the most appropriate statistical method to use in analyzing the data from the choices a–i that follow. Each choice may be used more than once.
　　a. Independent-groups *t* test
　　b. Chi-square test
　　c. Wilcoxon rank sum test
　　d. Pearson correlation
　　e. Analysis of variance
　　f. Mantel–Haenszel chi-square
　　g. Multiple regression
　　h. Paired *t* test
　　i. Odds ratio

66. Investigating average body weight before and after a supervised exercise program

67. Investigating gender of the head of household in families of patients whose medical costs are covered by insurance, Medicaid, or self

68. Investigating a possible association between exposure to an environmental pollutant and miscarriage

69. Investigating blood cholesterol levels in patients who follow a diet either low or moderate in fat

Table 13–11. Result of multivariate analysis.

Variable	Regression Coefficient	SE	P	R	Relative Risk
No severe pain	−1.1975	0.4881	0.01	−0.2007	0.3020
Living with partner	−0.6614	0.3087	0.03	−0.1612	0.5161
Comorbidity	0.7856	0.2673	0.003	0.2580	2.1937

Source: Reproduced, with permission, from Table 5 in Bajwa K et al: A prospective study of risk factors and decision making in discontinuation of dialysis. *Arch Intern Med* 1996;**156:**2571–2577.

Table 13–12. Patients seen in emergency department.

Age (years)	Severity of Problem			Total
	Low	Medium	High	
<5	1100	300	200	1600
5–14	500	900	300	1700
>14	600	500	600	1700
Total	2200	1700	1100	5000

Table 13–13. Logistic-regression model to predict aspirin therapy before infarction.

Variable	Odds Ratio (95% CI)
PTCA before MI	2.66 (1.57–4.51)
Catheterization before MI	2.22 (1.59–3.10)
Previous MI	1.95 (1.49–2.54)
CABG before MI	1.80 (1.27–2.55)
White race	1.47 (0.97–2.23)
Randomization after 1/28/88	1.43 (1.11–1.85)
Angina before MI	1.22 (0.94–1.60)
Hypertension	1.19 (0.95–1.50)
Male sex	1.19 (0.86–1.64)
Married status	1.03 (0.79–1.35)
Age	1.02 (1.01–1.04)
Education after high school	0.97 (0.77–1.22)
Orthopedic disease	0.97 (0.55–1.69)
Type of hospital (academic vs community)	0.92 (0.71–1.18)
Diabetes	0.83 (0.62–1.08)

Abbreviations: CI = confidence interval; PTCA = percutaneous transluminal coronary angioplasty; MI = myocardial infarction; CABG = coronary-artery bypass grafting.
Source: Adapted and used, with permission, from Table 2 in Lamas GA et al: Do the results of randomized clinical trials of cardiovascular drugs influence medical practice? *N Engl J Med* 1992;**327**:241–247.

and who take either a drug to lower cholesterol or a placebo
70. Investigating physical functioning in patients with diabetes on the basis of demographic characteristics and level of diabetic control

Questions 71–75: These questions constitute a set of multiple true–false items. For each of the statements, determine whether the statement is true or false.

Table 13–13 contains the variables used by Lamas and colleagues (1992) to predict aspirin therapy before myocardial infarction (MI). Refer to the table to answer the following questions.
71. Patients who had had a previous MI were significantly more likely to take aspirin.
72. Race was a more significant predictor of aspirin therapy than age.
73. Older patients were significantly more likely to take aspirin.
74. Diabetic patients were significantly less likely to take aspirin.
75. The type of hospital was significantly associated with aspirin use.

Glossary

absolute risk reduction (ARR) The reduction in risk with a new therapy compared with the risk without the new therapy; it is the absolute value of the difference between the experimental event rate and the control event rate (|EER − CER|).

absolute value The positive value of a number, regardless of whether the number is positive or negative. The absolute value of *a* is symbolized |a|.

actuarial analysis See *life table analysis*.

adjusted rate A rate adjusted so that it is independent of the distribution of a possible confounding variable. For example, age-adjusted rates are independent of the age distribution in the population to which they apply.

age-specific mortality rate The mortality rate in a specific age group.

alpha (α) error See *type I error*.

alpha value The level of alpha (α) selected in a hypothesis test.

alternative hypothesis The opposite of the null hypothesis. It is the conclusion when the null hypothesis is rejected.

analysis of covariance (ANCOVA) A special type of analysis of variance or regression used to control for the effect of a possible confounding factor.

analysis of residuals In regression, an analysis of the differences between *Y* and *Y'* to evaluate assumptions and provide guidance on how well the equation fits the data.

analysis of variance (ANOVA) A statistical procedure that determines whether any differences exist among two or more groups of subjects on one or more factors. The *F* test is used in ANOVA.

backward elimination A method to select variables in multiple regression that enters all variables into the regression equation and then eliminates the variable that adds the least to the prediction, followed by the other variables one at a time that decrease the multiple *R* by the least amount until all statistically significant variables are removed from the equation.

bar chart or bar graph A chart or graph used with nominal characteristics to display the numbers or percentages of observations with the characteristic of interest.

Bayes' theorem A formula for calculating the conditional probability of one event, $P(A|B)$, from the conditional probability of the other event, $P(B|A)$.

bell-shaped distribution A term used to describe the shape of the normal (gaussian) distribution.

beta (β) error See *type II error*.

bias The error related to the ways the targeted and sampled populations differ; also called measurement error, it threatens the validity of a study.

binary observation a nominal measure that has only two outcomes (examples are gender: male or female; survival: yes or no).

binomial distribution The probability distribution that describes the number of successes *X* observed in *n* independent trials, each with the same probability of occurrence.

bivariate plot A two-dimensional plot or scatterplot of the values of two characteristics measured on the same set of subjects.

blind study An experimental study in which subjects do not know the treatment they are receiving; investigators may also be blind to the treatment subjects are receiving; see also *double-blind trial*.

block design In analysis of variance, a design in which subjects within each block (or stratum) are assigned to a different treatment.

Bonferroni *t* A method for comparing means in analysis of variance; also called the Dunn multiple-comparison procedure.

box plot A graph that displays both the frequencies and the distribution of observations. It is useful for comparing two distributions.

box-and-whisker plot The same as box plot.

canonical correlation analysis An advanced statistical method for examining the relationships between two sets of interval or numerical measurements made on the same set of subjects.

case–control An observational study that begins with patient cases who have the outcome or disease being investigated and control subjects who do not have the outcome or disease. It then looks backward to identify possible precursors or risk factors.

case–series study A simple descriptive account of interesting or intriguing characteristics observed in a group of subjects.

categorical observation A variable whose values are categories (an example is type of anemia). See also *nominal scale*.

cause-specific mortality rate The mortality rate from a specific disease.

cell   A category of counts or value in a contingency table.

censored observation   An observation whose value is unknown, generally because the subject has not been in the study long enough for the outcome of interest, such as death, to occur.

central limit theorem   A theorem that states that the distribution of means is approximately normal if the sample size is large enough ($n \geq 30$), regardless of the underlying distribution of the original measurements.

chance agreement   A measure of the proportion of times two or more raters agree in their measurement or assessment of a phenomenon.

chi-square (χ^2) distribution   The distribution used to analyze counts in frequency tables.

chi-square (χ^2) test   The statistical test used to test the null hypothesis that proportions are equal or, equivalently, that factors or characteristics are independent or not associated.

classes or class limits   The subdivisions of a numerical characteristic (or the widths of the classes) when it is displayed in a frequency table or graph (an example is ages by decades).

clinical trial   An experimental study of a drug or procedure in which the subjects are humans.

cluster analysis   An advanced statistical method that determines a classification or taxonomy from multiple measures of a set of objects or subjects.

cluster random sample   A two-stage sampling process in which the population is divided into clusters, a random sample of clusters is chosen, and then random samples of subjects within the clusters are selected.

coefficient of determination (r^2)   The square of the correlation coefficient. It is interpreted as the amount of variance in one variable that is accounted for by knowing the second variable.

coefficient of variation (CV)   The standard deviation divided by the mean (generally multiplied by 100). It is used to obtain a measure of relative variation.

cohort   A group of subjects who remain together in the same study over time.

cohort study   An observational study that begins with a set of subjects who have a risk factor (or have been exposed to an agent) and a second set of subjects who do not have the risk factor or exposure. Both sets are followed prospectively through time to learn how many in each set develop the outcome or consequences of interest.

complementary event   An event opposite to the event being investigated.

computer package   A set of statistical computer programs for analyzing data.

concurrent controls   Control subjects assigned to a placebo or control condition during the same period that an experimental treatment or procedure is being evaluated.

conditional probability   The probability of an event, such as A, given that another event, such as B, has occurred, denoted $P(A|B)$.

confidence bands   Lines on each side of a regression line or curve that have a given probability of containing the line or curve in the population.

confidence interval (CI)   The interval computed from sample data that has a given probability that the unknown parameter, such as the mean or proportion, is contained within the interval. Common confidence intervals are 90%, 95%, and 99%.

confidence limits   The limits of a confidence interval. These limits are computed from sample data and have a given probability that the unknown parameter is located between them.

confounded   A term used to describe a study or observation that has one or more nuisance variables present that may lead to incorrect interpretations.

confounding variable   A variable more likely to be present in one group of subjects than another that is related to the outcome of interest and thus potentially confuses, or "confounds," the results.

conservative   A term used to describe a statistical test if it reduces the chances of a type I error.

construct validity   A demonstration that the measurement of a characteristic is related to similar measures of the same characteristic and not related to measures of other characteristics.

content validity   A measure of the degree to which the items on a test or measurement scale are representative of the characteristic being measured.

contingency table   A table used to display counts or frequencies for two or more nominal or quantitative variables.

continuity correction   An adaptation to a test statistic when a continuous probability distribution is used to estimate a discrete probability distribution; eg, using the chi-square distribution for analyzing contingency tables.

continuous scale   A scale used to measure a numerical characteristic with values that occur on a continuum (an example is age).

control event rate (CER)   The number of subjects in the control group who develop the outcome being studied.

control subjects   In a clinical trial, subjects assigned to the placebo or control condition; in a case–control study, subjects without the disease or outcome.

controlled for   A term used to describe a confounding variable that is taken into consideration in the design or the analysis of the study.

controlled trial   A trial in which subjects are assigned to a control condition as well as to an experimental condition.

corrected chi-square test   A chi-square test for a 2×2 table that uses Yates' correction, making it more conservative.

correlation coefficient r   A measure of the linear

relationship between two numerical measurements made on the same set of subjects. It ranges from −1 to +1, with 0 indicating no relationship. Also called the Pearson product moment.

cost-effectiveness analysis A quantitative method to evaluate the cost of a procedure or management strategy that takes into account the outcome as well.

covariate A potentially confounding variable controlled for in analysis of covariance.

Cox's regression A regression method used when the outcome is censored. The regression coefficients are interpreted as adjusted relative risk or odds ratios.

criterion validity An indication of how well a test or scale predicts another related characteristic, ideally a "gold standard" if one exists.

criterion variable The outcome (or dependent variable) that is predicted in a regression problem.

critical ratio The term for the z score used in statistical tests.

critical region The region (or set of values) in which a test statistic must occur for the null hypothesis to be rejected.

critical value The value that a test statistic must exceed (in an absolute value sense) for the null hypothesis to be rejected.

crossover study A clinical trial in which each group of subjects receives two or more treatments, but in different sequences.

cross-product ratio See *relative risk.*

cross-sectional study An observational study that examines a characteristic (or set of characteristics) in a set of subjects at one point in time; a "snapshot" of a characteristic or condition of interest; also called survey or poll.

cross-validation A procedure for applying the results of an analysis from one sample of subjects to a new sample of subjects to evaluate how well they generalize. It is frequently used in regression.

crude rate A rate for the entire population that is not specific or adjusted for any given subset of the population.

cumulative frequency or **percentage** In a frequency table, the frequency (or percentage) of observations having a given value plus all lower values.

curvilinear relationship (between X and Y) A relationship that indicates that X and Y vary together, but not in constant increments.

decision analysis A formal model for describing and analyzing a decision; also called medical decision making.

decision tree A diagram of a set of possible actions, with their probabilities and the values of the outcomes listed. It is used to analyze a decision process.

degrees of freedom A parameter in some commonly used probability distributions; eg, the t distribution and the chi-square distribution.

dependent groups or **samples** Samples in which the values in one group can be predicted from the values in the other group.

dependent variable The variable whose values are the outcomes in a study; also called response or criterion variable.

dependent-groups t test See *paired* t *test.*

descriptive statistics Statistics, such as the mean, the standard deviation, the proportion, and the rate, used to describe attributes of a set of data.

dichotomous observation A nominal measure that has only two outcomes (examples are gender: male or female; survival: yes or no); also called *binary.*

directional test See *one-tailed test.*

discrete scale A scale used to measure a numerical characteristic that has integer values (an example is number of pregnancies).

discriminant analysis A regression technique for predicting a nominal outcome that has more than two values; a method used to classify subjects or objects into groups; also called discriminant function analysis.

distribution The values of a characteristic or variable along with the frequency of their occurrence. Distributions may be based on empirical observations or may be theoretical probability distributions (eg, normal, binomial, chi-square).

dot plot A graphic method for displaying the frequency distribution of numerical observations for one or more groups.

double-blind trial A clinical trial in which neither the subjects nor the investigator(s) know which treatment subjects have received.

dummy coding A procedure in which a code of 0 or 1 is assigned to a nominal predictor variable used in regression analysis.

Dunnett's procedure A multiple-comparison method for comparing multiple treatment groups with a single control group following a significant F test in analysis of variance.

effect or effect size The magnitude of a difference or relationship. It is used for determining sample sizes and for combining results across studies in meta-analysis.

error mean square The mean square in the denominator of F in ANOVA.

estimation The process of using information from a sample to draw conclusions about the values of parameters in a population.

event A single outcome (or set of outcomes) from an experiment.

evidence-based medicine (EBM) The application of the evidence based on clinical research and clinical expertise to decide optimal patient management.

expected frequencies In contingency tables, the frequencies observed if the null hypothesis is true.

expected value Used in decision making to denote the probability of a given outcome over the long run.

experiment (in probability) A planned process of data collection.

experimental event rate (EER) The number of subjects in the experimental or treatment group who develop the outcome being studied.

experimental study A comparative study involving an intervention or manipulation. It is called a trial when human subjects are involved.

explanatory variable See *independent variable.*

exponential probability distribution A probability distribution used in models of survival or decay.

F distribution The probability distribution used to test the equality of two estimates of the variance. It is the distribution used with the *F* test in ANOVA.

F test The statistical test for comparing two variances. It is used in ANOVA.

factor A characteristic that is the focus of inquiry in a study; used in analysis of variance.

factor analysis An advanced statistical method for analyzing the relationships among a set of items or indicators to determine the factors or dimensions that underlie them.

factorial design In ANOVA, a design in which each subject (or object) receives one level of each factor.

false-negative A test result that is negative in a person who has the disease.

false-positive A test result that is positive in a person who does not have the disease.

first quartile The 25th percentile.

Fisher's exact test An exact test for 2×2 contingency tables. It is used when the sample size is too small to use the chi-square test.

Fisher's z transformation A transformation of the correlation coefficient so that it is normally distributed.

forward selection A model-building method in multiple regression that first enters into the regression equation the variable with the highest correlation, followed by the other variables one at a time that increase the multiple *R* by the greatest amount, until all statistically significant variables are included in the equation.

frequency The number of times a given value of an observation occurs. It is also called counts.

frequency distribution In a set of numerical observations, the list of values that occur along with the frequency of their occurrence. It may be set up as a frequency table or as a graph.

frequency polygon A line graph connecting the midpoints of the tops of the columns of a histogram. It is useful in comparing two frequency distributions.

frequency table A table showing the number or percentage of observations occurring at different values (or ranges of values) of a characteristic or variable.

functional status A measure of a person's ability to perform his or her daily activities, often called activities of daily living.

game theory A process of assigning subjective probabilities to outcomes from a decision.

gaussian distribution See *normal distribution.*

Gehan's test A statistical test of the equality of two survival curves.

generalized Wilcoxon test See *Gehan's test.*

geometric mean The *n*th root of the product of *n* observations, symbolized *GM* or *G*. It is used with logarithms or skewed distributions.

gold standard In diagnostic testing, a procedure that always identifies the true condition—diseased or disease-free—of a patient.

hazard function The probability that a person dies in a certain time interval, given that the person has lived until the beginning of the interval. Its reciprocal is mean survival time.

hierarchical regression A logical model-building method in multiple regression in which the investigators group variables according to their function and add them to the regression equation as a group or block.

histogram A graph of a frequency distribution of numerical observations.

historical cohort study A cohort study that uses existing records or historical data to determine the effect of a risk factor or exposure on a group of patients.

historical controls In clinical trials, previously collected observations on patients that are used as the control values against which the treatment is compared.

homogeneity The situation in which the standard deviation of the dependent (*Y*) variable is the same, regardless of the value of the independent (*X*) variable; an assumption in ANOVA and regression.

homoscedasticity See *homogeneity.*

hypothesis test An approach to statistical inference resulting in a decision to reject or not to reject the null hypothesis.

incidence A rate giving the proportion of people who develop a given disease or condition within a specified period of time.

independent events Events whose occurrence or outcome has no effect on the probability of the other.

independent groups or samples Samples for which the values in one group cannot be predicted from the values in the other group.

independent observations Observations determined at different times or by different individuals without knowledge of the value of the first observation.

independent variable The explanatory or predictor variable in a study. It is sometimes called a factor in ANOVA.

independent-groups *t* test See *two-sample t test.*

index of suspicion See *prior probability.*

inference (statistical) The process of drawing conclusions about a population of observations from a sample of observations.

intention-to-treat (principle) The statistical analysis of all subjects according to the group to which they were originally assigned or belonged.

interaction A relationship between two independent variables such that they have a different effect on the dependent variable; ie, the effect of one level of a factor *A* depends on the level of factor *B*.

intercept In a regression equation, the predicted value of *Y* when *X* is equal to zero.

internal consistency (reliability) The degree to which the items on an instrument or test are related to each other and provide a measure of a single characteristic.

interquartile range The difference between the 25th percentile and the 75th percentile.

interrater reliability the reliability between measurements made by two different persons (or raters).

intervention The maneuver used in an experimental study. It may be a drug or a procedure.

intrarater reliability The reliability between measurements made by the same person (or rater) at two different points in time.

joint probability The probability of two events both occurring.

Kaplan–Meier product limit method A method for analyzing survival for censored observations. It uses exact survival times in the calculations.

kappa (κ) A statistic used to measure interrater or intrarater agreement for nominal measures.

length of time to event A term used in outcome and cost-effectiveness studies; it measures the length of time from a treatment or assessment until the outcome of interest occurs.

level of significance The probability of incorrectly rejecting the null hypothesis in a test of hypothesis. Also see *alpha value* and *P value*.

Levene's test A test of the equality of two variances. It is less sensitive to departures from normality than the *F* test and is often recommended by statisticians.

life table analysis A method for analyzing survival times for censored observations that have been grouped into intervals.

likelihood ratio In diagnostic testing, the ratio of true-positives to false-positives.

linear combination A weighted average of a set of variables or measures. For example, the prediction equation in multiple regression is a linear combination of the predictor variables.

linear regression (of *Y* on *X*) The process of determining a regression or prediction equation to predict *Y* from *X*.

linear relationship (between *X* and *Y*) A relationship indicating that *X* and *Y* vary together according to constant increments.

logarithm (ln) The exponent indicating the power to which *e* (2.718) is raised to obtain a given number; also called the natural logarithm.

logistic regression The regression technique used when the outcome is a binary, or dichotomous, variable.

log-linear analysis A statistical method for analyzing the relationships among three or more nominal variables. It may be used as a regression method to predict a nominal outcome from nominal independent variables.

logrank test A statistical method for comparing two survival curves when censored observations occur.

longitudinal study A study that takes place over an extended period of time.

Mann–Whitney–Wilcoxon test See *Wilcoxon rank sum test*.

Mantel–Haenszel chi-square test A statistical test of two or more 2 × 2 tables. It is used to compare survival distributions or to control for confounding factors.

marginal frequencies (probabilities) The row and column frequencies (or probabilities) in a contingency table; ie, the frequencies listed on the margins of the table.

matched-groups *t* test See *paired t test*.

matching (or matched groups) The process of making two groups homogeneous on possible confounding factors. It is sometimes done prior to randomization in clinical trials.

McNemar's test The chi-square test for comparing proportions from two dependent or paired groups.

mean The most common measure of central tendency, denoted by μ in the population and by $\overline{X}$ in the sample. In a sample, the mean is the sum of the *X* values divided by the number *n* in the sample ($\Sigma X/n$).

mean square among groups An estimate of the variation in analysis of variance. It is used in the numerator of the *F* statistic.

mean square within groups An estimate of the variation in analysis of variance. It is used in the denominator of the *F* statistic.

measurement error The amount by which a measurement is incorrect because of problems inherent in the measuring process; also called bias.

measures of central tendency Index or summary numbers that describe the middle of a distribution. See *mean, median,* and *mode*.

measures of dispersion Index or summary numbers that describe the spread of observations about the mean. See *range; standard deviation*.

median (M or Md) A measure of central tendency. It is the middle observation; ie, the one that divides the distribution of values into halves. It is also equal to the 50th percentile.

medical decision making or analysis The application of probabilities to the decision process in medicine. It is the basis for cost-benefit analysis.

MEDLINE A system that permits search of the bibliographic database of all articles in journals included in *Index Medicus*. Articles that meet specific criteria or contain specific key words are extracted for the researcher's perusal.

meta-analysis A method for combining the results from several independent studies of the same outcome so that an overall P value may be determined.

modal class The interval (generally from a frequency table or histogram) that contains the highest frequency of observations.

mode The value of a numerical variable that occurs the most frequently.

model or modeling A statistical statement of the relationship among variables.

morbidity rate The number of patients in a defined population who develop a morbid condition over a specified period of time.

mortality rate The number of deaths in a defined population over a specified period. It is the number of people who die during a given period of time divided by the number of people at risk during the period.

multiple comparisons Comparisons resulting from many statistical tests performed for the same observations.

multiple R In multiple regression, the correlation between actual and predicted values of Y (ie, $r_{YY'}$).

multiple regression A multivariate method for determining a regression or prediction equation to predict an outcome from a set of independent variables.

multiple-comparison procedure A method for comparing several means.

multivariate A term that refers to a study or analysis involving multiple independent or dependent variables.

multivariate analysis of variance (MANOVA) An advanced statistical method that provides a global test when there are multiple dependent variables and the independent variables are nominal. It is analogous to analysis of variance with multiple outcome measures.

mutually exclusive events Two or more events for which the occurrence of one event precludes the occurrence of the others.

Newman–Keuls procedure A multiple-comparison method for making pairwise comparisons between means following a significant F test in analysis of variance.

nominal scale The simplest scale of measurement. It is used for characteristics that have no numerical values (examples are race and gender). It is also called a categorical or qualitative scale.

nondirectional test See *two-tailed test.*

nonmutually exclusive events Two or more events for which the occurrence of one event does not preclude the occurrence of the others.

nonparametric method A statistical test that makes no assumptions regarding the distribution of the observations.

nonprobability sample A sample selected in such a way that the probability that a subject is selected is unknown.

nonrandomized trial A clinical trial in which subjects are assigned to treatments on other than a randomized basis. It is subject to several biases.

normal distribution A symmetric, bell-shaped probability distribution with mean μ and standard deviation σ. If observations follow a normal distribution, the interval ($\mu \pm 2\sigma$) contains 95% of the observations. It is also called the gaussian distribution.

null hypothesis The hypothesis being tested about a population. *Null* generally means "no difference" and thus refers to a situation in which no difference exists (eg, between the means in a treatment group and a control group).

number needed to treat (NNT) The number of patients that need to be treated with a proposed therapy in order to prevent or cure one individual; it is the reciprocal of the absolute risk reduction (1/ARR).

numerical scale The highest level of measurement. It is used for characteristics that can be given numerical values; the differences between numbers have meaning (examples are height, weight, blood pressure level). It is also called an interval or ratio scale.

objective probability An estimate of probability from observable events or phenomena.

observational study A study that does not involve an intervention or manipulation. It is called case–control, cross-sectional, or cohort, depending on the design of the study.

observed frequencies The frequencies that occur in a study. They are generally arranged in a contingency table.

odds The probability that an event will occur divided by the probability that the event will not occur; ie, odds = $P/(1 - P)$, where P is the probability.

odds ratio (OR) An estimate of the relative risk calculated in case–control studies. It is the odds that a patient was exposed to a given risk factor divided by the odds that a control was exposed to the risk factor.

one-tailed test A test in which the alternative hypothesis specifies a deviation from the null hypothesis in one direction only. The critical region is located in one end of the distribution of the test statistic. It is also called a directional test.

ordinal scale Used for characteristics that have an underlying order to their values; the numbers used are arbitrary (an example is Apgar scores).

orphan P A P value given without reference to the statistical method used to determine it.

outcome (in an experiment) The result of an experiment or trial.

outcome assessment The process of including quality-of-life or physical-function variables in clinical outcomes. Studies that focus on outcomes often emphasize how patients view and value their health, the care they receive, and the results or outcomes of this care.

outcome variable The dependent or criterion variable in a study.

***P* value** The probability of observing a result as extreme as or more extreme than the one actually observed from chance alone (ie, if the null hypothesis is true).

paired *t* test The statistical method for comparing the difference (or change) in a numerical variable observed for two paired (or matched) groups. It also applies to before- and after-measurements made on the same group of subjects.

parameter The population value of a characteristic of a distribution (eg, the mean μ).

patient satisfaction Refers to outcome measures of patient's liking and approval of health care facilities and operations, providers, and other components of the entities that provide patient care.

percentage A proportion multiplied by 100.

percentile A number that indicates the percentage of a distribution that is less than or equal to that number.

person-years Found by adding the length of time subjects are in a study. This concept is frequently used in epidemiology but is not recommended by statisticians because of difficulties in interpretation and analysis.

piecewise linear regression A method used to estimate sections of a regression line when a curvilinear relationship exists between the independent and dependent variables.

placebo A sham treatment or procedure. It is used to reduce bias in clinical studies.

point estimate A general term for any statistic (eg, mean, standard deviation, proportion).

Poisson distribution A probability distribution used to model the number of times a rare event occurs.

polynomial regression A special case of multiple regression in which each term in the equation is a power of the independent variable X. Polynomial regression provides a way to fit a regression model to curvilinear relationships and is an alternative to transforming the data to a linear scale.

pooled standard deviation The standard deviation used in the independent-groups *t* test when the standard deviations in the two groups are equal.

population The entire collection of observations or subjects that have something in common and to which conclusions are inferred.

post hoc comparisons Methods for comparing means following analysis of variance.

posterior probability The conditional probability calculated by using Bayes' theorem. It is the predictive value of a positive test (true-positives divided by all positives) or a negative test (true-negatives divided by all negatives).

posttest odds In diagnostic testing, the odds that a patient has a given disease or condition after a diagnostic procedure is performed and interpreted. They are similar to the predictive value of a diagnostic test.

power The ability of a test statistic to detect a specified alternative hypothesis or difference of a specified size when the alternative hypothesis is true (ie, $1 - \beta$, where β is the probability of a type II error). More loosely, it is the ability of a study to detect an actual effect or difference.

predictive value of a negative test The proportion of time that a patient with a negative diagnostic test result does not have the disease being investigated.

predictive value of a positive test The proportion of time that a patient with a positive diagnostic test result has the disease being investigated.

pretest odds In diagnostic testing, the odds that a patient has a given disease or condition before a diagnostic procedure is performed and interpreted. They are similar to prior probabilities.

prevalence The proportion of people who have a given disease or condition at a specified point in time. It is not truly a rate, although it is often incorrectly called prevalence rate.

prior probability The unconditional probability used in the numerator of Bayes' theorem. It is the prevalence of a disease prior to performing a diagnostic procedure. Clinicians often refer to it as the index of suspicion.

probability The number of times an outcome occurs in the total number of trials. If A is the outcome, the probability of A is denoted $P(A)$.

probability distribution A frequency distribution of a random variable, which may be empirical or theoretical (eg, normal, binomial).

product limit method See *Kaplan–Meier product limit method.*

progressively censored A situation in which patients enter a study at different points in time and remain in the study for varying lengths of time. See *censored observation.*

proportion The number of observations with the characteristic of interest divided by the total number of observations. It is used to summarize counts.

proportional hazards model See *Cox's regression.*

prospective study A study designed before data are collected.

qualitative observations Characteristics measured on a nominal scale.

quality of life (QOL) A measure of a person's subjective assessment of the value of his or her health and functional abilities.

quantitative observations Characteristics measured on a numerical scale; the resulting numbers have inherent meaning.

quartile The 25th percentile or the 75th percentile, called the first and third quartiles, respectively.

random assignment The use of random methods to assign different treatments to patients or vice versa.

random error or **variation** The variation in a sample that can be expected to occur by chance.

random sample A sample of n subjects (or objects) selected from a population so that each has a known chance of being in the sample.

random variable A variable in a study in which subjects are randomly selected or randomly assigned to treatments.

randomization The process of assigning subjects to different treatments (or vice versa) by using random numbers.

randomized clinical trial An experimental study in which subjects are randomly assigned to treatment groups.

range The difference between the largest and the smallest observation.

rank-order scale A scale for observations arranged according to their size, from lowest to highest or vice versa.

ranks A set of observations arranged according to their size, from lowest to highest or vice versa.

rate A proportion associated with a multiplier, called the base (eg, 1000, 10,000, 100,000), and computed over a specific period.

ratio A part divided by another part. It is the number of observations with the characteristic of interest divided by the number without the characteristic.

regression (of Y on X) The process of determining a prediction equation for predicting Y from X.

regression coefficient The b in the simple regression equation $Y = a + bX$. It is sometimes interpreted as the slope of the regression line. In multiple regression, the bs are weights applied to the predictor variables.

regression toward the mean The phenomenon in which a predicted outcome for any given person tends to be closer to the mean outcome than the person's actual observation.

relative risk (RR) The ratio of the incidence of a given disease in exposed or at-risk persons to the incidence of the disease in unexposed persons. It is calculated in cohort or prospective studies.

relative risk reduction (RRR) The reduction in risk with a new therapy relative to the risk without the new therapy; it is the absolute value of the difference between the experimental event rate and the control event rate divided by the control event rate (|EER − CER|/CER).

reliability A measure of the reproducibility of a measurement. It is measured by kappa for nominal measures and by correlation for numerical measures.

repeated-measures design A study design in which subjects are measured at more than one time. It is also called a split-plot design in ANOVA.

representative population (or sample) A population or sample that is similar in important ways to the population to which the findings of a study are generalized.

residual The difference between the predicted value and the actual value of the outcome (dependent) variable in regression.

response variable See *dependent variable*.

retrospective cohort study See *historical cohort study*.

retrospective study A study undertaken in a post hoc manner, ie, after the observations have been made.

risk factor A term used to designate a characteristic that is more prevalent among subjects who develop a given disease or outcome than among subjects who do not. It is generally considered to be causal.

risk ratio See *relative risk*.

robust A term used to describe a statistical method if the outcome is not affected to a large extent by a violation of the assumptions of the method.

ROC (receiver operating characteristic) curve In diagnostic testing, a plot of the true-positives on the Y-axis versus the false-positives on the X-axis; used to evaluate the properties of a diagnostic test.

sample A subset of the population.

sampled population The population from which the sample is actually selected.

sampling distribution (of a statistic) The frequency distribution of the statistic for many samples. It is used to make inferences about the statistic from a single sample.

scale of measurement The degree of precision with which a characteristic is measured. It is generally categorized into nominal (or categorical), ordinal, and numerical (or interval and ratio) scales.

scatterplot A two-dimensional graph displaying the relationship between two numerical characteristics or variables.

Scheffé's procedure A multiple-comparison method for comparing means following a significant F test in analysis of variance. It is the most conservative multiple-comparison method.

self-controlled study A study in which the subjects serve as their own controls, achieved by measuring the characteristic of interest before and after an intervention.

sensitivity The proportion of time a diagnostic test is positive in patients who have the disease or condition. A sensitive test has a low false-negative rate.

sensitivity analysis In decision analysis, a method for determining the way the decision changes as a function of probabilities and utilities used in the analysis.

sign test The nonparametric test used for testing a hypothesis about the median in a single group.

simple random sample A random sample in which each of the n subjects (or objects) in the sample has an equal chance of being selected.

skewed distribution A distribution in which a few outlying observations occur in one direction only. If the outlying observations are small, the distribution is skewed to the left, or negatively skewed; if they are large, the distribution is skewed to the right, or positively skewed.

slope (of the regression line) The amount Y changes for each unit that X changes. It is designated by b in the sample.

Spearman's rank correlation (rho) A nonparametric correlation that measures the tendency for two measurements to vary together.

specific rate A rate that pertains to a specific group or segment of the observations (examples are age-specific mortality rate and cause-specific mortality rate).

specificity The proportion of time that a diagnostic test is negative in patients who do not have the disease or condition. A specific test has a low false-positive rate.

standard deviation (SD) The most common measure of dispersion or spread, denoted by σ in the population and SD or s in the sample. It can be used with the mean to describe the distribution of observations. It is the square root of the average of the squared deviations of the observations from their mean.

standard error (SE) The standard deviation of the sampling distribution of a statistic.

standard error of the estimate A measure of the variation in a regression line. It is based on the differences between the predicted and actual values of the dependent variable Y.

standard error of the mean The standard deviation of the mean in a large number of samples.

standard normal distribution The normal distribution with mean 0 and standard deviation 1, also called the z distribution.

standardized regression coefficient A regression coefficient that has the effect of the measurement scale removed so that the size of the coefficient can be interpreted.

statistic A summary number for a sample (eg, the mean), often used as an estimate of a parameter in the population.

statistical significance Generally interpreted as a result that would occur by chance, eg, 1 time in 20, with a P value less than or equal 0.05. It occurs when the null hypothesis is rejected.

statistical test The procedure used to test a null hypothesis (eg, t test, chi-square test).

stem-and-leaf plot A graphic display for numerical data. It is similar to both a frequency table and a histogram.

stepwise regression In multiple regression, a sequential method of selecting the variables to be included in the prediction equation.

stratified random sample A sample consisting of random samples from each subpopulation (or stratum) in a population. It is used so that the investigator can be sure that each subpopulation is appropriately represented in the sample.

subjective probability An estimate of probability that reflects a person's opinion or best guess from previous experience.

sums of squares Quantities calculated in analysis of variance and used to obtain the mean squares for the F test.

suppression of zero A term used to describe a misleading graph that does not have a break (a jagged line) in the Y-axis to indicate that part of the scale is missing.

survey An observational study that generally has a cross-sectional design; a commonly used design to collect opinions.

survival analysis The statistical method for analyzing survival data when there are censored observations.

symmetric distribution A distribution that has the same shape on both sides of the mean. The mean, median, and mode are all equal. It is the opposite of a skewed distribution.

systematic error A measurement error that is the same (or constant) over all observations. See also *bias.*

systematic random sample A random sample obtained by selecting each kth subject or object.

t **distribution** A symmetric distribution with mean zero and a standard deviation larger than that for the normal distribution for small sample sizes. As n increases, the t distribution approaches the normal distribution.

t **test** The statistical test for comparing a mean with a norm or for comparing two means with small sample sizes ($n \leq 30$). It is also used for testing whether a correlation coefficient or a regression coefficient is zero.

target population The population to which the investigator wishes to generalize.

test statistic The specific statistic used to test the null hypothesis (eg, the t statistic or chi-square statistic).

testing threshold In diagnostic testing, the point at which the optimal decision is to perform a diagnostic test.

test–retest (reliability) A measure of the degree to which an instrument or test provides a consistent measure of a characteristic on different occasions.

third quartile The 75th percentile.

threshold model A model for deciding when a diagnostic test should be ordered, as opposed to doing nothing or treating the patient without performing the test.

transformation A change in the scale for the values of a variable.

treatment threshold In diagnostic testing, the point at which the optimal decision is to treat the patient without first performing a diagnostic test.

trial An experiment involving humans, commonly called a clinical trial. It is also a replication (repetition) of an experiment.

true-negative A test result that is negative in a person who does not have the disease.

true-positive A test result that is positive in a person who has the disease.

Tukey's HSD (honestly significant difference) test A post hoc test for making multiple pairwise comparisons between means following a significant F test in analysis of variance. It is a method highly recommended by statisticians.

two-sample t test The statistical test used to test the null hypothesis that two independent (or unrelated) groups have the same mean.

two-tailed test A test in which the alternative hypothesis specifies a deviation from the null hypothesis in either direction. The critical region is located in both ends of the distribution of the test statistic. It is also called a directional test.

two-way analysis of variance ANOVA with two independent variables.

type I error The error that results if a true null hypothesis is rejected or if a difference is concluded when no difference exists.

type II error The error that results if a false null hypothesis is not rejected or if a difference is not detected when a difference exists.

unbiasedness (of a statistic) A term used to describe a statistic whose mean based on a large number of samples is equal to the population parameter.

uncontrolled study An experimental study that has no control subjects.

utility The value of different outcomes in a decision tree.

validity The property of a measurement that indicates how well it measures the characteristic.

variable A characteristic of interest in a study that has different values for different subjects or objects.

variance The square of the standard deviation.

variation (within subject) The variability in measurements of the same object or subject. It may occur naturally or may represent an error.

vital statistics Mortality and morbidity rates used in epidemiology and public health.

weighted average A number formed by multiplying each number in a set of numbers by a value called a weight, adding the resulting products, and then dividing by the sum of the weight.

Wilcoxon rank sum test A nonparametric test for comparing two independent samples with ordinal data or with numerical observations that are not normally distributed.

Wilcoxon signed ranks test A nonparametric test for comparing two dependent samples with ordinal data or with numerical observations that are not normally distributed.

Yates' correction The process of subtracting 0.5 from the numerator at each term in the chi-square statistic for 2×2 tables prior to squaring the term.

z approximation (to the binomial) The z test used to test the equality of two independent proportions.

z distribution The normal distribution with mean 0 and standard deviation 1. It is also called the standard normal distribution.

z ratio The test statistic used in the z test. It is formed by subtracting the hypothesized mean from the observed mean and dividing by the standard error of the mean.

z score The deviation of X from the mean divided by the standard deviation.

z test The statistical test for comparing a mean with a norm or comparing two means for large samples ($n \geq 30$).

z transformation A transformation that changes a normally distributed variable with mean $\overline{X}$ and standard deviation SD to the z distribution with mean 0 and standard deviation 1.

References

ARTICLES PUBLISHED
IN THE MEDICAL LITERATURE

Alderman EL et al: Ten-year follow-up of survival and my-ocardial infarction in the randomized Coronary Artery Surgery Study. *Circulation* 1990;**82:**1629–1640.

Alexandrov AV et al: Correlation of peak systolic velocity and angiographic measurement of carotid stenosis revisited. *Stroke* 1997;**28:**339–342.

Anasetti C et al: Marrow transplantation for severe aplastic anemia. *Ann Intern Med* 1986;**104:**461–466.

Avis M, Bond M, Arthur A: Exploring patient satisfaction with out-patient services. *J Nurs Manag* 1995; **3:**59–65.

Bajwa K, Szabo E, Kjellstrand CM: A prospective study of risk factors and decision making in discontinuation of dialysis. *Arch Intern Med* 1996;**156:**2571–2577.

Bale P, Bradbury D, Colley E: Anthropometric and training variables related to 10 km running performance. *Br J Sports Med* 1986;**20:**170–173.

Ballard RA et al: Antenatal thyrotropin-releasing hormone to prevent lung disease in preterm infants. *N Engl J Med* 1998;**338:**493–498.

Barker DJP: Rise and fall of Western diseases. *Nature* 1989;**338:**371–372.

Bartle WR, Gupta AK, Lazor J: Nonsteroidal anti-inflammatory drugs and gastrointestinal bleeding. *Arch Intern Med* 1986;**146:**2365–2367.

Benson JT, Lucente V, McClellan E: Vaginal versus abdominal reconstructive surgery for treatment of pelvic support defects: A prospective randomized study with long-term outcome evaluation. *Am J Obstet Gynecol* 1996;**175:**1418–1422.

Borowitz KC, Glascoe FP: Sensitivity of the Denver Developmental Screening Test in speech and language. *Pediatrics* 1986;**78:**1075–1078.

Bossi P et al: Acquired hemophilia due to Factor VIII inhibitors in 34 patients. *Am J Med* 1998;**105:**400–408.

Brandeau ML, Eddy DM: The workup of the asymptomatic patient with a positive fecal occult blood test. *Med Decis Making* 1987;**7:**32–46.

Brown AD, Garber AM: Cost-effectiveness of 3 methods to enhance the sensitivity of Papanicolaou testing. *JAMA* 1999;**281:**347–353.

Buchsbaum DG et al: Screening for alcohol abuse using CAGE scores and likelihood ratios. *Ann Intern Med* 1991;**115:**774–777.

Buckley WE: Concussions in college football. *Am J Sports Med* 1988;**16:**51–56.

Bush B et al: Screening for alcohol abuse using the CAGE questionnaire. *Am J Med* 1987;**82:**231–235.

Camitta BM et al: A prospective study of androgens and bone marrow transplantation for treatment of severe aplastic anemia. *Blood* 1979;**53:**504–514.

CASS Principal Investigators and Associates: Coronary Artery Surgery Study (CASS): A randomized trial of coronary bypass surgery. *Circulation* 1983;**68:**951–960.

Chassin MR et al: Does inappropriate use explain geographic variations in the use of health care services? *JAMA* 1987;**258:**2533–2537.

Colditz GA et al: A prospective study of parental history of myocardial infarction and coronary heart disease in women. *N Engl J Med* 1987;**316:**1105–1110.

Colquitt WL, Smith IP, Killian CD: Specialty selection and success in obtaining choice of residency training among 1987 US medical graduates by race-ethnicity and gender. *Acad Med* 1992;**67:**660–671.

Cooley TP et al: Once-daily administration of 2′,3′-dideoxyinosine (ddI) in patients with the acquired immunodeficiency syndrome or AIDS-related complex. *N Engl J Med* 1990;**322:**1340–1345.

Crook JM et al: Radiotherapy for localized prostate carcinoma. *Cancer* 1997;**79:**328–336.

D'Angio CT, Maniscalco WM, Pichichero ME: Immunologic responses of extremely premature infants to tetanus, *Haemophilus influenzae,* and polio immunizations. *Pediatrics* 1995;**96:**18–22.

Dennis N. Consumer audit in the NHS. *Br J Hosp Med* 1995;**53:**532–534.

Dennison BA, Rockwell HL, Baker SL: Excess fruit juice consumption by preschool-aged children is associated with short stature and obesity. *Pediatrics* 1997;**99:** 15–22.

Detsky AS. Predicting cardiac complication in patients undergoing non-cardiac surgery. *J Gen Intern Med* 1986;**1:**211–219.

Deyo R, Rainville J, Kent DL: What can the history and physical examination tell us about low back pain? *JAMA* 1992;**268:**760–765.

Diermayer M et al: Epidemic serogroup B meningococcal disease in Oregon: The evolving epidemiology of the ET-5 strain. *JAMA* 1999;**281:**1493–1497.

Doll R, Hill AB: Smoking and carcinoma of the lung. *Br Med J* 1950;**2:**739–748.

Doll R, Peto R: Mortality in relation to smoking: 20 years' observations on male British doctors. *Br Med J* 1976; **2(6051):**1525–1536.

Dowling PT: Return of tuberculosis: Screening and preventive therapy. *Am Fam Pract* 1991;**43:**457–467.

Eddy DM: Screening for colorectal cancer. *Ann Intern Med* 1990;**113:**373–384.

Einarsson K et al: Influence of age on secretion of cholesterol and synthesis of bile acids by the liver. *N Engl J Med* 1985;**313:**277–282.

Fletcher EC et al: Undiagnosed sleep apnea in patients with essential hypertension. *Ann Intern Med* 1985; **103:**190–195.

Francis PT et al: Neurochemical studies of early-onset Alzheimer's disease. *N Engl J Med* 1985;**313:**7–11.

Funkhouser AW et al: Estimated effects of a delay in the recommended vaccination schedule for diphtheria and tetanus toxoids and pertussis vaccine. *JAMA* 1987;**257:** 1341–1346.

Gage TP: Managing the cancer risk in chronic ulcerative colitis. *J Clin Gastroenterol* 1986;**8:**50–57.

Garneau RA et al: Glenoid labrum: Evaluation with MR imaging. *Radiology* 1991;**179:**519–522.

Gelber DA et al: Cardiovascular autonomic nervous system tests: Determination of normative values and effect of confounding variables. *J Auton Nerv Syst* 1997; **62:**40–44.

Gelkopf M, Sigal M, Kramer R: Therapeutic use of humor to improve social support in an institutionalized schizophrenic inpatient community. *J Soc Psychol* 1994; **134:**175–182.

Gold MR et al (editors). *Cost-Effectiveness in Health and Medicine.* Oxford University Press, 1996.

Goldman L. Cardiac risk in noncardiac surgery: An update. *Anesth Analg* 1995;**80:**810–820.

Goldman L et al: Multifactorial index of cardiac risk in non-cardiac surgical procedures. *N Engl J Med* 1977; **297:**845–850.

Goldsmith AM et al: Sequential clinical and immunologic abnormalities in hemophiliacs. *Arch Intern Med* 1985;**145:**431–434.

Gonzalo MA et al: Glucose tolerance, insulin secretion, insulin sensitivity and glucose effectiveness in normal and overweight hyperthyroid women. *Clin Endocrinol* 1996;**45:**689–697.

Good DC et al: Sleep-disordered breathing and poor functional outcome after stroke. *Stroke* 1996;**27:**252–259.

Gordon T, Kannel WB: The Framingham, Massachusetts, Study twenty years later. In Kessler IJ, Levin ML (editors): *The Community as an Epidemiologic Laboratory.* Johns Hopkins Press, 1970.

Gordon T et al: Some methodologic problems in the long term study of cardiovascular disease: Observations on the Framingham Study. *J Chronic Dis* 1959;**10:**186–206.

Gotto AM. The Multiple Risk Factor Intervention Trial (MRFIT): A return to a landmark trial. *JAMA* 1997;**277:** 595–597.

Greene MF, Benacerraf BR: Prenatal diagnosis in diabetic gravidas: Utility of ultrasound and maternal serum alpha-fetoprotein screening. *Obstet Gynecol* 1991; **77:**520–523.

Greenfield S et al: Variations in resource utilization among medical specialties and systems of care. *JAMA* 1992;**267:**1624–1630.

Greenwood M: The natural duration of cancer. *Rep Public Health Med Subjects* 1926;**33:**1–26.

Haddow JE et al: Screening of maternal serum for fetal Down's syndrome in the first trimester. *N Engl J Med* 1998;**338:**955–961.

Haider AW et al: The association of chronic cough with the risk of myocardial infarction: The Framingham Heart Study. *Am J Med* 1999;**106:**279–284.

Hall JA, Milburn MA, Epstein AM. A causal model of health status and satisfaction with medical care. *Med Care* 1993;**31:**84–94.

Harper DM. Paracervical block diminishes cramping associated with cryotherapy. *J Fam Pract* 1997;**44:**71–75.

Hartz AJ et al: The association of smoking with cardiomyopathy. *N Engl J Med* 1984;**311:**1201–1206.

He J et al: Aspirin and risk of hemorrhagic stroke. *JAMA* 1998;**280:**1930–1935.

Hébert R, Brayne C, Spiegelhalter D: Incidence of functional decline and improvement in a community-dwelling very elderly population. *Am J Epidemiol* 1997;**145:**935–944.

Helmrich SP et al: Venous thromboembolism in relation to oral contraceptive use. *Obstet Gynecol* 1987;**69:**91–95.

Henderson AS et al: The course of depression in the elderly: A longitudinal community-based study in Australia. *Psychol Med* 1997;**27:**119–129.

Hillner BE, Smith TJ: Efficacy and cost effectiveness of adjuvant chemotherapy in women with node-negative breast cancer. *N Engl J Med* 1991;**324:**160–168.

Hindmarsh PC, Brook CGD: Final height of short normal children treated with growth hormone. *Lancet* 1996; **348:**13–16.

Hodgson LG, Cutler SJ: Anticipatory dementia and well-being. *Am J Alzheimer's Dis* 1997;**12:**62–66.

Horvath EP Jr et al: Effects of formaldehyde on the mucous membranes and lungs. *JAMA* 1988;**259:**701–707.

Horwitz RI et al: Developing improved observational methods for evaluating therapeutic effectiveness. *Am J Med* 1990;**89:**630–638.

Ingelfinger JA: Routine testing for chlamydial cervical infections. (Letter to editor.) *Ann Intern Med* 1988; **108:**153.

Ioannidis JPA, Cappelleri JC, Lau J: Issues in comparisons between meta-analyses and large trials. *JAMA* 1998; **279:**1089–1093.

Irwin M et al: Life events, depressive symptoms, and immune function. *Am J Psychiatry* 1987;**144:**437–441.

Kaku DA, Lowenstein DH: Emergency of recreational drug abuse as a major risk factor for stroke in young adults. *Ann Intern Med* 1990;**113:**821–827.

Kalichman MW, Friedman PJ: A pilot study of biomedical trainees' perceptions concerning research ethics. *Acad Med* 1992;**67:**769–775.

Kalman CM, Laskin OL: Herpes zoster and zosteriform herpes simplex virus infections in immunocompetent adults. *Am J Med* 1986;**81:**775–778.

Kassebaum DG, Szenas PL: Specialty preferences of graduating medical students: 1992 update. *Acad Med* 1992;**67:**800–806.

Kassirer JP. The quality of care and the quality of measuring it. *N Engl J Med* 1993;**329:**1263–1265.

Kellermann AL et al: Suicide in the home in relation to gun ownership. *N Engl J Med* 1992;**327:**467–472.

Kilbourne EM et al: Clinical epidemiology of toxic-oil syndrome. *N Engl J Med* 1983;**309:**1408–1414.

Kind P. The EuroQol instrument: An index of health-related quality of life. In Spilker B (editor): *Quality of Life and Pharmacoeconomics in Clinical Trials,* 2nd ed., pp. 191–201. Lippincott-Raven, 1996.

Knutson RA et al: Use of sugar and providone-iodine to enhance wound healing: Five years' experience. *South Med J* 1981;**74:**1329–1335.

Kremer JM et al: Fish-oil fatty acid supplementation in active rheumatoid arthritis. *Ann Intern Med* 1987; **106:**497–503.

Lamas GA et al: Do the results of randomized clinical trials of cardiovascular drugs influence medical practice? *N Engl J Med* 1992;**327**:241–247.

Langlois JA et al: Association between insulin-like growth factor I and bone mineral density in older women and men: The Framingham Heart Study. *J Clin Endocrinol Metab* 1998;**83**:4257–4262.

Lash TL, Aschengrau A: Active and passive cigarette smoking and the occurrence of breast cancer. *Am J Epidemiol* 1999;**149**:5–12.

Lawrie GM, Morris GC, Earle N: Long-term results of coronary bypass surgery. *Ann Surg* 1991;**213**:377–385.

LeLorier K et al: Discrepancies between meta-analysis and subsequent large randomized, controlled trials. *N Engl J Med* 1997;**337**:536–542.

Leveno KJ et al: A prospective comparison of selective and universal electronic fetal monitoring in 34,995 pregnancies. *N Engl J Med* 1986;**315**:615–619.

Levine MN et al: A bedside decision instrument to elicit a patient's preference concerning adjuvant chemotherapy for breast cancer. *Ann Intern Med* 1992;**117**:53–58.

Levinsky RJ et al: Circulating immune complexes in steroid-responsive nephrotic syndrome. *N Engl J Med* 1978;**298**:126–129.

Lissner L et al: Variability of body weight and health outcomes in the Framingham population. *N Engl J Med* 1991;**324**:1839–1844.

Lledo R et al. Information as a fundamental attribute among out-patients attending the nuclear medicine service of a university hospital. *Nucl Med Commun* 1995;**16**:76–83.

Lord SR, Clark RD, Webster IW: Postural stability and associated physiological factors in a population of aged persons. *J Gerontol* 1991;**44**:M60–76.

MacMahon B, Yen S, Trichopoulos D: Coffee and cancer of the pancreas. *N Engl J Med* 1981;**304**:630-633.

Maki DG et al: Prevention of central venous catheter-related bloodstream infection by use of an antiseptic-impregnated catheter: A randomized, controlled trial. *Ann Intern Med* 1997;**127**:257–266.

Marwick TH et al: The noninvasive prediction of cardiac mortality in men and women with known or suspected coronary artery disease. *Am J Med* 1999;**106**:172–178.

Maulik D et al: Comparative efficacy of umbilical arterial Doppler indices for predicting adverse perinatal outcome. *Am J Obstet Gynecol* 1991;**164**:1434–1440.

Maxwell MH et al: Error in blood-pressure measurement due to incorrect cuff size in obese patients. *Lancet* 1982;**2(8288)**:33–36.

McDowell I, Newell C. *Measuring Health: A Guide to Rating Scales and Questionnaires,* 2nd ed. Oxford University Press, 1996.

Meier P: The biggest public health experiment ever. In Tanur JM et al (editors): *Statistics: A Guide to the Unknown,* 3rd ed. Brooks/Cole, 1989.

Moertel CG et al: High-dose vitamin C versus placebo in the treatment of patients with advanced cancer who have had no prior chemotherapy. *N Engl J Med* 1985;**312**:137–141.

Moore JG et al: Age does not influence acute aspirin-induced gastric mucosal damage. *Gastroenterology* 1991;**100**:1626–1629.

Multiple Risk Factor Intervention Trial Research Group: Multiple risk factor intervention trial. *JAMA* 1982;**248**:1465–1477.

Murphy JL et al: Energy content of stools in normal healthy controls and patients with cystic fibrosis. *Arch Dis Child* 1991;**66**:495–500.

Nathan DM et al: The clinical information value of the glycosylated hemoglobin assay. *N Engl J Med* 1984;**310**:341–346.

Nelson KB, Ellenberg JH: Antecedents of cerebral palsy. *N Engl J Med* 1986;**315**:81–86.

Nesselroad JM et al: Accuracy of automated finger blood pressure devices. *Fam Med* 1996;**28**:189–192.

O'Connor SJ, Shewchuk RM, Carney LW. The great gap. Physicians' perceptions of patient service quality expectations fall short of reality. *J Health Care Marketing* 1994;**14**:32–39.

O'Malley MS, Fletcher SW: Screening for breast cancer with breast self examination. *JAMA* 1987;**257**:2196–2203.

Phillips R et al: Should tests for *Chlamydia trachomatis* cervical infection be done during routine gynecologic visits? *Ann Intern Med* 1987;**107**:188–194.

Poikolainen K et al: Alcohol intake: A risk factor for psoriasis in young and middle aged men? *Br Med J* 1990:**300**:780–783.

Ransohoff DF, Lang CA: Screening for colorectal cancer. *N Engl J Med* 1991;**325**:37–41.

Raskin IE, Maklan CW: Medical treatment effectiveness research. *Eval Health Prof* 1991;**14**:161–186.

Robin ED: The cult of the Swan-Ganz catheter: Overuse and abuse of pulmonary flow catheters. *Ann Intern Med* 1985;**103**:445–449.

Roethlisberger FJ, Dickson WJ, Wright HA: *Management and the Worker.* Harvard Univ Press, 1946.

Rogers WJ et al: Ten-year follow-up of quality of life in patients randomized to receive medical therapy or coronary artery bypass graft surgery. The Coronary Artery Surgery Study. *Circulation* 1990;**82**:1647–1658.

Rubin HR et al. Patients' ratings of out-patient visits in different practice settings: Results from the medical outcomes study. *JAMA* 1993;**270**:835–840.

Schulman et al: The duration of oral anticoagulant therapy after a second episode of venous thromboembolism. *N Engl J Med* 1997;**336**:393–398.

Sempos CT et al: The influence of cigarette smoking on the association between body weight and mortality. The Framingham Heart Study revisited. *Ann Epidemiol* 1998;**8**:289–300.

Serrano CW, Wright JW, Newton ER: Surgical glove perforation in obstetrics. *Obstet Gynecol* 1991;**77**:525–528.

Shipley WU et al: Radiation therapy for clinically localized prostate cancer: A multi-institutional pooled analysis. *JAMA* 1999;**281**:1598–1604.

Shlipak MG et al: Should the electrocardiogram be used to guide therapy for patients with left bundle-branch block and suspected myocardial infarction? *JAMA* 1999;**281**:714–719.

Singh JP et al: Blood pressure response during treadmill testing as a risk factor for new-onset hypertension: The Framingham Heart Study. *Circulation* 1999;**99**:1831–1836.

Society of Actuaries and Association of Life Insurance Medical Directors of America: *Blood Pressure Study 1979.* Recording & Statistical Corporation, 1980.

Soderstrom CA et al: Predictive model to identify trauma patients with blood alcohol concentrations ≥ 50 mg/dl. *J Trauma Injury Infec Crit Care* 1997;**42**:67–73.

Spilker B (editor): *Quality of Life and Pharmacoeconomics in Clinical Trials,* 2nd ed. Lippincott-Raven, 1996.

Steere AC et al: Successful parenteral penicillin therapy of established Lyme arthritis. *N Engl J Med* 1985;**312**:869–874.

Steering Committee of the Physicians' Health Study Research Group: Final report on the aspirin component of the ongoing Physicians' Health Study. *N Engl J Med* 1989;**321:**129–135.

Steinberg EP et al: A case study of physicians' use of liver-spleen scans. *Arch Intern Med* 1986;**146:**253–258.

Stewart AL et al. Functional status and well-being of patients with chronic conditions. *JAMA* 1989;**262:**907–913.

Stewart AL, Hays RD, Ware JE Jr. The MOS short-form general health survey. *Med Care* 1988;**26:**724–735.

Tan EM et al: The 1982 revised criteria for the classification of systemic lupus erythematosus. *Arthritis Rheum* 1982;**25:**1271–1277.

Tarlov AR et al. The Medical Outcomes Study: An application of methods for monitoring the results of medical care. *JAMA* 1989;**262:**925–930.

Tirlapur VG, Mir MA: Effect of low calorie intake on abnormal pulmonary physiology in patients with chronic hypercapneic respiratory failure. *Am J Med* 1984;**77:**987–994.

Ulrich CD, Rosner B, Sturmer T: An epidemiologic study of abuse of analgesic drugs. *N Engl J Med* 1991;**324:**155–160.

Users' Guides to the Medical Literature
  I.   Oxman AD, Sackett DL, Guyatt GH: How to get started. *JAMA* 1993;**270:**2093–2095.
  II. Guyatt GH, Sackett DL, Cook DJ: How to use an article about therapy or prevention: A. Are the results of the study valid? *JAMA* 1993;**270:**2598–2601.
  II. Guyatt GH, Sackett DL, Cook DJ: How to use an article about therapy or prevention; B. What were the results and will they help me in caring for my patients? *JAMA* 1994;**271:**59–63.
  III. Jaeschke R, Guyatt GH, Sackett DL: How to use an article about a diagnostic test: A. Are the results of the study valid? *JAMA* 1994;**271:**389–391.
  III. Jaeschke R, Guyatt GH, Sackett DL: How to use an article about a diagnostic test: B. What are the results and will they help me in caring for my patients? *JAMA* 1994;**271:**703–707.
  IV. Levine M et al: How to use an article about harm. *JAMA* 1994;**271:**1615–1619.
  V.   Laupacis A et al: How to use an article about progress. *JAMA* 1994;**272:**234–237.
  VI. Oxman AD, Cook DJ, Guyatt GH: How to use an overview. *JAMA* 1994;**272:**1367–1371.
  VII. Richardson WS, Detsky AS: How to use a clinical decision analysis: A. Are the results of the study valid? *JAMA* 1995;**273:**1292–1295.
  VII. Richardson WS, Detsky AS: How to use a clinical decision analysis: B. What are the results and will they help me in caring for my patients? *JAMA* 1995;**273:**1610–1613.
  VIII. Hayward RSA et al: How to use clinical practice guidelines: A. Are the recommendations valid? *JAMA* 1995;**274:**570–574.
  VIII. Hayward RSA et al: How to use clinical practice guidelines: B. What are the recommendations and will they help you in caring for your patients? *JAMA* 1995;**274:**1630–1632.
  IX. Guyatt GH et al: A method for grading health care recommendations. *JAMA* 1995;**274:**1800–1804.
  X.   Naylor D, Guyatt GH: How to use an article reporting variations in the outcomes of health services. *JAMA* 1996;**275:**554–558.
  XI. Naylor D, Guyatt GH: How to use an article about a clinical utilization review. *JAMA* 1996;**275:**1435–1439.
  XII. Guyatt GH et al: How to use articles about health-related quality of life. *JAMA* 1997;**277:**1232–1237.
  XIII. Drummond MF et al: How to use an article on economic analysis of clinical practice: A. Are the results of the study valid? *JAMA* 1997;**277:**1552–1557.
  XIII. O'Brien BJ et al: How to use an article on economic analysis of clinical practice: B. What are the results and will they help me in caring for my patients? *JAMA* 1997;**277:**1802–1806.
  XIV. Dans AL et al: How to decide on the applicability of clinical trial results to your patient. *JAMA* 1998;**279:**545–549.
  XV. Richardson WS et al: How to use an article about disease probability for differential diagnosis. *JAMA* 1999;**281:**1214–1219.
  XVI. Guyatt GH et al: How to use a treatment recommendation. *JAMA* 1999;**281:**1836–1843.
  XVII. Barratt A et al: How to use guidelines and recommendations about screening. *JAMA* 1999;**281:**2029–2034.

van Crevel H, Habbema JDF, Braakman R: Decision analysis of the management of incidental intracranial saccular aneurysms. *Neurology* 1986;**36:**1335–1339.

Veenstra DL et al: Efficacy of antiseptic-impregnated central venous catheters in preventing catheter-related bloodstream infection. *JAMA* 1999;**281:**261–267.

Ware JE et al: Comparison of health outcomes at a health maintenance organization with those of fee-for-service care. *Lancet* 1986;**1(8488)**:1017–1022.

Ware JE et al: Health Outcomes for Adults in Prepaid and Fee-for-service Systems of Care. The RAND Corporation, 1987.

Ware JE Jr. Conceptualizing and measuring generic health outcomes. *Cancer* 1991;**67**(suppl 3):774–779.

Ware JE Jr, Davies AR. *Monitoring Health Outcomes from the Patients' Point of View: A Primer.* Integrated Therapeutics Group, March 1995.

Ware JE Jr et al. Differences in 4-year outcomes for elderly and poor, chronically ill patients treated in HMO and fee for service systems. *JAMA* 1995;**276:**1039–1047.

Weingarten SR et al. A study of patient satisfaction and adherence to preventive care practice guidelines. *Am J Med* 1995;**99:**590–596.

Weinstein JN: Clinical crossroads: A 45-year-old man with low back pain and a numb left foot. *JAMA* 1998;**280:**730–736.

Wenstrom KD et al: Maternal serum alpha-fetoprotein and dimeric inhibin A detect aneuploidies other than Down syndrome. *Am J Obstet Gynecol* 1998;**179:**966–970.

Willett WC et al: Relative and absolute excess risks of coronary heart disease among women who smoke cigarettes. *N Engl J Med* 1987;**317:**1303–1309.

Wilson IB, Cleary PD. Linking clinical variables with health-related quality of life. *JAMA* 1995;**273:**59–65.

Woolson ST, Watt JM: Intermittent pneumatic compression to prevent proximal deep venous thrombosis during and after total hip replacement. *J Bone Joint Surg* 1991;**73-A:**507–511.

MEDICAL STATISTICS, EPIDEMIOLOGY, DECISION MAKING, & EVIDENCE-BASED MEDICINE

Abramson JH: *Survey Methods in Community Medicine: Epidemiologic Studies,* 5th ed. Churchill-Livingstone, 1999.

Albert DA: Decision theory in medicine: A review and critique. *Millbank Mem Fund Q* 1978;**56**:362–401.

Altman DG: *Practical Statistics for Medical Research.* Chapman & Hall, 1991a.

Altman DG: Statistics in medical journals: Developments in the 1980s. *Stat Med* 1991b;**10**:1897–1913.

Altman DG et al: Review of survival analysis published in cancer journals. *Br J Cancer* 1995;**72**:511–518.

Armitage P: *Statistical Methods in Medical Research,* 2nd ed. Blackwell Scientific, 1987.

Avram M et al: Statistical methods in anesthesia articles: An evaluation of two American journals during two six-month periods. *Anesth Analg* 1985;**64**:604–611.

Bailar JC, Mosteller F (editors): *Medical Uses of Statistics,* 2nd ed. Massachusetts Medical Society, 1992.

Bar-Hillel M: The base-rate fallacy in probability judgments. *Acta Psychol* 1980;**44**:211–233.

Bartko JJ: Rationale for reporting standard deviations rather than standard errors of the mean. *Am J Psychiatry* 1985;**142**:1060.

Berkson J: Limitations of the application of four-fold table analyses to hospital data. *Biometrics Bull* 1946;**2**:47–53.

Breslow NE, Day NE (editors): *Statistical Methods in Cancer Research: Volume I—The Analysis of Case–Control Studies.* Published by the International Agency for Research on Cancer, Lyon, France. Distributed by Oxford University Press. 1993.

Breslow NE, Day NE (editors): *Statistical Methods in Cancer Research: Volume II—The Design and Analysis of Cohort Studies.* Published by the International Agency for Research on Cancer, Lyon, France. Distributed by Oxford University Press. 1987.

Byrt T. How good is that agreement? (Letter to editor) *Epidemiology* 1996;**7**:561.

Chalmers TC: A challenge to clinical investigators. *Gastroenterology* 1969;**57**:631–635.

Clancey WJ, Shortliffe EH: Introduction: Medical artificial intelligence programs. In Clancey WJ, Shortliffe EH (editors): *Readings in Medical Artificial Intelligence,* pp. 1–17. Addison-Wesley, 1984.

Clancy CM, Eisenberg JM: Outcomes research at the Agency for Health Care Policy and Research. *Dis Management Clin Outcomes* 1997;**1**:72–80.

Collett D: *Modelling Survival Data in Medical Research.* Chapman & Hill, 1994.

Colton T: *Statistics in Medicine.* Little, Brown, 1974.

Cox DR: Regression models and life tables. *J R Stat Soc Series B* 1972;**34**:187–220.

Cutler S, Ederer F: Maximum utilization of the lifetable method in analyzing survival. *J Chronic Dis* 1958;**8**:699–712.

Daniel WW. *Biostatistics: A Foundation for Analysis in the Health Sciences,* 7th ed. Wiley, 1998.

Davidoff F: In the teeth of the evidence: The curious case of evidence-based medicine. *Mt Sinai J Med* 1999;**66**:75–83.

DerSimonian R et al: Reporting on methods in clinical trials. *N Engl J Med* 1982;**306**:1332–1337.

Doubilet PM: Statistical techniques for medical decision making: Applications to diagnostic radiology. *Am J Radiol* 1988;**150**:745–750.

Eddy DM: *Clinical Decision Making: From Theory to Practice: A Collection of Essays.* Jones & Bartlett, 1996.

Elveback LR, Guillier CL, Keating FR: Health normality, and the ghost of Gauss. *JAMA* 1970;**211**:69–75.

Emerson JD, Colditz GA: Use of statistical analysis in the *New England Journal of Medicine. N Engl J Med* 1983;**309**:709–713.

Eraker SA et al: To test or not to test—To treat or not to treat. *J Gen Intern Med* 1986;**1**:177–182.

Fagan TJ: Nomogram for Bayes' theorem. *N Engl J Med* 1975;**293**:257.

Feinstein AR: *Clinical Epidemiology: The Architecture of Research.* Saunders, 1985.

Feinstein AR, Sosin DM, Wells CK: The Will Rogers phenomenon. *N Engl J Med* 1985;**312**:1604–1608.

Feltovich PJ, Ford KM, Hoffman RR: *Expertise in Context: Human and Machine.* MIT Press, 1997.

Fisher LD, van Belle G. *Biostatistics: A Methodology for Health Sciences.* Wiley, 1993.

Fleiss JL: *Statistical Methods for Rates and Proportions,* 2nd ed. Wiley, 1981.

Fleiss JL: *Design and Analysis of Clinical Experiments.* Wiley, 1999.

Fletcher RH, Fletcher SW, Wagner EH: *Clinical Epidemiology,* 2nd ed. Williams & Wilkins, 1988.

Freedman LS, Parmar MKB, Baker SG: The design of observer agreement studies with binary assessments. *Stat Med* 1993;**12**:165–179.

Freiman JA et al: The importance of beta, the Type II error and sample size in the design and interpretation of the randomized control trial. *N Engl J Med* 1978;**299**:690–694.

Fromm BS, Snyder VL: Research design and statistical procedures used in the *Journal of Family Practice. J Fam Pract* 1986;**23**:564–566.

Garb JL: *Understanding Medical Research.* Little, Brown, 1996.

Gardner MJ, Altman DG: Confidence intervals rather than *P* values: Estimation rather than hypothesis testing. *Br Med J* 1986;**292**:746–750.

Gardner MJ, Altman DG: *Statistics with confidence. Br Med J,* 1989.

Garfunkle JM: Analysis of statistical analysis. (Editor's column.) *J Pediatr* 1986;**109**:827.

Gillings D, Koch G: The application of the principle of intention-to-treat to the analysis of clinical trials. *Drug Information J* 1991;**25**:411–424.

Glass GV: Integrating findings: The meta-analysis of research. In Shulman LS (editor): *Review of Research in Education.* pp. 351–379, Peacock, 1977.

Glasziou P et al. Applying the results of trials and systematic reviews to individual patients. *ACP J Club* 1998;**129**:A15–A16.

Gordon T et al: Some methodologic problems in the long term study of cardiovascular disease: Observations on the Framingham Study. *J Chronic Dis* 1959;**10**:186–206.

Greenberg RS: Retrospective studies. In Kotz S, Johnson NL (editors): *Encyclopedia of Statistical Sciences,* Vol 8, pp 120–124. Wiley, 1988.

Greenberg RS et al: Prospective studies. In Kotz S, Johnson NL (editors): *Encyclopedia of Statistical Sciences,* Vol 7, pp 315–319. Wiley, 1986.

Greenberg RS, et al: *Medical Epidemiology,* 2nd ed. Appleton & Lange, 1996.

Greenhalgh T: How to read a paper: Papers that report diagnostic or screening tests. *Br Med J* 1997a;**315:**540–543.

Greenhalgh T: *How to Read a Paper: The Basics of Evidence Based Medicine.* BMJ Publishing Group, 1997b.

Griner PF et al: Selection and interpretation of diagnostic tests and procedures. *Ann Intern Med* 1981;**94:**553–600.

Hanley JA, McNeil BJ: A method of comparing the areas under receiver operator characteristic curves derived from the same cases. *Radiology* 1983;**148:**839–843.

Haynes RB et al: More informative abstracts revisited. *Ann Intern Med* 1990;**113:**69–76.

Hershey JC, Cebul RD, Williams SV: The importance of considering single testing when two tests are available. *Med Decis Making* 1987;**7:**212–219.

Hokanson JA, Luttman DJ, Weiss GB: Frequency and diversity of use of statistical techniques in oncology journals. *Cancer Treat Rep* 1986a;**70:**589–594.

Hokanson JA et al: Spectrum and frequency of use of statistical techniques in psychiatric journals. *Am J Psychiatry* 1986b;**143:**1118–1125.

Hokanson JA et al: Statistical techniques reported in pathology journals during 1982–1985. *Arch Pathol Lab Med* 1987a;**111:**202–207.

Hokanson J et al: The reporting of statistical techniques in otolaryngology journals. *Arch Otolaryngol Head Neck Surg* 1987b;**113:**45–50.

Hosmer DW, Lemeshow S: *Applied Logistic Regression.* Wiley, 1989.

Hulley SB, Cummings SR: *Designing Clinical Research.* Williams & Wilkins, 1988.

Ingelfinger JA et al: *Biostatistics in Clinical Medicine,* 3rd ed. Macmillan, 1993.

International Committee of Medical Journal Editors: Uniform requirements for manuscripts submitted to biomedical journals. *Can Med Assoc J* 1988;**138:**321–328.

Kahneman D, Tversky A: On prediction and judgment. *Oregon Res Inst Bull* 1972;**12(4):**1–30.

Kalbfleisch JD, Prentice RL: *The Statistical Analysis of Failure Time Data.* Wiley, 1980.

Kane RL: *Understanding Health Care Outcomes Research.* Aspen Publishers, 1997.

Kassirer JP, Koppelman RI: *Learning Clinical Reasoning.* Lippincott, Williams & Wilkins, 1991.

Kassirer JP et al: Decision analysis: A progress report. *Ann Intern Med* 1987;**106:**270–291.

Katz MH: *Multivariable Analysis: A Practical Guide for Clinicians.* Cambridge University Press, 1999.

Kleinbaum DG. *Logistic Regression: A Self-Learning Text.* Springer, 1994.

Kleinbaum DG. *Survival Analysis: A Self-Learning Text.* Springer, 1996.

L'Abbé KA, Detsky AS, O'Rourke K: Meta-analysis in clinical research. *Ann Intern Med* 1987;**107:**224–233.

Lee ET: *Statistical Methods for Survival Data Analysis,* 2nd ed. Lifetime Learning, 1992.

Lerman J. Study design in clinical research: Sample size estimation and power analysis. *Can J Anaesth* 1996;**43:**184–191.

Locket T: *Evidence-Based and Cost-Effective Medicine for the Uninitiated.* Radcliff Medical Press, 1997.

Marks RG et al: Interactions between statisticians and biomedical journal editors. *Stat Med* 1988;**7:**1003–1011.

Matthews DE, Farewell VT: *Using and Understanding Medical Statistics,* 3rd ed. Karger, 1996.

McMaster University Health Sciences Centre, Department of Clinical Epidemiology and Biostatistics: Clinical disagreement, I: How it occurs and why. *Can Med Assoc J* 1980a;**123:**499–504.

McMaster University Health Sciences Centre, Department of Clinical Epidemiology and Biostatistics: Clinical Disagreement, II: How to avoid it and learn from it. *Can Med Assoc J* 1980b;**123:**613–617.

Moses LE, Emerson JD, Hosseini H: Analyzing data from ordered categories. *N Engl J Med* 1984;**311:**442–448.

Murphy EA: *Biostatistics in Medicine.* Johns Hopkins Press, 1982.

Norman GR, Streiner DL: *PDQ Statistics,* 2nd ed. Decker, 1996.

Pauker SG, Kassirer JP: The threshold approach to clinical decision making. *N Engl J Med* 1980;**302:**1109–1117.

Pauker SG, Kassirer JP: Decision analysis. *N Engl J Med* 1987;**316:**250–258.

Pocock SJ, Hughes MD, Lee RJ: Statistical problems in the reporting of clinical trials. *N Engl J Med* 1987; **317:**426–432.

Raiffa H: *Decision Analysis.* McGraw-Hill, 1997.

Reznick RK, Dawson-Saunders B, Folse JR: A rationale for the teaching of statistics to surgical residents. *Surgery* 1987;**101:**611–617.

Sackett DL: Bias in analytic research. *J Chronic Dis* 1979; **32:**51–63.

Sackett DL, Haynes RB, Tugwell P: *Clinical Epidemiology: A Basic Science for Clinical Medicine,* 2nd ed. Little, Brown, 1991.

Sackett DL et al: *Evidence-Based Medicine.* Churchill-Livingstone, 1998.

Sacks H, Chalmers TC, Smith H: Randomized versus historical controls for clinical trials. *Am J Med* 1982;**72:** 233–240.

Sacks HS et al: Meta-analysis of randomized controlled trials. *N Engl J Med* 1987;**316:**450–455.

Schlesselman JJ. *Case-Control Studies: Design, Conduct, Analysis.* Oxford, 1982.

Simon R: A decade of progress in statistical methodology for clinical trials. *Stat Med* 1991;**10:**1789–1817.

Sokal RR, Rohlf FJ: *Biometry,* 3rd ed. Freeman, 1994.

Solomon DH et al: Techniques to improve physicians' use of diagnostic tests. *JAMA* 1998;**280:**2020–2027.

Sonnenberg FA, Kassirer JP, Kopelman RI: An autopsy of the clinical reasoning process. *Hosp Pract* 1986; **21:**45–56.

Sox HC: Probability theory in the use of diagnostic tests. *Ann Intern Med* 1986;**104:**60–66.

Sox HC et al: *Medical Decision Making.* Butterworth-Heinemann, 1988.

Thompson SG, Pocock SJ: Can meta-analyses be trusted? *Lancet* 1991;**338:**1127–1130.

Weinstein MC et al: *Clinical Decision Analysis.* Saunders, 1980.

Welch GE II, Gabbe SG. Review of statistics usage in the *American Journal of Obstetrics and Gynecology. Am J Obstet Gynecol* 1996;**175:**1138–1141.

Williams JL et al: Lower power, type II errors, and other statistical problems in recent cardiovascular research. *Am J Physiol* 1997;**273**(*Heart Circ Physiol* 42):H487–H493.

Williamson JW, Goldschmidt PG, Colton T: The quality of

medical literature: An analysis of validation assessments. In Bailar JC, Mosteller F (editors): *Medical Uses of Statistics.* Massachusetts Medical Society, 1986.

Zelen M: Guidelines for publishing papers on cancer clinical trials: Responsibilities of editors and authors. *J Clin Oncol* 1983;**1:**164–169.

GENERAL STATISTICS AND MISCELLANEOUS READINGS

Anastasi A: *Psychological Testing,* 7th ed. Macmillan, 1997.

Box GEP: Non-normality and tests on variance. *Biometrika* 1953;**40:**318–335.

Box GEP: Some theorems on quadratic forms applied in the study of the analysis of variance. *Ann Math Stat* 1954; **25:**290–302.

Briscoe MH: *Preparing Scientific Illustrations: A Guide to Better Posters, Presentations, and Publications,* 2nd ed. Springer-Verlag, 1996.

Browne RH: On visual assessment of the significance of a mean difference. *Biometrics* 1979;**35:**657–665.

Chatfield C: *Problem Solving: A Statistician's Guide.* Chapman & Hall, 1988.

Cleveland WS: *The Elements of Graphing Data.* Duxbury Press, 1985.

Cohen J: *Statistical Power Analysis for the Behavioral Sciences,* 2nd ed. Academic Press, 1988.

Conover WJ: *Practical Nonparametric Statistics.* Wiley, 1998.

Conover WJ, Iman RL: Rank transformations as a bridge between parametric and nonparametric statistics. *Am Stat* 1981;**35:**124–129.

Dawson-Saunders B et al: The instruction of biostatistics in medical school. *Am Stat* 1987;**41:**263–266.

Dunn OJ, Clark VA: *Applied Statistics: Analysis of Variance and Regression,* 2nd ed. Wiley, 1987.

Freund JE: *Introduction to Probability.* Dover, 1993.

Gehan EA: A generalized Wilcoxon test for comparing arbitrarily singly-censored samples. *Biometrika* 1965; **52:**15–21.

Glass GV, Stanley JC: *Statistical Methods in Education and Psychology.* Prentice Hall, 1970.

Grizzle JE: Continuity correction in the χ^2-test for 2×2 tables. *Am Stat* 1967;**21:**28–32.

Hays WL: *Statistics for the Social Sciences,* 5th ed. Holt, Rinehart and Winston, 1997.

Hollander M, Wolfe DA. *Nonparametric Statistical Methods,* 2nd ed. Wiley, 1998.

Hotelling H: The selection of variates for use in prediction with some comments on the problem of nuisance parameters. *Ann Math Stat* 1940;**11:**271–283.

Iman RL: Use of a *t*-statistic as an approximation to the exact distribution of the Wilcoxon signed ranks test statistic. *Comm Stat* 1974;**3:**795–806.

Iman RL: Graphs for use with the Lilliefors test for normal and exponential distributions. *Am Stat* 1982;**36:**109–112.

Kirk RE: *Experimental Design: Procedures for the Behavioral Sciences,* 3rd ed. Brooks/Cole, 1995.

Kleinbaum DG et al: *Applied Regression Analysis and Other Multivariable Methods,* 3rd ed. Duxbury Press, 1997.

Levy PS, Lemeshow S: *Sampling of Populations.* Wiley, 1999.

Pedhazur EJ: *Multiple Regression in Behavioral Research,* 3rd ed. Holt, Rinehart and Winston, 1997.

Peto R, Peto J: Asymptotically efficient rank invariant test procedures (with discussion). *J R Stat Soc Series A* 1972; **135:**185–206.

Snedecor GW, Cochran WG. *Statistical Methods,* 8th ed. Iowa State University Press, 1989.

Spirer HF, Spirer L, Jaffe AJ. *Misused Statistics.* Marcel Dekker, 1998.

Stoline MR: The status of multiple comparisons: Simultaneous estimation of all pairwise comparisons in one-way ANOVA designs. *Am Stat* 1981;**35:**134–141.

Tarone RE, Ware J: On distribution-free tests for equality of survival distributions. *Biometrika* 1977;**64:**156–160.

Tukey J: *Exploratory Data Analysis.* Addison-Wesley, 1977.

Wainer H: How to display data badly. *Am Stat* 1984; **38:**137–147.

Wainer H: Understanding graphs and tables. *Educ Researcher* 1992;**21:**14–23.

Walker H: *Studies in the History of Statistical Method.* Williams & Wilkins, 1931.

Yates F: Tests of significance for 2×2 contingency tables. *J R Stat Soc Series A* 1984;**147:**426–463.

SOFTWARE

General Statistical Software

Decision Analysis by TreeAge, Version 3.0.13. TreeAge. Williamstown, MA, 1997.

JMP, Version 3.2.1. SAS Institute Inc. Cary, NC, 1997.

NCSS (Number Cruncher Statistical System), Version 2000. J Hintze. Kaysville, UT, 1999.

SPSS, Version 10.0. SPSS Inc. Chicago, IL, 1999.

SYSTAT, Version 8.0. SPSS Inc. Chicago, IL, 1998.

Power Analysis Programs

nQuery Advisor, Version 3.0. Statistical Solutions. Saugus, MA, 1997.

PASS (Power Analysis and Sample Size), Version 6.0. J Hintze. Kaysville, UT, 1997.

Sample Power, Version 1.0. SPSS Inc. Chicago, IL, 1997.

Programs for Teaching and Conceptualizing Statistics

ConStatS, Version 1 (Conceptual Software for Conceptualizing Statistics). Tufts College. Boston, MA, 1992.

Visual Statistics, Version 1. McGraw-Hill Companies. New York, NY, 1997.

Internet Web Site

The following Web site was established for readers of this book:

http://www.clinicalbiostatistics.com

Appendix A:
Tables

Table A–1. Random numbers.

927415	956121	168117	169280	326569	266541
926937	515107	014658	159944	821115	317592
867169	388342	832261	993050	639410	698969
867169	542747	032683	131188	926198	371071
512500	843384	085361	398488	774767	383837
062454	423050	670884	840940	845839	979662
806702	881309	772977	367506	729850	457758
837815	163631	622143	938278	231305	219737
926839	453853	767825	284716	916182	467113
854813	731620	978100	589512	147694	389180
851595	452454	262448	688990	461777	647487
449353	556695	806050	123754	722070	935916
169116	586865	756231	469281	258737	989450
139470	358095	528858	660128	342072	681203
433775	761861	107191	515960	759056	150336
221922	232624	398839	495004	881970	792001
740207	078048	854928	875559	246288	000144
525873	755998	866034	444933	785944	018016
734185	499711	254256	616625	243045	251938
773112	463857	781983	078184	380752	492215
638951	982155	747821	773030	594005	526828
868888	769341	477611	628714	250645	853454
611034	167642	701316	589251	330456	681722
379290	955292	664549	656401	320855	215201
411257	411484	068629	050150	106933	900095
407167	435509	578642	268724	366564	511815
895893	438644	330273	590506	820439	976891
986683	830515	284065	813310	554920	111395
335421	814351	508062	663801	365001	924418
927660	793888	507773	975109	625175	552278
957559	236000	471608	888683	146821	034687
694904	499959	950969	085327	352611	335924
863016	494926	871064	665892	076333	990558
876958	865769	882966	236535	541645	819783
619813	221175	370697	566925	705564	472934
476626	646911	337167	865652	195448	116729
578292	863854	145858	206557	430943	591126
286553	981699	232269	819656	867825	890737
819064	712344	033613	457019	478176	342104
383035	043025	201591	127424	771948	762990
879392	378486	198814	928028	493486	373709
924020	273258	851781	003514	685749	713570
502523	157212	472643	439301	718562	196269
815316	651530	080430	912635	820240	533626
914984	444954	053723	079387	530020	703312
312248	619263	715357	923412	252522	913950
030964	407872	419563	426527	565215	243717
870561	984049	445361	315827	651925	464440
820157	006091	670091	478357	490641	082559
519649	761345	761354	794613	330132	319843

Table A–2. Areas under the standard normal curve.[a]

z	Area Between −z & +z	Area in Two Tails (< −z & > +z)	Area in One Tail (< −z or > +z)
0.00	0.000	1.000	0.500
0.05	0.040	0.960	0.480
0.10	0.080	0.920	0.460
0.15	0.119	0.881	0.440
0.20	0.159	0.841	0.421
0.25	0.197	0.803	0.401
0.30	0.236	0.764	0.382
0.35	0.274	0.726	0.363
0.40	0.311	0.689	0.345
0.45	0.347	0.653	0.326
0.50	0.383	0.617	0.309
0.55	0.418	0.582	0.291
0.60	0.451	0.549	0.274
0.65	0.484	0.516	0.258
0.70	0.516	0.484	0.242
0.75	0.547	0.453	0.227
0.80	0.576	0.424	0.212
0.85	0.605	0.395	0.198
0.90	0.632	0.368	0.184
0.95	0.658	0.342	0.171
1.00[b]	0.683	0.317	0.159
1.05	0.706	0.294	0.147
1.10	0.729	0.271	0.136
1.15	0.750	0.250	0.125
1.20	0.770	0.230	0.115
1.25	0.789	0.211	0.106
1.28[b]	0.800	0.200	0.100
1.30	0.806	0.194	0.097
1.35	0.823	0.177	0.089
1.40	0.838	0.162	0.081
1.45	0.853	0.147	0.074
1.50	0.866	0.134	0.067
1.55	0.879	0.121	0.061
1.60	0.890	0.110	0.055
1.645[b]	0.900	0.100	0.050
1.65	0.901	0.099	0.049
1.70	0.911	0.089	0.045
1.75	0.920	0.080	0.040
1.80	0.928	0.072	0.036
1.85	0.936	0.064	0.032
1.90	0.943	0.057	0.029
1.95	0.949	0.051	0.026
1.96[b]	0.950	0.050	0.025
2.00	0.954	0.046	0.023
2.05	0.960	0.040	0.020
2.10	0.964	0.036	0.018
2.15	0.968	0.032	0.016
2.20	0.972	0.028	0.014
2.25	0.976	0.024	0.012
2.30	0.979	0.021	0.011
2.326[b]	0.980	0.020	0.010
2.35	0.981	0.019	0.009
2.40	0.984	0.016	0.008
2.45	0.986	0.014	0.007
2.50	0.988	0.012	0.006
2.55	0.989	0.011	0.005
2.575[b]	0.990	0.010	0.005
2.60	0.991	0.009	0.005
2.65	0.992	0.008	0.004
2.70	0.993	0.007	0.003
2.75	0.994	0.006	0.003

(continued)

Table A–2. Areas under the standard normal curve.[a] (continued)

z	Area Between −z & +z	Area in Two Tails (< −z & > +z)	Area in One Tail (< −z or > +z)
2.80	0.995	0.005	0.003
2.85	0.996	0.004	0.002
2.90	0.996	0.004	0.002
2.95	0.997	0.003	0.002
3.00	0.997	0.003	0.001

[a]Adapted and reproduced, with permission, from Table 1 in Pearson ES, Hartley HO (editors): *Biometrika Tables for Statisticians,* 3rd ed, Vol 1. Cambridge University Press, 1966. Used with the kind permission of the Biometrika trustees.
[b]Commonly used values are underlined.

Table A–3. Percentage points or critical values for the *t* distribution corresponding to commonly used areas under the curve.[a]

	Area in 1 Tail				
	0.05	0.025	0.01	0.005	0.0005
	Area in 2 Tails				
Degrees of Freedom	0.10	0.05	0.02	0.01	0.001
1	6.314	12.706	31.821	63.657	636.62
2	2.920	4.303	6.965	9.925	31.598
3	2.353	3.182	4.541	5.841	12.924
4	2.132	2.776	3.747	4.604	8.610
5	2.015	2.571	3.365	4.032	6.869
6	1.943	2.447	3.143	3.707	5.959
7	1.895	2.365	2.998	3.499	5.408
8	1.860	2.306	2.896	3.355	5.041
9	1.833	2.262	2.821	3.250	4.781
10	1.812	2.228	2.764	3.169	4.587
11	1.796	2.201	2.718	3.106	4.437
12	1.782	2.179	2.681	3.055	4.318
13	1.771	2.160	2.650	3.012	4.221
14	1.761	2.145	2.624	2.977	4.140
15	1.753	2.131	2.602	2.947	4.073
16	1.746	2.120	2.583	2.921	4.015
17	1.740	2.110	2.567	2.898	3.965
18	1.734	2.101	2.552	2.878	3.922
19	1.729	2.093	2.539	2.861	3.883
20	1.725	2.086	2.528	2.845	3.850
21	1.721	2.080	2.518	2.831	3.819
22	1.717	2.074	2.508	2.819	3.792
23	1.714	2.069	2.500	2.807	3.767
24	1.711	2.064	2.492	2.797	3.745
25	1.708	2.060	2.485	2.787	3.725
26	1.706	2.056	2.479	2.779	3.707
27	1.703	2.052	2.473	2.771	3.690
28	1.701	2.048	2.467	2.763	3.674
29	1.699	2.045	2.462	2.756	3.659
30	1.697	2.042	2.457	2.750	3.646
40	1.684	2.021	2.423	2.704	3.551
60	1.671	2.000	2.390	2.660	3.460
120	1.658	1.980	2.358	2.617	3.373
∞	1.645	1.960	2.326	2.576	3.291

[a]Adapted and reproduced, with permission, from Table 12 in Pearson ES, Hartley HO (editors): *Biometrika Tables for Statisticians,* 3rd ed, Vol 1. Cambridge University Press, 1966. Used with the kind permission of the Biometrika Trustees.

Table A–4. Percentage points or critical values for the *F* distribution corresponding to areas of 0.05 and 0.01 under the upper tail of the distribution.[a]

Degrees of Freedom, Denominator	Area	Degrees of Freedom, Numerator									
		1	2	3	4	5	6	7	8	9	10
1	0.05	161.4	199.5	215.7	224.6	230.2	234.2	236.8	238.9	240.5	241.9
	0.01	4052	4999.5	5403	5625	5764	5859	5928	5981	6022	6056
2	0.05	18.51	19.00	19.16	19.25	19.30	19.33	19.35	19.37	19.38	19.40
	0.01	98.50	99.00	99.17	99.25	99.30	99.33	99.36	99.37	99.39	99.40
3	0.05	10.13	9.55	9.28	9.12	9.01	8.94	8.89	8.85	8.81	8.79
	0.01	34.12	30.82	29.46	28.71	28.24	27.91	27.67	27.49	27.35	27.23
4	0.05	7.71	6.94	6.59	6.39	6.26	6.16	6.09	6.04	6.00	5.96
	0.01	21.20	18.00	16.69	15.98	15.52	15.21	14.98	14.80	14.66	14.55
5	0.05	6.61	5.79	5.41	5.19	5.05	4.95	4.88	4.82	4.77	4.74
	0.01	16.26	13.27	12.06	11.39	10.97	10.67	10.46	10.29	10.16	10.05
6	0.05	5.99	5.14	4.76	4.53	4.39	4.28	4.21	4.15	4.10	4.06
	0.01	13.75	10.92	9.78	9.15	8.75	8.47	8.26	8.10	7.98	7.87
7	0.05	5.59	4.74	4.35	4.12	3.97	3.87	3.79	3.73	3.68	3.64
	0.01	12.25	9.55	8.45	7.85	7.46	7.19	6.99	6.84	6.72	6.62
8	0.05	5.32	4.46	4.07	3.84	3.69	3.58	3.50	3.44	3.39	3.35
	0.01	11.26	8.65	7.59	7.01	6.63	6.37	6.18	6.03	5.91	5.81
9	0.05	5.12	4.26	3.86	3.63	3.48	3.37	3.29	3.23	3.18	3.14
	0.01	10.56	8.02	6.99	6.42	6.06	5.80	5.61	5.47	5.35	5.26
10	0.05	4.96	4.10	3.71	3.48	3.33	3.22	3.14	3.07	3.02	2.98
	0.01	10.04	7.56	6.55	5.99	5.64	5.39	5.20	5.06	4.94	4.85
12	0.05	4.75	3.89	3.49	3.26	3.11	3.00	2.91	2.85	2.80	2.75
	0.01	9.33	6.93	5.95	5.41	5.06	4.82	4.64	4.50	4.39	4.30
15	0.05	4.54	3.68	3.29	3.06	2.90	2.79	2.71	2.64	2.59	2.54
	0.01	8.68	6.36	5.42	4.89	4.56	4.32	4.14	4.00	3.89	3.80
20	0.05	4.35	3.49	3.10	2.87	2.71	2.60	2.51	2.45	2.39	2.35
	0.01	8.10	5.85	4.94	4.43	4.10	3.87	3.70	3.56	3.46	3.37
24	0.05	4.26	3.40	3.01	2.78	2.62	2.51	2.42	2.36	2.30	2.25
	0.01	7.82	5.61	4.72	4.22	3.90	3.67	3.50	3.36	3.26	3.17
30	0.05	4.17	3.32	2.92	2.69	2.53	2.42	2.33	2.27	2.21	2.16
	0.01	7.56	5.39	4.51	4.02	3.70	3.47	3.30	3.17	3.07	2.98
40	0.05	4.08	3.23	2.84	2.61	2.45	2.34	2.25	2.18	2.12	2.08
	0.01	7.31	5.18	4.31	3.83	3.51	3.29	3.12	2.99	2.89	2.80
60	0.05	4.00	3.15	2.76	2.53	2.37	2.25	2.17	2.10	2.04	1.99
	0.01	7.08	4.98	4.13	3.65	3.34	3.12	2.95	2.82	2.72	2.63
120	0.05	3.92	3.07	2.68	2.45	2.29	2.17	2.09	2.02	1.96	1.91
	0.01	6.85	4.79	3.95	3.48	3.17	2.96	2.79	2.66	2.56	2.47
∞	0.05	3.84	3.00	2.60	2.37	2.21	2.10	2.01	1.94	1.88	1.83
	0.01	6.63	4.61	3.78	3.32	3.02	2.80	2.64	2.51	2.41	2.32

(continued)

Table A–4. Percentage points or critical values for the F distribution corresponding to areas of 0.05 and 0.01 under the upper tail of the distribution.[a] (continued)

Degrees of Freedom, Denominator	Area	Degrees of Freedom, Numerator								
		12	15	20	24	30	40	60	120	∞
1	0.05	243.9	245.9	248.0	249.1	250.1	251.1	252.2	253.3	254.3
	0.01	6106	6157	6209	6235	6261	6287	6313	6339	6366
2	0.05	19.41	19.43	19.45	19.45	19.46	19.47	19.48	19.49	19.50
	0.01	99.42	99.43	99.45	99.46	99.47	99.47	99.48	99.49	99.50
3	0.05	8.74	8.70	8.66	8.64	8.62	8.59	8.57	8.55	8.53
	0.01	27.05	26.87	26.69	26.60	26.50	26.41	26.32	26.22	26.13
4	0.05	5.91	5.86	5.80	5.77	5.75	5.72	5.69	5.66	5.63
	0.01	14.37	14.20	14.02	13.93	13.84	13.75	13.65	13.56	13.46
5	0.05	4.68	4.62	4.56	4.53	4.50	4.46	4.43	4.40	4.36
	0.01	9.89	9.72	9.55	9.47	9.38	9.29	9.20	9.11	9.02
6	0.05	4.00	3.94	3.87	3.84	3.81	3.77	3.74	3.70	3.67
	0.01	7.72	7.56	7.40	7.31	7.23	7.14	7.06	6.97	6.88
7	0.05	3.57	3.51	3.44	3.41	3.38	3.34	3.30	3.27	3.23
	0.01	6.47	6.31	6.16	6.07	5.99	5.91	5.82	5.74	5.65
8	0.05	3.28	3.22	3.15	3.12	3.08	3.04	3.01	2.97	2.93
	0.01	5.67	5.52	5.36	5.28	5.20	5.12	5.03	4.95	4.86
9	0.05	3.07	3.01	2.94	2.90	2.86	2.83	2.79	2.75	2.71
	0.01	5.11	4.96	4.81	4.73	4.65	4.57	4.48	4.40	4.31
10	0.05	2.91	2.85	2.77	2.74	2.70	2.66	2.62	2.58	2.54
	0.01	4.71	4.56	4.41	4.33	4.25	4.17	4.08	4.00	3.91
12	0.05	2.69	2.62	2.54	2.51	2.47	2.43	2.38	2.34	2.30
	0.01	4.16	4.01	3.86	3.78	3.70	3.62	3.54	3.45	3.36
15	0.05	2.48	2.40	2.33	2.29	2.25	2.20	2.16	2.11	2.07
	0.01	3.67	3.52	3.37	3.29	3.21	3.13	3.05	2.96	2.87
20	0.05	2.28	2.20	2.12	2.08	2.04	1.99	1.95	1.90	1.84
	0.01	3.23	3.09	2.94	2.86	2.78	2.69	2.61	2.52	2.42
24	0.05	2.18	2.11	2.03	1.98	1.94	1.89	1.84	1.79	1.73
	0.01	3.03	2.89	2.74	2.66	2.58	2.49	2.40	2.31	2.21
30	0.05	2.09	2.01	1.93	1.89	1.84	1.79	1.74	1.68	1.62
	0.01	2.84	2.70	2.55	2.47	2.39	2.30	2.21	2.11	2.01
40	0.05	2.00	1.92	1.84	1.79	1.74	1.69	1.64	1.58	1.51
	0.01	2.66	2.52	2.37	2.29	2.20	2.11	2.02	1.92	1.80
60	0.05	1.92	1.84	1.75	1.70	1.65	1.59	1.53	1.47	1.39
	0.01	2.50	2.35	2.20	2.12	2.03	1.94	1.84	1.73	1.60
120	0.05	1.83	1.75	1.66	1.61	1.55	1.50	1.43	1.35	1.25
	0.01	2.34	2.19	2.03	1.95	1.86	1.76	1.66	1.53	1.38
∞	0.05	1.75	1.67	1.57	1.52	1.46	1.39	1.32	1.22	1.00
	0.01	2.18	2.04	1.88	1.79	1.70	1.59	1.47	1.32	1.00

[a]Adapted and reproduced, with permission, from Table 18 in Pearson ES, Hartley HO (editors): *Biometrika Tables for Statisticians,* 3rd ed, Vol 1. Cambridge University Press, 1966. Used with the kind permission of the Biometrika Trustees.

Table A–5. Percentage points or critical values for the χ^2 distribution corresponding to commonly used areas under the curve.[a]

Degrees of Freedom	Area in Upper Tail			
	0.10	0.05	0.01	0.001
1	2.706	3.841	6.635	10.828
2	4.605	5.991	9.210	13.816
3	6.251	7.815	11.345	16.266
4	7.779	9.488	13.277	18.467
5	9.236	11.071	15.086	20.515
6	10.645	12.592	16.812	22.458
7	12.017	14.067	18.475	24.322
8	13.362	15.507	20.090	26.125
9	14.684	16.919	21.666	27.877
10	15.987	18.307	23.209	29.588
11	17.275	19.675	24.725	31.264
12	18.549	21.026	26.217	32.909
13	19.812	22.362	27.688	34.528
14	21.064	23.685	29.141	36.123
15	22.307	24.996	30.578	37.697
16	23.542	26.296	32.000	39.252
17	24.769	27.587	33.409	40.790
18	25.989	28.869	34.805	42.312
19	27.204	30.144	36.191	43.820
20	28.412	31.410	37.566	45.315
21	29.615	32.671	38.932	46.797
22	30.813	33.924	40.289	48.268
23	32.007	35.173	41.638	49.728
24	33.196	36.415	42.980	51.179
25	34.382	37.653	44.314	52.620
26	35.563	38.885	45.642	54.052
27	36.741	40.113	46.963	55.476
28	37.916	41.337	48.278	56.892
29	39.088	42.557	49.588	58.302
30	40.256	43.773	50.892	59.703
40	51.805	55.759	63.691	73.402
50	63.167	67.505	76.154	86.661
60	74.397	79.082	88.379	99.607
70	85.527	90.531	100.425	112.317
80	96.578	101.879	112.329	124.839
90	107.565	113.145	124.116	137.208
100	118.498	124.342	135.807	149.449

[a]Adapted and reproduced, with permission, from Table 8 in Pearson ES, Hartley HO (editors): *Biometrika Tables for Statisticians,* 3rd ed, Vol 1. Cambridge University Press, 1966. Used with the kind permission of the Biometrika Trustees.

Table A–6. z Transformation[a] of the correlation coefficient.[b]

r	z	r	z
0.00	0.000	0.50	0.549
0.01	0.010	0.51	0.563
0.02	0.020	0.52	0.576
0.03	0.030	0.53	0.590
0.04	0.040	0.54	0.604
0.05	0.050	0.55	0.618
0.06	0.060	0.56	0.633
0.07	0.070	0.57	0.648
0.08	0.080	0.58	0.663
0.09	0.090	0.59	0.678
0.10	0.100	0.60	0.693
0.11	0.110	0.61	0.709
0.12	0.121	0.62	0.725
0.13	0.131	0.63	0.741
0.14	0.141	0.64	0.758
0.15	0.151	0.65	0.775
0.16	0.161	0.66	0.793
0.17	0.172	0.67	0.811
0.18	0.182	0.68	0.829
0.19	0.192	0.69	0.848
0.20	0.203	0.70	0.867
0.21	0.213	0.71	0.887
0.22	0.224	0.72	0.908
0.23	0.234	0.73	0.929
0.24	0.245	0.74	0.951
0.25	0.255	0.75	0.973
0.26	0.266	0.76	0.996
0.27	0.277	0.77	1.020
0.28	0.288	0.78	1.045
0.29	0.299	0.79	1.071
0.30	0.310	0.80	1.099
0.31	0.321	0.81	1.127
0.32	0.332	0.82	1.157
0.33	0.343	0.83	1.188
0.34	0.354	0.84	1.221
0.35	0.365	0.85	1.256
0.36	0.377	0.86	1.293
0.37	0.388	0.87	1.333
0.38	0.400	0.88	1.376
0.39	0.412	0.89	1.422
0.40	0.424	0.90	1.472
0.41	0.436	0.91	1.528
0.42	0.448	0.92	1.589
0.43	0.460	0.93	1.658
0.44	0.472	0.94	1.738
0.45	0.485	0.95	1.832
0.46	0.497	0.96	1.946
0.47	0.510	0.97	2.092
0.48	0.523	0.98	2.298
0.49	0.536	0.99	2.647

[a]$z = 1/2\{\ln[(1 + r)/(1 - r)]\}$.

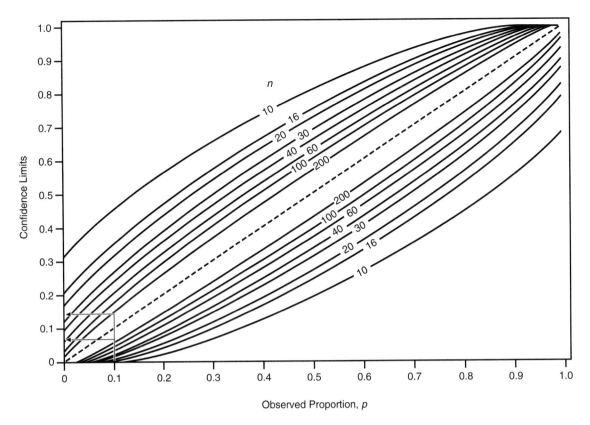

Figure A–1. 95% Confidence intervals for population proportion. (Adapted and reproduced, with permission, from Pearson ES, Hartley HO (editors): *Biometrika Tables for Statisticians,* 3rd ed., Vol. 1. Cambridge University Press, 1966.)

Appendix B: Answers to Exercises

CHAPTER 2

1. This is a classic example of a crossover clinical trial in which patients receive one treatment and then cross over to the second treatment. See Figure B–1 for an illustration of how the authors described the study decision.

2. This study looks at the rate of seroconversion among adult providers who were negative at the beginning of the study; therefore it qualifies as a cohort study. It is based on only six centers, however, and the results should be accepted with caution because of the wide variability among centers.

3. This article examines cross-sectional information collected at the same time; because no specific mention is made of quantitatively combining results across studies, we classify it simply as a review and not as a meta-analysis.

4. The study is observational and evaluates the history of patients with the symptoms and persons without the symptoms to identify possible exposure or risk factors; therefore, it is a classic case–control study.

5. Because a treatment, sugar and providone-iodine, was used, the study qualifies as a clinical trial. The controls were concurrent; that is, the standard therapy and the treatment with sugar and providone-iodine were evaluated during the same time. There is no indication that the patients were randomly assigned to treatment and standard therapy; thus, the study is a nonrandomized clinical trial.

6. The group of subjects was identified and initial data collection occurred in 1976; the same subjects were followed up in future years. The study design is therefore best described as a cohort or prospective study to identify risk factors.

7. This study begins with patients with acute nonvariceal upper gastrointestinal tract bleeding and control subjects and examines their histories for information on nonsteroidal antiinflammatory drug use—a typical case–control study.

8. This study evaluates a group of patients who were referred to these investigators. It sounds like they took all patients and examined the diagnosis closely. There are no controls, and there doesn't appear to be any follow-up through time. We therefore classify this as a case–series.

9. The best design is cohort study, which follows a group of subjects over time to see whether bile supersaturation with cholesterol increases as they grow older; however, this study design would take several years to complete. To avoid the extended time period, these investigators collected data on cholesterol saturation levels and ages of a group of healthy subjects at one point and examined the relationship between these two factors—a typical cross-sectional study.

10. Several study designs are possible, but the most realistic is an observational study. A case–control study provides information faster, but several case–control studies are required; a group of cases for each cause of death and type of cardiovascular morbidity needs to be identified. A cohort study is the best study design and actually was performed by Ulrich and colleagues (1991). We suggest you obtain a copy of this study and read and discuss the pros and cons of how the study was done.

CHAPTER 3

1.
$$\sum \frac{(X - \overline{X})}{n} = \frac{\Sigma X}{n} - \frac{\Sigma \overline{X}}{n}$$
$$= \overline{X} - \frac{n\overline{X}}{n}$$
$$= \overline{X} - \overline{X} = 0$$

2. The lower norm is the value represented by the 14.5th person [580 subjects $\times$ 0.025 (the 2½ percentile) = 14.5]. The upper norm is the value represented by the 565.5th subject [580 $\times$ 0.975 (the 97½ percentile) = 565.5]. We generated a stem-and-leaf plot and then counted in from both ends to obtain approximately 12 for the lower norm and 103 for the upper norm. Alternatively, you might generate a frequency distribution and find the values defined by the 2½ and 97½ per-

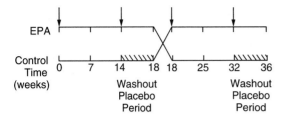

EPA

Control
Time
(weeks)

0   7   14   18 18   25   32   36

Washout
Placebo
Period

Washout
Placebo
Period

Figure B–1. Illustration of study design (Adapted and reproduced, with permission, from Kremer JM et al: Fish-oil fatty acid supplementation in active rheumatoid arthritis: A double-blinded, controlled, crossover study. *Ann Intern Med* 1987;**106:**497–503.)

centiles. These values differ only slightly from the values of 12.8 and 103.5 published by the authors; the discrepancy is due to interpolation by the authors.

3. The mean age for the 490 patients must be estimated using the weighted means formula. It is found by multiplying the midpoint of each age interval by the count:

$$(52 \times 15.5) + (162 \times 25.5) + (144 \times 35.5) + (78 \times 45.5)$$
$$+ (20 \times 55.5) + (23 \times 65.5) + (11 \times 75.5) = 34.8$$

The mean heart rate variation is estimated by multiplying the count by the mean in each age group:

$$(52 \times 63.0) + (162 \times 57.6) + (144 \times 51.1) + (78 \times 39.6)$$
$$+ (20 \times 34.0) + (23 \times 29.1) + (11 \times 16.8) = 50.2$$

The means calculated from the raw data are 34.5 years and 50.2 heart rate variation. The heart rate variation is a very good estimate because the means in each age group are used. The age is a good estimate because this table follows the rules for good frequency construction by choosing class limits so that most of the observations in the class are closer to the midpoint of the class than to either end of the class.

4. **a.** $10 - 7 - 5 + 3 = 1$; therefore, the deviation for patient 5 is -1, because $\Sigma(X - \overline{X}) = 0$.

    b. 50, 33, 35, 43, 39.

5. **a.** Bimodal with one peak in the early 20s and with a smaller peak in the 40s and 50s.

    b. Skewed positively, with many physicians delivering 30–60 babies (family or general practitioners) and fewer delivering 200–250 (obstetricians); the distribution might also be bimodal with one mode at 50 babies and another at 225.

    c. Probably bell-shaped, with a few hospitals referring a very small number of patients and a few referring a very large number of patients, but with the majority referring moderate numbers of patients.

6. See Figure B–2.

7.
$$SD = \sqrt{\frac{\Sigma X^2 - [(\Sigma X)^2/n]}{n-1}}$$
$$= \sqrt{\frac{52,461.14 - [(877.80)^2/18]}{18-1}}$$
$$= \sqrt{567.87} = 23.83$$

8. **a.** Both measures are numerical, and the desire

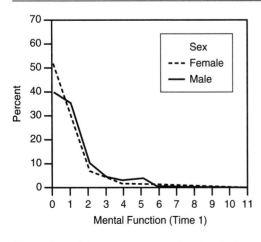

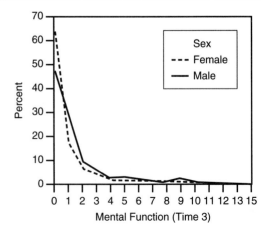

Figure B–2. A larger percentage of women had very low scores at both times, but, overall, the distributions are very similar. Both men and women had higher scores at time 3. (Data, used with permission, from Hébert R et al: Incidence of functional decline and improvement in a community-dwelling very elderly population. *Am J Epidemiol* 1997;**145:**935–944. Graphs produced using SPSS, used by permission.)

is to exhibit the relationship between them; therefore, a scatterplot with neutrophil leukotriene B_4 production on the X-axis and number of tender joints on the Y-axis is appropriate.

b. A reasonable approach in a problem like this is to illustrate the distribution of cases across time with a histogram for each subset of patients. In this study, the authors drew three histograms: for patients with self-limited illness, patients with subsequent neuromuscular illness, and patients with intermediate illness. Figure B–3 reproduces the authors' figure. Note that time is displayed along the X-axis and the number of patients along the Y-axis.

c. The table presented in Bartle and colleagues (1986) is reproduced here in Table B–1. This table clearly communicates the information.

9. a. Salaries probably do not follow a bell-shaped curve; they tend to have a positive skew, with a few physicians making relatively larger salaries. The median and either the range or the interquartile range are therefore best.

b. Standardized ability and achievement tests administered to large numbers of examinees tend to follow a bell-shaped curve; therefore, the mean and the standard deviation are appropriate.

c. A bell-shaped distribution is a reasonable assumption, so the mean and the standard deviation are used.

d. The number of tender joints probably has a positively skewed distribution, so the median and the range or interquartile range are appropriate.

e. Presence of diarrhea either occurs or does not; therefore, this is a nominal characteristic, and proportions or percentages are correct.

f. This ordinal scale calls for the use of the median and the range; alternatively, proportions or percentages may be used.

g. Somewhat negatively skewed, with the majority of females developing the disease at

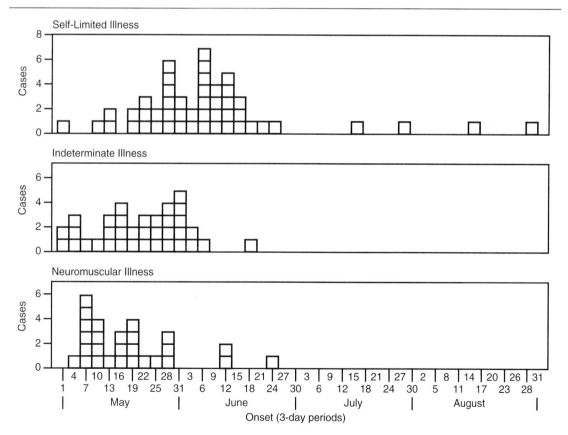

Figure B–3. Histogram illustrating onset and progression of disease. (Adapted and reproduced, with permission, from Kilbourne EM et al: Clinical epidemiology of toxic-oil syndrome: Manifestations of a new illness. *N Engl J Med* 1983;**309**:1408–1414.)

Table B–1. Patients in nonsteroidal antiinflammatory drug use group.

	Number of Subjects	Number of Patients Taking Acetylsalicylic Acid	Number of Patients Taking Nonacetylsalicylic Acid NSAID	Total	
				Number	(Percent)
AUGIB group	57	14	10	24	(42.1)[a]
Control group	123	16	7	23	(18.1)

Abbreviation: AUGIB = acute upper GI bleeding.
[a] χ^2 equals 11.05, $P < 0.005$.
Source: Reproduced, with permission, from Table 1 in Bartle WR, Gupta AK, Lazor J: Nonsteroidal anti-inflammatory drugs and gastrointestinal bleeding. *Arch Intern Med* 1986;**146**:2365–2367.

ages 50–70 years, so the median and range are appropriate.

   h. Assuming compliance is fairly good, the distribution has a positive skew, with most patients having a low pill count, and the median and range may be used.

10. The rate of coronary heart disease (CHD) increases with age, regardless of cigarettes per day. The rate of CHD also increases with number of cigarettes per day in women age 40 years or more; in women age 30 to 39 years, the relationship between rate of CHD and number of cigarettes per day is inconsistent.

11. The mean heart rate variation appears to become smaller as subjects age. A correlation is best for measuring the relationship between two numerical measures; the correlation between age and heart rate variation is −0.45.

12. A correlation of −0.45 indicates a negative relationship between age and heart rate variation: As subjects get older, their heart rate variation decreases. A correlation of this magnitude indicates a fair degree of relationship, and it indicates that having norms for each age group is a good idea if the number of subjects is sufficient. Unfortunately, the number of subjects in each age group is not large enough to permit the calculation of age-adjusted norms.

13. a. Approximately 25 lb, or 11.5 kg.
    b. Approximately 18.5 in., or 42 cm.
    c. Approximately 13 lb, or 6 kg.

14. The coefficient of variation for men is 10.75/7.27, or 147.9%; for women it is 7.22/6.11, or 118.2%. Therefore, in this small sample, men had more variability in their red blood cell counts than did women.

15. a. The risk ratio using person-years of observation is

$$RR = \frac{139/54,560.0}{239/54,355.7}$$
$$= \frac{0.0025}{0.0044} = 0.579$$

The risk ratio for person-years is similar in

size to the value based on subjects because both the aspirin and control groups were observed for similar periods of time. They differ if one group is followed for a substantially longer period than the other.

   b. This statistical adjustment (described in Chapters 8 and 10) controls for differences in age and use of beta-carotene in the aspirin and control groups by calculating the value of the relative risk that would occur if no differences existed.

   c. It is possible to speculate that the subjects in this study, all physicians who agreed to participate in the study, are more health-conscious than the general public. If so, the effects of aspirin and beta-carotene, when added to the already healthy life-style factors, might have a smaller incremental effect than in the general population.

16. The odds that a person with a stroke abuses drugs are

$$\frac{(73/214)}{(141/214)} = \frac{73}{141}$$
$$= 0.518$$

The odds that a person without a stroke abuses drugs are

$$\frac{(18/214)}{(196/214)} = \frac{18}{196} = 0.092$$

Therefore, the odds ratio is 0.518/0.092 = 5.64; that is, a person in this study who abuses drugs is more than five times more likely to have a stroke.

17. a. The purpose of the study was to learn about acute effects of acetylsalicylic acid (ASA) on the gastroduodenal mucosa in young and old healthy men.

   b. The study design was an experiment because a manipulation was made, and each subject was used as his own control; therefore, it is a self-controlled clinical trial.

   c. Two groups were used because part of the

purpose was to determine if differences existed between young and old men.

d. Figure 1 in Moore et al (1991) indicates that a dose-response relationship exists between the total number of lesions observed on endoscopic study: The smallest number was observed under the placebo condition, and the largest number when subjects received 1300 mg aspirin. The long whiskers and dots representing the extreme values when subjects received 1300 mg aspirin show that considerable variability exists between subjects in the total number of lesions observed.

e. Figure 2 in Moore et al (1991) indicates that significantly more variability occurs between subjects at the higher ranges of pH values than at the lower ranges. The figure legend points out that the median or middle value for three of the plots is at the very bottom of the plot; this means that half of the men had pH values under 1.0.

CHAPTER 4

1. **a.** To show that gender and blood type are independent, we must show that

$$P(A) \, P(B) = P(A \text{ and } B)$$

for each cell in the table:

$$0.42 \times 0.50 = 0.21$$
$$0.43 \times 0.50 = 0.215$$
$$0.11 \times 0.50 = 0.055$$
$$0.04 \times 0.50 = 0.02$$

b.
$$P(\text{male and type O}) = P(\text{male} \mid \text{type O}) \times P(\text{type O})$$
$$= \frac{0.21}{0.42} \times \frac{0.42}{1.00}$$
$$= (0.50) \times (0.42) = 0.21$$

This demonstrates that $P(\text{male} \mid \text{type O}) = P(\text{male})$ when these are independent.

2. Assuming 47 patients were in the study,

a.
$$P(\text{chronic}) = \frac{7 + 8 + 2}{47}$$
$$= 0.36$$

b.
$$P(\text{acute}) = \frac{6 + 2 + 2}{47} = 0.21$$

c.
$$P(\text{acute} \mid \text{seroconvert}) = \frac{2}{18} = 0.11$$

d.
$$P(\text{seropositive} \mid \text{died}) = \frac{2}{8} = 0.25$$

e.
$$P(\text{seronegative}) = \frac{17}{47} = 0.36$$

Using the binomial distribution, we get

$$P(4 \text{ out of } 8) = \frac{8!}{4!\,4!}(0.36)^4(0.64)^4$$
$$= \frac{40,320}{(24)(24)}(0.0168)(0.1678)$$
$$= 0.1973, \text{ or } 0.20$$

3. **a.**
$$P(\text{sepsis at only site}) = \frac{66}{150}$$
$$= 0.44$$

b. $P(\text{sepsis at one of the sites}) = \dfrac{66 + 36}{150}$
$$= 0.68$$

c. $(78/150)\,(120/150)\,(150) = (0.52)\,(0.80)\,(150)$
$$= 62.4$$

4. Use the binomial distribution.
   a. $P(\text{infection}) = 0.30$

$$P(1 \text{ infection in 8 patients}) = \frac{8!}{1!\,7!}(0.30)^1(0.70)^7$$
$$= 8(0.30)\,(0.0824)$$
$$= 0.1977, \text{ or } 0.20$$

b.
$P(\text{survival}) = 0.80$

$P\left(\begin{array}{c}7 \text{ survivals} \\ \text{in 8 patients}\end{array}\right) = \dfrac{8!}{7!\,1!}(0.80)^7(0.20)^1$
$$= 8(0.2097)\,(.020) = 0.3355, \text{ or } 0.34$$

5. $\lambda = 1487/390 = 3.81$. The probability of exactly five hospitalizations is

$$P(X = 5) = (3.81^5)\,\frac{e^{-3.81}}{5!}$$
$$= \frac{(802.83)(0.022)}{120} = 0.147$$

6. **a.** The probability that a normal healthy adult has a serum sodium above 147 mEq/L is $P(z > 2) = 0.023$.
   b. $P[z < (130 - 141)/3] = P(z < -3.67) < 0.001$

   c.
   $$P\left[\frac{132 - 141}{3} < z < \frac{150 - 141}{3}\right]$$
   $$= P(-3 < z < +3) = 0.997$$

   d. The top 1% of the standard normal distribution is found at $z = 2.326$; therefore, $2.326 = (X - 141)/3$, or $X = 147.98$. So a serum sodium level of approximately 148 mEq/L puts a patient in the upper 1% of the distribution.

e. The bottom 10% of the standard normal distribution is found at $z = -1.28$; therefore, $-1.28 = (X - 141)/3$, or $X = 137.16$. So a serum sodium level of approximately 137 mEq/L puts a patient in the lower 10% of the distribution.

7. The distributions are given in Table B–2. Thus,

$$P(X = 4 \text{ when } \pi = 0.3) = \left[\frac{6!}{(4! \times 2!)} \right] (0.3)^4 (0.7)^2$$

$$= \left[\frac{720}{(24 \times 2)} \right] (0.008)(0.49)$$

$$= 0.060$$

Graphs of the preceding distributions illustrate that the binomial distribution is quite skewed when the proportion is 0.1 (as well as when the proportion is close to 1.0, such as 0.9 and 0.8). When the proportion is near 0.5, the distribution is nearly symmetric—perfectly so at 0.5.

8. a.

$$\text{Mean number of months} = \frac{(12 + 13 + 14 + 15 + 16)}{5}$$

$$= \frac{70}{5} = 14.0$$

and the standard deviation is

$$\sqrt{\frac{(12 - 14)^2 + (13 - 14)^2 + (14 - 14)^2 + (15 - 14)^2 + (16 - 14)^2}{5}} = 1.41$$

(Note that the standard deviation uses 5 in the denominator instead of 4 because we are assuming that these 5 observations make up the entire population.)

Table B–2. Binomial distributions for different values of the parameter, π.

Probability	$\pi = 0.1$	$\pi = 0.3$	$\pi = 0.5$
$P(X = 0)$	0.531	0.118	0.016
$P(X = 1)$	0.354	0.303	0.094
$P(X = 2)$	0.098	0.324	0.234
$P(X = 3)$	0.015	0.185	0.313
$P(X = 4)$	0.001	0.060	0.234
$P(X = 5)$	<0.001	0.010	0.094
$P(X = 6)$	<0.001	0.001	0.016

b.

$$\text{The mean of the mean number of months} = \frac{(12 + 12.5 + \cdots + 15.5 + 16)}{25}$$

$$= \frac{350}{5} = 14.0$$

and the standard deviation of the mean (or the standard error of the mean, SE) is

$$\sqrt{\frac{(12 - 14)^2 + (12.5 - 14)^2 + \cdots + (15.5 - 14)^2 + (16 - 14)^2}{25}} = 1.0$$

Note that the mean of the means found in part b is the same as the mean found in part a, and the SE is the same as

$$\frac{\sigma}{\sqrt{n}} = \frac{1.41}{\sqrt{2}}$$

$$= 1.0$$

9. a. This question refers to individuals and is equivalent to asking what proportion of the area under the curve is greater than $(103 - 100)/3 = +1.00$ and less than $(97 - 100)/3 = -1.00$, using the z distribution; the area is 0.317, or 31.7%, from Table A–2.

b. This question concerns means. The standard error with $n = 36$ is $3/6 = 0.5$. The critical ratio for a mean equal to 99 is $(99 - 100)/0.5 = -2.00$ and for 101 is $+2.00$. The area below -2.00 and above $+2.00$ is 0.046; therefore, 4.6% of the *means* are outside the limits of 99 and 101.

10. a. The standard deviation is

$$\sqrt{n}(SE) = \sqrt{131} \,(6.2)$$

$$= (11.45)(6.2) = 71.0$$

Then the probability that a patient is intoxicated more than 102 times per year is

$$P(X > 102) = P\left[z > \frac{(102 - 61.6)}{71} \right]$$

$$= P(z > 0.567)$$

From Table A–2, the $P(z > 0.55)$ is 0.291, so we know the probability is slightly less.

b. From Table A–2, the value of z that separates the upper 5% of the distribution from the lower 95% is 1.645. We need to find X so that

$$P[(X - \mu)/\sigma > 1.645] = 0.05$$

Solving for X gives $X = (1.645 \times 71.0) + 61.6 = 178.4$, or approximately 179 times a year.

CHAPTER 5

1. **a.** Wider.
   b. Increase the sample size to obtain a narrower confidence interval.
   c. Narrower.
2. The P value is listed as 0.000. It is customary, however, to report such a P value as $P < 0.001$; computer programs typically print out only three decimal places and the probability would be given as greater than 0 were it not for this limitation. The 95% confidence interval does not contain zero, so we know the P value is <0.05. We can request a 99.9% confidence interval if we want more precision, as illustrated in the lower part of Table B–3, produced using SYSTAT.
3. The two-tailed z value for α of 0.05 is ± 1.96, and the lower one-tailed z value related to $\beta = 0.80$ is approximately -0.84. With a standard deviation of 3 and a 2-oz difference, the sample size is approximately 18. This is much less than the sample needed to find a 1-oz difference.

$$n = \left\{ \frac{[1.96 - (-0.84)]\, 3}{2} \right\}^2$$
$$= \left[\frac{(1.96 + 0.84)\, 3}{2} \right]^2$$
$$= \left(\frac{8.40}{2} \right)^2 = 17.64, \text{ or } 18$$

4. If we assume 20% instead of 30% as the norm and want to detect a difference between 10% observed in the study and the norm, we need a sample of 108. The number of patients needed to detect a difference between 10% and an assumed norm of 30% was 34, so a larger sample is needed when the difference is smaller.

$$n = \left[\frac{1.96\sqrt{0.20 \times 0.80} - (-0.84)\sqrt{0.10 \times 0.90}}{0.20 - 0.10} \right]^2$$
$$= \left(\frac{1.036}{0.10} \right)^2$$
$$= 10.36^2 = 107.33, \text{ or } 108$$

Table B–3. Hypothesis test and confidence interval for mean soda consumption among 2-year-old children.

Data for the following results were selected according to:
(AGE2_5 = 2) / COMPLETE
One-sample t test of SODA with 94 cases; H_0: Mean = 0.000

Mean = 1.167	95.00% CI = 0.865 to 1.469
SD = 1.473	t = 7.679
df = 93	Probability = 0.000
	99.90% CI = 0.651 to 1.683

Source: Dennison BA et al: Excess fruit juice consumption by preschool-aged children is associated with short stature and obesity. *Pediatrics* 1997;**99**:15–22. Table produced with SYSTAT, used with permission.

5. Our power calculations assumed $SD = 3$ oz, and Dennison and coworkers (1997) had an SD of 4.77. This illustrates the role of the standard deviation in finding the sample size.

6.
$$n = \left[\frac{(z_\alpha - z_\beta)\, \sigma}{\mu_1 - \mu_0} \right]^2$$
$$\text{or } 10 = \left\{ \frac{[1.96 - (-0.84)]\, 2.1}{X} \right\}^2$$
$$= \left[\frac{(2.8)\, 2.1}{X} \right]^2$$
$$= \left(\frac{5.88}{X} \right)^2 \text{ or } 10 = \frac{35}{X^2}$$

Solving for X:
$$X^2 = \frac{35}{10} = 3.5$$
$$\text{and } X = \sqrt{3.5} = 1.87$$

7. See Table B–4.
   They agree by chance that $30/50 = 60\% \times 35/50 = 70\%$ or 42% were positive and $40\% \times 30\%$ or 12% were negative, for a total of 54% of the mammograms. They actually agreed on $25 + 10$ or 35 of 50, or 70%.

$$\kappa = \left(\frac{\text{Observed} - \text{Expected agreement}}{1 - \text{Expected agreement}} \right)$$
$$= \frac{0.70 - 0.54}{1 - 0.54}$$
$$= \frac{0.16}{0.46} = 0.348$$

8. **a.** A histogram using NCSS is reproduced in Figure B–4 and indicates that the distribution is fairly normal, so we will proceed with the t test.
   b. Selected output from the NCSS procedure for the paired t test is reproduced in Table B–5. Note that the mean in the one-sample test is the same as the mean difference in the paired t test, as the t Value and the Probability Level. The two approaches therefore give identical results.
9. **a.** A histogram of the change in depression scores in Figure B–5 shows a fairly normal distribution, so it is appropriate to use the paired t test to learn if the change is significantly different from zero.

Table B–4. Classification of a sample of 50 mammograms by two physicians.

	Physician 2		
Physician 1	**Negative**	**Positive**	
Negative	25	5	30
Positive	10	10	20
	35	15	50

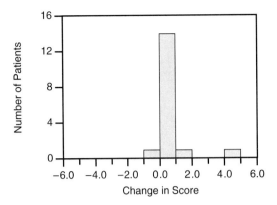

Figure B–4. Staff support in neutral-film group. (Data, used with permission, from Gelkopf M, Sigal M, Kramer R: Therapeutic use of humor to improve social support in an institutionalized schizophrenic inpatient community. *J Soc Psychol* 1994;**134(2)**:175–182. Analyzed with NCSS 97, a registered trademark of the Number Cruncher Statistical System; used with permission.)

    b. The McNemar statistic indicates no change in the proportion of people who were depressed. See Table B–6.

    c. Both the paired *t* test and the McNemar test lead to the same conclusion.

10. a. The distribution of ounces is skewed to the right (see Figure B–6). A nonparametric procedure is therefore recommended.

    b. Selected output from the NCSS One-Sample *t* Test is reproduced in Table B–7. The observed value of the *t* test is 9.7483 with a *P* value of 0.000 (although we know the value should be reported as *P* < 0.001), and the decision is to reject the null hypothesis that the mean daily juice consumption in 5-year-old children is equal to zero. The probability for the sign test is also given as 0.000; thus, in this example, the two procedures lead to the same conclusion.

    c. The box plots in Figure B–7 show that the distribution of juice consumption is slightly less among 5-year-olds. It does not appear to be a lot less, however. Exercise 14 in Chapter 6 asks you to perform the statistical test to compare the two groups of children.

CHAPTER 6

1. The critical value of *t* is smaller, 2.01, and the standard error must be recalculated. The 95% confidence interval is

$$-19.15 \pm (2.01) (42.38) \sqrt{\frac{1}{25} + \frac{1}{25}} = -19.15 \pm 24.09$$

or −43.24 to 4.94

Table B–5. Equivalence of results from paired *t* test and one-sample *t* test on differences in number of staff rated as supportive.

Variable	Count	Mean	Standard Deviation	Standard Error	95% Lower Confidence Limit of Mean	95% Upper Confidence Limit of Mean
STAF_PST	17	0.9411765	1.43486	0.3480047	0.2034395	1.678913
STAF_PRE	17	0.7058824	1.159995	0.2813401	0.109468	1.302297
Difference	17	0.2352941	1.032558	0.2504322	−0.2955983	0.7661865

t Test for Difference between Means Section

Alternative Hypothesis	t Value	Probability Level	Decision (5%)
STAF_PST-STAF_PRE<>0	0.9396	0.361416	Accept H₀

Variable	Count	Mean	Standard Deviation	Standard Error	95% Lower Confidence Limit of Mean	95% Upper Confidence Limit of Mean
staffdiff	17	1.032558 0.7661865	0.2504322	0.2352941 −0.2955983		

t Test for Difference between Mean and Value Section

Alternative Hypothesis	t Value	Probability Level	Decision (5%)
staffdiff<>0	0.9396	0.361416	Accept H₀

Source: Data used, with permission, from Gelkopf M, Sigal M, Kramer R: Therapeutic use of humor to improve social support in an institutionalized schizophrenic inpatient community. *J Soc Psychol* 1994;**134(2)**:175–182. Output produced with NCSS; used with permission.

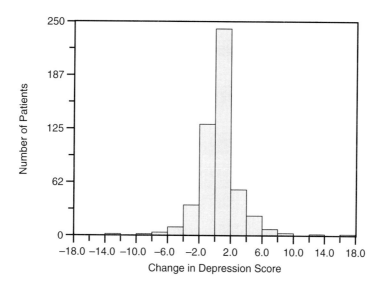

Figure B–5. Histogram of depression score changes. (Data, used with permission, from Henderson AS et al: The course of depression in the elderly: A longitudinal community-based study in Australia. *Psychol Med* 1997;**27**:119–129. Output produced using NCSS; used with permission.)

Table B–6. Equivalence of results from paired *t* test on the mean difference and the McNemar test for paired proportions of number of depressive symptoms.

Descriptive Statistics Section

Variable	Count	Mean	Standard Deviation	95% Lower Confidence Limit of Mean	95% Upper Confidence Limit of Mean
DPSCALE2	517	1.862669	2.514011	1.645964	2.079375
DPSCALE1	517	1.814313	2.156734	1.628405	2.000222
Difference	517	0.0483559	2.505726	−0.1676355	0.264347
t for Confidence Limits = 1.9600					

t Test for Difference between Means Section

Alternative Hypothesis	*t* Value	Probability Level	Decision
DPSCALE2–DPSCALE1<>0	0.4388	0.660994	Accept H_0

Counts Section

Depressed at Time 1	Depressed at Time 2		
	No	Yes	Total
No	486	15	501
Yes	14	2	16
Total	500	17	517

Chi-Square Statistics Section

McNemar's test statistic	0.034483
McNemar's degrees of freedom	1.000000
McNemar's probability level	0.852684
WARNING: At least one cell had an expected value less than 5.	

Source: Data, used with permission, from Henderson AS et al: The course of depression in the elderly: A longitudinal community-based study in Australia. *Psychol Med* 1997;**27**:119–129. Table produced using NCSS; used with permission.

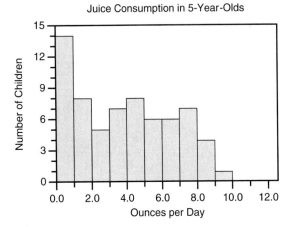

Figure B–6. Juice consumption in 5-year-olds. (Data, used with permission, from Dennison BA et al: Excess fruit juice consumption by preschool-aged children is associated with short stature and obesity. *Pediatrics* 1997; **99**:15–22. Output produced using NCSS; used with permission.)

This confidence interval is wider than the one in Section 6.2 and now contains zero. We therefore conclude that no difference exists in operating room times if only 25 women were in each group.

2. $SD_p = \sqrt{\dfrac{(45 - 1)(28.11)^2 + (39 - 1)(28.45)^2}{45 + 39 - 2}}$

       $= 28.27$

3. **a.** The group with DI < 10 and the group with DI ≥ 10 are two independent groups. A confidence interval for the difference in Barthel

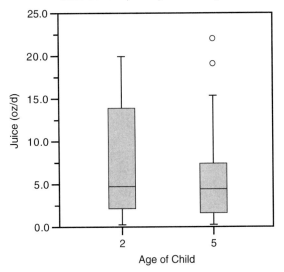

Figure B–7. Juice consumption by 2- and 5-year-olds. (Data, used with permission, from Dennison BA et al: Excess fruit juice consumption by preschool-aged children is associated with short stature and obesity. *Pediatrics* 1997;**99**:15–22. Output produced using NCSS; used with permission.)

Index therefore uses degrees of freedom equal to the sum of the sample sizes minus 2. Table B–8 shows the output from NCSS.

Because the interval contains zero, it is possible that the difference is zero and thus that the two groups do not differ on BI at discharge.

b. Answering this question requires us to look

Table B–7. Equivalence of results from *t* test and sign test for juice consumption in 5-year-old children.

Variable	Count	Mean	Standard Deviation	Standard Error	95% Lower Confidence Limit of Mean	95% Upper Confidence Limit of Mean
JUICE	74	4.968	4.384	0.510	3.952	5.984

Tests of Assumptions Section

Assumption	Value	Probability	Decision (5%)
Skewness Normality	4.4035	0.000011	Reject normality
Kurtosis Normality	3.2358	0.001213	Reject normality
Omnibus Normality	29.8610	0.000000	Reject normality

***t* Test for Difference between Mean and Value Section**

Alternative Hypothesis	*t* Value	Probability Level	Decision
JUICE<>0	9.7483	0.0000	Reject H$_0$

Nonparametric Tests Section
Quantile (Sign) Test

Hypothesis Value	Quantile	Number Lower	Number Higher	Probability Lower	Probability Higher	Probability Both
0	0.5	0	67	0.000	0.000	0.000

Table B–8. Confidence limits for the difference in mean Barthel Index.

Variable	Count	Mean	Standard Deviation
DI ≥ 10	32	63.28125	18.25489
DI < 10	15	50.66667	23.96923

at the same group (all the patients) twice, so the analytic method is the paired t. From NCSS, the mean difference in BI from admission to discharge is −26.81, and the standard deviation is 12.49.

$$95\% \text{ Confidence interval} = \text{Difference} \pm t_{(47-1)} \times \frac{SD \text{ difference}}{\sqrt{47}}$$

$$= -26.81 \pm 2.02 \times \frac{12.49}{\sqrt{47}}$$

$$= -26.81 + 3.68$$

$$= -30.49 \text{ to } -23.13$$

or −30.4745 to −23.14252 using NCSS. Because the interval does not contain zero, it is unlikely that the difference in BI from admission to discharge is zero. In fact, we can be 95% sure it has increased between approximately 23 and 30 points.

4. If sample sizes are equal, $n_1 = n_2$, so we can use simply n in the formula for pooled SD. The result is that the pooled SD is the square root of the mean of SD_1^2 and SD_2^2.

$$\frac{(n_1 - 1)\, SD_1^2 + (n_2 - 1)\, SD_2^2}{n_1 + n_2 - 2}$$

$$= \frac{(n - 1)\, SD_1^2 + (n - 1)\, SD_2^2}{n + n - 2}$$

$$= \frac{(n - 1)\,(SD_1^2 + SD_2^2)}{2n - 2}$$

$$= \frac{(n - 1)\,(SD_1^2 + SD_2^2)}{2(n - 1)}$$

$$= \frac{SD_1^2 + SD_2^2}{2}$$

5.

Step 1. H_0: Operating room times were the same; that is,

$$\mu_1 = \mu_2 \quad \text{or} \quad \mu_1 - \mu_2 = 0$$

H_1: Operating room times were not the same; that is,

$$\mu_1 \neq \mu_2 \quad \text{or} \quad \mu_1 - \mu_2 \neq 0$$

Step 2. The t test can be used for this research question.

Step 3. Use an α of 0.05 so results can be compared with the 95% confidence interval.

Step 4. The degrees of freedom are

$$(n_1 + n_2 - 2) = 48 + 40 - 2 = 86$$

The critical value is approximately ±2.00.

Step 5. The pooled standard deviation, found in Section 6.2, is 42.38. So the t statistic is

$$t_{(48+40-2)} = \frac{(195.63 - 217.78)}{42.38\sqrt{[(1/48) + (1/40)]}}$$

$$= \frac{-22.15}{9.07} = -2.44$$

Step 6. The absolute value of t, |−2.44|, is 2.44, greater than the critical value of 2.00, so we reject the null hypothesis and conclude that, on the average, women who had a vaginal procedure were in the operating room a significantly shorter time than women who had the abdominal procedure. This conclusion is consistent with the confidence limits that did not contain zero.

6. **a.** Table B–9 shows the output from NCSS. Because the chi-square value is not significant, we conclude that no association exists.

b.

$$RR = \frac{[a/(a + b)]}{[c/(c + d)]}$$

$$= \frac{(33/68)}{(6/16)}$$

$$= \frac{0.485}{0.375}$$

$$= 1.29$$

An odds ratio of 1.29 indicates that women who experience either pain or cramping are 29% more likely not to have had a paracervical block. Based on the chi-square test, we expect that this value of the odds ratio is not significant. Chapter 8 presents confidence intervals for the odds ratio.

7. Let N be the total number of observations, A the

Table B–9. Results of chi-square test for association between the occurrence of pain and cramping and having a paracervical block.

Block	Pain or Cramping		Total
	Both	**Not Both**	
No	33	6	39
Yes	35	10	45
Total	68	16	84
Chi-square	0.633484		
Degrees of freedom	1.000000		
Probability level	0.426080		Accept H_0

Table B–10. Contingency table with two rows and three columns.

	*		A
			B
J	K	L	N

number of observations in a given row, and K the number of observations in a given column. For example, for a table with two rows and three columns, we have Table B–10, in which we want to find the expected value for the cell with the asterisk (*).

The probability that an observation occurs in row A, $P(A)$, is A/N, and the probability that an observation occurs in column K, $P(K)$, is K/N. The null hypothesis being tested by chi-square is that the events represented by the rows and columns are independent. Using the multiplication rule for independent events, the probability that an observation occurs in row A *and* column K is $P(A)P(K) = A/N \times K/N = AK/N^2$. Multiplying this probability by the total number of observations N gives the number of observations that occur in both row A and column K; that is, $AK/N^2 \times N = AKN/N^2 = AK/N$ or the row total $\times$ the column total $\div$ the grand total.

8. The rule of thumb for α equal to 0.05 and power equal to 0.80 has $z_\alpha = 1.96$ and $z_\beta = -1.28$ for all computations; that is, only σ and $(\mu_0 - \mu_1)$ change. Therefore,

$$n = 2\left[\frac{(z_\alpha - z_\beta)\,\sigma}{\mu_1 - \mu_2}\right]^2$$

$$= 2\left\{\frac{[1.96 - (-1.28)]\,\sigma}{\mu_1 - \mu_2}\right\}^2$$

$$= 2\left[\frac{(3.24)\,\sigma}{\mu_1 - \mu_2}\right]^2$$

$$= 2 \times 10.5\left(\frac{\sigma}{\mu_1 - \mu_2}\right)^2$$

9. Output from PASS (Table B–11) indicates that 35 patients are needed in each group for 80% power.

10. The 95% confidence interval from Section 6.2.1 was $-19.15 \pm (1.99)(9.07) = -19.15 \pm 18.05$ or -37.20 to -1.10. To have 90% and 99% confidence intervals, only the value for t with 86 degrees of freedom needs to be changed.

The 90% CI is

$$-19.15 \pm (1.67)\,(9.07) = -19.15 \pm 15.15 \text{ or } -34.30 \text{ to } -4.00$$

The 99% CI is

$$-19.5 \pm (2.64)\,(9.07) = -19.15 \pm 23.94 \text{ or } -43.09 \text{ to } +4.79$$

Lower confidence gives a narrower interval, and higher confidence gives a wider interval.

11. Chances are good that more variation exists in the number of procedures done in the midsized centers. The t test requires that the variances (or standard deviations) not be different in the two groups. Because the sample sizes are quite different, 60 compared with 25, it is possible that violating the assumption of equal variances resulted in a nonsignificant t test.

12. The z test, confidence limits for the difference in two proportions, or the chi-square test may be used for each question. We illustrate the use of each.
    a. The cesarean rate is $1777/17,409 = 0.1021$ with selective monitoring and $1933/17,586 = 0.1099$ with universal monitoring. For a z test, the pooled proportion is

$$P = \frac{(1777 + 1933)}{(17,409 + 17,586)}$$
$$= 0.1060$$

Then,

$$z = \frac{(0.1021 - 0.1099)}{\sqrt{(0.106)(1 - 0.106)[(1/17,409) + (1/17,586)]}}$$
$$= \frac{-0.0078}{0.0033} = -2.36$$

which is significant ($P < 0.02$) from Table A–2. A statistically significant difference therefore exists in cesarean rates with selective versus universal electronic fetal monitoring. We should note, however, that the sample sizes in this study are very large, and it is always important for clinicians to ask about the clinical significance of the difference.

    b. The proportions are $196/7330 = 0.0267$ and $551/7288 = 0.0756$, respectively. The pooled proportion is 0.0511. A 99% confidence interval for the difference in proportions is

$$(0.0267 - 0.0756) \pm (2.575)$$
$$\sqrt{(0.0511)(1 - 0.0511)\left(\frac{1}{7330} + \frac{1}{7288}\right)}$$
$$= -0.0489 \pm 0.0094$$

Table B–11. Power analysis using NCSS.

Power	N_1	N_2	P_1	P_2	Alpha (α)	Beta (β)
0.80641	35	35	0.85000	0.55000	0.05000	0.19359

Table B–12. Contingency table of observed and expected frequencies of neonatal deaths in low-risk pregnancies.

	Selective	Universal	Total
Deaths	5	4	9
	(4.51)	(4.49)	
Live Births	7325	7284	14,609
	(7325.49)	(7283.51)	
Total	7330	7288	14,618

or (−0.0583, −0.0395). Because the 99% CI does not contain zero, we can be 99% sure that the difference between the proportions with abnormal fetal heart rate in low-risk pregnancies is greater than 0. Stated another way, there appears to be evidence ($P < 0.01$) that the two proportions are different, with fewer patients with abnormal fetal heart rates with selective monitoring.

c. A chi-square test is illustrated here; expected values are in parentheses (Table B–12):

$$\chi^2 = \frac{(5 - 4.51)^2}{4.51} + \frac{(4 - 4.49)^2}{4.49}$$
$$+ \frac{(7325 - 7325.49)^2}{7325.49} + \frac{(7284 - 7283.51)^2}{7283.51}$$
$$= 0.107$$

which is not significant. The difference in death rates is therefore not statistically significant.

d. Although universal monitoring has no effect on the neonatal death rate among low-risk pregnancies, it is associated with an increased cesarean rate and with a higher proportion of infants with abnormal heart rates. The authors' conclusions therefore seem to be justified.

13. a. The numbers are too small to use with the z approximation; $n(1 - p) = 2$ for responders. The chi-square test can be used, but Fisher's exact test is the optimal method.

b. The same reasoning as in part a applies, except the problem occurs with the nonresponders.

c. If the number of months follows a normal distribution, the independent two-group t test may be used; if not, the Wilcoxon rank sum test is appropriate with sample sizes under 30.

d. Use the same reasoning as in part c.

14. Selected output from the NCSS program for the two-group t test is given in Table B–13. Because the 95% confidence limits include zero (−0.410 to 2.417), we conclude that no difference exists in juice consumption between 2- and 5-year-olds.

CHAPTER 7

1. The ANOVA results are given in Table B–14. The observed value for the F ratio is 6.83, with 2 and 34 degrees of freedom. The critical value from Table A–4 with 2 and 30 degrees of freedom (the closest value) is 5.39 at $P = 0.01$; therefore, there is sufficient evidence to conclude that the mean scores on the Hamilton Depression Rating Scale are not the same for all three groups of women.

2. The critical value for the Tukey HSD test is

$$\text{HSD} = (\text{multiplier from Table 7–7}) \times \sqrt{MS_E n}$$
$$= 4.42 \times \sqrt{\frac{42.83}{12}}$$
$$= 8.35$$

assuming 12 patients in each group. The differences between the means are (1) moderate minus low = 11.98 − 5.34 = 6.64; (2) high minus low = 14.71 − 5.34 = 9.37; and (3) high minus moderate = 14.71 − 11.98 = 2.84. Only the high and

Table B–13. t Test comparing mean daily juice consumption by 2- and 5-year-old children.

Descriptive Statistics Section

	Count	Mean	Standard Deviation
AGE2_5=2	94	5.971415	4.773115
AGE2_5=5	74	4.968149	4.384122

Confidence Limits of Difference Section

	df	Mean Difference	Standard Deviation	Standard Error	95% Lower Confidence Limit of Mean	95% Upper Confidence Limit of Mean
Equal	166	1.003	4.606	0.716	−0.410	2.417
Unequal	162.05	1.003	6.481	0.709	−0.396	2.403

Note: t alpha (Equal) = 1.9744, t alpha (Unequal) = 1.9747

Source: Data, used with permission, from Dennison BA et al: Excess fruit juice consumption by preschool-aged children is associated with short stature and obesity. *Pediatrics* 1997;**99**:15–22. Output produced using NCSS; used with permission.

Table B–14. ANOVA table.

Source of Variation	Sum of Squares	df	Mean Square	F	P
Among groups	584.93	2	292.47	6.83	0.01
Within groups	1456.24	34	42.83		
Total	2041.18				

low groups are significantly different because their difference is greater than 8.35.

The critical value for the Scheffé procedure, using the value for the contrast found in Section 7.4.2.b, is

$$S = \sqrt{(j-1) \times \text{(Multiplier)}} \sqrt{MS_E \times \text{(Contrast)}}$$
$$= \sqrt{2 \times 5.31}\sqrt{42.83 \times 0.167}$$
$$= 3.259 \times 2.674$$
$$= 8.72$$

Again, only the difference between the high and low groups surpasses 8.72, so they are the only two groups that differ significantly on the Hamilton Depression Scale, according to Scheffé's procedure. The conclusions in this example are the same using the Tukey and the Scheffé procedures.

3. Two comparisons are independent if they use nonoverlapping information.

  a. Independent because each comparison uses different data.

  b. Dependent because data on physicians are used in each comparison.

  c. Independent because each comparison uses different data.

  d. None of these three comparisons are independent from the other two because they all use data on medical students.

4. The grand mean is

$$\frac{[(34)\,(3.9) + (32)\,(4.7) + (14)\,(16.4)]}{80} = 6.4$$

Therefore, the estimate of the mean square among groups is

$$34(3.9 - 6.4)^2 + 32(4.7 - 6.4)^2 + 14(16.4 - 6.4)^2 = 1705$$

divided by the number of groups minus 1, or 852.5. The estimate of the mean square error from the pooled variances is

$$\frac{[33(4.7)^2 + 31(3.9)^2 + 13(10.1)^2]}{33 + 31 + 13} = 32.8$$

Thus, the F ratio is $852.5/32.8 = 25.99$, significant at $P < 0.01$ when compared with the critical value of 4.98 (with 2 and 60 degrees of freedom in Table A–4). The conclusion is that a significant difference exists in the mean total number of minutes of disordered breathing among controls, hypertensive patients with apnea, and hypertensive patients without apnea. The assumption of equal (homogeneous) variances is violated, however, which is a problem when sample sizes are not equal. A possible way to deal with this problem is to use a logarithmic transformation of the total number of minutes.

5. a. This is a one-way or one-factor ANOVA because only one nonerror term occurs, the among-groups term.

  b. Total variation is 2000.

  c. There were 4 groups of patients because the degrees of freedom are 3. There were 40 patients because $n - 4 = 36$.

  d. The F ratio is $(800/3)/33.3 = 8.01$.

  e. The critical value with 3 and 30 degrees of freedom is 4.51; with 3 and 40 degrees of freedom is 4.31; interpolating for 3 and 36 degrees of freedom gives 4.39.

  f. Reject the null hypothesis of no difference and conclude that mean blood pressure differs in groups that consume different amounts of alcohol. A post hoc comparison is necessary to determine specifically which of the four groups differ.

6. a. Time of onset (early or late) and disease status (Alzheimer's or control) are the two main factors.

  b. It is possible that an interaction occurs in serotonin, norepinephrine, and 3-methoxy-4-hydroxy-phenylglycol. In the first two, mean values were higher for early-onset controls and lower for late-onset controls, whereas means were lower for early-onset patients and higher for late-onset patients. The reverse is the case for 3-methoxy-4-hydroxy-phenylglycol.

  c. The authors used the least significant difference test to make pairwise comparisons.

  d. Sample sizes are not equal; they vary from 14 in younger controls to 29 in older patients. If sample sizes are not equal, the analysis must be modified.

7. a. The P value for the interaction between thyroid status and weight is 0.728; therefore, it makes sense to continue to examine the main effects of thyroid and weight.

  b. The P value for thyroid status is 0.54 and for weight is 0.50.

  c. The conclusion is: The observed differences in glucose level were not large enough to conclude that hyperthyroid patients differed from controls, that overweight patients differed from normal weight patients, or that an interaction occurred between thyroid and weight status. We can therefore conclude that the four groups had similar mean levels of glucose.

CHAPTER 8

1. a.
$$r = \frac{16.65}{\sqrt{(533.20)\,(2.91)}}$$
$$- 0.42$$

The correlation of 0.42 indicates a fair degree of relationship between daily stool lipid content and energy.

b. Figure 8–19 was presented to show the relationship between fecal lipid level and fecal energy in the cystic fibrosis patients and the difference between the relationship in these patients and the relationship in control children. The correlation in control patients appears to be stronger than in the cystic fibrosis patients and to have a more positive slope.

2. a.
$$\chi^2 = \frac{(260 - 256.9)^2}{256.9} + \frac{(132 - 135.1)^2}{135.1}$$
$$+ \frac{(244 - 247.1)^2}{247.1} + \frac{(133 - 129.9)^2}{129.9}$$
$$= 0.22$$

where 132 and 133 are found by subtracting 260 and 244 from the total number of infants at risk in the TRH and placebo groups, respectively.

With 1 degree of freedom, this value is much smaller than the 3.841 associated with $P = 0.05$. We conclude that the evidence is insufficient to conclude that a significant relationship exists between TRH and the development of respiratory distress.

b. The odds ratio for risk of death among infants not at risk is

$$\frac{(2/171)}{(1/194)} = \frac{0.0117}{0.0052}$$
$$= 2.269$$

The 95% CI is

$$\exp\left[\ln(2.269) \pm 1.96\sqrt{\frac{1 - (2/171)}{2} + \frac{1 - (1/194)}{1}} \right]$$
$$= \exp(0.819 \pm 2.39)$$
$$= \exp(-1.57, +3.21)$$
$$= 0.21 \text{ to } 10.91$$

Because the confidence interval contains 1, the odds ratio could be 1; therefore, the

evidence is insufficient to conclude that a significant risk of death exists in infants who were given TRH.

3.
$$r = b \times \left(\frac{s_x}{s_y}\right)$$
$$= -0.043 \times \left(\frac{3.82}{0.30}\right)$$
$$= -0.043 \times 12.73$$
$$= -0.547, \text{ or } -0.55$$

4. a. Both the ratio of OKT4 to OKT8 cells and the lifetime concentrate use have skewed distributions, and the logarithmic transformation makes them more closely resemble the normal distribution.

b. $r = -0.453$ indicates a fair to moderate inverse (or negative) relationship; r^2 indicates that approximately 21% of the variation in one measure is accounted for by knowing the other.

c. The 95% confidence bands are specified as being related to single observations; therefore, 95% of predicted log(OKT4/OKT8) falls within these lines. Note also the appropriate slight curve of the bands.

5. a. Case–control.

b. The odds ratio is $(20 \times 1157)/(41 \times 121) = 4.66$; 95% confidence limits are the antilogarithms of

$$\exp\left[\ln(4.66) \pm 1.96\sqrt{\frac{1}{20} + \frac{1}{41} + \frac{1}{1157} + \frac{1}{121}} \right]$$
$$= \exp(0.97, 2.11)$$
$$= 2.65 \text{ to } 8.21$$

c. The age-adjusted odds ratio is an estimate of the value of the odds ratio if the cases and controls had identical age distributions. Because the age adjustment increases the odds ratio from 4.66 to 8.1, the cases represented a younger group of women than the controls, and the age adjustment compensates for this difference. Thus, controlling for age, we have 95% confidence that the interval from 3.7 to 18 contains the true increase in risk of deep vein thrombosis (pulmonary embolism) with the use of oral contraceptives.

6. a. Bile acid synthesis, because the absolute value of the correlation is the highest.

b. Bile acid synthesis, because it has the highest correlation.

c. The relationships between age and bile acid synthesis look as if they are relatively similar for men and women; however, the relationship between cholesterol secretion and age appears to be more positive in women than in men, and the relationship between age and pool-size cholic acid appears to be more negative in women than men (because the slopes are steeper in women).

7. The residuals are given in Figure B–8. The residuals most resemble Figure 8–14B and indicate a linear relationship.

8. The regression line goes through the point $(\overline{X}, \overline{Y})$; therefore, the point at which X intersects the regression line, when projected onto the Y axis, is $\overline{Y}' = \overline{Y}$.

9. A positive correlation indicates that the values of X and Y vary together; that is, large values of X are associated with large values of Y, and small values of X are associated with small values of Y. A positive slope of the regression line indicates that each time X increases by 1, Y increases by the amount of the slope, thereby pairing small values of X with small values of Y; a similar statement holds for large values.

10. a. The questions addressed by the study were: Is the pathogenesis of steroid-responsive nephritis syndrome (SRNS) immune-complex-mediated? Does the clinical activity of the disease relate to the presence of circulatory immune complexes?

b. Preexisting groups were used, patients with SRNS and patients with systemic lupus erythematosus (SLE), so the study was not randomized. No treatment was administered, so it was not a clinical trial. The observations on the variables of interest, IgG-containing complexes and C1q binding, were obtained at the same time, and the study question focused on "What is happening?" This study is therefore best described as cross-sectional.

c. Patients with and without evidence of active disease were studied. Patients with SLE were also studied because immune complexes are known to have a pathogenetic role in this disease.

d. According to Figure 8–22, the correlation between C1q-binding and IgG complexes for SLE patients is significant, $r = 0.91$, but this result in and of itself does not establish a cause-and-effect relationship. The correlation is not significant for patients with SRNS, but the sample size is relatively small, indicating low power to detect a significant relationship.

e. Authors state that the lines are 95% confidence limits for the patients with lupus. The lines are parallel, however, instead of curved, as they should be. They probably relate to individuals, because (1) of the way they are described in the legend, and (2) limits for the mean would probably be closer to the regression line.

f. It's not possible to tell for sure; however, it looks as if they might. First, the correlation for SRNS patients is not significantly different from 0 and the correlation for SLE patients is 0.91; if correlations are different, so are the regression lines. The sample size of SRNS patients is very small, however, and may keep us from detecting a statistically significant difference.

g. No. The study population must be carefully defined to reduce the likelihood that patients with other disease processes are not included.

CHAPTER 9

1. a. See Table B–15 for the arrangements of the observations according to the length of time patients were in the study and survival probabilities.

b. The survival curve, produced with NCSS, is given in Figure B–9.

c. Information for the logrank statistic is as shown in Table B-16.

2. a. There appears to be no difference in survival among those receiving PO, IM, or no androgen. (In fact, this conclusion is correct, from statistical tests summarized by the authors.) Furthermore, the greatest mortality rates occur early in the study.

b. It appears that the transplanted group has higher survival rates than the nontransplanted group; however, no statistical results are given in Figure 9–11.

c. The median survival in transplanted patients cannot be determined because more than half of the patients are still alive. In nontrans-

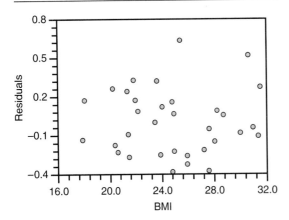

Figure B–8. A plot of residuals. (Data, used with permission of the author and the publisher, from Gonzalo MA et al: Glucose tolerance, insulin secretion, insulin sensitivity and glucose effectiveness in normal and overweight hyperthyroid women. *Clin Endocrinol* 1996;**45**:689–697. Output produced using NCSS; used with permission.)

Table B–15. Kaplan–Meier tables for patients who had kidney transplantation.

Treatment = azathioprine

Rank	Sample Size	Time	Survivorship $S(t)$
1	31	1.0	0.967742
2	30	1.0	0.935484
3	29	1.0	0.903226
4	28	1.0+	
5	27	1.0+	
6	26	2.0	0.868486
7	25	2.0+	
8	24	3.0	0.832299
9	23	3.0	0.796112
10	22	3.0	0.759926
11	21	4.0+	
12	20	5.0	0.721929
13	19	5.0+	
14	18	5.0+	
15	17	8.0+	
16	16	8.0+	
17	15	8.0+	
18	14	10.0+	
19	13	10.0+	
20	12	12.0+	
21	11	12.0+	
22	10	13.0+	
23	9	14.0+	
24	8	15.0+	
25	7	17.0	0.618797
26	6	18.0+	
27	5	18.0+	
28	4	19.0+	
29	3	20.0+	
30	2	23.0+	
31	1	23.0+	

Treatment = cyclosporine

Rank	Sample Size	Time	Survivorship $S(t)$
1	21	1.0	0.952381
2	20	6.0	0.904762
3	19	8.0	0.857143
4	18	12.0+	
5	17	12.0+	
6	16	12.0+	
7	15	13.0+	
8	14	14.0+	
9	13	15.0+	
10	12	15.0+	
11	11	16.0+	
12	10	17.0+	
13	9	17.0+	
14	8	18.0+	
15	7	19.0+	
16	6	19.0+	
17	5	20.0+	
18	4	21.0+	
19	3	22.0+	
20	2	22.0+	
21	1	22.0+	

Source: Data courtesy of Dr. Alan Birtch; used with permission. Output produced with NCSS; used with permission.

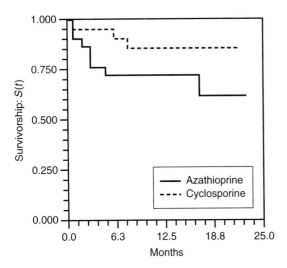

Figure B–9. Kaplan–Meier survival curves for patients who had kidney transplantations. (Data courtesy of Dr. Alan Birtch; used with permission. Figure produced with NCSS; used with permission.)

planted patients, median survival appears to be approximately 4 months; that is, 50% of these patients survive 4 months or less.

   d. (1) Recall the "eyeball" test from Chapter 6 in which we stated that two groups are significantly different if their individual 95% confidence limits do not overlap. Based on this rule, the two groups differ significantly ($P < 0.05$) at 6 months. (2) A more likely explanation is that the number of patients in the study beyond 6 months is not large enough to result in statistical significance, that is, a problem of low power exists.

   e. Although the authors do not state so, the small dots represent survival times of the 33 transplanted and 22 nontransplanted patients who survived at least 6 months.

3. a. There appears to be no difference in the lengths of time until disease progression in the vitamin C and placebo groups. In fact, the curve for vitamin C is lower than the curve for placebo at all points, indicating shorter times prior to disease progression in the vitamin C group.

   b. Median time to disease progression was approximately 3 months in the vitamin C group and 4.5 months in the placebo group.

   c. As you probably suspect, the authors found no significant differences in survival between patients receiving the vitamin C and those receiving placebo.

4. a. The survival curves are given in Figure B–10. It appears that survival rates for the two treatment methods were similar. After 2 years, survival was slightly better in the group on traditional hemodialysis, but a statistical test is needed to learn if this slight difference is significant or could occur by chance.

   b. The logrank statistic is 0.92. Because this is a chi-square statistic with 1 degree of freedom, we know that the value does not reach statistical significance. We therefore conclude that these observations do not provide sufficient evidence for a difference in survival in the two treatment groups.

   c. This study was not randomized. We therefore do not know the basis for choosing continuous ambulatory peritoneal dialysis or traditional hemodialysis. As a result, no conclusions should be drawn about any differences in treatment.

Table B–16. Information on the logrank statistic.

Treatment Value	Failed Count	Censored Count	Total Count
Azathioprine	9	22	31
Cyclosporine	3	18	21
Chi-square = 2.38	$df = 1$	$P = 0.12$	

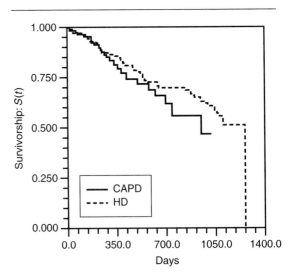

Figure B–10. Kaplan–Meier survival curve comparing continuous ambulatory peritoneal dialysis to hemodialysis. (Data, used with permission, from Bajwa K, Szabo E, Kjellstrand CM: A prospective study of risk factors and decision making in discontinuation of dialysis. *Arch Intern Med* 1996; **156:**2571–2577. Figure produced with NCSS; used with permission.)

5. It is possible to estimate median survival for two of the groups. The patients with tumor stage T2b–c have a median survival of approximately 50 months. Those with a tumor stage of T3 or T4 have a median survival of a little less than 40 months.

6. The Mantel–Haenszel is an excellent procedure to compare two distributions. Note that it is possible to estimate the Mantel–Haenszel statistic from the study's Figure 2.

CHAPTER 10

1. For smokers, the adjusted mean is the mean in smokers, 3.33, minus the product of the regression coefficient, 0.0113, and the difference between the occlusion score in smokers and the occlusion score in the entire sample (estimated from Figure 10–2); that is,

$$-[0.0113 \times (198.33 - 151.67)] = 2.80$$

Similarly, the adjusted mean in nonsmokers is

$$1.00 - [0.0113 \times (105.00 - 151.67)] = 1.53$$

These are the same values we found (within round-off error) in Section 10.3.

2. **a.** With 400 variables, a substantial number can be expected to be significant merely by chance. The requirement for R^2 to increase 5% assures us that variables in the equation have clinical as well as statistical significance.

   b. The nursery period, because it has the highest R^2; however, none of the values for R^2 are very large, indicating that cerebral palsy is difficult to predict, at least from the variables considered in this study.

   c. Neonatal seizures, because it has a predicted risk of 9.6%.

   d. A good question, and the answer is not obvious. It could be that these variables were included because previous reports had indicated them to be of interest. It is also possible that the univariate a priori tests were one-tailed with $\alpha = 0.05$, but the 95% confidence limits in Table 10–9 are equivalent to a one-tailed test for $\alpha = 0.025$ instead of 0.05.

3. Predicted value for a 27-year-old Caucasian man who comes to the emergency department on Saturday night with BAC $\geq$ 50 mg/dL:

$$
\begin{aligned}
\text{Predicted value} &= -0.80 - 1.84 \text{ (if daytime)} \\
&+ 0.66 \text{ (if Fri.–Sun.)} \\
&+ 0.28 \text{ (if Caucasian)} \\
&- 0.11 \text{ (if 40 or older)} \\
&= -0.80 + 0.66 + 0.28 \\
&= +0.08
\end{aligned}
$$

and

$$
\begin{aligned}
P_x &= \frac{1}{1 + \exp[-(0.08)]} \\
&= \frac{1}{1 + 0.923} = 0.52
\end{aligned}
$$

Therefore, there is more than a 50–50 chance that this man has an elevated blood alcohol level.

4. The chance agreement that a male is not intoxicated (rounding to whole-number percentages) is $0.82 \times 0.74 = 0.61$; the chance agreement for intoxication is $0.18 \times 0.26 = 0.05$. Thus the agreement beyond chance is $0.77 - (0.61 + 0.05) = 0.11$. To find kappa, divide by 1 minus the chance agreement $(1 - 0.66 = 0.34)$ to obtain $0.11/0.34 = 0.32$, or 32%. Based on the guidelines suggested by Sackett and colleagues (1991), a kappa between 0.21 and 0.40 indicates only slight agreement.

5. If the investigators want to distinguish among three groups of runners, using the numerical anthropometric measures, discriminant analysis should be used. Multiple regression can be used, however, if the actual running time of each runner was used instead of dividing the runners into three groups; in this situation, the outcome measure is numerical.

6. The regression equation is

$$
\begin{aligned}
&0.613 - (0.0002 \times 80) - (0.00006 \times 80) \\
&- (0.002 \times 75) - (0.0001 \times 70) - (0.021 \times 10) \\
&+ (0.002 \times 1) - (0.003 \times 1) - (0.105 \times 14) = 1.694
\end{aligned}
$$

which gives 1.694 predicted bed-days during a 30-day period.

7. R^2 with the blood glucose test results is 0.58^2, or 0.336; without the blood glucose testing, it is 0.39^2, or 0.152; therefore, an additional $0.336 - 0.152 = 0.184$, or approximately 18%, of the variation in physicians' estimates is accounted for with this information. This finding implies (perhaps not surprisingly) that physicians depend more on blood glucose test information than on the other variables in estimating a patient's blood glucose level.

8. **a.** Yes, with a reported P value of 0.0000.

   b. TUMSTAGE(2) and TUMSTAGE(3), the T classification for T2b–c and T3–4, and pretreatment PSA are both statistically significant.

   c. exp (1.4588) = 4.3008. The 95% confidence interval goes from approximately 1.45 to 12.73; therefore, we can be 95% confident that the true odds ratio in the population falls within this range. This interval does not contain 1, so the odds ratio is statistically significant (consistent with the *P* value).

d. The pretreatment PSA, which was not significant when posttreatment PSA was included, is now significant. In addition, the *t* classification T2b–c is significant.

9. a. Your regression results should resemble those we produced in Table 10–14.

b. Father's height was the variable included in model 1. Stepwise regression begins with the independent variable that has the highest correlation with the outcome, so father's height had the highest correlation with the child's final height.

c. Mother's height, height for chronologic age, and dose are in the final model. Based on the standardized coefficients, the variable making the largest contribution is height for chronologic age.

d. After the other variables entered the equation in model 4, the father's height was no longer significant. This can occur when the other variables are predicting the same portion of the outcome that father's height was predicting, once the values of all other variables are held constant.

e.
$$-1.138 + (-0.575 \times -2.20)$$
$$+ (1.325 \times -3.07) + (0.121 \times 20)$$
$$= -1.138 + 1.265 - 4.068 + 2.42$$
$$= -1.52$$

This child's final height is therefore predicted to be −1.52, compared with the child's actual height of −2.18.

CHAPTER 11

1. a. With a baseline of 2% and 95% sensitivity, $0.95 \times 20 = 19$ true-positives; with 50% sensitivity, the false-positive rate is 50% and $0.50 \times 980 = 490$ false-positives occur. The probability of lupus with a positive test is TP/(TP + FP) = 19/509 = 3.7%.

b. With a baseline of 20%, 190 true-positives occur. Similarly, with 50% specificity, 400 false-positives occur. The chances of lupus with this index of suspicion is therefore 190/590 = 32.2%.

2. Using Bayes' theorem with *D* = lupus and *T* = test, we have

$$P(D^-|T^-) = \frac{P(T^-|D^-)\,P(D^-)}{P(T^-|D^-)\,P(D^-) + P(T^-|D^+)\,P(D^+)}$$
$$= \frac{0.50 \times 0.98}{(0.50 \times 0.98) + (0.05 \times 0.02)}$$
$$= \frac{0.49}{0.49 + 0.001} = 0.998$$

Using the likelihood ratio method requires us to redefine the pretest odds as the odds of *no* disease, that is, 0.98/(1 − 0.98) = 49. The likelihood ratio for a negative test is the specificity divided by the false-negative rate (ie, the likelihood of a negative test for persons without the disease versus persons with the disease); therefore, the likelihood ratio is 0.50/0.05 = 10. Multiplying, we get $49 \times 10 = 490$, the posttest odds. Reconverting to the posttest probability, or the predictive value of a negative test, gives 490/(1 + 490) = 0.998, the same result as with Bayes' theorem.

3. See Table B–17.

Therefore, when the witness says green, he or she is correct 12 out of 12 + 17 times, or 41%.

4. a. Positive results occurred 138 times in 150 known diabetics = 138/150 = 92% sensitivity.

b. 150 − 24 = 126 negative results in 150 persons without diabetes gives 126/150 = 84% specificity.

c. The false-positive rate is 24/150, or 100% − specificity = 16%

d. 80% sensitivity in 150 persons with diabetes gives 120 true-positives. 4% false-positives in 150 persons without diabetes is 6 persons. The chances of diabetes with a positive fasting blood sugar is thus 120/126 = 95.2%.

e. 80% sensitivity in 90 (out of 100) patients with diabetes = 72 true-positives; 4% false-positive rate in 10 patients without diabetes = 0.4 false-positive. Therefore, 72/72.4 = 0.9945, or 99.45%, of patients like this man who have a positive fasting blood sugar actually have diabetes.

5. a. Using Bayes' theorem with prior probability of 0.30; we have

$P(\text{mitral valve prolapse} \mid \text{positive echocardiogram})$
$$= \frac{(0.90)\,(0.30)}{[(0.90)\,(0.30) + (0.05)\,(0.70)]}$$
$$= \frac{0.27}{(0.27 + 0.035)}$$
$$= 0.885$$

that is, an 88.5% chance.

Table B–17. Contingency table for finding the probability the errant cab was green.

Witness	Actual Color	
	Green	Blue
Says green	12	17
Says blue	3	68

b.

P (no mitral valve prolapse | negative echocardiogram)

$$= \frac{(0.95)\,(0.70)}{[(0.95)\,(0.70) + (0.10)\,(0.30)]}$$

$$= \frac{0.665}{(0.665 + 0.03)}$$

$$= 0.957$$

or a 95.7% chance.

6. **a.** This is not the information we need. To use Table 11–9, we must assume that the children identified as having a language deficit by the PLS were the same ones identified by the DDST; even then, only sensitivity can be evaluated. For example, on *articulation*, the DDST correctly identified 28 of 60, or 47%, of those identified by the PLS. We do not know, however, whether the DDST produces any false-positives; that is, did any of the 11 children who passed the PLS fail the DDST? We cannot therefore evaluate the specificity of the DDST. In fairness to the investigators, the title of the article referred only to the sensitivity of the DDST; however, as we learned in this chapter, sensitivity alone is not sufficient to evaluate a diagnostic procedure.

   b. The authors stated that the Wilcoxon matched pairs rank sign test was used; probably meaning the Wilcoxon matched pairs sign ranks test. Of more importance, however, is that the children either passed or failed each test, according to the article; and the results in the table are given as proportions. Pass or fail is, of course, a nominal scale. Although the investigators correctly recognized the need for a matched (or paired) nonparametric test, they used the test for ordinal observations or numerical observations that are not normally distributed. The appropriate test is the McNemar chi-square test for matched (or paired) proportions.

7. With low prevalence, a positive result on a diagnostic test does not provide a great deal of information, even when the test is very accurate. On the other hand, a negative test in a low-prevalence situation is quite useful, especially if the test is accurate. As the prevalence or index of suspicion increases, however, the results of either a positive or a negative test that is accurate are useful.

8. **a.** There are $80 \times 0.19 = 15.2$ true-positives, and $80 - 15.2 = 64.8$ false-negatives; $20 \times 0.82 = 16.4$ true-negatives and $20 - 16.4 = 3.6$ false-positives. Therefore, the probability of an MI with a positive ECG is $15.2/(15.2 + 3.6) = 80.9\%$.

   b. The probability of an MI even if the test is negative is $64.8/(64.8 + 16.4) = 79.8\%$.

   c. These calculations illustrate the uselessness of this criterion (ST elevation ≥ 5 mm in discordant leads) in diagnosing MI.

   d. The likelihood ratio is TP/FP or $19/18 = 1.06$.

   e. The pretest odds are $80/20$, or 4 to 1. The posttest odds are $4 \times 1.06 = 4.24$. As you can see, the test does very little to change the index of suspicion.

9. **a.** The best test to rule in is the one with the highest specificity to minimize the number of false-positives: ankle dorsiflexion weakness.

   b. The best test to rule out is the one with the highest sensitivity to minimize the number of false-negatives: ipsilateral straight-leg raising.

CHAPTER 12

1. A patient's preference may change depending on the value of the outcome; that is, a patient who chooses surgical over medical treatment to avoid almost certain death without the surgery may opt for medical treatment if the outcome without surgery is mild to moderate disability instead of death. Another factor affecting a patient's preference is the risk of the procedure or treatment, for instance, weighing the risk of morbidity and mortality associated with carotid endarterectomy versus the risk of stroke if the procedure is not performed. A patient's preference can also be affected by the timing of the outcome; an elderly patient may make one decision to avoid immediate major disability and a different decision if the disability is more likely to occur in 5–10 years.

2. At approximately 42%, where the lines for culture and rapid test cross.

3. For a sensitivity of 0.60 and a specificity of 0.98 from Section 12.3.2, with 7% prevalence, there are 4.2 true-positives and $0.02 \times 93 = 1.86$ false-positives. Therefore, PV+ $= 4.2/(4.2 + 1.86) = 0.693$, or 69%.

4. **a.** 0.20, seen on the top branch.

   b. No, this is not obvious. Although the author provides the proportion of patients who have a positive examination, 0.26 (and negative examination, 0.74), these numbers include false-positives (and false-negatives) as well as true-positives (and true-negatives). The author also gives the predictive value of a positive test, 0.78 (and of a negative test, 0.997); and by using quite a bit of algebra, we can work backward to obtain the estimates of 0.989 for sensitivity and 0.928 for specificity. Readers of the article should not be expected to do these manipulations, however; authors should give precise values used in any analysis.

c. For no test or therapy: $(0.20)(48) + (0.80)(100) = 89.6$; for colectomy: $(0.03)(0) + (0.97)[(0.20)(78) + (0.80)(100)] = 92.7$. Therefore, colonoscopy is the arm with the highest utility, at 94.6.

5. a. The incidence of pertussis and the incidence of severe adverse effects believed to be attributable to the vaccine, such as encephalopathy, seizures, and HHE, are the most important assumptions.

b. The current schedule is better, because the proposed schedule would result in a 42% increase in the incidence of pertussis.

c. No difference occurs as far as attributable events are concerned, but the rate of chance events is higher under the proposed schedule. Although a larger number of deaths occurs under the present schedule, approximately 50% more seizures would occur under the proposed schedule. The proposed schedule, therefore, appears to be preferable if the overall desire is to decrease deaths from pertussis.

CHAPTER 13

1. C
2. A
3. D
4. D
5. D
6. B
7. E
8. A
9. C
10. E
11. C
12. B
13. A
14. B
15. E
16. B
17. E
18. C
19. C
20. A
21. E
22. B
23. C
24. A
25. C
26. D
27. D
28. C
29. A
30. D
31. B
32. C
33. A
34. E
35. D
36. A
37. D
38. B
39. E
40. D
41. D
42. C
43. G
44. A
45. C
46. A
47. B
48. B
49. A
50. B
51. C
52. C
53. B
54. D
55. E
56. A
57. E
58. B
59. C
60. B
61. B
62. E
63. A
64. A
65. B
66. H
67. B
68. I
69. E
70. G
71. T
72. F
73. T
74. F
75. F

Appendix C:
Flowcharts for Relating Research Questions to Statistical Methods

Flowchart to Use	Research Question
C-1	Is there a difference in means or medians (ordinal or numerical measures)?
C-2	Is there a difference in means or medians (ordinal or numerical measures, three or more groups)?
C-3	Is there a difference in proportions (nominal measures)?
C-4	Is there an association?
C-5	Is there a difference in measures of association?
C-6	Are there two or more independent variables?

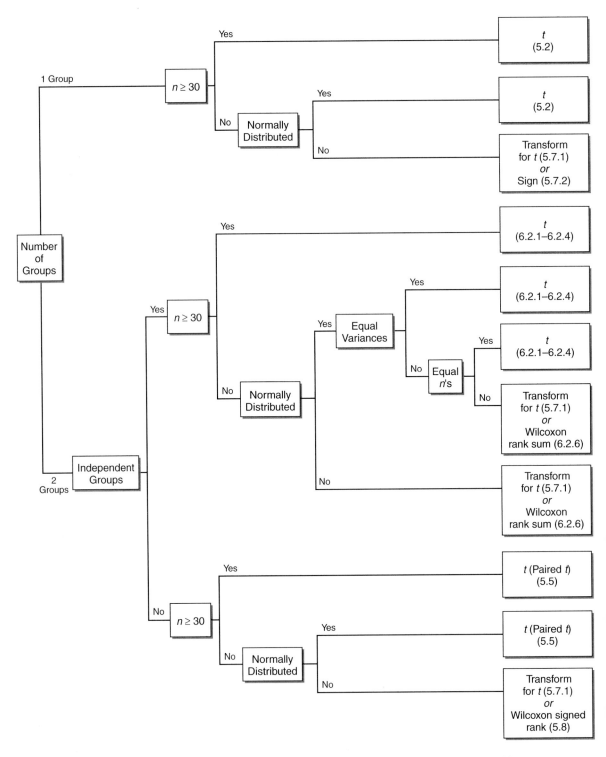

Figure C–1. Is there a difference in means or medians (ordinal or numerical measures)?

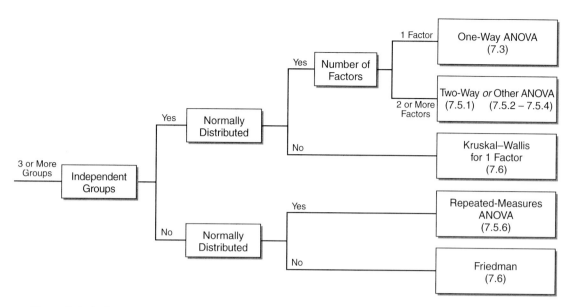

Figure C–2. Is there a difference in means or medians (ordinal or numerical measures, three or more groups)?

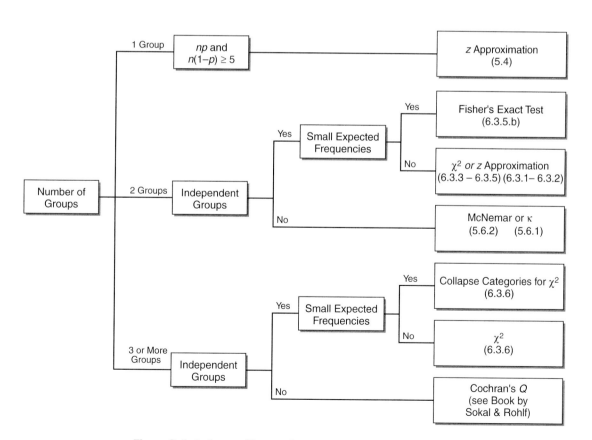

Figure C–3. Is there a difference in proportions (nominal measures)?

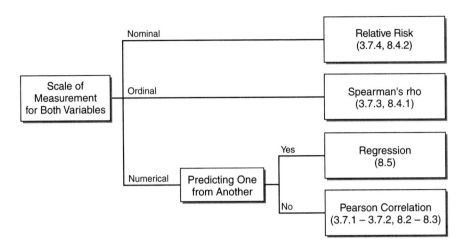

Figure C–4. Is there an association?

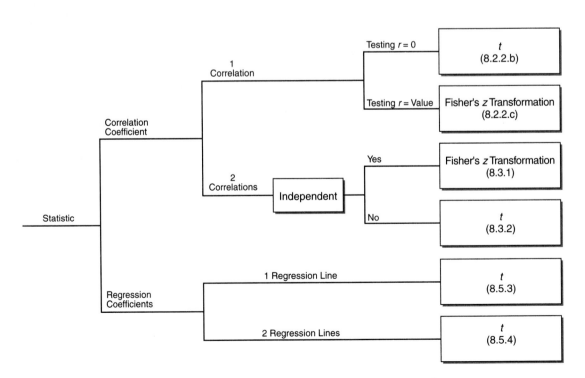

Figure C–5. Is there a difference in measures of association?

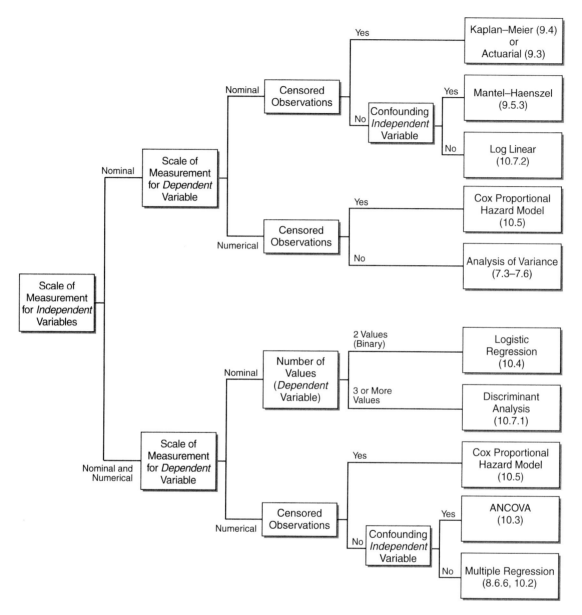

Figure C-6. Are there two or more independent variables?

Index

Page numbers followed by *t, f* or *b* denote tables, figures or boxes, respectively.

ISBN 0-8385-0510-4